THE SCIENCE OF

THE SCIENCE OF HUMAN NUTRITION

JUDITH E. BROWN
University of Minnesota

HBJ
HARCOURT BRACE JOVANOVICH, PUBLISHERS
AND ITS SUBSIDIARY, ACADEMIC PRESS
San Diego New York Chicago Austin Washington, D.C.
London Sydney Tokyo Toronto

To Joe. Thanks for making it easy.

Cover Credit: © John Martin/The Image Bank, Inc.

ISBN: 0-15-578687-3

Library of Congress Catalog Card Number: 89-85852

Printed in the United States of America.

PREFACE

My goals for *The Science of Human Nutrition* were clearly in mind before I wrote the first word. I knew the book should be a friendly, up-to-date, beautifully illustrated, interesting, and accurate textbook for students taking their first course in nutrition. It should focus on normal human nutrition and the role of nutrition in promoting and maintaining health, and it should foster an appreciation for the scientific bases that provide the foundation for our understanding of nutrition. The book should convey state-of-the-art information about nutrition issues of current concern, while making the complexity of these issues understandable. It should be a book that students use for reference long after they experience their first nutrition course. And now that the book has been written, analyzed by many helpful colleagues, and modified, I feel confident that it meets these goals.

During the past 20 years, both scientists and consumers have been bombarded with information about nutrition. The information has taken a variety of forms, from that which is based on scientific study, to that which is useless or even dangerous. Students who take a college course in human nutrition must learn to evaluate this information. *The Science of Human Nutrition* is an attempt to help students to do just that by providing a solid scientific foundation. By promoting an understanding of the role of nutrition in maintaining health, the book will help students make informed decisions about nutrition as knowledge continues to expand and as new issues arise.

ORGANIZATION

The Science of Human Nutrition is presented in three parts. Part One provides students with the "Basic Knowledge of Human Nutrition." After an introduction, Chapter 2 presents eleven principles that establish the scientific foundation for the rest of the book. The next two chapters go on to discuss such fundamental topics as food, energy, and energy balance (Chapter 3) and food intake, body weight, and health (Chapter 4).

Part Two is concerned with "The Nutrients"—chemical substances that are at the very heart of nutrition. Chapters 5 through 7 deal with carbohydrates, proteins, and fats. Chapter 8 provides an introduction and overview to vitamins and minerals, and these topics are discussed in greater depth in Chapters 9 and 10 (vitamins) and Chapters 11 and 12 (minerals). Chapter 13 deals with that most basic of nutrients, water.

Part Three, "Nutrition and the Life Course," addresses those topics that undoubtedly draw most students to the study of nutrition in the first place.

Now that a proper foundation has been laid, students can begin to learn about nutrition and reproduction (Chapter 14), nutrition for growth and development (Chapter 15), and nutrition for adulthood (Chapter 16).

PEDAGOGY

Several features of this book facilitate learning and make it enjoyable to study. The book design is attractive and colorful, and photographs, illustrations, marginal notes, and tables reinforce textual explanations. It uses boxed inserts, cartoons, and examples to illuminate important concepts and provide interesting background information. Because students in introductory nutrition courses vary widely in academic experience, important scientific terms are printed in boldface and defined in context. The terms are also defined in the margin near where they appear in the text and in the glossary at the back of the book.

Review questions provide a means of assessing student comprehension of the chapter material, and answers to those questions provide immediate feedback. Student activities that call for independent discovery about personal nutrition and other factors that can affect health are provided in the "Putting Nutrition Knowledge to Work" sections. Such activities foster learning by doing. The "Notes" sections provide documentation for the facts presented throughout the chapter and serve as sources for further reading.

Expanded discussions of digestion, absorption, and metabolism appear as appendixes at the back of the book. These appendixes are intended for instructors and students who want additional coverage of these topics. Other appendixes contain food exchange lists, food composition tables, sources of reliable nutrition information, "The Dietary Guidelines for Americans," and other useful information.

SUPPLEMENTS

Computer Software

To enrich independent student learning, computer software for dietary analysis, calculation of total caloric need, and determination of energy expenditure from physical activities is available. This easy-to-use software provides students with opportunities to relate nutrition concepts to their own lives.

Student Study Guide

A *Student Study Guide* has been developed by a gifted teacher, Catherine Breedon. The *Guide* presents interesting learning exercises and clever alternate explanations of nutrition concepts.

Instructor's Manual with Tests

An *Instructor's Manual* provides a course syllabus, detailed lecture outlines, a student knowledge pre-test, notes, exam policies and procedures, and more than 1600 test questions (with the difficulty of each indicated).

Computerized Test Bank

The test questions in the *Instructor's Manual* are also available in a computerized format.

Transparencies

Acetate transparencies of text illustrations are available to instructors for classroom use.

ACKNOWLEDGMENTS

I must thank many people for their help in creating this book—the hundreds of instructors who took the time to respond to our questionnaire about the features they desire in an introductory nutrition text, those instructors who reviewed my outline, and those instructors who reviewed one or more drafts of the manuscript. I gratefully acknowledge the contributions of Martha S. Brown of Eastern Illinois University, Deirdre Michael-Mechelke, and Catherine H. Breedon. They have been "students" of this book and were the sources of many terrific ideas on how to make a textbook teach. In addition, a number of other reviewers helped to shape the final product. They are Mary Head, West Virginia University; Bettylu Kessler, El Camino College; E. Elaine Boston, Tulane University; LaRose Ketterling, University of North Dakota; Billie H. Wood, Daytona Beach Community College; Catherine Justice, Purdue University; Sylvia E. Gartung, Michigan State; Sheron Sunmer, University of North Carolina–Greensboro; Ellen Parham, Northern Illinois University; Lavon Bartel, University of Vermont; Paul V. Benko, Sonoma State University; Nancy Betts, University of Nebraska; Joanne Curran-Cellantano, University of New Hampshire; June Frederickson, North Central Technical Institute; Deon Gines, Louisiana Technical University; Marianne Krismer, Cincinnati Technical College; and Eleanor Roman, Otterbein College. I also thank the students in my introductory nutrition classes. They have taught me much about teaching and writing.

Jan Gangelhoff, a wizard of microcomputer software, processed and reprocessed the works that formed the manuscripts. Her undaunted enthusiasm and support for the project and her willingness to deliver typed manuscript pages to my home at 3:00 A.M. kept me going.

There is no one person an author relates to more closely while writing a book than the editor. I was lucky to have Jeff Holtmeier as my editor. He has given constant support and enthusiasm, and he has been my trusted advisor. For her calls to Australia to find a photograph of a green plum and other calls to Japan to identify a picture of a commonly eaten puffer fish, I thank Candace Young, the art editor. Carole Reagle edited my manuscript and transformed it into a text worthy of students. Brett Smith was the able production editor who provided work, energy, and support. Kay Faust has provided a beautiful design and unwavering enthusiasm for the project. There have been many behind-the-scenes heroes connected with this book, but Lynne Bush requires special recognition. Lynne had the thankless job of overseeing the budget and schedule. On both fronts, she exceeded our most enthusiastic expectations. All of the Harcourt Brace Jovanovich professionals have spoken with a common, helpful, encouraging voice. Thanks to you all.

Finally, I thank my children Amanda and Max for not scribbling on the manuscript pages and for allowing me to sleep late on weekends. This book will show them what I was doing all those nights I stayed up late.

Writing this book has been a long, difficult task, but it has also been fun. I have had many hours of pleasure assembling it, and I am dedicated to making it a pleasure for you to use. Please let me know how I can improve the book in future printings or editions. I am not eager to find errors in the presentation, but I know that it is inevitable that some mistakes will sneak through in a work of this size. The publisher and I will do everything possible to keep the book up to date and correct. Any feedback will be appreciated.

Judith E. Brown

CONTENTS

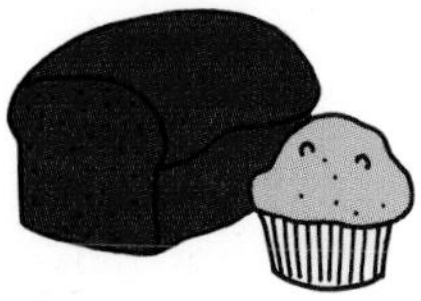

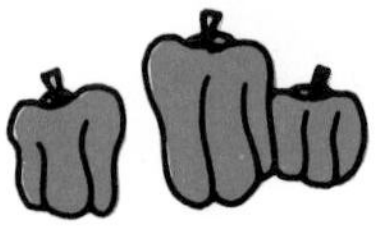

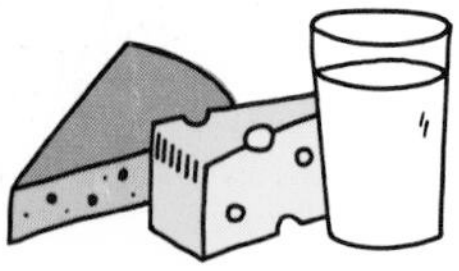

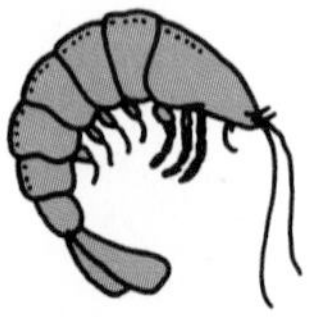

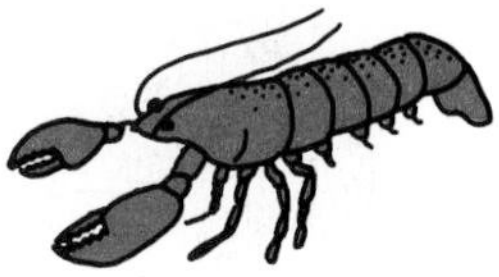
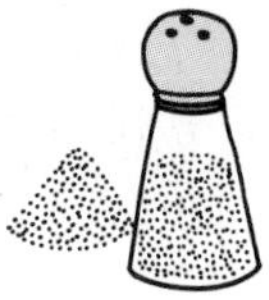
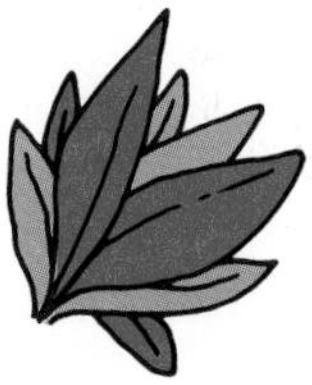
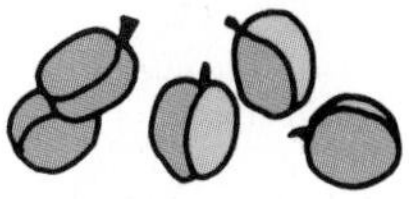
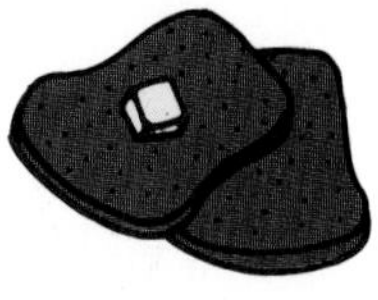
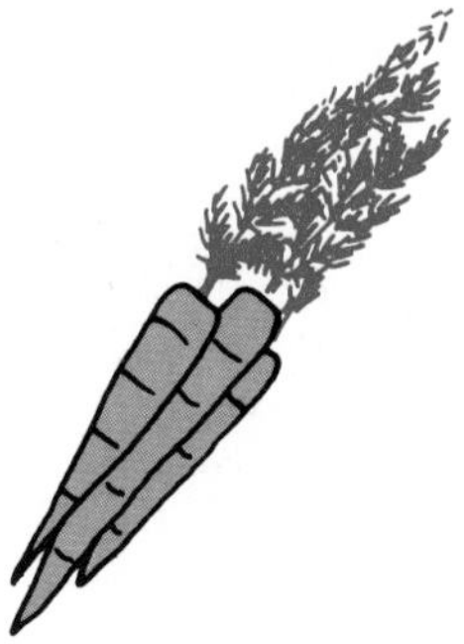

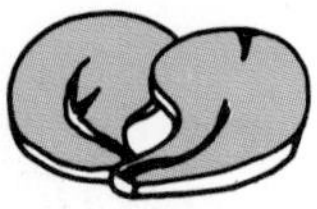

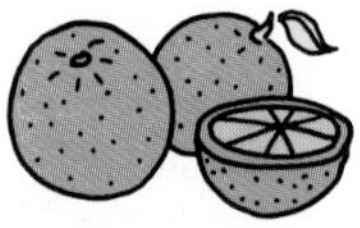

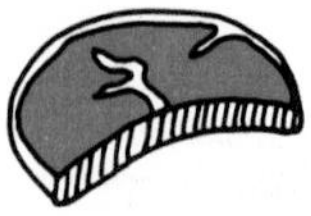

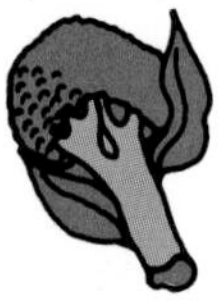

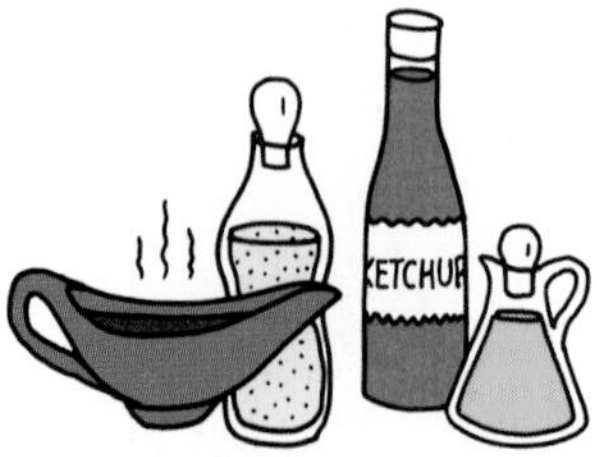

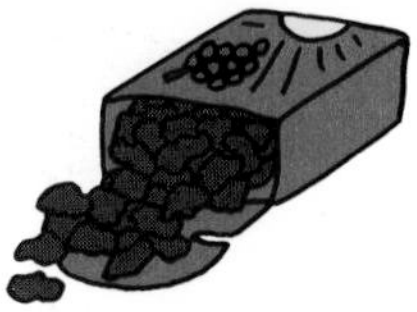
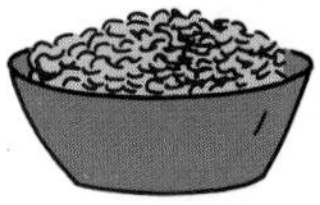
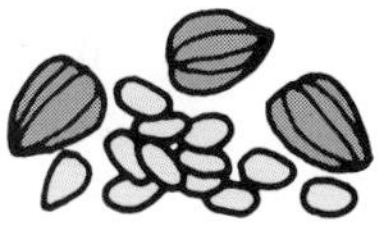
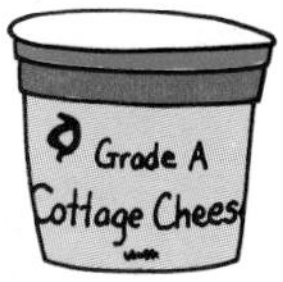
Grade A
Cottage Chees
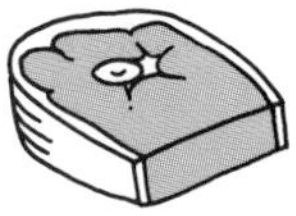
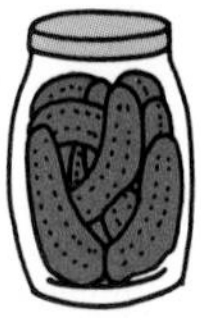
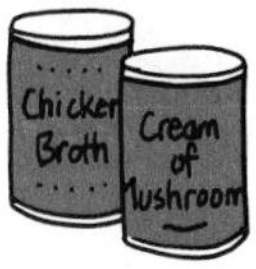
Chicken Broth
Cream of Mushroom

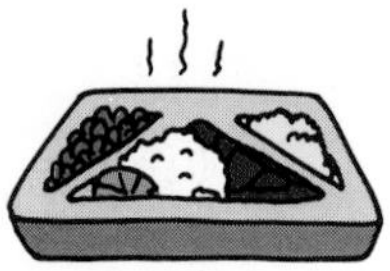

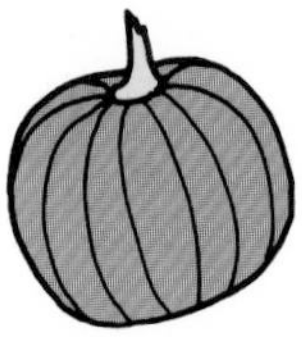

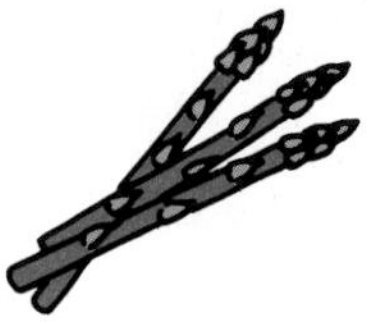

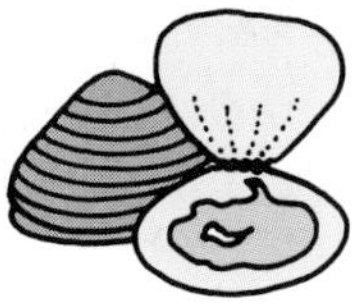

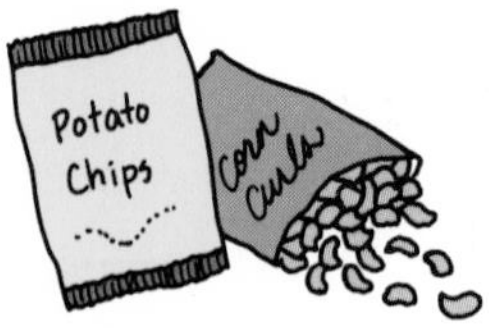
Potato Chips
Corn Curls

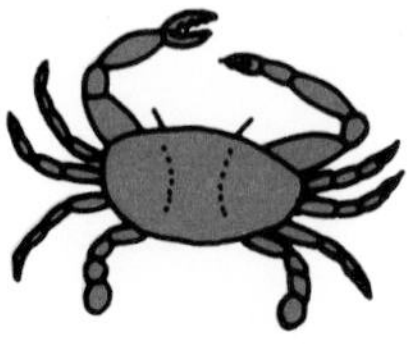

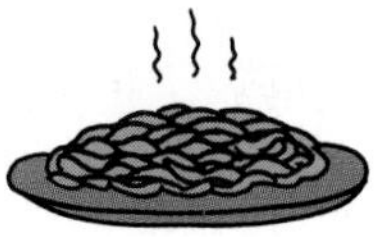

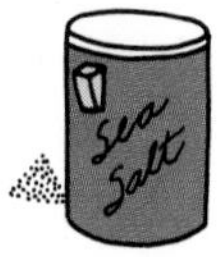
Sea Salt

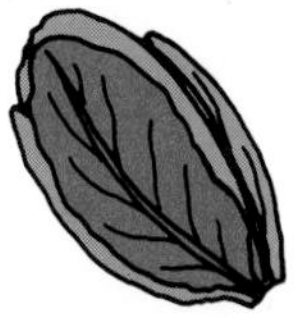

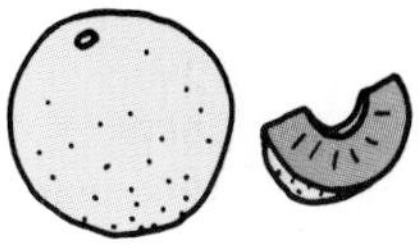

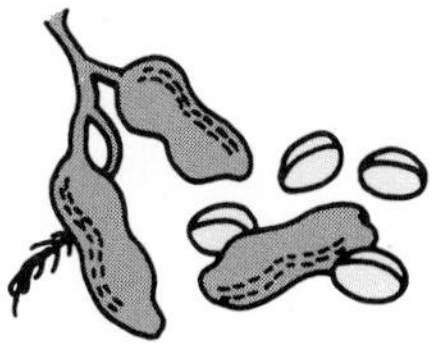

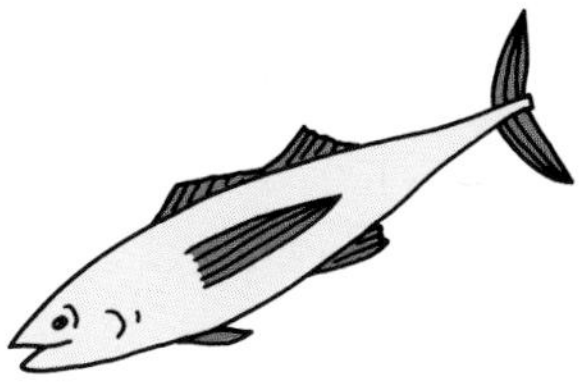

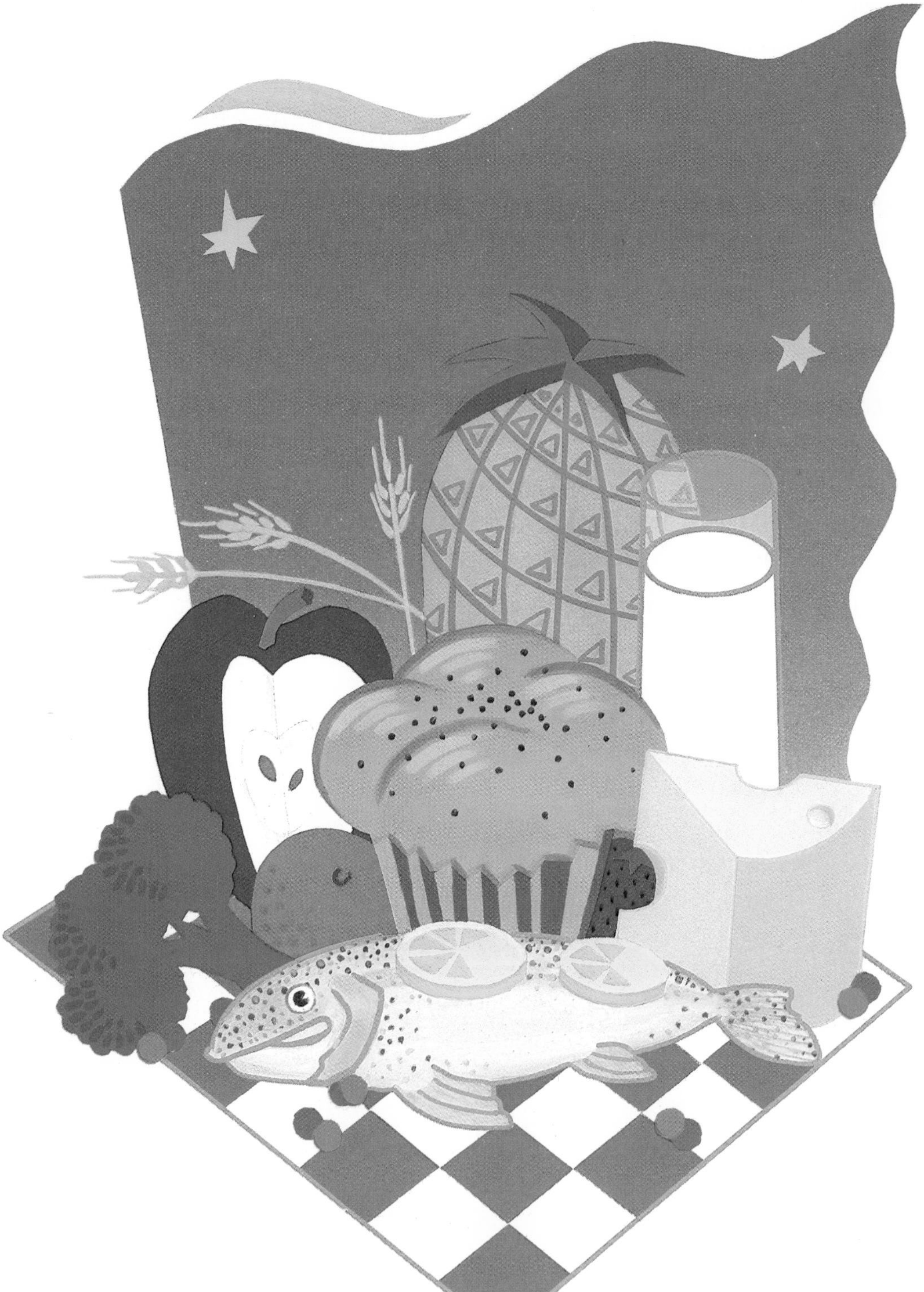

PART ONE

BASIC KNOWLEDGE OF HUMAN NUTRITION

CHAPTER 1

INTRODUCTION TO THE STUDY OF NUTRITION

Your health primarily depends on the genes you received from your parents and the environment in which you live. Of all the environmental factors that affect health, diet is probably the most important.

nutrition: Simply stated, the study of the effects of substances in food on the body and health.

Nutrition* is a subject that touches everyone. It is the study of how the substances in food affect our bodies and our health. The study of nutrition is broadly defined as the science of food, the nutrients and other substances therein, their actions, interactions, and balance in relation to health and disease; and the processes by which the organism ingests, digests, absorbs, transports, utilizes, and excretes food substances.

This book will broaden and deepen your understandings about foods, nutrition, and health. You will learn the principles of nutrition and apply them as you study the relationships between diet and health. You will become acquainted with important research in the field of human nutrition. This book—along with this course—will probably change your life, because it will show you that health and quality of life are related to the foods you eat.

■ ■ ■

HISTORICAL PERSPECTIVE OF HUMAN NUTRITION

Biologically modern humans have walked the earth for about 40,000 years. For 30,000 of those years, humans survived by hunting wild animals and gathering plants. Early humans were constantly on the move, either pursuing wild game or following the seasonal maturation of fruits and vegetables. Animal and plant foods obtained from successful hunting and gathering journeys spoiled quickly, so they had to be consumed within a short time. Very often, feasts were followed by periods of famine. Refined sugar, salt,

*Words in bold type are defined in the margin of the page on which they are discussed, as well as in the glossary, Appendix I at the end of the book.

alcohol, food additives, and oils, margarine, and butter—common components of our **diets**—were unknown to early humans. These things came with civilization.

diet: Foods and fluids regularly consumed in the course of living.

The bodies of biologically modern humans adapted to diets of wild game and fresh fruits and vegetables, alternating periods of feasting and famine, and physically demanding lifestyles. Our bodies are now exposed to different foods and different circumstances, however. The types of food available to people in the U.S. in the late twentieth century (Table 1-1) bear little resemblance to the foods available to our early ancestors. Periods of feasts are generally not followed by famines or periods of strenuous physical activity.

The human body developed biological mechanisms that facilitated the survival of the hunter–gatherers. One of these mechanisms stimulates hunger, even in the presence of excessive body stores of fat. Other mechanisms conserve the body's supply of sodium, confer an inborn preference for sweet-tasting foods, and cause the digestive system to function best on a high-fiber diet. These mechanisms served early humans very well, but they do not serve us well. Nonetheless, the mechanisms remain; they are part of the human genetic makeup. Although the human body has a remarkable ability to adapt to changes in diet, many health problems of modern civilization—heart disease, cancer, hypertension, and diabetes, for example—are thought to result partly from exposing the body to diets that are vastly different from those of our biological ancestors, the hunter–gatherers.[1,2] The diets to which we expose our 40,000-year-old biological systems continue to change, whereas the human body remains basically the same.

Diets Are Dynamic

When you were a child, did you eat the same foods that children eat today? Are the foods you eat today similar to those you ate when you were in high school? What foods would you eat if you could afford anything you wanted? People's diets are not stable; they change over time, for a variety of reasons.

(Below left) Foods representative of those consumed by today's hunter–gatherers. Do you recognize any of them? Included are birds' eggs, wild cucumbers, tubers, roots, nuts, berries, bulbs. Not shown are grubs and insects, which might be consumed as quickly as they are discovered.

(Below right) Two !Kung families go hunting and gathering. Today, only a few hunter–gatherer tribes exist in the world.

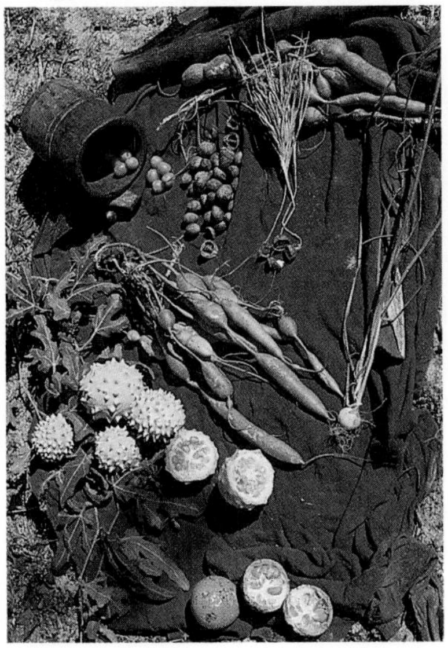

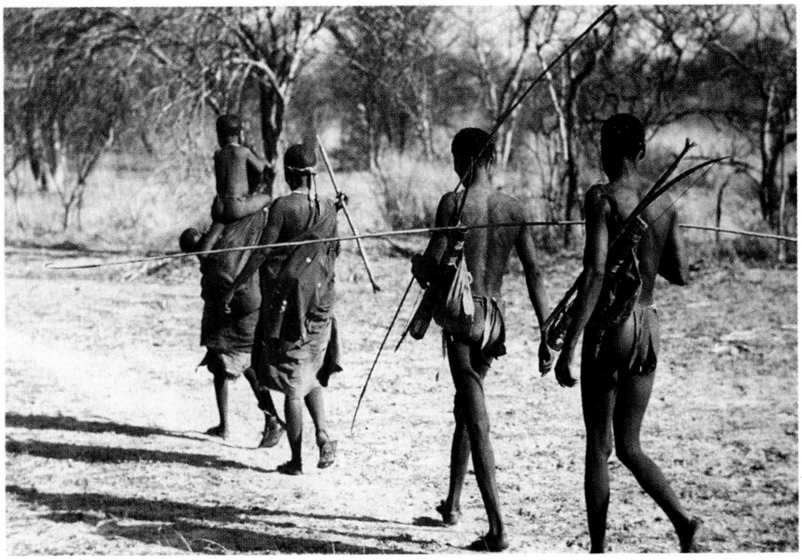

TABLE 1-1

U.S. average daily per capita food supply[3]

Food	Amount, pounds
beef	.21
pork	.19
poultry	.17
fish	.05
eggs	.09
whole milk	.47
lowfat milk	.29
cheese	.06
butter	.01
margarine, oils, shortening, lard	.15
citrus fruits	.21
other fruits:	
fresh	.29
canned, dried, etc.	.24
vegetables:	
tomatoes	.15
spinach, broccoli, carrots	.07
other (peas, green beans, corn)	.39
white potatoes	.31
sweet potatoes	.01
dried beans	.05
flour	.33
cornmeal	.02
table sugar	.24
syrups (corn syrup)	.15
coffee	.02
tea	.01

(Below left) Crackers and milk were often the daily lunch at this turn-of-the-century day nursery. How do the foods eaten as a child by a person now over 60 years old compare with the foods today's children eat?

(Below right) Would an adult enjoy cotton candy as much as this child does? People's food preferences change over time.

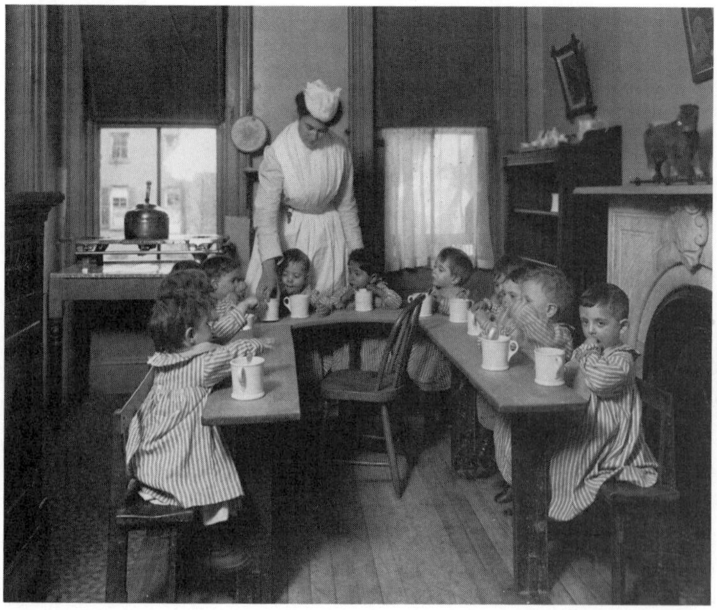

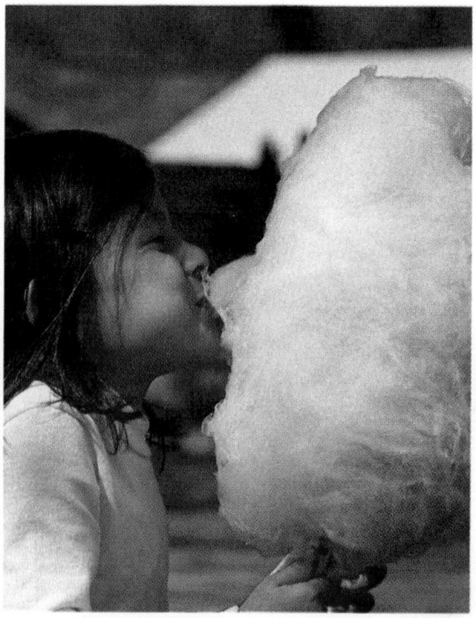

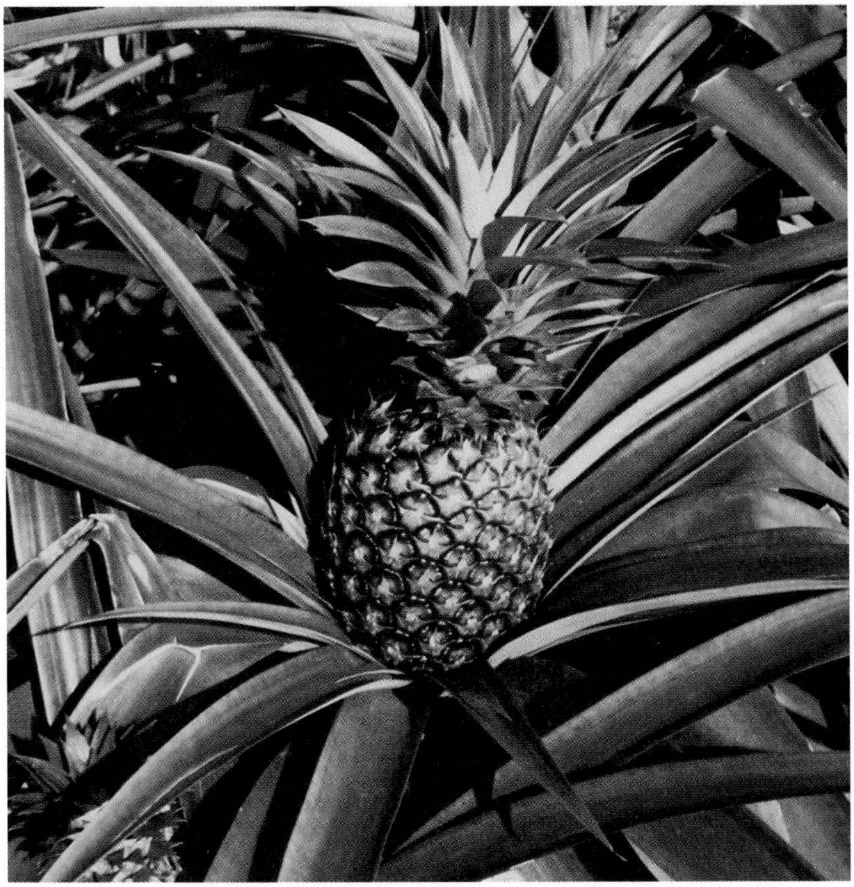

Although these pineapples are grown on the island of Maui, they can be found at grocery stores throughout the mainland U.S. on a regular basis.

Recent Changes in the U.S. Diet Many factors contribute to the changing U.S. diet: new methods of food production, transportation, preservation, and storage; increased income; the changing pace of life; shifting food preferences; and knowledge about diet–disease relationships. No longer do we primarily depend upon locally produced foods for our food supply. Supermarkets typically carry more than 15,000 food items, most of which are brought in from outside the local area. American families regularly dine on fish from the East Coast, vegetables from the West Coast, potatoes from Idaho, beef from the Midwest and South America, and fruits from islands in the Pacific. Modern food technology has expanded our options to include dehydrated, rehydrated, texturized, freeze-dried, irradiated, and low-fat and low-calorie foods. There are a lot more snack items on grocers' shelves than there used to be. Gone are the days when apples were the main snack food of Americans. Apples now compete with creme-filled cakes, candy, yogurt, granola bars, potato chips, and other prepared snacks. The popularity of fast-food hamburgers and fries and the increasing consumption of "low-cal" frozen entrées, artificial sweeteners, soft drinks, bottled waters, pasta salads, and ethnic foods illustrate food-preference shifts that contribute to changes in diets.

Changes in diets are also related to people's concerns about good health. Information about sweets and tooth decay, cholesterol and heart disease, low-fiber diets and colon cancer, calcium and osteoporosis, and the effects of too much caffeine have influenced people's food choices. Current trends in U.S. diets are toward less consumption of sugar, beef, eggs, salt, and caffeine, and greater consumption of cheese, fruits, chicken, vegetables, whole-grain products, and low-fat dairy products.[3,4]

New foods are being introduced to the market in response to these changes in consumer preferences. Of growing impact on the U.S. diet is the increasing availability of "designer foods"—foods that are developed to have specific characteristics. Examples of these include low-cholesterol eggs, low-fat pork and beef, nonfat yogurt, oat-bran muffins and high-fiber breakfast cereals, low-salt soups, and artificial sweeteners and fats. The demand for designer foods is expected to increase as more Americans attempt to change their diets in order to improve their health.

Changes in the Health Status of Americans Along with changes in food intake, major shifts have occurred in the causes of illness and death among Americans during this century. Before 1950 the major causes of death in the U.S. were infectious diseases such as influenza, pneumonia, and tuberculosis. Today those diseases account for fewer than 3 percent of deaths.[5] The major nutrition problems in the U.S. before 1950 were dietary deficiencies of calories and certain vitamins and minerals. These deficiencies contributed to the development and spread of the infectious diseases.[6] Since 1950, the major causes of illness and death have been long-term, chronic diseases such as heart disease, cancer, and diabetes (Figure 1-1). Chronic diseases accounted for only 14 percent of deaths in 1900; today they account for over 75 percent.

Chronic diseases develop over time and are probably caused by multiple environmental and genetic factors. Although they are generally noninfectious, their increasing incidence is related to "contagious" changes in lifestyle. Environmental factors such as what and how much we eat, smoking, drinking too much alcohol, level of physical activity, and amount of psychological stress largely determine whether we are promoting good health or contributing to the development of chronic disease.[7] The manner in which we live our day-to-day lives strongly influences our long-term health.

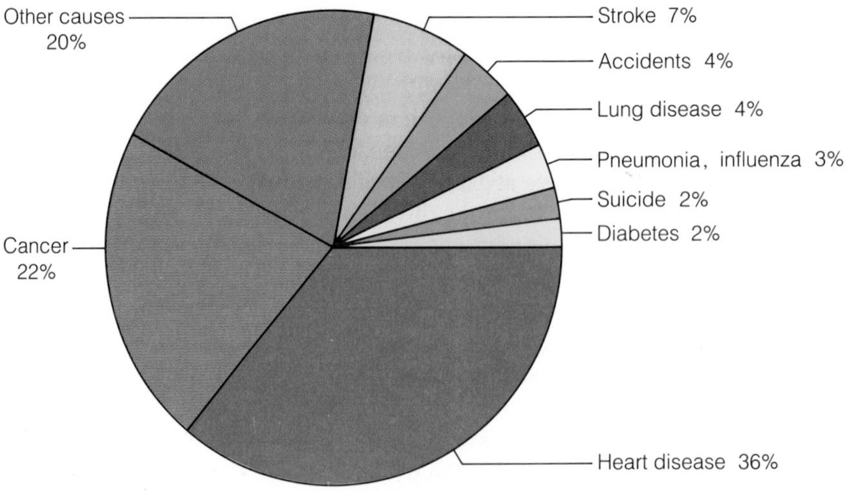

FIGURE 1-1
Leading causes of death in the United States.

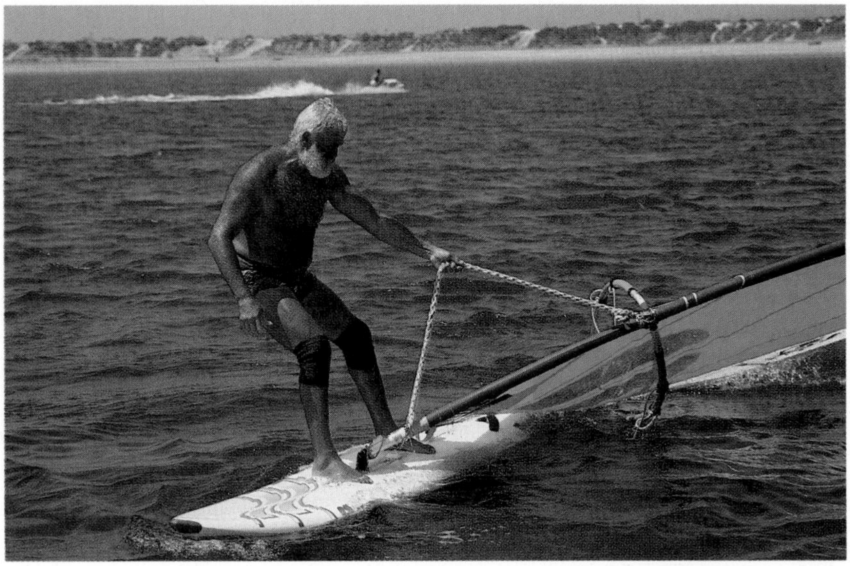

As exemplified by today's vigorous elderly, the manner in which we live our lives from day to day can strongly influence our long-term health.

Interest in preventing chronic diseases through dietary and other lifestyle improvements is stronger today than ever before. The costs of poor health in terms of illness care, human productivity, and quality of life are becoming unbearably high in this and many other countries. Between 1960 and 1985, U.S. expenditures for health care increased twelvefold. (It is predicted that the yearly total may be one and a half trillion dollars by the year 2000.[8]) During that fifteen years, however, life expectancy in the U.S. increased by 5 years, or 7 percent.[9] Reductions achieved in infant and early childhood deaths accounted for most of the gain in life expectancy.[10] It is expected that future gains in life expectancy will largely stem from lifestyle improvements that help to prevent chronic disease.[6,7]

IDENTIFYING DIET–DISEASE RELATIONSHIPS

The links between diet and heart disease, cancer, hypertension, and other chronic health problems are not clear-cut **cause-and-effect relationships**. Rather than directly causing chronic disorders, dietary factors, along with a number of other factors, are **associated** with their development. The causes of most chronic diseases now prevalent in the U.S. are yet to be identified. A number of conditions associated with their development have been identified, however.

Nutrition Risk Factors

Dietary patterns associated with the development of a disease or disorder are referred to as nutrition **risk factors**. The presence of these risk factors increases the likelihood that a person will develop a particular disease or condition. For example, diets that are high in animal fat have been shown to increase the risk of heart disease and certain types of cancer. People who

cause-and-effect relationship: Relationship that exists when one condition produces another. For example, bacteria *cause* wounds to become infected, and vitamin C deficiency *causes* scurvy.

association: Relationship that exists when one condition accompanies another condition. An association does not show a cause-and-effect relationship. High-fat diets, high blood pressure, and smoking are all *associated* with the development of heart disease, for example, but it is not clear at this time that any of them *causes* heart disease.

risk factors: Conditions that increase the likelihood that a particular disease or condition will develop. For example, since diets that are high in animal fat have been found to increase the likelihood of developing heart disease, they are said to be a risk factor for heart disease.

consume high-fat diets may not develop heart disease or cancer, but their chances of developing one or the other are higher than those of people who consume less fat.

Heart disease and cancer cause over half of all deaths in the U.S., so nutrition risk factors associated with their development have received a great deal of attention. Nutrition risk factors have also been identified for a variety of other diseases and disorders. A summary of nutrition risk factors associated with the development of a number of diseases and disorders is given in Table 1-2. Although not all-inclusive, the information presented gives a good indication of the broad influence of nutrition on the development of health problems.

Many nutrition risk factors for chronic disease development can be reduced or eliminated. When the risk factors are reduced, the likelihood of developing those diseases is decreased. The declining incidence of heart

TABLE 1-2

Nutrition risk factors associated with the development of diseases and disorders[11–14]

Disease or Disorder	Nutrition Risk Factors
Heart disease and atherosclerosis ("hardening of the arteries")	diets high in animal fat and cholesterol; obesity
Cancer*	diets high in fat and low in vitamin A, beta-carotene, dietary fiber, and certain types of vegetables
Diabetes (in adults)	obesity
Cirrhosis of the liver	excessive alcohol consumption, malnutrition
Infertility	underweight, obesity, zinc deficiency (in men)
Health problems of pregnant women and newborns	maternal underweight, obesity, malnutrition, and excessive use of vitamin and mineral supplements or alcohol
Growth retardation in children	diets low in calories, protein, iron, zinc
Tooth decay	frequent consumption of sweets, diets low in fluoride
Iron-deficiency anemia	diets low in iron
Constipation	diets low in fiber and fluids
Obesity	excessive calorie intake
Underweight	deficient calorie intake
Hypertension	diets high in sodium, excessive alcohol consumption, obesity
Osteoporosis	diets low in calcium and vitamin D

*The development of most types of cancer, notably excluding leukemia, have been associated with nutrition risk factors.

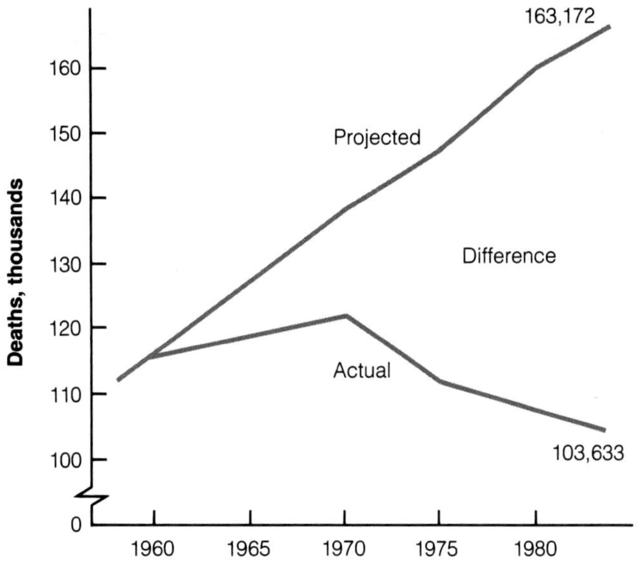

FIGURE 1-2
Projected and actual deaths due to heart disease for persons 55–64 years of age in the United States, 1960–1982.

disease in the U.S. is a good example of this. The rates of death from heart disease in the U.S. since 1960 are considerably lower than they were projected to be (Figure 1-2). The reduced intake of animal fat and cholesterol in the past 30 years is strongly associated with the decreased death rates from heart disease.[15,16] A reduction in the percentage of males who smoke has also contributed to the decline.[15] Although the treatments for heart disease have improved, the decline in deaths from the disease is primarily related to the reduction in the percentage of people who are at risk of developing it.

Unfortunately, dietary habits that have contributed to the development of heart disease in the U.S. are also being adopted by people in other industrialized countries. Since 1964, the rate of heart disease in the Soviet Union, Yugoslavia, Italy, Poland, and a number of other countries has increased. The increases in these countries are associated with higher animal fat and cholesterol intakes and with increasing use of tobacco.[17]

Achieving dietary changes that reduce nutrition risk factors is a major goal of health programs in this country. It is an ambitious, important goal. Such dietary habits as overeating, excessive consumption of fat, high cholesterol intake, excessive salt intake, and inadequate consumption of fiber tend to represent the all-American diet. They are risk factors that are shared by the majority of Americans.[11]

NUTRITION RESEARCH

Limitations

All diseases and disorders have causes, but the causes can be so complex and difficult to study that they escape identification. Yet to be identified, for example, are the causes of most cases of heart disease, cancer, diabetes, hypertension, arthritis, obesity, and depression. The lack of absolute knowledge about the causes of these diseases and disorders leaves the door wide open for speculation. In the area of nutrition, such speculation often turns into widely publicized controversies: Can vitamin supplements help you live longer? Is obesity inherited? Do large doses of vitamin C cure the common cold? Does sugar cause hyperactivity in children? Do food additives cause cancer? The existence of nutrition controversies makes perfectly obvious the gaps in our knowledge about nutrition and health relationships.

The complexity of nutrition and health relationships and the present limitations of research into human nutrition make for large gaps in knowledge. The variety of conditions that researchers must consider if the actual nutrition and health relationships are to be identified with absolute certainty is enormous.

Most foods we eat contain hundreds to thousands of chemical components (see Figure 1-3), and there are thousands of foods. There are about 40,000 edible plants, for example, and most contain chemical components yet to be identified. Each chemical component of food may have different effects on body processes. Between two billion and ten billion chemical reactions occur inside the body, and each reaction may play a role in how the food we eat ultimately affects our health. Along with these considerations, research needs to assess the potential influence of existing diseases, physical activity, psychological factors, genetic characteristics, age, occupation, and other factors. Further complicating the search for definitive knowledge about the relationships between nutrition and health is the fact that nutrition-related health problems often take many years to develop. Moreover, human nutrition research is generally very expensive to conduct and must be limited in ways so as not to endanger the health of the human subjects.

Given these constraints, it is unlikely that science will be able to explain with absolute certainty how dietary factors cause health problems. Thus we must take action, in the form of nutrition guidance and programs, before we know all the details. We cannot afford to wait for absolute certainty, because it may never exist and we may miss important opportunities to improve life through better health.

The methods used for determining the truth about suspected relationships between nutrition and health are specific and rigorous. Nutrition truths cannot be based on personal experience, opinions, or assumptions; they must be demonstrated through research studies that employ the scientific method.

The Scientific Method

The scientific method is the basic approach to identifying the truth in many areas of scientific research. It consists of seven steps:

1. Statement of the question to be answered by the research
2. Formulation of a **hypothesis** to be tested by the research
3. Development of a design for the research (a plan for how the study will be carried out) that will succeed in testing the hypothesis
4. Implementation of the research design
5. Collection and analysis of data
6. Interpretation of the results
7. Acceptance or rejection of the hypothesis

hypothesis: (hī päth′ ə sis) An educated guess about the anticipated result of an experiment. A hypothesis is formulated during the planning stage of a research study to focus the research on a specific issue. The research then proves or disproves the hypothesis.

Toast and Coffee Cake:
Gluten
Amino acids
Amylose
Starches
Dextrins
Sucrose
Pentosans
Hexosans
Triglycerides
Mono- and diglycerides
Sodium chloride
Phosphorus
Calcium
Iron
Thiamin (vitamin B_1)
Riboflavin (vitamin B_2)
Niacin
Pantothenic acid
Vitamin D
Methyl ethyl ketone
Acetic acid
Propionic acid
Butyric acid
Valeric acid
Caproic acid
Acetone
Diacetyl
Maltol
Ethyl acetate
Ethyl lactate

Chilled Cantaloupe:
Starches
Cellulose
Pectin
Fructose
Sucrose
Glucose
Malic acid
Citric acid
Succinic acid
Anisyl propionate
Amyl acetate
Ascorbic acid (vitamin C)
β-carotene (vitamin A)
Riboflavin (vitamin B_2)
Thiamin (vitamin B_1)
Niacin
Phosphorus
Potassium

Tea:
Caffeine
Tannin
Butanol
Isoamyl alcohol
Hexanol
Phenyl ethyl alcohol
Benzyl alcohol
Geraniol
Quercetin
3-Galloyl epicatechin
3-Galloyl epigallocatechin

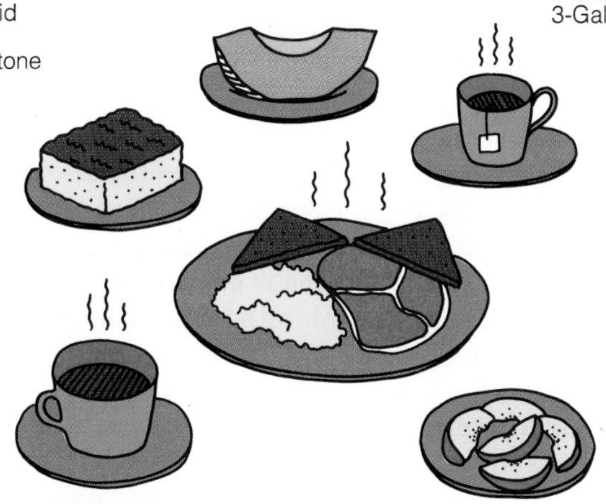

Cinnamon Apple Chips:
Pectin
Hemicellulose
Cellulose
Starches
Sucrose
Glucose
Fructose
Malic acid
Lactic acid
Citric acid
Succinic acid
Ascorbic acid (vitamin C)
β-carotene (vitamin A)
Cinnamyl alcohol
Cinnamic aldehyde
Potassium
Phosphorus
Acetaldehyde
Amyl formate
Amyl acetate
Amyl caproate
Geraniol

Coffee:
Caffeine
Methanol
Ethanol
Butanol
Methylbutanol
Acetaldehyde
Methyl formate
Dimethyl sulfide
Propionaldehyde
Pyridine
Acetic acid
Furfural
Furfuryl alcohol
Acetone
Methyl acetate
Furan
Methylfuran
Diacetyl
Isoprene
Guaiacol
Hydrogen sulfide

Scrambled Eggs:
Ovalbumin
Conalbumin
Ovomucoid
Mucin
Globulins
Amino acids
Lipovitellin
Livetin
Cholesterol
Lecithin
Choline
Lipids (fats)
Fatty acids
Lutein
Zeaxanthine
Vitamin A
Biotin
Pantothenic acid
Riboflavin (vitamin B_2)
Thiamin (vitamin B_1)
Niacin
Pyridoxine (vitamin B_6)
Folic acid (folacin)
Cyanocobalamin (vitamin B_{12})
Sodium chloride
Iron
Calcium
Phosphorus

Sugar-Cured Ham:
Myosin
Actomyosin
Myoglobin
Collagen
Elastin
Amino acids
Creatine
Lipids (fats)
Linoleic acid
Oleic acid
Lecithin
Cholesterol
Sucrose
Glucose
Pyroligneous acid
Phosphorus
Thiamin (vitamin B_1)
Riboflavin (vitamin B_2)
Niacin
Cyanocobalamin (vitamin B_{12})
Pyridoxine (vitamin B_6)
Sodium chloride
Iron
Magnesium
Potassium

FIGURE 1-3
Chemical breakfast. The chemicals shown are some of those found naturally in these foods.

An Application of the Scientific Method

The Question Let's imagine that a team of nutrition researchers wanted to determine if vitamin C supplements prevent the common cold. According to the rules of the scientific method, they would first pose the question to be answered by the research. In this case, it might be "Do vitamin C supplements prevent the common cold?" In an actual study, the question would be made more specific by adding such details as the amount of supplemental vitamin C to be tested, the duration of the use of the supplement, and a precise description of "common cold" for use in identifying cases of the illness.

The Hypothesis The next step would be to formulate a hypothesis about the effect of vitamin C on the prevention of the common cold. Let's say the hypothesis is "People who take vitamin C supplements experience significantly fewer episodes of the common cold than people who do not take vitamin C supplements."

The Design Then the researchers would develop a "design" for the study—a set of procedures for testing the hypothesis. As part of the study design, the researchers would calculate statistically how many subjects (people) are needed in the study in order to give them the certainty they desire. They would also specify who is eligible to participate in the study based on such factors as age, sex, health status, history of colds, and so on. The design would call for the formation of an "experimental group" (subjects who would receive vitamin C tablets) and a "control group" (subjects who would receive a **placebo**—in this case, a tablet that does *not* contain vitamin C). In well-designed studies, neither the subjects nor the researchers know which subjects are the "experimentals" and which are the "controls." Such a design is called a "double-blind" study. It has the advantage of avoiding the **placebo effect**, which commonly results when people think the substance they are given will produce particular changes. This design might test the hypothesis by comparing the occurrence of the common cold in subjects taking the supplement with the occurrence among subjects who do not receive vitamin C. It's not quite that simple, however.

placebo: (plə sē′ bō) A substance having no medical properties that is used as a control in an experiment to test the effects of a biologically active substance. Also, a "sugar pill" or other substance with no medicinal effect that is given to a patient as though it were a medication.

placebo effect: An improvement in physical health or sense of well being in response to the use of a placebo. It is often observed among control subjects in experiments that employ placebos.

Designing the study is often the most challenging part of a research project, especially in research with human subjects. Humans vary in many, many respects in addition to the difference introduced by an experiment. In the case of our imaginary study, some of the differences may influence subjects' susceptibility to the common cold apart from any effect of vitamin C. The study subjects will experience different levels of exposure to germs that cause the common cold and will vary in their eating patterns and other lifestyle habits that may influence their susceptibility to colds. Each of these conditions, as well as the use of vitamin C supplements, must be assessed if a unique effect of vitamin C supplements in preventing the common cold is to be identified. Due to time, money, and other constraints, human studies cannot assess all of the conditions that may influence the results. Consequently, the results of most human studies show relationships rather than definite proofs.

Implementation, Analysis, Interpretation After the study was designed, it would be implemented, and data would be collected on each subject. Data would be analyzed for the presence of a "statistically significant" difference (a difference that is not due to chance) between the number of episodes of the common cold in the experimental group and the control group.

Acceptance/Rejection If the experimental group experienced significantly fewer colds than the control group, then the proposed hypothesis would be accepted by the researchers. If not, the hypothesis would be rejected; it would be concluded that vitamin C supplements do not reduce the incidence of colds. Now, even if the hypothesis—that vitamin C supplements do significantly reduce the incidence of the common cold—were accepted, it would not mean that vitamin C supplements had been shown to prevent the common cold in *all people*. It would mean that the occurrence of the common cold among a group of people is less frequent if vitamin C supplements are taken than if they are not. The results would not guarantee that vitamin C supplements would prevent the common cold in everyone who takes them.

Experiments similar to the one just discussed have been carried out, and the results have not always been the same. Contradictory results of studies that investigate the same question can be due to differences in the designs of the experiments. For example, the results of studies may differ due to the use of a double-blind design, the use of a control group, and different numbers of subjects.

Establishing Nutrition Truths

The decisions scientists make about nutrition and health relationships are based on the results of studies that employed designs best-suited for testing particular hypotheses. When well-designed research studies consistently show the same result, the result becomes generally accepted as representing the truth. It is at this point that scientists make recommendations aimed at improving health. Most dietary changes recommended to the public by groups of scientists have the support of at least 90 percent of the nutrition science community.[18] Though based on less than 100-percent certainty, the dietary recommendations identified have generally led to improvements in health. For example, far more people have benefited than have been harmed from the recommendations to enrich grain products with certain vitamins and iron and to reduce fat and salt intakes if they are high.

An unavoidable problem is connected with human nutrition research. Basing dietary recommendations on less-than-perfect data about nutrition and health relationships automatically leaves room for criticism about the reliability of the conclusions and for confusion about what the truth is. Some opinions that differ with those of the majority of scientists are based on scholarly scientific disagreement. Sometimes it isn't the research results that are at the heart of a dispute, but rather what to *do* about the results. For example, should it be recommended that *all* Americans reduce total fat intake, or just those who show signs of developing heart disease or cancer? Furthermore, decisions about which diets and foods are "good" or "bad" can have profound effects within the food industry and other industries. Consequently, special-interest groups are drawn into nutrition controversies because they have a product to protect.

PROPHETS, PROFITS, AND PROOF: AN EXAMINATION OF NUTRITION SENSE AND NONSENSE

Are brown eggs more nutritious than white eggs?
Does bee pollen increase strength?
Is honey better for you than table sugar?
Does garlic unplug arteries?
Do extra B vitamins give you energy?

Unfortunately, the gaps in knowledge about nutrition and health have left room for unscientific conclusions about the causes of some diseases. All too often, nutrition quacks have stepped in to fill the gaps in scientific knowledge. Unlike careful, methodical scientists, nutrition quacks are not deterred by a lack of scientific data to support their contentions. They skillfully select information that supports their views—and the products they sell—while ignoring evidence to the contrary. They specialize in making misinformation believable.

Nutrition information and products represent big business in this country and throughout the world. Whether you want to lower your weight, raise your I.Q., grow stronger fingernails, or protect yourself from the "poisons" in food, there are claims that certain foods or dietary supplements can do it. The selling of nutrition information, "health" foods, and other products is a multibillion dollar business in the U.S. The claims made for various foods and supplements help keep business healthy.

A lot of nutrition information is available, and much of it is erroneous. At best, nutrition misinformation and quackery may benefit health by coincidence. Most often they are simply useless and expensive. At worst, they damage health. For example, a number of deaths have been directly associated with liquid protein diets and potassium supplements.[19,20] Lead poisoning has resulted from the use of "natural" calcium supplements that naturally contain lead.[20] Reports of overdoses of vitamin and mineral supplements are increasingly common.

Why is so much nutrition misinformation available to consumers? Because there is no law against fiction. Purveyors of nutrition misinformation are protected under the First Amendment of the Constitution, which guarantees freedom of speech. As long as no direct connection is made between a false or deceptive nutrition claim and a specific product, books, flyers, magazines, newspapers, and radio and television talk show personalities can claim anything about nutrition. In most states, any food may be labeled as "organic," "natural," or "health," and any substance may be sold as a "vitamin" or "dietary supplement." (See Box 1-1.) Vitamins and other dietary supplements do not have to contain ingredients that are useful or necessary for health. Sawdust could be sold as a dietary supplement!

The opportunities for proliferating nutrition misinformation are also enhanced by the fact that people do not have to have credentials to call themselves nutritionists. Until laws are passed that change this situation, anyone may take the title "nutritionist" or "nutrition expert." Bogus nutrition credentials can easily be purchased. (See Box 1-2.) Only the designation *Registered Dietitian* carries a guarantee that a person has expertise in nutrition. Registered Dietitians have successfully completed at least a bachelor's degree, approved college courses, and supervised work experience and have passed a national qualifying examination.

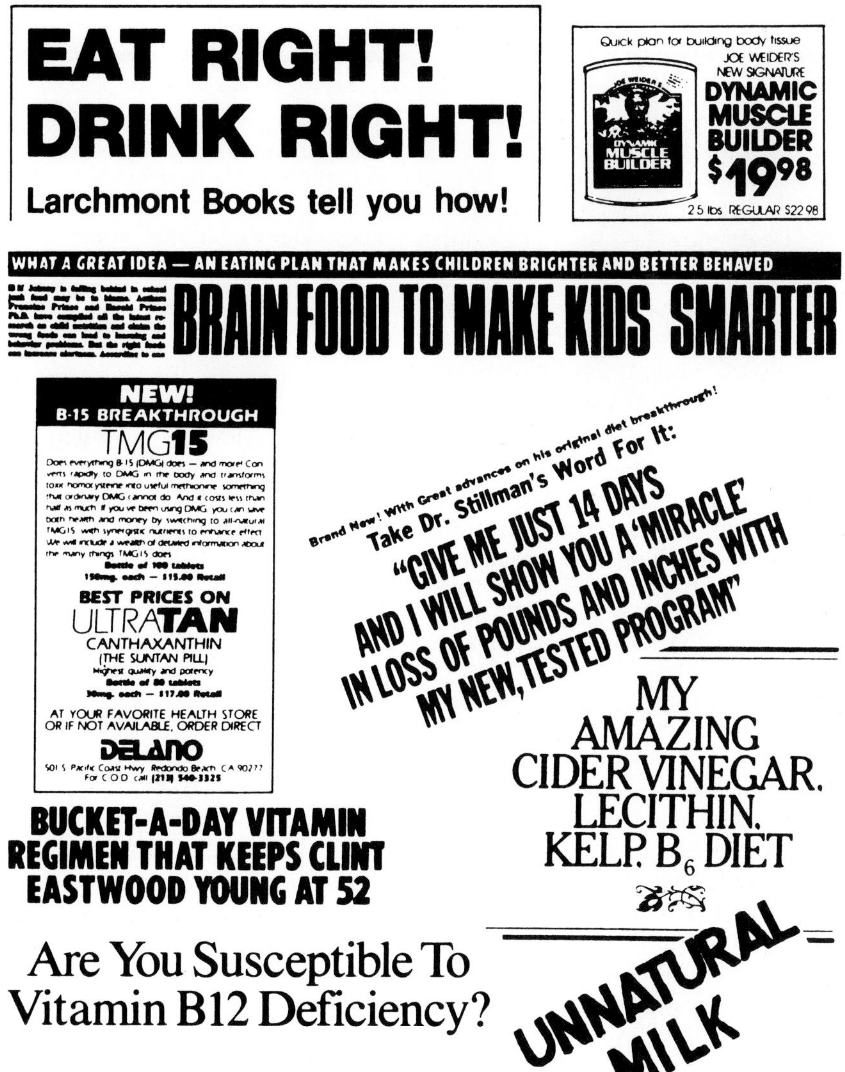

BIOTICS & BIOLOGICALS

Product Description	Size	Wholesale Unit Price	Suggested Retail Price
ADRENAL GLANDS (Lyophilized) Granular Form	$ 15 gm 50 gm	$ 6.75 16.00	$ 13.50 30.00
BUFFERED VITAMIN C (Effervescent) with Ca, Mg: Carbonates & Potassium Bicarbonate	100 gm 250 gm	5.00 10.00	10.00 20.00
dl-CARNITINE HCl – 250 mg tablets 500 mg capsules (Discontinued until further notice)			
HAIR FOLLICLE STIMULATOR SOLUTION No. I – Dropper Bottle " " " " No. II – Bottle	15 ml 30 ml 1 pint	4.00 6.00 7.00	7.95 10.50 15.00
DIGESTIVE MIXTURE containing Gastric Factors, Intestinal Factors & Thymus	80 gm	20.00	38.00

"I shall begin, my friends, with a definition of a pseudoscience. A pseudoscience consists of a nomenclature, with a self-adjusting arrangement, by which all positive evidence, or such as favors its doctrines, is admitted, and all negative evidence, or such as tells against it, is excluded. It is invariably connected with some lucrative practical application. . . ." (O. W. Holmes in *The Professor at the Breakfast Table*)

The burden is on consumers to decide if what they read or hear about nutrition is true, and distinguishing nutrition facts from fiction is not easy. The nutrition misinformation business is sophisticated, and it uses convincing selling techniques. Nevertheless, its ploys have a pattern, and you can often distinguish nutrition fact from fiction by examining how the information is presented.

BOX 1-1

WHAT ARE *ORGANIC, NATURAL,* AND *HEALTH* FOODS?

Are "organic," "natural," or "health" foods better for you than other foods? Are these products superior to other products on the supermarket shelves? These questions are at the heart of disputes about what these terms mean.

"Organic" foods are generally thought of as those that were grown using only fertilizers and pesticides of animal or vegetable origin. Not all foods labeled as "organic" are grown organically, however. Organic foods have been found to be just as likely to contain potentially harmful pesticide residues as similar foods not labeled "organic."[21] To many people, "natural" foods are those that are unprocessed and additive-free. Few foods labeled "natural" meet these qualifications. "Natural" foods are products of nature, but then so are all other foods; there are no "unnatural" or "inorganic" foods. Similarly, there are no "health" foods. There are, however, unhealthy *diets.*

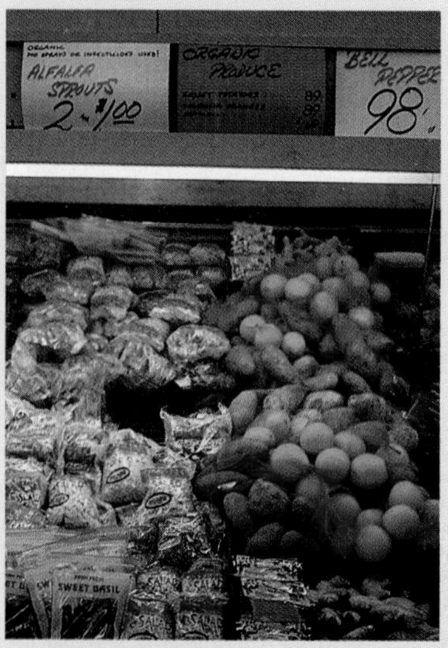

An unhealthy diet is one that contains foods that do not help the particular person to maintain health. No single food can be identified as "healthy" or "unhealthy." Matching what you eat with what your body needs for health is what makes for a healthy diet. Sherbet, for example, contains mostly water and sugar. If a serving of sherbet is consumed by a child who needs additional calories, then the sherbet contributes to a healthy diet. If eaten by a child who consumes too many calories, sherbet would be a detriment to a healthy diet. So, sherbet, like other foods, cannot be considered "healthy" or "unhealthy" in itself.

"Organic," "natural," and "health" foods have not been found to be better for health than foods without these labels. In addition, these labels do not guarantee that the foods are free of harmful pesticides or additives.

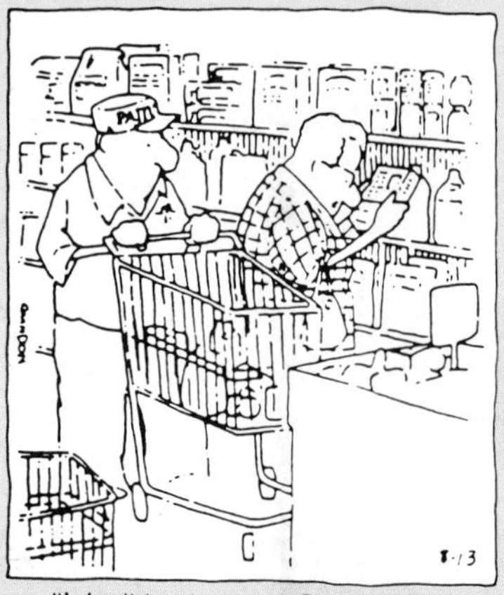

"I don't trust natural. People die all the time from natural causes."

Characteristics of Nutrition Misinformation

The Money Motive The most common feature of nutrition misinformation is the goal of selling something. Products, services, or programs are offered that promise a new, unique approach to treating ailments and diseases. (Otherwise, why would you need it?) Nutrition misinformation is used liberally to convince customers of the effectiveness of the product being sold.

To circumvent truth-in-advertising laws, the benefits of special foods and dietary supplements may be promoted in articles that are interspersed with advertisements. Although they are careful to avoid making health claims on the labels of their products, peddlers of nutrition nonsense can say whatever they want in magazine and newspaper articles. For example, here is a

NUTRITION CREDENTIALS FOR SALE

How easy is it to obtain certification as a nutrition expert? Very easy. All it takes is money and a filled-out application. The applicant needn't even be human.

To demonstrate how easily nutritionist certification can be obtained, Dr. Victor Herbert, a well-known and respected scientist, applied for certification for his cat. In response to an advertisement, he sent in fifty dollars and an application in his cat's name. Several weeks later, his cat received a signed and embossed certificate verifying her affiliation with the International Academy of Nutritional Consultants.[22]

This cat, Charlie Herbert, is a certified nutritional consultant.

portion of an article that appeared in a popular magazine. (The advertisements that surrounded the article were for zinc and other supplements.)

> *Zinc is without a doubt crucial to a healthy sex life. The scientific awareness of zinc's importance grew out of observations made by Dr. Prasad, M.D., Ph.D., in the 1960s. Dr. Prasad and other pioneers conducted studies with undernourished, sexually underdeveloped dwarfs in the Middle East that showed that the cause of those men's sexual retardation was zinc deficiency.*
>
> *Researchers in this country now use zinc to treat sexual problems.*

Dr. Ananda Prasad is a respected medical and nutrition scientist who might have been surprised to see his work reported in this way. His research showed that zinc supplements fostered normal sexual maturation in

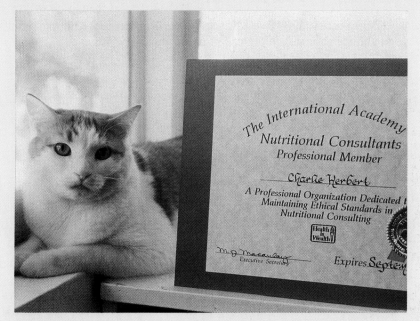

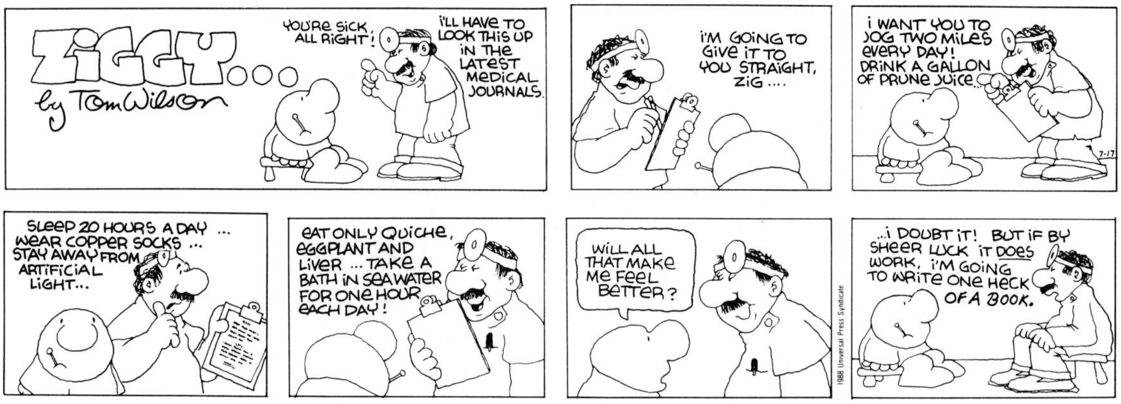

zinc-deficient males; no more than that. Here is an excerpt from the results Prasad and his co-workers published regarding zinc deficiency:

> *In recent years a syndrome of severe iron-deficiency anemia, hepatosplenomegaly,* hypogonadism, hyperpigmentation, and dwarfism in Iranian and Egyptian dwarfs has been attributed to primary zinc deficiency. Geophagia is common in the Iranian dwarfs, and it was suggested that zinc deficiency may have resulted from excessive consumption of a cereal diet containing large amounts of phytate, which inhibits zinc absorption. Upon treatment with supplemental zinc salts a striking response in growth and development of secondary sex characteristics was observed.*[23]

Nothing prevents purveyors of nutrition misinformation from misinterpreting research results and drawing their own conclusions in their effort to make money.

Cures for Common Problems Overweight? Under stress? Losing your hair? Tire easily? Getting wrinkles?

Nutrition misinformation and trendy products are usually aimed at relieving common problems that are difficult to treat or currently untreatable. The "safe, easy, and effective" approaches offered for solving problems are frequently irresistible, although one may suspect that they are probably too good to be true. As with other huckster pitches, if it sounds too good to be true, it probably is. If the purported cures really worked, the problems would have been solved and there would be no market for the products. Yet, there is always a new fad diet, "miracle" vitamin or mineral supplement, or new nutrition gimmick on the market, because those that went before have failed.

Creative Credibility Marketers of nutrition misinformation and products are aware of the need to appear credible, and they attempt to fill in credibility gaps in various ways. One means they use is hiring an M.D., Ph.D., or a superstar athlete to endorse the information or product. Informed consumers know that such nutrition endorsements cannot be trusted.

**Hepatosplenomegaly* means enlarged liver and spleen; *hypogonadism* is the term for immature sex glands; *hyperpigmentation* is abnormal skin color; and *geophagia* means the eating of dirt or clay.

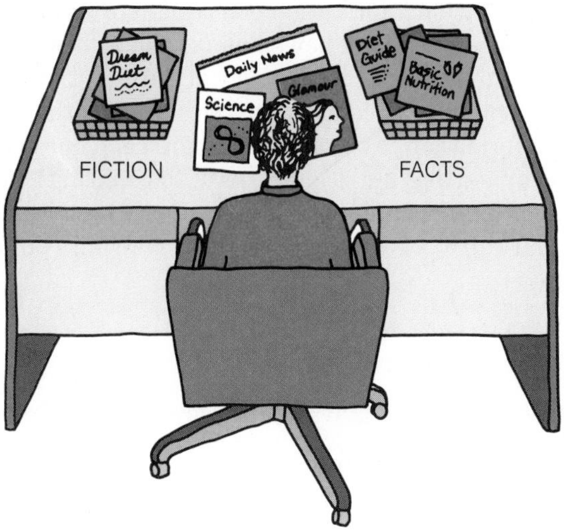

It's important to distinguish nutrition facts from nutrition fiction.

Individuals with impeccable credentials—including Nobel Prize–winning scientists, renowned surgeons, and Olympic gold medal winners—have been known to promulgate nutrition schemes. One dietary supplement company that freely promoted nutrition misinformation went so far as to enlist the services of fifteen internationally known scientists and physicians to serve on its "scientific advisory board." All were well respected in their fields and were employed by such honorable institutions as Harvard Medical School, the University of Washington, the National Institute of Mental Health, and the University of California at Berkeley. None, however, was an expert on *nutrition*. Their affiliation with this company that sold "revolutionary, breakthrough nutrition products for weight loss, protection against cancer and heart disease, and sustained energy" sent shock waves through the scientific community. This reaction was followed by aftershocks when it was learned that many of the members of the "scientific advisory board" had been awarded $100,000 research grants by the company whose products they were endorsing.[24]

Testimonials with the theme, "if it worked for me, it will work for you," are another common ploy used to make nutrition misinformation seem credible. They come in very handy when formal tests of a product's effectiveness have not been carried out, or when research results are unlikely to support the case being made. The use of testimonials to support a nutrition claim is a dead giveaway to false or deceptive information.

Examining the Source

Awareness of the source of nutrition information can sometimes help you judge its credibility. Some newspapers (particularly "tabloids"), talk shows, and magazines regularly present nutrition information because their audience surveys indicate strong interest in the topic. The more spectacular or controversial the information, the more likely it is to be presented. (News about rose-colored glasses suppressing appetite or of a superstar fighting cancer with fish oils, for example, will attract attention.) For these publications and broadcasts, it matters little if the information is drawn from nutrition fantasyland or scientific reports.

Not all of the nutrition information you read in print or hear on the radio or television is nonsense. Many newspapers, magazines, and broadcasting companies are cautious about the accuracy of the nutrition information they present. They exercise this caution by investigating the reliability of the sources of the information, by presenting more than one side of controversial topics, and by getting nutrition experts to confirm the conclusions before presenting the information. Some print and broadcasting companies have policies that reject advertisements that make false or deceptive nutrition claims.

Reliable Sources of Nutrition Information

Reliable nutrition information is available from a number of sources, including:

- government health publications
- information produced by scientifically recognized professional organizations such as the American Dietetic Association, the American Institute of Nutrition, and the Society for Nutrition Education
- scientific journals devoted to the publication of research studies
- college nutrition course textbooks

A listing of reliable sources of nutrition information on topics ranging from nutrition education to diet and cancer is given in Appendix B.

Other sources of reliable nutrition information exist, but it is impossible to give them blanket approval because the quality of the information pre-

TABLE 1-3
Evaluating nutrition information

The Quick List	yes	no
1. Is something being sold?	____	____
2. Does the information offer a solution to common problems for which there is no easy or available cure?	____	____
3. Are testimonials included?	____	____
4. Does the information sound too good to be true?	____	____
5. Does the information present a new, unique, or breakthrough method for solving a health problem?	____	____
Other Considerations		
1. Are quick, easy results promised?	____	____
2. Are endorsements by experts or public figures used to support the effectiveness of the product being promoted?	____	____
3. Did you read the information in a tabloid newspaper, magazine, advertisement, or popular book or hear it promoted on a talk show?	____	____

sented varies. For example, popular nutrition books written by people with impressive credentials may or may not be reliable. You can't tell by the credentials of the author alone. Nor can you always trust the information in "educational" publications produced by the food and dietary supplement industry. Infant formula companies, food-industry organizations (such as those representing the meat, wheat, potato, and dairy industries), manufacturers of vitamin and mineral supplements, and a host of other organizations publish nutrition information as a public service. Sometimes the nutrition information conveyed is accurate, but often it is slanted in favor of the organization's products. Advertisements often accompany the articles on nutrition, and the topics selected for coverage commonly relate only to the products of the sponsoring organization.

Table 1-3 summarizes our guidelines for judging the credibility of nutrition information. It can serve as a checklist.

COMING UP IN CHAPTER 2

Chapter 2 begins our discussion of the scientific principles of human nutrition. The eleven principles presented will provide you with the basics of the science.

REVIEW QUESTIONS

1. What are the seven steps of the scientific method?
   a. What is the purpose of a control group?
   b. What is a double-blind study design?
   c. What is the placebo effect?
2. What is the difference between a cause-and-effect relationship and an association? Cite three or more reasons why it is difficult to show cause-and-effect relationships in human nutrition studies.
3. Name four common chronic diseases or disorders, and list one or more nutrition risk factors for each.

Answers

1. Refer to the discussion of the scientific method.
2. See the "Identifying Diet–Disease Relationships" section.
3. See Table 1-2.

PUTTING NUTRITION KNOWLEDGE TO WORK

1. Compare a day in your life—what you eat, your level of physical activity, how you spend your time—with the diet, eating patterns, and lifestyle of your biological ancestors, the hunter–gatherers.

FIGURE 1-4

'Brain Fuel'

Do you have trouble remembering or concentrating?

Do you feel mentally fatigued often?

Do you have fear of becoming SENILE?

Do you have a lack of confidence?

Do you have trouble in making decisions?

It could be that you are lacking the proper balance of "BRAIN FUEL" in the form of Hematinics, Nutrients, Amino Acids, Vitamins and Minerals.

The brain, which is made up of more than 50 billion cells, directs all bodily functions including MEMORY and CONCENTRATION. To carry on this function, the brain needs a balanced quantity of FUEL to FUNCTION PROPERLY.

Total Research, Inc. has a capsule which contains 35 Hematinics, Nutrients, Amino Acids, Vitamins and Minerals.

These capsules are safe. Use 10 capsules: If you are not satisfied with the capsules return the unused portion for a full refund.

Along with the capsules comes the booklet, "Brain Fuel".

50 capsules $7.50; And 100 capsules $13.50. Or for a SUPER SAVINGS order 200 capsules for only $20.00. Canadians add $1.

2. Ask someone over sixty years of age about the types of food he or she ate as a child. What did he or she eat for breakfast, for lunch, for dinner, and for snacks? Contrast those foods with what you ate as a child. What are the differences? Speculate about the reasons for them.

3. How does your lifestyle shape up? Get an idea of how your lifestyle may be affecting your longevity by taking this quiz.* Check all questions with "yes" answers and use the table below to evaluate your lifestyle.

   _____ 1. Do you smoke cigarettes?
   _____ 2. Are you overweight?
   _____ 3. Do you generally skip breakfast?
   _____ 4. Do you usually snack between meals?
   _____ 5. Are you physically inactive?
   _____ 6. Do you generally drink three or more alcoholic beverages a day?
   _____ 7. Do you generally get fewer than 7–8 hours of sleep a day?

Number of Yes Responses	Change in Average Life Expectancy in Years
0 or 1	+10
2	0
3	−6
4	−13

4. Read the tabloid article in Figure 1-4 (which is actually an advertisement). Then apply the "Quick List" test of nutrition misinformation. (Apply this test to *all* nutrition information you read and hear.)
   1. Is something being sold?
   2. Does the information offer a solution to problems for which there is no easy or available cure?
   3. Are testimonials included?
   4. Does the information sound too good to be true?
   5. Does the information present a new, unique, or breakthrough method for solving a health problem?

5. What's wrong with this story?

   After four days of feeling unusually weak and tired, Amanda decided to take a B-complex vitamin supplement to help "pick her up." The day after taking the supplement, she felt like her old self again, full of energy and alert. She couldn't wait to tell her friends what she'd discovered. Did the B-complex supplement cure Amanda's "blahs"? (To help you decide, review the discussion of the scientific method.)

*Adapted from "The Future of Public Health," an address given by L. Breslow at a national workshop in Washington, D.C., October 1987.

NOTES

1. A. S. Truswell and J. D. L. Hansen, Medical research among the !Kung, in *Kalahari Hunter–Gatherers*, eds. R. B. Lee and I. DeVore (Cambridge, Mass.: Harvard University Press, 1976), 166–194.
2. D. Velican and C. Velican, Atherosclerotic involvement of the coronary arteries of adolescents and young adults, *Atherosclerosis* 36 (1980): 449–460.
3. S. O. Welsh and R. M. Marston, Review of trends in food use in the United States, 1909 to 1980, *Journal of the American Dietetic Association* 81 (1982): 120–125.
4. *Nutrition monitoring in the United States*, DHHS publication no. (PHS) 86-1255 (Hyattsville, Md.: July 1986).
5. *Prevention '82*, DHHS publication no. (PHS) 82-50157 (Washington, D.C.: Office of Disease Prevention and Health Promotion, 1982).
6. T. McKeown, *The role of medicine: Dream, mirage, or nemesis* (London: Nuffield Provencial Hospitals Trust, 1976).
7. A. Califano, Jr., America's health care revolution: Health promotion and disease prevention, *Journal of the American Dietetic Association* 87 (1987): 437–440.
8. *Medicine and Health Perspectives*, 41 (June 22, 1987): 3.
9. *Charting the Nation's Health Trends since 1960*, DHHS publication no. (PHS) 85–125 (Washington, D.C.: National Center for Health Statistics, 1985).
10. M. I. Roemer, The value of medical care for health promotion, *American Journal of Public Health* 74 (1984): 243–248.
11. B. Friend, Changes in nutrients in the U.S. diet caused by alternations in food intake patterns, Paper presented to The Changing Food Supply in America Conference, Washington, D.C., May 1974.
12. H. E. Sauberlich, Implications of nutritional status on human biochemistry, *Clinical Biochemistry* 17 (1984): 132–142.
13. J. E. Brown, Nutrition services for pregnant women, infants, children, and adolescents, *Clinical Nutrition* 3 (1984): 100–108.
14. M. Cornblath and N. Kretchmer, Research needs in human nutrition, in *Infant and Child Feeding* (New York: Academic Press, 1981), 453–465.
15. D. M. Berleson and J. Stambler, Epidemiology of the killer chronic diseases, in *Nutrition and the Killer Diseases*, ed. M. Winick (New York: John Wiley and Sons, 1981), 17–55.
16. M. L. Slattery and D. E. Randell, Trends in coronary heart disease mortality and food consumption in the United States between 1909 and 1980, *American Journal of Clinical Nutrition* 47 (1988): 1060–1067.
17. H. Blackburn and R. Luepker, Heart Disease, in *Health and Preventive Medicine*, 12th ed., ed. J. Last (Norwalk, Conn.: Appleton-Century-Croft, 1985), 1159–1193.
18. A. Forbes, Government regulations and nutrition alternatives, *Proceedings* of Conference on Balancing the Balanced Diet (Port St. Lucie, Fla.: Vitamin Information Service, 1981), 24–32.
19. V. P. Frattali, Deaths associated with the liquid protein diet, *FDA By-Lines* 9 (1979): 179.
20. The confusing world of health foods. *FDA Consumer*, DHEW publication no. (FDA) 79-2108 (Washington, D.C.: Food and Drug Administration, 1980).
21. S. P. Gourdine, W. W. Traiger, and D. S. Cohen, Health food stores investigation, *Journal of the American Dietetic Association* 83 (1983): 285–290.
22. *U.S. News and World Report*, 15 February 1988, 86.
23. A. S. Prasad, A. Miale, Z. Farid, et al., Zinc metabolism in patients with the syndrome of iron deficiency anemia, hepatosplenomegaly, dwarfism, and hypogonadism, *Journal of Laboratory Clinical Medicine* 61 (1963): 537–541.
24. F. J. Stare, Marketing a nutritional "revolutionary breakthrough," *New England Journal of Medicine* 315 (1986): 971–973.

CHAPTER

2

SCIENTIFIC PRINCIPLES OF HUMAN NUTRITION

What are human beings? They are a set of complex chemical reactions.

At the heart of the science of nutrition is a set of eleven principles. These principles represent basic "truths" that serve as the core of our understanding about normal nutrition, and as the foundation for growth in knowledge. This chapter is devoted to a discussion of the principles and to building a framework for understanding the relationships between human nutrition and health that are presented in later chapters.

PRINCIPLE 1: FOOD IS A BASIC NEED OF HUMANS

The first principle is very straightforward: humans need food to live.

PRINCIPLE 2: FOODS PROVIDE NUTRIENTS NEEDED FOR LIFE AND HEALTH

nutrients: Chemical substances found in food that are used by the body to maintain health. The six categories of nutrients are carbohydrates, proteins, fats, vitamins, minerals, and water.

Our need for food is based on the body's requirement for **nutrients** found in food. Nutrients are chemical substances needed by the body for health and growth. There are six categories of nutrients:

- carbohydrates
- proteins
- fats

TABLE 2-1
The nutrients and their functions

Nutrient	Function
Carbohydrates	energy
Proteins	structure, energy
Fats	energy
Vitamins	regulation
Minerals	structure, regulation
Water	regulation, structure

- vitamins
- minerals
- water

Each category of nutrient performs one or more of the three basic functions of nutrients:

- provide energy
- serve as components of body structures
- regulate body processes

Carbohydrates, proteins, and fats provide energy. They are the only nutrients that can supply energy to the body. *Structural* functions are primarily performed by proteins, minerals, and water. These nutrients serve as the major constituents of muscle, bone, blood, and all other body tissues. Vitamins, minerals, and water perform *regulatory* functions—body processes that control energy formation and storage, bone and muscle development, repair of damaged tissues, and other processes that maintain health.

carbohydrates, proteins, and fats are the body's sole sources of energy.

Each nutrient is a unique chemical substance, and its role in the body is dictated by its chemical characteristics. The chemical characteristics of nutrients allow them to be used by, and become part of living tissue. Whether nutrients are obtained from foods or are manufactured in a laboratory makes no difference to the roles they perform in the body. There is a major advantage to getting your nutrients from foods rather than from a laboratory, however. Nature does not "package" nutrients individually; nutrients occur in combinations in foods. A manufactured vitamin C supplement, for example, cannot replicate the nutrients contained in an orange. In addition to vitamin C, oranges contain carbohydrates, B-complex vitamins, potassium, and other minerals.

The Nutrient Composition of Foods

The plants and animal products that fulfill the nutrient requirements of humans have their own genetically determined requirements for nutrients. Without adequate levels of required nutrients, plants and animals fail to grow normally and generally do not become part of our food supply. It is assumed that the plants and animal products we consume contain the variety and level of nutrients that were required for their growth and survival.

The nutrition content of vegetables partly depends on the nutrient content of the soil in which they were grown.

Consequently, specific foods tend to have a constant composition of certain nutrients. They may contain other nutrients as well, however.

The nutrients contained in plants and animal products vary because of differences in growing conditions and processing methods. The particular nutrients present in soil and water, the fertilizers that are used, the nutrient composition of animal feed, and food preparation and storage methods all influence the nutrient content of the foods we eat. For example, plants grown in soils that are rich in iodine contain higher levels of iodine than plants grown in other soils. Although plants grown in different soils have different nutrient contents, they look the same; iodine-rich spinach does not have a particular appearance. Oysters harvested from the shores off the East Coast may contain four times as much zinc as oysters from the West Coast. The difference in zinc content is due to the greater concentration of zinc in the Atlantic coastal waters. Beef from grass-fed cattle contains more polyunsaturated fats than does beef from grain-fed cattle.

Because of the variation in the composition of foods, nutrient levels reported in food tables are averages based on analyses of multiple samples of the foods. The averages represent the best estimates of the nutrient compositions of specific foods. A table of the nutrient composition of foods appears in Appendix H.

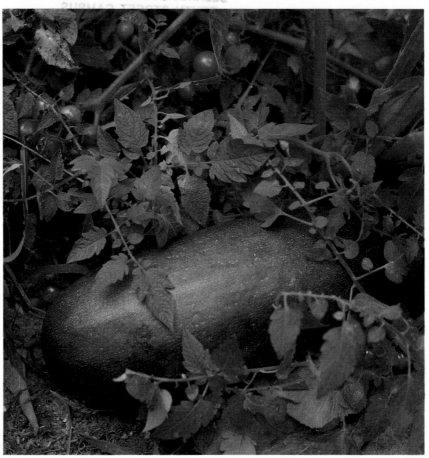

■ ■ ■

PRINCIPLE 3: SOME NUTRIENTS MUST BE PROVIDED BY THE DIET

Many nutrients are required for growth and health. Some of these can be manufactured in the body from the raw materials supplied by food, whereas others must be directly provided in food. Nutrients that the body cannot manufacture, or manufacture in sufficient quantities, are referred to as **essential nutrients**. The essential nutrients must be supplied by the diet. Vitamin C, iron, and calcium are examples of essential nutrients. On the other hand, fructose, lecithin, cholesterol, and glucose are **nonessential nutrients**; they may be present in food and used by the body, but they are not required in the diet because the body can produce them from substances found in food.

Both essential and nonessential nutrients are required for life and health. The difference between them is whether we need *dietary* sources of them. A continuing dietary deficiency of an essential nutrient will cause a specific deficiency symptom or disease. So far, 40 essential nutrients have been identified. Some others that are required in extremely small amounts may be recognized as essential nutrients in years to come. A list of essential nutrients is given in Table 2-2. Noted in the table are the potentially prob-

essential nutrients: Substances required by the body for normal growth and health that cannot be manufactured in sufficient amounts by the body; they must be obtained in the diet.

nonessential nutrients: Nutrients the body can manufacture in sufficient quantities from components of the diet.

■

TABLE 2-2

Essential nutrients for humans

Energy Nutrients	Minerals
proteins[1]	calcium*
fats[2],**	chloride
Water-Soluble Vitamins	chromium
thiamin (B_1)	copper
riboflavin (B_2)	fluoride*
niacin (B_3)	iodine**
pantothenic acid	iron*
folacin	magnesium
biotin	manganese
vitamin B_6 (pyroxidine)	molybdenum
vitamin B_{12}	phosphorus
vitamin C* (ascorbic acid)	potassium
Fat-Soluble Vitamins	selenium*
vitamin A*	sodium**
vitamin D	zinc*
vitamin E	**Water**
vitamin K	

[1]Proteins supply essential amino acids.
[2]Fats supply linoleic acid, an essential nutrient.
*Nutrients most likely to be low in U.S. diets.
**Nutrients most likely to be excessive in U.S. diets.

EXPLANATION OF THE MEASUREMENT UNITS USED IN THIS BOOK

Property	Unit	Abbreviation	Approximate Equivalents
Length	meter	m	1 m = 1.09 yd = 3.28 ft
	millimeter	mm	1 mm = 0.04 in
Volume	liter	L	1 L = 1.06 qt = 1,000 ml
	milliliter	ml	1 ml = 0.2 t
	teaspoon	t or tsp	1 t = 5 ml
	tablespoon	T	1 T = 3 t = 15 ml
	cup	c	1 c = 16 T = 8 oz (fluid)
	quart	qt	1 qt = 4 c = 32 oz (fluid) = 0.95 L
Weight	kilogram	kg	1 kg = 2.2 lb = 1,000 g
	gram	g	1 g = 0.04 oz = 1,000 mg
	milligram	mg	1 mg = 1,000 mcg = 0.00004 oz
	microgram	mcg or μg	1 mcg = 0.00000004 oz
	ounce	oz	1 oz = 28.35 g
	pound	lb	1 lb = 16 oz = 454 g
Energy	calorie (Calorie)	cal	1 cal = 1 kcal = 4.18 kilojoules
Temperature	degree Celsius (centigrade)	°C	°C = 5/9 (°F − 32)
	degree Fahrenheit	°F	°F = 9/5 (°C + 32)

Some Approximate Equivalents

5 grams = the weight of 1 teaspoon of salt = the weight of a nickel
1 ounce = 28 grams = the weight of a slice of bread
1 kilogram = the weight of 2 pounds plus 4/5 stick of margarine or butter

lematic nutrients—those that Americans are most likely to consume too much or too little of in their diets.[1]

The amounts of essential nutrients needed each day by humans vary greatly, from cups to micrograms. (Micrograms and other units of measure used in this book are explained in Box 2-1.) Generally speaking, humans need to consume about 10 cups of water from fluids and foods, 9 tablespoons of protein, and one-fourth teaspoon of calcium, but only one-thousandth teaspoon (a 3-microgram speck) of vitamin B_{12} each day.[2]

Individual Variation in Nutrient Need

We all need the same nutrients, but not always in the same amounts. The amounts needed vary among people depending upon a person's:

- age
- sex
- growth status
- genetic traits
- physical activity level

and the presence of conditions such as:

- pregnancy
- breast feeding
- illness
- drug use
- exposure to environmental contaminants

Each of these factors, and others, influence nutrient requirements. General recommendations for diets that provide all the essential nutrients usually make allowances for the major factors that influence level of nutrient need, but they cannot allow for all of the factors. The **recommended dietary allowances (RDAs)** are the most widely used standards for adequate intake levels of essential nutrients. This set of standards applies to healthy people, and the recommendations are categorized by age and gender, and whether women are pregnant or breast-feeding.

Recommended Dietary Allowances: Specified levels of intake of essential nutrients, considered on the basis of available scientific evidence, to be adequate to meet the known nutritional needs of practically all healthy people.

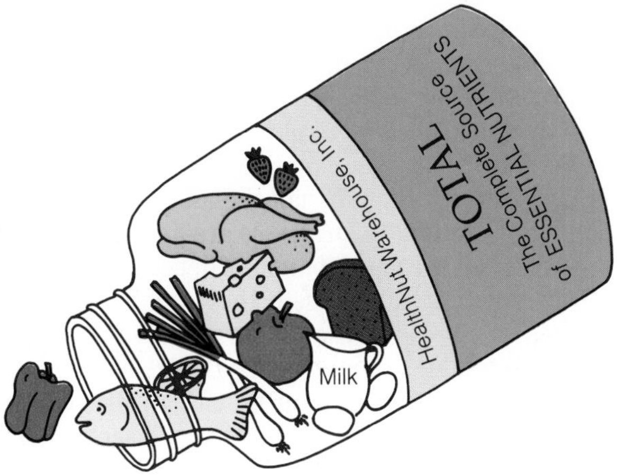

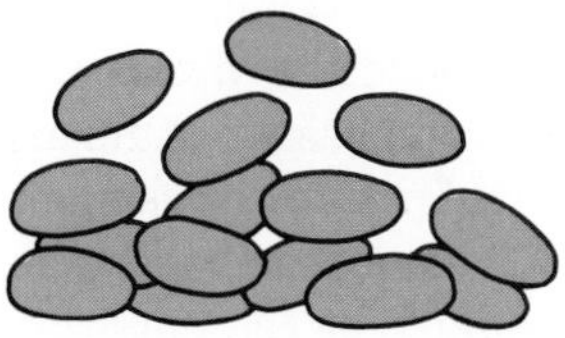

Foods: The real, complete source of essential nutrients.

BOX 2-2

CONTROVERSY SURROUNDING THE RDAs

The RDAs were first published in 1943 and have been revised every six to ten years since then. Publication of revised RDA tables has been postponed twice due to scientific controversies. The most recent controversy resulted in the failure to release the 1985 revision. The disagreement centered around the RDA levels proposed for vitamins A and C. On one side of the controversy were scientists who recommended that the levels be decreased to more closely reflect what is required to maintain normal nutrient functions. On the other side were those who thought that greater levels should be recommended because they may provide people with a degree of protection against chronic diseases. Whether the RDAs should be based on levels needed for normal nutrient function or levels associated with optimal health and chronic disease prevention is expected to remain the subject of debate for some time to come.

The unofficial 1985 RDA values have been published and are referred to as *Recommended Dietary Intakes (RDIs)*, rather than *RDAs*. The (1985) RDIs are not widely used; the 1980 RDAs are, however.

The RDAs

Recommended levels of intake have been established for 17 of the 40 essential nutrients, and estimates of safe and adequate intakes have been defined for 13 others. Because they are referred to frequently, these RDA tables are printed inside the covers of this text. The RDAs indicate neither the required level of nutrient intake nor the minimal levels of nutrient need. Rather, they are estimates, based on the best available scientific data, of the levels of essential nutrients that would meet the needs of 95 percent of all healthy Americans. In calculating the RDAs, a "margin of safety" is added to the average nutrient intake level required for the maintenance of the nutrient's functions. For example, the adult RDA for protein is set at a level that is 30 percent higher than the amount needed to maintain the normal functions of protein.[2] RDA levels are generally set well above the amounts associated with the development of deficiency diseases. Although the RDAs are widely accepted and used, they are not without controversy. Box 2-2 discusses recent controversies surrounding the RDAs.

A major assumption underlying the RDAs is that *foods* are the sources of essential nutrients. It is assumed that foods containing adequate amounts of nutrients with established RDAs will also contain adequate amounts of essential nutrients for which there are no RDAs.

U.S. RDAs: Standards by which the nutrient composition of food products are assessed and reported on food labels. They are based on the 1968 RDA table.

The U.S. RDAs An offshoot of the RDAs, the **U.S. RDAs**, were introduced in 1971 to help inform consumers about the nutrient values of foods and supplements. These standards are used to determine the values you sometimes see listed in the nutrition information labels on breakfast cereal boxes, milk containers, and other food packages as well as on supplement bottles. The Food and Drug Administration (F.D.A.) established the U.S. RDAs for the sole purpose of providing a legal standard for the nutrition labeling of foods and supplements. Four sets of U.S. RDAs were identified based on the 1968 RDA tables—sets for:

- infants
- children one to four years of age
- children four years and over and adults
- pregnant and breast-feeding women

The set of values for children four years and over and adults is the one most commonly used on nutrition information labels.

It is important not to confuse the U.S. RDAs, which are used for labeling purposes, with the RDAs. The U.S. RDAs may not accurately reflect variations in nutrient needs related to a person's gender and age. They are based on the 1968 RDAs, not the RDAs that are currently in use.

You can get an idea of the differences between the U.S. RDAs and the RDAs by reviewing the information given in Table 2-3. The table lists the 11 required and 12 optional components of a nutrition label, and gives the U.S. RDAs for children aged 4 and over and adults and the 1980 RDAs for adult males (23 to 50 years of age) and for children aged 4 to 6. Notice that the U.S. RDAs and the RDAs are the same for vitamin D, but they range from slightly different to vastly different for the 19 other nutrients. The table presents recommendations for just one of the 4 U.S. RDA groups and just two of the 30 RDA groups, but the differences in the recommended levels are representative. Bear this in mind when you read a nutrition label. Remember that the standards set for the U.S. RDAs tend to be high.

The Old MDRs Prior to the introduction of U.S. RDAs, standards called **Minimum Daily Requirements (MDRs)** were used for food and supplement labels. They represented the minimum amount of nutrients needed to prevent deficiency diseases. The MDRs are two to six times lower than the U.S. RDAs and are no longer recognized as appropriate standards for food and supplement labeling. (You may still see the MDRs on some supplement labels, but they should not be there; the U.S. RDAs are now required by federal regulation.)

Minimum Daily Requirements (MDRs): Standards of nutrient intake levels based on amounts of nutrients needed to prevent deficiency diseases. *These standards are no longer recognized as appropriate for labeling purposes.*

Nutrition Labeling

Federal regulations requiring that food labels state ingredients were established as early as 1938. In 1973 the regulations were expanded to include requirements for reporting the nutrient content of foods and supplements on product labels. Nutrition labeling is voluntary except for products that make claims about nutrient content, such as "high in iron" or "protein-rich," and for products containing added nutrients, such as fortified breakfast cereals and fruit drinks. The packaging of vitamin and mineral supplements also must contain nutrition information. The nutrition labels on supplements must provide comparisons between the amounts of vitamins and minerals in one dose and the U.S. RDAs.

Regulations specify the type of information that is allowed on nutrition information labels. At a minimum, a label must include the following infor-

TABLE 2-3
Selected comparisons of U.S. RDAs with 1980 RDAs

Nutrient	U.S. RDAs for Children (aged four years and older) and adults	1980 RDAs	
		Adult males 23–50 years old	Children 4–6 years old
Required to Be Listed on Nutrition Labels			
Calories	—	—	—
Carbohydrates	—	—	—
Fats	—	—	—
Protein		56 g	30 g
animal sources	45 g		
vegetable sources	65 g		
Vitamin A	5,000 IU	5,000 IU	2,500 IU
Vitamin C	60 mg	60 mg	45 mg
Thiamin (vitamin B_1)	1.5 mg	1.4 mg	0.9 mg
Riboflavin (vitamin B_2)	1.7 mg	1.6 mg	1.0 mg
Niacin (vitamin B_3)	20 mg	18 mg	11 mg
Calcium	1,000 mg	800 mg	800 mg
Iron	18 mg	10 mg	10 mg
Allowed to Be Listed on Nutrition Labels			
Vitamin D	400 IU	400 IU	400 IU
Vitamin E	30 IU	15 IU	9 IU
Vitamin B_6	2.0 mg	2.2 mg	1.3 mg
Folic acid (folacin)	400 mcg	400 mcg	200 mcg
Vitamin B_{12}	6 mcg	3 mcg	2 mcg
Phosphorus	1,000 mg	800 mg	800 mg
Iodine	150 mcg	150 mcg	90 mcg
Magnesium	400 mg	350 mg	200 mg
Zinc	15 mg	15 mg	10 mg
Copper	2 mg	2–3 mg	1.5–2.0 mg
Biotin	300 mcg	100–200 mcg	85 mcg
Pantothenic acid	10 mg	4–7 mg	3–4 mg

mation about the content of a standard portion (one serving) of the food product:

- calories
- grams of protein, carbohydrate, and fat
- percent of the U.S. RDAs for 5 vitamins and 2 minerals

The percent of the U.S. RDAs provided in one serving of the food for 7 other vitamins and 5 other minerals may also be listed on the label. All of these "optional" nutrients must be listed on the label if any of them are. Table 2-3 lists the nutrients whose listing is required and optional on nutrition labels.

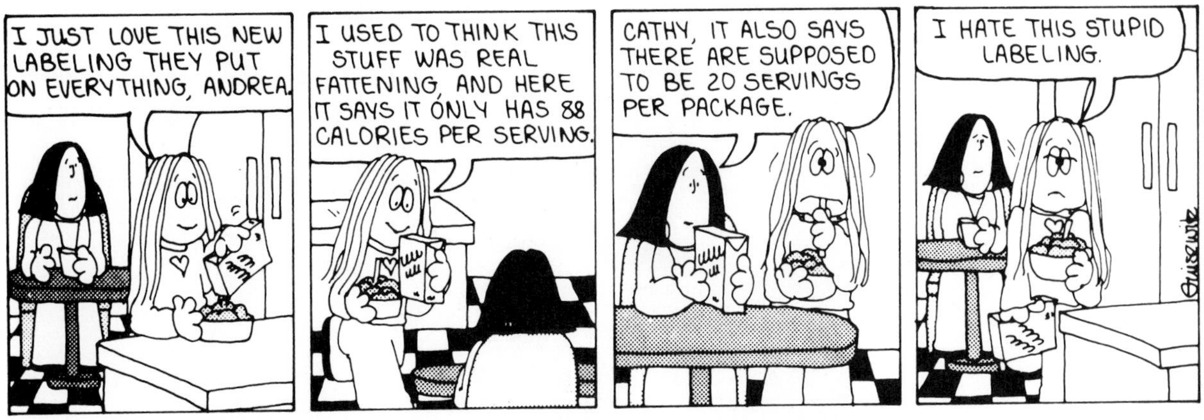

If you're a nutrition label reader, you have probably noticed that some food packages include information about sodium, sucrose, fiber, and cholesterol content. There are no rules that require the routine inclusion of information about these substances, and none of them has been assigned a U.S. RDA. Information about these nutrients is required only if a claim is made about them on the package. If they are listed on a label, the amounts in one serving must be given in milligrams or grams. The next time you see a food package that announces the product is "low in sodium" or "high in fiber," check the nutrition label for more specific information.

Some food companies appear to have taken undue advantage of the option of including information about a food's sodium, sucrose, fiber, and cholesterol content. Foods that naturally contain little sodium or no cholesterol are being promoted as "low-sodium" or "no-cholesterol" foods. Bananas, for example, are being advertised as "low in sodium." Margarines made from vegetable oils that are cholesterol-free anyway are being promoted as "no-cholesterol" on their packaging. The purpose of nutrition labeling is to inform consumers about the nutrients contained in food products, not to misguide people about the usual nutrient content of foods.

PRINCIPLE 4: MOST HEALTH PROBLEMS RELATED TO NUTRITION ORIGINATE WITHIN CELLS

The main employers of nutrients are cells (Figure 2-1). All of the processes for which nutrients are required occur within cells or in the fluid that surrounds them. There are more than one hundred trillion (100,000,000,000,000) cells in the human body, each of which is a living unit fueled and maintained by the supply of nutrients it receives.

Cells are the building blocks of tissues (such as muscles and bones), organs (the kidney, heart, and liver, for example), and systems (such as the digestive, reproductive, circulatory, and nervous systems). Normal cell functioning and health are maintained when cells receive the nutrients and other substances they need and are free from harmful substances. Disruptions in the availability of nutrients or the presence of harmful substances in the environment of cells can initiate diseases and disorders that eventually

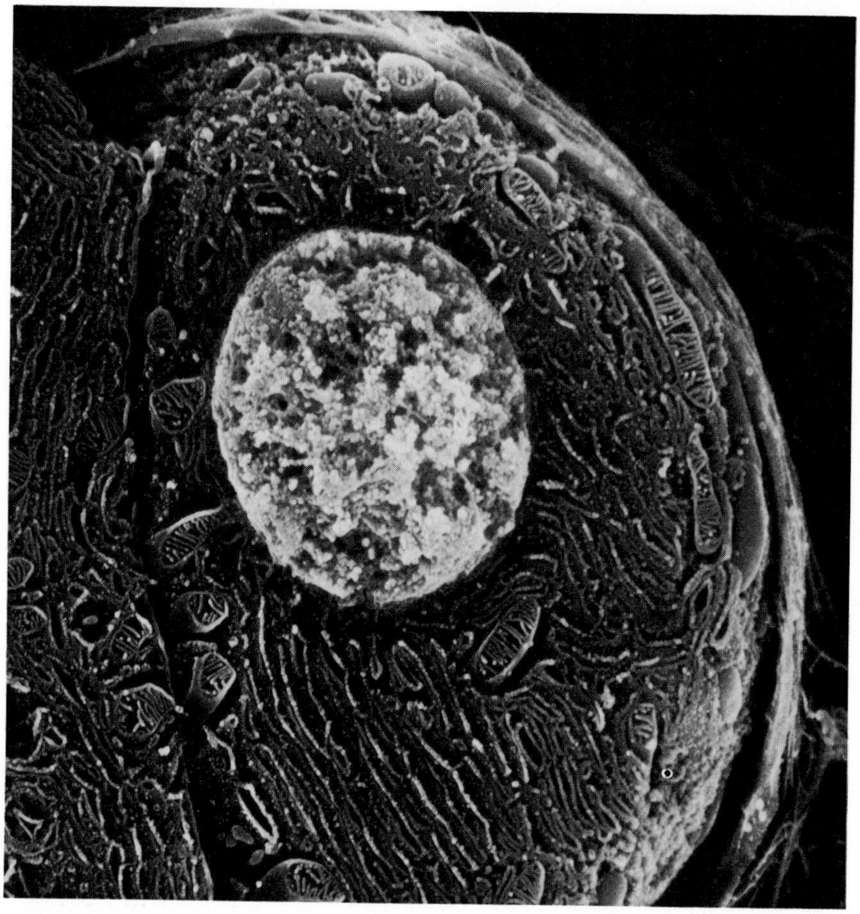

FIGURE 2-1
Scanning electron micrograph of a human cell.

affect tissues, organs, and systems. Health problems in general begin with disruptions in the normal activities of cells.

The types and amounts of foods consumed by people affect the environment of cells and their ability to function normally. Excessive and inadequate supplies of nutrients and other chemical substances produce the disruptions in cell functions that ultimately become identified as a health problem. Quite simply, humans are as healthy as their cells.

PRINCIPLE 5: POOR NUTRITION CAN RESULT FROM EITHER INADEQUATE OR EXCESSIVE LEVELS OF NUTRIENT INTAKE

For each nutrient, for each individual, there is an optimal range of intake for cell and body functioning.[3] Above and below the optimal range are levels of intake associated with impaired body functioning. (This concept is illustrated in Figure 2-2.) Inadequate essential nutrient intake, if prolonged, results in obvious deficiency diseases. Marginally deficient diets cause subtle changes in behavior or in physical condition. If the optimal intake range is exceeded, then mild to severe changes in mental and physical functions

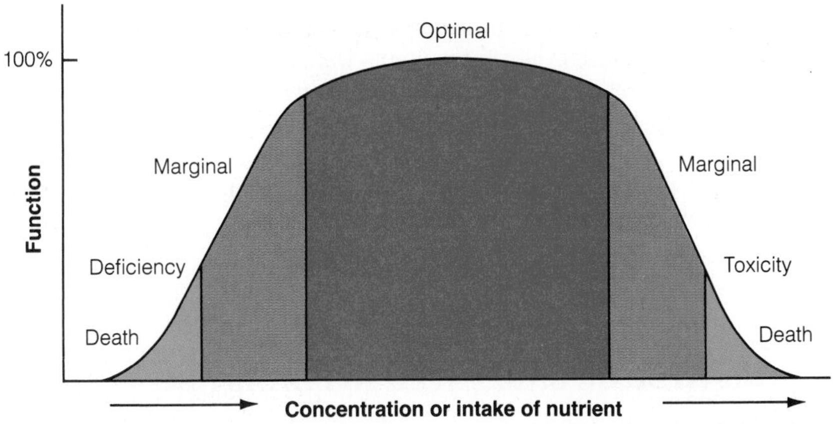

FIGURE 2-2
How much is enough? The body's response to nutrients varies depending on tissue concentration and intake level of the nutrients. The optimal range of nutrient intake varies for each nutrient and is affected by many individual and environmental factors.

occur, depending on the amount of the excess and the nutrient.[4] Severe vitamin C deficiency, for example, produces bleeding gums, pain upon being touched, and a failure of bone to grow. A marginal deficiency may cause wounds to heal slowly. On the excessive side, high intakes of vitamin C may contribute to the development of diarrhea and kidney stones.[5]

Severe consequences of deficient and excessive nutrient intakes are rare in the U.S., but marginally inadequate and excessive intakes of some nutrients are probably quite common.[3] Nearly all cases of vitamin and mineral overdose are due to excessive use of supplements; they are almost never caused by excessive intake of foods containing the particular nutrient. (Box 2-3 discusses an exception—a food that can cause vitamin A overdose.)

Nutrient Deficiencies Are Often Multiple

Most foods contain many nutrients, so inadequate diets usually affect the level of intake of more than a single nutrient. Inadequate diets generally produce a spectrum of signs and symptoms related to deficiencies of several nutrients. For example, protein, vitamin B_{12}, iron, and zinc occur together

BOX 2-3

A FOOD THAT CAUSES VITAMIN A OVERDOSE

There is a well-known exception to the general rule that nutrient toxicities result from the excessive use of supplements. Be careful not to eat too much polar bear or seal liver, lest you overdose on vitamin A. Folklore handed down by Eskimos and Arctic explorers for centuries (which has been confirmed by research) has warned that a dreadful, mysterious disease results from eating too much polar bear or seal liver.[6] It is said that even sled dogs hesitate to eat the liver. A half-pound of polar bear liver may provide up to 2,600 times the adult RDA for vitamin A. Symptoms of acute (rapid-onset) vitamin A toxicity may appear within eight hours after eating a polar bear liver meal and persist for a few days to several weeks.[8] The symptoms include cracking and peeling skin, headache, bone and joint pain, blurred vision, and hair loss.[7,8]

in many high-protein foods. Therefore, diets that are low in protein are likely to be low in these other nutrients as well.

Dietary changes can affect body levels of many nutrients. Switching from a high-fat diet to a low-fat diet, for instance, generally results in reduced intakes of calories, cholesterol, and vitamin E as well. Thus, dietary changes introduced to improve a person's intake of a particular nutrient may produce a ripple effect on the intake of other nutrients.

PRINCIPLE 6: MALNUTRITION MAY BE DIRECTLY RELATED OR UNRELATED TO DIETARY INTAKE

Malnutrition means a state of poor nutrition and applies to problems such as obesity and vitamin overdoses as well as to underweight and vitamin deficiencies. It can result from poor diets *or* from conditions that interfere with the utilization of nutrients by cells. Malnutrition that results directly from inadequate or excessive intakes is referred to as **primary malnutrition**. When the basic cause of malnutrition is the abnormal utilization of nutrients by cells, it is classified as **secondary malnutrition**. Although they have different causes, both types of malnutrition produce similar consequences to health. The consequences range from mild to severe, depending upon which nutrients are involved and how long the problem exists.

malnutrition: "Poor" nutrition caused by an inadequate or excessive intake of calories or one or more nutrients. Protein–calorie malnutrition is caused by a lack of protein and calories. Obesity is a form of malnutrition related to excessive intake of calories.

primary malnutrition: Malnutrition directly resulting from inadequate or excessive dietary intakes; vitamin A deficiency and toxicity are examples.

secondary malnutrition: Malnutrition resulting from a condition not directly related to dietary intake; weight loss due to a gastrointestinal-tract infection is an example.

Primary Malnutrition

Inadequate and excessive dietary intakes and the use of large doses of vitamin and mineral supplements are the most common causes of primary malnutrition. Vegetarians who develop deficiency diseases because they fail to consume enough vitamin B_{12} and zinc and children who become overloaded with iron when they accidentally ingest too many iron pills are victims of primary malnutrition.

Primary malnutrition develops in stages, and the further it progresses the more serious are the consequences to health. The stages in the development of primary malnutrition are outlined in Figure 2-3. We'll start with a discussion of how nutrient deficiencies develop and then address nutrient overdoses. As you can observe from the figure, the stages involved in the development of nutrient deficiencies and nutrient overdoses are similar.

Nutrient Deficiency Primary malnutrition in the form of a nutrient deficiency begins with a period of deficient intake of an essential nutrient. After several weeks to months of deficient intake, tissue reserves of the nutrient become depleted. Blood levels of the nutrient then decrease because there are no reserves for replenishing the blood supply. Without an adequate supply of the nutrient in the blood, cells get short-changed; they no longer receive the nutrients needed for maintaining normal cell functions. If the dietary deficiency is prolonged, the malfunctioning cells cause sufficient impairment to produce physically obvious signs of a deficiency disease. Eventually, some problems produced by the deficiency may no longer be repairable, and permanent changes in health and function may occur. In most cases, the problems resulting from the deficiency can be reversed if the nutrient is supplied before this final stage occurs. A specific example of the

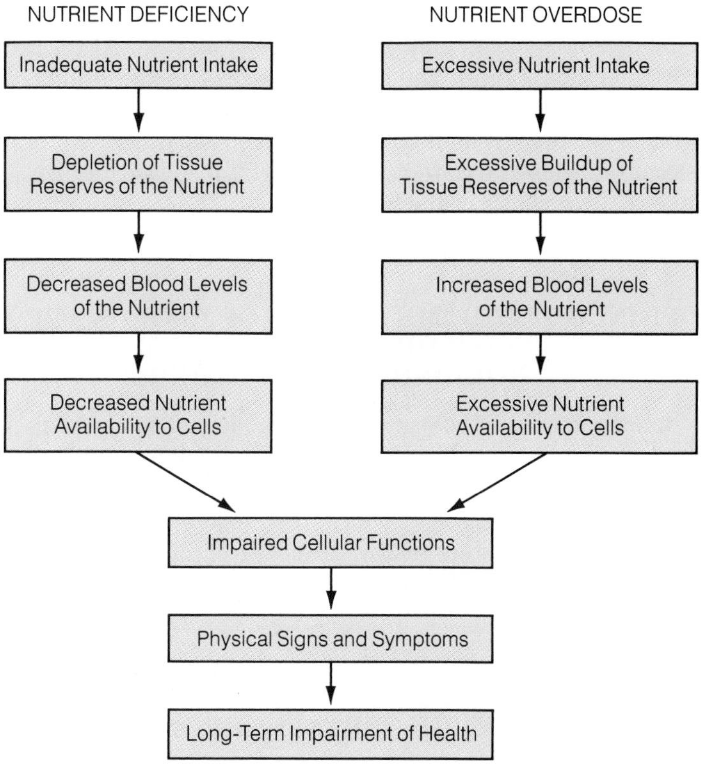

FIGURE 2-3
The usual sequences of events in the development of nutrient deficiencies and overdoses.

progression and consequences of a deficiency disease is included in the discussion of vitamin A in Chapter 10.

Nutrient Overdose Malnutrition due to overdoses of nutrients begins with excessive intakes of nutrients that are readily absorbed into the blood stream. If the high levels of intake persist, tissues become saturated with the nutrients. After the tissues are filled, incoming supplies of the nutrients remain in the blood for a time and cause blood levels of the nutrients to rise. This causes cells to become oversupplied with nutrients. The high nutrient loads upset the balance needed for normal cell functioning. The changes in cell functions lead to the signs and symptoms of nutrient overdose diseases.

The severity and duration of the health consequences of nutrient overdoses partly depend on how rapidly the body can lower blood levels by excreting nutrient excesses in the urine. The body can eliminate excesses of some nutrients, such as vitamin C and the B-complex vitamins, in a matter of weeks. Elimination of excesses of vitamin D and iron, on the other hand, takes much longer, because they are not readily excreted in the urine.

The best time to correct a developing deficiency or overdose disease is before tissue stores are depleted or exceeded. If that is accomplished, no harmful effects on cell functions and health occur; they are prevented.

Secondary Malnutrition

Ingested nutrients have many possible fates. They can only be used to nourish cells if they are absorbed into the bloodstream and made available to cells. The extent to which nutrients are absorbed and used by the body can be affected by the types of foods included in a meal, drugs and medications the person is using, and the presence of disease. Alcoholism, AIDS, diabetes, diarrhea, cancer, and kidney disease are some of the health problems that affect nutrient absorption and utilization.

Secondary malnutrition is the ninth-ranked cause of death in America.[9] It generally is closely related to the effects of a disease such as cancer, pneumonia, or cirrhosis of the liver.

PRINCIPLE 7: SOME GROUPS OF PEOPLE ARE AT GREATER RISK OF BECOMING INADEQUATELY NOURISHED THAN OTHERS

Every human requires the same nutrients but not in the same amounts. Pregnant and breast-feeding women, growing children, and persons who are ill or recovering from illness have greater requirements for nutrients than other people. In cases of widespread food shortages, such as those induced by natural disasters or war, the health of these nutritionally vulnerable groups is compromised most by inadequate diets.

PRINCIPLE 8: MALNUTRITION CAN CONTRIBUTE TO THE DEVELOPMENT OF CERTAIN CHRONIC DISEASES

The consequences of poor nutrition are not limited to nutrient deficiency and overdose diseases. Poor nutrition in the form of overeating and of excess consumption of animal fat, cholesterol, sodium, alcohol, or sugars, and underconsumption of calcium or fiber, for example, all can contribute to the development of chronic diseases. Malnutrition due to faulty diets appears to play an important role in the development of heart disease, hypertension, cancer, osteoporosis, dental disease, and a number of other chronic problems.

PRINCIPLE 9: IN ADDITION TO NUTRIENTS, FOODS CONTAIN OTHER SUBSTANCES THAT MAY AFFECT HEALTH

Nutrients come packaged in foods along with thousands of other chemical substances that may affect health. The health effects of these "extra" substances are far from completely known, but evidence indicates that some of these substances can be harmful and others, beneficial to health. Most of them, however, appear to have little effect on human health. Chemical substances in food (other than nutrients) that may affect health can be classified into three groups:

- naturally occurring toxicants
- environmental contaminants
- food additives

Table 2-4 provides examples of these substances and their effects on human health.

BOX 2-4

PUFFER FISH POISONING

The puffer fish must taste very good. One wrong stroke of a knife blade during cleaning can transform it from a delicacy to a deadly poison. Yet people still insist on eating it.

The poison of the puffer fish lies in its internal organs and skin. These parts must be removed carefully so as not to leave even a trace of the poison on the flesh. Although it is highly prized and very expensive, people gamble with their lives each time they eat it. Several hundred Japanese die each year from puffer fish poisoning.

A report in the scientific literature gives a very clear picture of just how toxic this food toxin is. It describes the experience of four soldiers who came upon a bonfire where fishermen had roasted some puffer fish earlier. The fishermen had carefully removed the internal organs and skin of the fish and laid the discarded parts out on shells. Despite the fishermen's warnings, the soldiers decided to try some puffer fish liver. One soldier, who ate a small amount of the liver, died within a half-hour. The others, who had chewed small amounts but had not swallowed any of the liver, all died within twenty-four hours.[10]

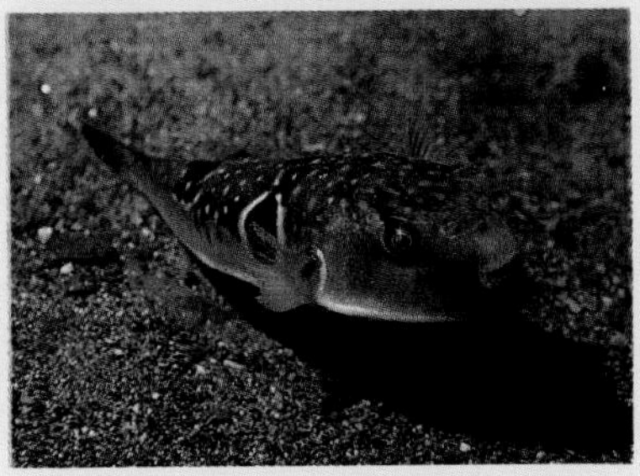

Puffer fish (*Takifugu rupribes*) is a prized delicacy in Japan, although it contains a poison.

Virtually every substance we ingest is **toxic** at some level of consumption. Whether substances we consume in foods pose a hazard to our health primarily depends upon how toxic they are and the amount of them that we consume. Humans can tolerate large or moderate amounts of weak toxins, but only small amounts of strong toxins. Just exposing the tongue to poisonous parts of a puffer fish, for example, is enough to cause death within hours. (The puffer fish is a sometimes-deadly Japanese delicacy. Read about it in Box 2-4.) Several ounces of oxalic acid, a chemical found in some dark green, leafy vegetables, must be consumed before signs of a toxic reaction occur. Some people have gotten oxalic-acid poisoning from eating raw rhubarb.

toxic: Poisonous; harmful to the body.

We are exposed to potential toxins in foods every day, but our level of exposure to toxins is rarely high enough to cause problems. Most overdoses of toxins in food result from consuming foods that contain strong toxins or those that have been contaminated.

Naturally Occurring Toxicants

naturally occurring toxicants: Substances that are a natural part of foods that can have a harmful effect on health if consumed in excessive quantities.

Have you ever noticed a bright green area right beneath the skin of a potato or on the edge of a potato chip? The greenish area contains a very small amount of solanine, a poisonous substance. Solanine is colorless but it generally occurs in the green areas sometimes found in and under potato peels. The substance has a slightly bitter flavor and it can cause nausea, headache, and other problems if ingested in sufficient quantity. The risk of ingesting too much solanine can be avoided by not eating the green portions of potatoes.[11] Phytates are a natural part of whole grains that attach firmly to calcium, zinc, and other minerals in foods. The tightness of the bond between phytates and certain minerals causes them to be excreted rather than absorbed into the bloodstream. The simultaneous consumption of inky-cap mushrooms and alcohol turns the body of the drinker purplish red.[12] Per-

TABLE 2-4

Examples of naturally occurring toxicants, environmental contaminants, and food additives

Substance	Some Sources	Possible Effects of Excessive Intake
Naturally Occurring Toxicants		
Allergens	wheat gluten, cow's milk protein	diarrhea and rash in genetically susceptible people
Avidin	raw egg whites	inhibition of biotin (a B vitamin) absorption
Goitrogens	cabbage, turnips, kale, brussels sprouts, rutabaga	goiter (enlarged thyroid)
Oxalic acid	spinach, Swiss chard, beet greens, rhubarb	oxalic-acid poisoning, the symptoms of which include gastrointestinal upset and convulsions
Phytic acid	whole grains	inhibition of absorption of calcium, zinc, and other minerals
Tryramine	aged cheese and wine, some chocolates, tofu, soy sauce	severe hypertension and headaches among people taking certain anti-depressant drugs
Fish toxins	toxins in puffer fish, dinoflagellates, others	wide range of effects including gastrointestinal upset, paralysis, coma
Environmental Contaminants		
Aflatoxin	moldy grains, beans, peas, and peanuts	liver damage
Bacteria	chicken, salads, honey, cheese, and other foods contaminated with bacteria	"food poisoning"
Lead	lead-base-paint flakes, car exhaust, plants grown in contaminated soil	anemia, mental retardation from lead poisoning
Mercury	industrial pollution of water and fish	numbness, loss of coordination, visual disturbances
Radioactive particles	fall-out from nuclear plant accidents, leakages of stored or discarded radioactive materials	gastrointestinal upset, cancer
Pesticides, herbicides	fruits and vegetables	wide range of effects including rash, numbness, headaches, birth defects
Food Additives, Intentional		
Flavoring agents: sugar, salt, herbs, sweeteners, more than 1,000 natural and artificial flavors	beverages, breakfast cereals, snack products, desserts, candy, bakery products	sticky sweets: tooth decay; salt: hypertension

TABLE 2-4, *continued*

Substance	Some Sources	Possible Effects of Excessive Intake
Food Additives, Intentional		
Flavor enhancers: MSG (trade names: Accent, Ajinomoto, Vestin)	Oriental foods, some processed meats	"Chinese-restaurant syndrome," characterized by temporary chest pain, headache, burning sensation, and sweating
Coloring agents: blue #1 and #2, green #3, red #3 and #40, yellow #5 and #6, carrot oil, dehydrated beets, caramel and other natural coloring agents	margarine, soft drinks, fruit drinks, candy, bakery products, ice cream, orange peel, cheese, and many other products	yellow dye #5: possible allergic reaction
Fortifying nutrients: ferrous sulfate (iron), reduced iron, thiamin hydrochloride, thiamin mononitrate (thiamin, B_1), riboflavin (B_2), niacinamide (niacin, B_3), calcium carbonate (calcium), sodium ascorbate (vitamin C), pyridoxine hydrochloride (B_6), vitamin A palmitate (vitamin A), zinc oxide (zinc), trisodium phosphate (phosphorus), iodine	refined flour and rice, bakery products, breakfast cereals, dairy products, beverages	Manufacturing errors that have led to excess levels of fortified nutrients have resulted in overdose diseases.
Preservatives: BHA/BHT, salt, citric acid, gamma radiation, sulfites (sulfur dioxide), sodium nitrite, sodium benzoate, vitamins C and E	breakfast cereals, bakery products, beverages, fruits, vegetables, bacon, sausage, ham, snack foods, salad dressings	Some preservatives (sodium nitrate, for example) are weakly linked with cancer. High salt (sodium) intakes may predispose some people to hypertension. Individuals sensitive to sulfites may react severely or die if they eat sulfite-containing food.
Texture enhancers: mono- and diglycerides, alginates, agar, gelation, gums, carrageenan, lecithin, starches	margarine, ice cream, frozen desserts, puddings, cheese spreads, gravies, bakery products	
Food Additives, Unintentional		
Iodine (iodide)	milk and bakery products	
Estrogen	meats	may increase the risk of cancer
Antibiotics	meats	may encourage development of susceptibility to certain bacteria
Vitamin B_{12}	microorganisms in food	
Lead	calcium supplements made from crushed bone or dolomite	lead poisoning
Mercury	fish from contaminated waters	mercury poisoning

Sign posted near oil depot in Searsport, Maine.

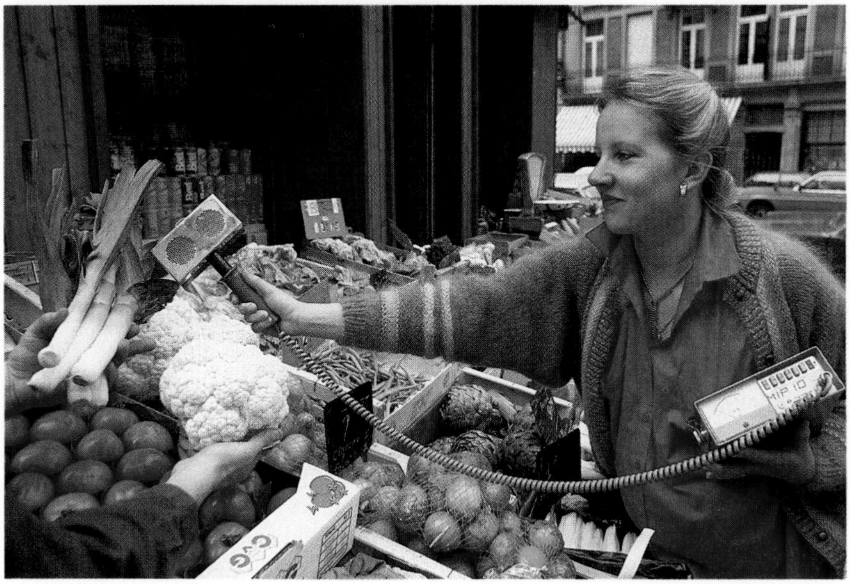

A woman in Western Europe checks produce for radioactivity after the Chernobyl nuclear power plant accident in 1987.

haps the most bizarre example of a naturally occurring toxin is one that has been identified in the brains of some people who have eaten their relatives. Kuru, a degenerative disorder of the central nervous system, is believed to be transmitted by cannibalism among close relatives of the Fore tribe in New Guinea. Other examples of naturally occurring toxicants are listed in Table 2-4.

Environmental Contaminants

Toxic chemicals can enter foods as a result of environmental contamination. Aflatoxin, a substance formed by molds allowed to grow on stored beans, grains, and some other foods, can cause liver damage. Aflatoxin poisoning is

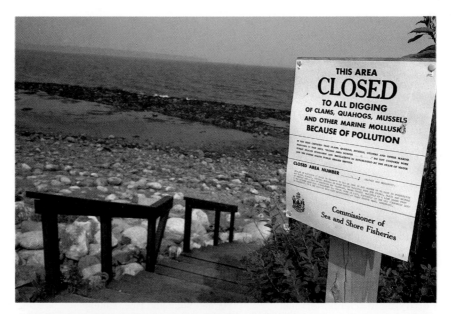

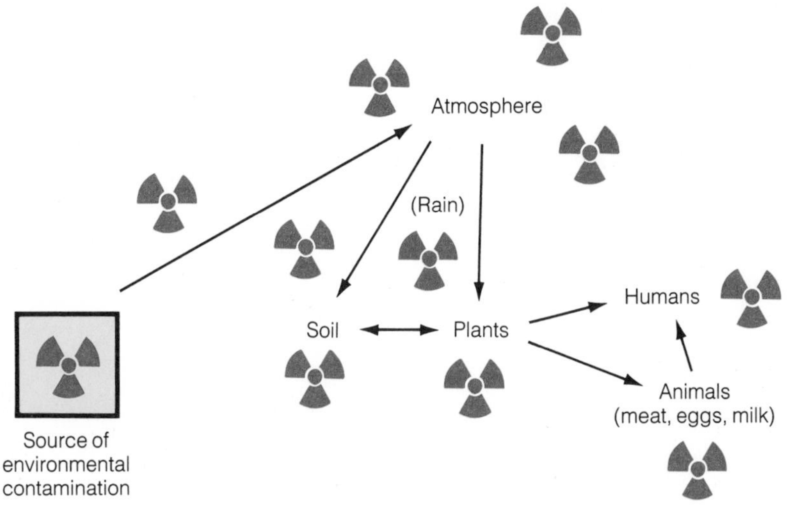

FIGURE 2-4
The major pathways by which humans consume radioactive particles. (Note the symbol for radioactive substances.)

considered a major cause of liver cancer in certain developing countries where stockpiles of grain commonly become contaminated during storage.[13]

Dangerously high levels of lead, mercury, **radioactive particles**, and other substances can end up in foods as a result of environmental contamination. Lead poisoning can result from the ingestion of lead-based-paint flakes, inhaling air that has a heavy concentration of car exhaust fumes, or eating plants grown in lead-contaminated soil. Mercury poisoning has occurred among people who have eaten fish from industrially contaminated water. Warnings not to eat the fish are generally posted by waters recognized as being contaminated with mercury and other toxic substances. Radioactive particles enter the atmosphere, groundwater, and soil as a result of nuclear weapon testing, nuclear power plant accidents, and other industrial- and toxic-waste-storage accidents. Food is the primary route of human exposure to radioactive particles.[14] The pathways by which humans ultimately consume radioactive particles are shown in Figure 2-4. It is generally agreed that health risks from radioactive-particle contamination of food are small except in areas where significant radioactive fallout has occurred. The amount of radioactive particles in the atmosphere has decreased in general since 1965, when nuclear-weapons testing was cut back dramatically.[14]

radioactive particles: Substances that emit rays of energy from their center (or nucleus). Atoms of iodine-131 (^{131}I), strontium-90 (^{90}Sr), and uranium are examples of radioactive particles; the energy emitted by the nuclei of these atoms can damage human cells.

Food Additives

Chemical substances that are intentionally or unintentionally added to foods are referred to as **food additives**. There are over 10,000 food additives. Some of the major ones are listed in Table 2-4.

food additive: Any substance put into a food that becomes part of the food and (or) affects the characteristics of the food. The term applies both to substances intentionally added to foods and to substances added inadvertently, such as packaging materials.

Intentional Food Additives Most additives are intentionally put into foods to improve their flavor, texture, color, appearance, nutrient value, or physical properties. The two most common intentional additives are sugar and salt. Of those that are used in smaller amounts, flavorings are by far the most common.

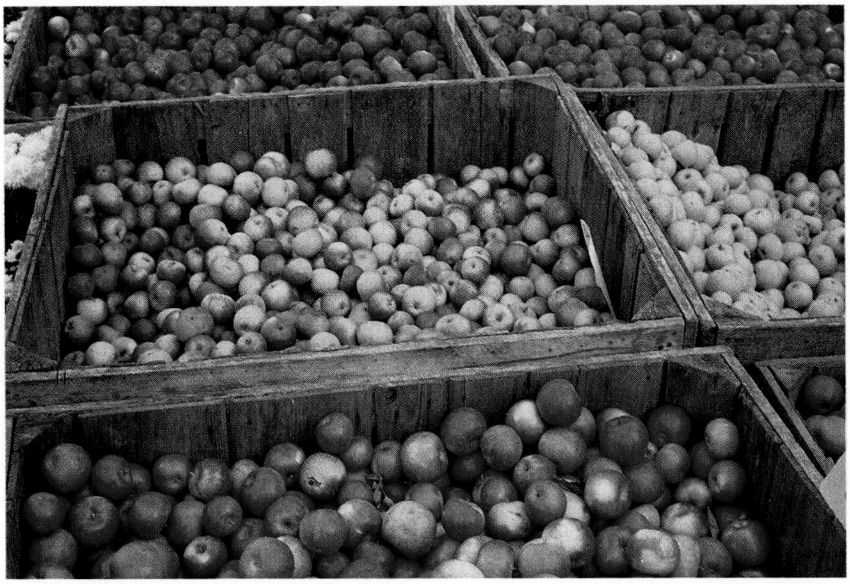

For many people across the country the thought of apples brings to mind Alar, a chemical growth regulator that some apple growers spray on apple trees to enhance the appearance of the apples and increase their shelf life. Because Alar is toxic in small amounts, its use is now closely monitored.

Intentional food additives:
flavorings
preservatives
coloring agents
nutrients
texture enhancers

Unintentional Food Additives Other additives incidentally end up in foods during processing or storage. For example, foods that are processed or stored in aluminum, tin, or copper containers may absorb small amounts of these minerals, which are then considered unintentional food additives. Iodine may be added unintentionally when foods such as milk, cheese, and bread are prepared in vats cleaned with an iodine solution.

The Safety of Food Additives Because food additives may affect health, their presence and use in foods are regulated by the Food and Drug Administration. Legislation passed in 1958 makes it the responsibility of food manufacturers to prove the safety of new or previously unapproved food additives before they use them. The Delaney Clause of this legislation requires that additives known to cause cancer in humans or animals be deemed unsafe. In addition, the legislation lists certain commonly used food additives that are "generally recognized as safe" (the **GRAS** list) and specifies that these additives need not be tested for safety before they are used in food. In 1969 the federal government began a major review of the safety of substances on the GRAS list. Because over 600 substances are on the list, the review is taking a long time to complete.

GRAS: "***G***enerally ***r***ecognized ***a***s ***s***afe," a category of food additives that have not been specifically tested for safety but are assumed to be safe because of their long-term use without apparent connections to health problems. The vast majority of food additives used today are on the GRAS list.

Relatively few of the enormous number of food additives currently in use are suspected of causing health problems. Concerns have been raised about the safety of sulfites, monosodium glutamate (MSG), nitrates, saccharin, aspartame, and some dyes.[20] Many consumers are questioning the need for particular additives, especially those used only to enhance the appearance of food such as dyes. As can be deduced from observing the wide variety of food labels brightly announcing "no preservatives" and "all natural flavors," food companies are listening to the consumers.

Food Irradiation Food irradiation is placed within the category of food additives by the Food and Drug Administration. The reason is that the process helps to preserve foods. It is unlike most other food additives, how-

BOX 2-5

THE SLOW ACCEPTANCE OF IRRADIATED FOODS IN THE U.S.

Frozen foods are antedated, ask for yours irradiated.
—Science Digest, *circa 1966*

The U.S. Army began testing irradiation on troop rations in the 1950s.[15] The Army discovered that irradiated meat held in airtight containers could be stored for years. Potatoes, soups, milk, and many other foods also were shown to last for previously unimagined lengths of time. The process was viewed as a revolution in food preservation. Some people envisioned that the need for refrigerators, freezers, canning plants, and many types of chemical preservatives would diminish greatly because the use of food irradiation would become widespread. That hasn't been the case.

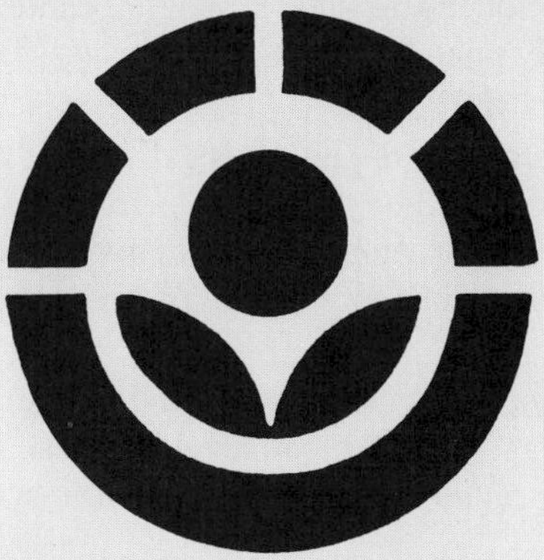

Labels of foods treated with irradiation must display the statement *Treated by Irradiation* and this symbol in the United States.

Food irradiation is slowly gaining acceptance in the U.S., although it is widely used to preserve foods in China and some other countries.[18] Only a very small percentage of the U.S. food supply is irradiated, and when the process is used, a special symbol and statement must appear on the food label.[15,19]

It has been suggested that the unenthusiastic reception in the U.S. is partly due to people's confusing irradiated foods with foods that are contaminated with radioactive particles. The nuclear accident in Chernobyl, USSR, and the resulting contamination of foods with radioactive particles probably strengthened this misconception.[18] Concerns about disposal of radioactive wastes and the potential for nuclear accidents also appear to affect sentiments about food irradiation. It appears that irradiation as a food preservation method will remain unpopular as long as such concerns abound.

ever, in that it is a *process* that adds no chemical substances permanently to foods. Food irradiation involves exposing foods, generally while they are frozen, to streams of powerful gamma rays. Produced by certain types of radioactive atoms, the rays vibrate intensely as they move through food. This destroys insects, bacteria, and other microorganisms in the food. Food irradiation also prevents vegetables such as potatoes and onions from sprouting, thus prolonging their shelf life.

Because the gamma rays used to irradiate foods completely pass through food, no radiation remains in the food after treatment. The process is somewhat similar to heating foods in a pan on the stove or in a microwave oven.[15] Some of the properties of the foods are changed by food irradiation, just as they are by cooking. However, since irradiation exposes foods to even higher levels of energy than heating does, it may cause greater destruction of vitamins.[16] When food irradiation is conducted according to the recommended guidelines, the loss in vitamin content is minimized.[17] As of 1988, the Food and Drug Administration has ruled that food irradiation is safe for spices, pork, and some types of fruits and vegetables given the use of specified doses of gamma rays.[18] Nonetheless, the process is not yet widely used in the U.S. Box 2-5 explains some reasons for the slow acceptance.

■ ■ ■

PRINCIPLE 10: HUMANS HAVE ADAPTIVE MECHANISMS FOR MANAGING FLUCTUATIONS IN DIETARY INTAKE

adaptive mechanisms: In the context of nutrition, body processes that act to maintain a constant supply of nutrients for cells.

Healthy humans possess a great number of **adaptive mechanisms**, some of which protect the body from malnutrition due to fluctuations in dietary intake. These adaptive mechanisms act to conserve energy and nutrients when dietary supply is low and to eliminate nutrients if they are present in excessively high amounts.

Here are some examples of how the body adapts to changes in dietary intake:

- When caloric intake is reduced by fasting, starvation, or dieting, the body adapts to the decreased supply by lowering energy expenditure. Decreases in body temperature and the capacity to do physical work act to reduce the body's need for calories. When caloric intake exceeds the body's need for energy, the excess is stored as fat to meet energy needs in the future.
- The ability of the gastrointestinal tract to absorb dietary iron increases when the body's stores of iron are low. The mechanisms that facilitate iron absorption in times of need rapidly shut down when enough iron has been absorbed. This helps prevent iron overload.
- The body has no absorption barriers for some vitamins, so the amount absorbed is directly related to the amount consumed. To avoid the toxic effects of high blood levels of these vitamins, excessive levels in the blood are rapidly cleared by the kidneys and excreted in the urine.

Although these built-in mechanisms do not protect humans from many of the consequences of poor diets, they do provide an important buffer against the development of malnutrition. They contribute to the body's ability to establish and maintain **homeostasis**.

Our bodies are capable of operating like finely tuned machines when the mechanisms that maintain homeostasis are allowed to operate.

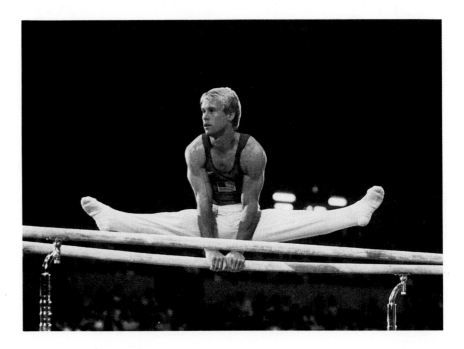

Homeostasis

Every process that occurs in the body is directed toward one goal: the maintenance of a state of balance in the body's internal environment. A balanced internal environment allows cells, tissues, and organs to function optimally. Homeostasis is maintained in healthy individuals by processes that make adjustments for changes that occur in the body's internal environment. These processes are continually underway because the body's internal environment is changing all the time. Eating, drinking, exercising, breathing, drugs, illnesses, exposure to varying external temperatures, and the thousands of chemical reactions that occur in the body all cause changes in the internal environment. Body processes act to maintain homeostasis by altering the rate at which reactions occur, modifying which reactions occur, causing excesses of certain chemical substances to be excreted, increasing the rate of breathing, regulating body temperature, and many other means. Malnutrition, disease states, and other disorders disrupt homeostasis. Our bodies function as well-tuned machines only when the mechanisms that serve to maintain homeostasis are allowed to operate normally.

homeostasis: (hō′ mē ō stā′ sis) The state of equilibrium of the body's internal environment. Homeostatic mechanisms act to maintain a constant balance among fluid, nutrients, and other substances in the body.

■ ■ ■

PRINCIPLE 11: BALANCE AND VARIETY CHARACTERIZE A HEALTHY DIET

All of the nutrients humans need for health are available from foods, and many different combinations of foods can lead to a healthy or **balanced diet**. A balanced diet contains a variety of foods that together provide calories

balanced diet: A diet that consists of a variety of foods that together provide calories and nutrients in amounts that promote health; it contains neither too little nor too much energy (calories), fat, protein, vitamins, minerals, water, and fiber.

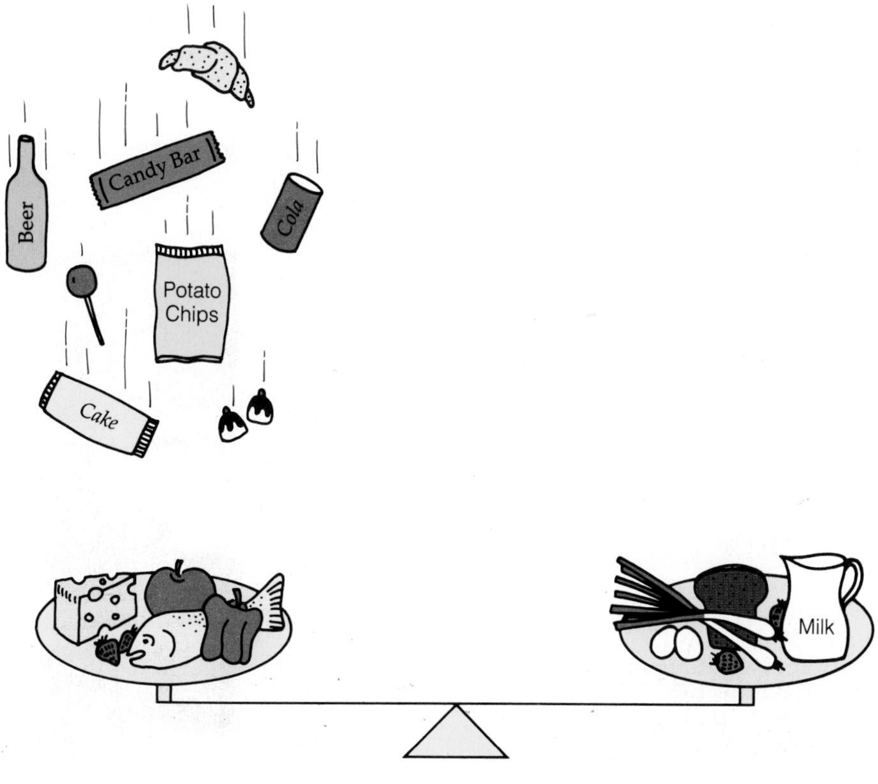

A healthy diet is a matter of balance.

and nutrients in amounts that promote health. All balanced diets, regardless of the specific foods they contain, have one property in common: they include a variety of foods.

Balanced diets require a variety of foods, because no one food—with the exception of breast milk for young infants—provides all the nutrients humans need. Few foods even come close. It matters little what specific foods go into a balanced diet. (A balanced diet may include ants, snails, and raw sea cucumbers.) What matters is that the caloric and nutrient composition of the foods complement each other and add up to a balanced diet.

Nutrient Density

Balanced diets are most easily achieved if the foods they contain are good sources of a number of nutrients and are not too high in calories. Foods that provide multiple nutrients in appreciable amounts relative to calories are described as **nutrient-dense**. Those that provide calories but few nutrients are referred to as **empty-calorie foods**. It is obviously easier to build a balanced diet around nutrient-dense foods such as fruits, vegetables, breads, cereals, lean meats, and milk than around such foods as soft drinks, candy, pastries, chips, and alcoholic beverages. Figure 2-5 illustrates this by comparing the nutrient compositions of skim milk and a cola soft drink.

nutrient-dense foods: Foods that contain relatively high amounts of nutrients compared to their content of calories. Broccoli, collards, bread, and cantaloupe are examples of nutrient-dense foods.

empty-calorie foods: Foods that provide an excess of calories in relation to nutrients. Soft drinks, candy, sugar, alcohol, and fats such as butter, margarine, and oil are considered empty-calorie foods.

Guides for Selecting a Balanced Diet

A number of guides have been developed to help people choose an assortment of foods that will make up a balanced diet. Some of these guides focus on dietary recommendations that may help prevent particular chronic diseases. An overview of dietary guides published in the U.S. is presented in Table 2-5. The number of recommendations given in the guides has grown

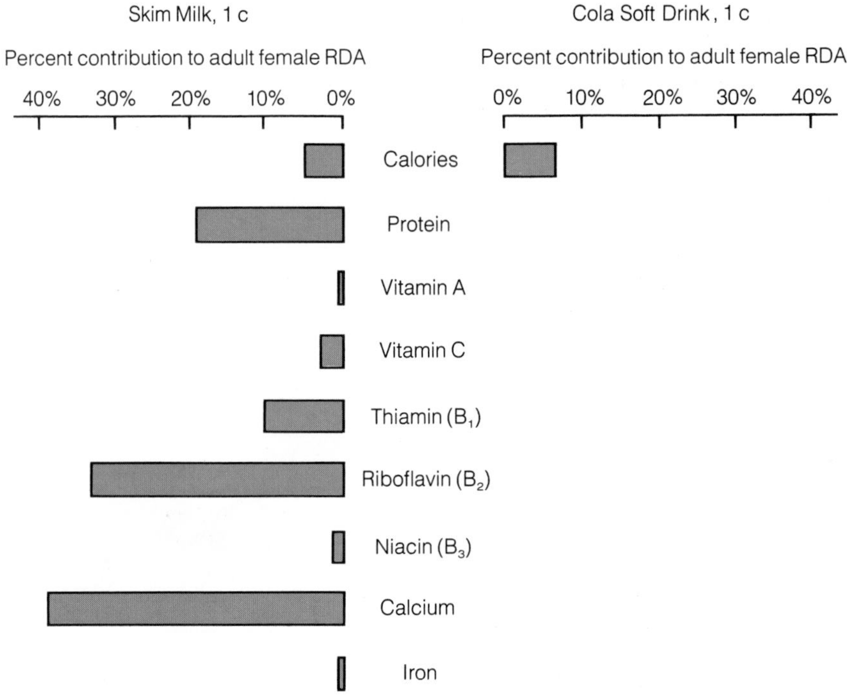

FIGURE 2-5
Examples of foods with high and low nutrient densities. Comparison of the nutrients provided by one cup (eight ounces) of skim milk and one cup of a cola soft drink. Percentages given represent percent contributions to adult female RDAs.

TABLE 2-5

Federal dietary recommendations for the general public, 1917–1988

Year	Agency[b]	Publication	Recommendation[a]							
			Variety	Maintain Ideal Body Weight	Include Starch and Fiber	Limit Sugar	Limit Fat	Limit Choles-terol	Limit Salt	Limit Alcohol
1917	USDA	What the Body Needs—Five Food Groups	+		+	*	*			
1942	USDA	Food for Freedom—Daily Eight	+		+		*			
1943	USDA	National Wartime Nutrition Guide—Basic Seven	+		+		*			
1946	USDA	National Food Guide—Basic Seven	+		+		*			
1946	USDA	Food for Growth—Four Food Groups	+		+					
1958	USDA	Food for Fitness—Four Food Groups	+		+					
1977	U.S. Senate	Dietary Goals for the U.S.		+	+	+	+	+	+	
1979	USDA	Building a Better Diet—Five Food Groups	+	+	+	+	+	+	+	+
1979	DHEW	Healthy People: The Surgeon General's Report on Health Promotion and Disease Prevention	+	+	+	+	+	+	+	+
1979	DHEW/ NCI	Statement on Diet, Nutrition, and Cancer—Prudent Interim Principles	+	+	+		+			+
1980	USDA/ DHHS	Dietary Guidelines for Americans	+	+	+	+	+	+	+	+
1980	DHHS	National 1990 Nutrition Objectives	+	+	+	+	+	+	+	+
1984	DHHS/ NHLBI	Recommendations for Control of High Blood Pressure		+			+		+	+
1985	USDA/ DHHS	Dietary Guidelines for Americans, 2nd edition	+	+	+	+	+	+	+	+
1986	DHHS/ NCI	Cancer Control Nutrition Objectives for the Nation: 1985–2000		+	+		+			+

continued

■
TABLE 2-5, *continued*

Year	Agency[b]	Publication	Recommendation[a] Variety	Maintain Ideal Body Weight	Include Starch and Fiber	Limit Sugar	Limit Fat	Limit Choles-terol	Limit Salt	Limit Alcohol
1987	DHHS/ NHLBI	National Cholesterol Education Program Guidelines	+	+	+		+	+		+
1988	DHHS/ NCI	Dietary Guidelines for Cancer Prevention	+	+	+		+		+	+

*Recommended for *inclusion* in the daily diet, as opposed to subsequent recommendations to *limit* intake.
[a]Other recommendations include: increased consumption of foods containing vitamins and minerals (USDA 1917–1958; NCI 1986), increased physical activity (USDA/DHHS 1980, 1985; DHHS 1980), and reduced intake of salt-cured or smoked foods (NCI 1988).
[b]USDA = U.S. Department of Agriculture, U.S. Senate = U.S. Senate Select Committee on Nutrition and Human Needs, DHEW = Department of Health, Education, and Welfare, DHHS = Department of Health and Human Services, NCI = National Cancer Institute, NHLBI = National Heart, Lung, and Blood Institute.
Source: *Surgeon General's Report*, 1988.

over the years as nutrition and health relationships have become more clear. The most comprehensive of these guides is the "Dietary Guidelines for Americans" published by the U.S. Department of Health and Human Services and the Department of Agriculture. The "Dietary Guidelines" are reprinted in Appendix A.

The "Dietary Guidelines for Americans"

The twenty-three-page pamphlet "Dietary Guidelines for Americans" was developed in response to consumers' concerns about what a healthy diet is. Consumers wanted to know what type of diet promotes health. The "Guidelines" center around seven recommendations:

- Maintain desirable weight.
- Eat a variety of foods.
- Eat foods with adequate starch and fiber.
- Avoid too much sodium.
- Avoid too much fat, saturated fat, and cholesterol.
- Avoid too much sugar.
- If you drink alcoholic beverages, do so in moderation.

Each recommendation reflects scientific conclusions about how Americans can improve their health through dietary changes. The "Dietary Guidelines" includes advice on how to reduce sugar, sodium, fats, and cholesterol in the diet, how to ensure adequate fiber and starch intake, and how to maintain normal weight.

At the core of the recommendations is a guide for choosing a balanced variety of foods based on the food groups listed in Table 2-6. Because of

■

TABLE 2-6

Food groups that serve as the foundation of a balanced diet

Food Group	Standard Serving Size	Recommended Minimum Number of Servings: Children	Teenagers	Adults[1]	Adult Vegetarians
Breads and Cereals		4	4	4	4
Whole-grain and enriched bread	1 slice or 1 oz				
English muffin	½				
Roll, biscuit, muffin	1				
Bagel	½				
Tortilla	1				
Noodles, macaroni	½ c				
Rice	½ c				
Ready-to-eat cereal	1 c or 1 oz				
Cooked cereal	½ c				
Crackers	4 squares				
Pancake	5″ × ½″				
Waffle	4″ × 4″ × ½″				
Vegetables and Fruits		4	4	4	4
		(at least one serving from each category)			
Vitamin A-rich					
Broccoli					
Carrots					
Collards					
Spinach	½ c				
Green peppers					
Sweet potatoes					
Winter squash					
Apricots	3				
Vitamin C-rich					
Cantaloupe	¼				
Orange/juice	1 or 6 oz				
Grapefruit/juice	½ or 6 oz				
Tomato/juice	1 or 1 c				
Strawberries	⅔ c				
Cabbage, raw	1 c				
Brussels sprouts	½ c				
Other					
Potatoes	1 med.				
Corn	½ c				
Peas	½ c				
Green beans	½ c				
Beets	½ c				
Banana	1				
Apple/juice	1 or 6 oz				

continued

TABLE 2-6, *continued*

Food Group	Standard Serving Size	Recommended Minimum Number of Servings: Children	Teenagers	Adults[1]	Adult Vegetarians
Vegetables and Fruits					
Other, *cont.*					
Pear	1				
Peach	1				
Grape/juice	1 or 6 oz				
Watermelon	1 c				
Milk and Milk Products (includes low-fat products)		3	4	2	2
Milk	1 c				
Soy "milk" (fortified)	1 c				
Yogurt	1 c				
Cheese	1½ oz				
Cottage cheese	1 c				
Pudding	1 c				
Ice cream	2 c				
Ice milk	1 c				
Meats and Meat Alternates		2	2	2	3[2] (vegetable protein sources)
Beef, fish, poultry, pork, and other meats (lean)	3 oz (½ c diced)				
Eggs	2				
Dried beans, cooked	1 c				
Peanut butter	4 T				
Nuts, seeds	½ c				
Tofu	½ c				
Miscellaneous (optional)		based on caloric need			
Fats (butter, margarine, oil, mayonnaise)	1 t				
Cream, whipped toppings	2 T				
Salad dressing	2 T				
Gravy, sauces	¼ c				
Bacon, sausage	1 oz				
Sweets (candy, sugar, soft drinks, fruit drinks, etc.)	1 oz solid or 8 oz beverage				
Alcoholic beverages	1 drink				

[1]Pregnant and breast-feeding women should consume two additional servings from the milk and milk products group and one more serving from the meat and meat alternates group. Women beyond the age of 50 may benefit from more than two daily servings of low-fat milk and milk products.
[2]Vegetable protein sources should be consumed along with grains.

BOX 2-6

THE FOOD EXCHANGE SYSTEM

The food exchange system is another aid in planning diets. The system is based on six "exchange lists," which group foods by similarity of calorie, carbohydrate, protein, and fat content. The exchange lists enable people to design diets that provide particular levels of calories and specified percentages of calories from carbohydrates, protein, and fats. Although the exchange system was initially developed as a meal planning guide for the dietary management of diabetes, it has become popular for planning weight-loss diets.

Additional information about the food exchange system, including how it can be used to plan diets and the food exchange lists, is presented in Appendix F.

the importance of variety in the diet, we will take a close look at the basic food groups and explain how they can be used in selecting a balanced diet. (Box 2-6 explains an alternate method for planning diets—the "food exchange" system.)

The Food-Group Approach to Selecting a Balanced Diet

You can almost tell a person's age by finding out the number of basic food groups he or she studied in school. Since 1916, food guides based on 4, 5, 7, 11, and even 16 food groups have been developed. The "basic food group" approach to balanced diets continues to be a cornerstone of nutrition education.

Foods are classified into groups primarily on the basis of their key nutrients; all foods within a particular group are good sources of the same set of nutrients. The key nutrient content of foods within the basic four food groups and the contributions of the "miscellaneous" group of foods are

A basic food group guide developed for Southeast Asians.

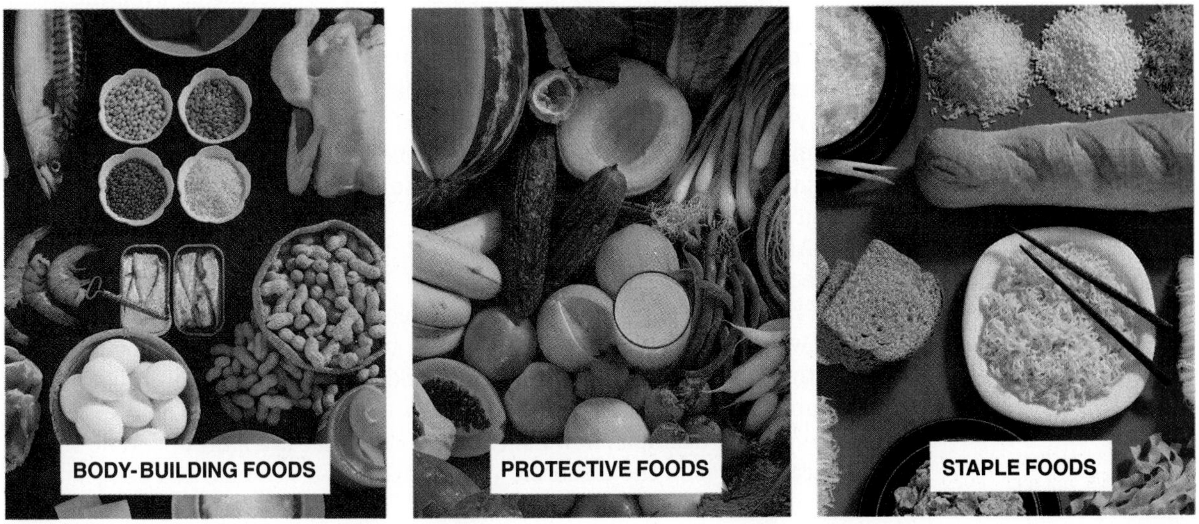

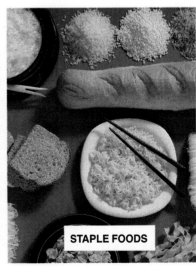

TABLE 2-7
Key nutrients of the food groups

Food Group	Key Nutrients
Breads and cereals	carbohydrates dietary fiber thiamin (B_1) riboflavin (B_2) niacin (B_3) iron
Vegetables and fruits	vitamin A vitamin C carbohydrates dietary fiber
Milk and milk products	calcium riboflavin (B_2) protein
Meat and meat alternates	protein fat iron zinc niacin (B_3)
Miscellaneous	fats carbohydrates (including sugars)

shown in Table 2-7. Diets containing the recommended number of servings of each food group tend to provide at least 80 percent of the RDAs of all nutrients. The caloric level of diets that just meet the minimum recommended number of servings, however, is generally on the low side. Calories can be increased by consuming more than the minimum number of servings and by including foods from the "miscellaneous" group.

Food-group approaches to food selection have endured over the years because they are quite easy to understand, they allow leeway for personal choices within each group, and they generally lead to an adequate intake of essential nutrients. The basic food groups have very practical applications; they are useful when making grocery lists, planning meals, and ordering from restaurant menus. They can also be used to estimate the adequacy of an individual diet. (Box 2-7 is an exercise in comparing your diet to the basic food group guide.)

Although time-tested and practical, the basic food group approach to selecting a balanced diet is not perfect. The food groups do not include the full range of food possibilities. Ethnic foods and mixed dishes such as tacos, chow mein, stews, and soups are not included in the basic food groups. Estimating serving sizes is not easy, and this can make it difficult to assign appropriate portions of a serving of a mixed dish to the respective food groups. For example, how many carrot sticks are in a half cup, or, how much macaroni was in the casserole you ate? (Box 2-8 will help you assign mixed

BOX 2-7

HOW DOES MY DIET COMPARE WITH THE BASIC FOOD GROUP GUIDE?

Compare one day of your diet with the Basic Food Group Guide. First, think about what you did and what you ate yesterday. Write down all the foods you ate and all the beverages you drank, beginning when you got up and ending when you went to bed.

After you have listed the foods and beverages, go back and estimate the amount of each that you consumed. Refer to food labels, measuring cups and spoons, and recipes for help in deciding amounts

If your diet failed to include at least the minimum number of servings from each group, how could it be modified to balance your intake? and ingredients if necessary. (If you need to assign mixed dishes to the food groups, Box 2-8 will help you.)

Compare your intake with the Basic Food Guide's minimum number of servings and serving sizes for each food group (Table 2-6), and with the U.S. average figures given in the table on page 61.

		Amount I Ate Compared to a Standard Serving						
			Vegetables and Fruits					
My Food and Beverage Intake	Amount	Breads and Cereals	Vitamin A-Rich	Vitamin C-Rich	Other	Milk and Milk Products	Meats and Alternates	Miscellaneous
Total number of servings								
Recommended minimum number of servings (adult)		4		4		2	2	
Difference (Total − Recommended)								Total:

ASSIGNING MIXED DISHES TO FOOD GROUPS

Real diets usually include mixed dishes, and they, too, can be assigned to food groups with a little work. They first must be broken down by their major ingredients, and then the amount of each major ingredient must be measured or estimated. For example, a cheese omelet that contains two eggs and one-half slice of presliced American cheese (1/2 ounce) would equal one serving of "meat and meat alternates" and one-third serving of "milk and milk products." Here are breakdowns of three other mixed dishes into their food-group components:

	Food Group					
		Vegetables and Fruits				
Mixed Dish	Breads and Cereals	Vitamin A-Rich	Vitamin C-Rich	Other	Milk and Milk Products	Meats and Alternates
Chili, 1 c						
hamburger, 1½ oz (¼ c)						½
tomatoes, ½ c			½			
kidney beans, ¼ c						¼
Pizza, 1 wedge						
crust, 1 wedge	1					
tomato sauce, ¼ c			½			
cheese, ½ oz					⅓	
sausage, ⅛ oz*						
Beef Stew, 1½ c						
chuck roast, 3 oz (½ c)						1
potatoes, ¼ c				1		
carrots, ¼ c		½				
gravy, ½ c*						

*"Miscellaneous" foods

dishes to food groups.) Furthermore, the basic-food-group approach totally ignores one essential nutrient—water.

It is also possible to end up low on calories and certain nutrients, or to formulate a diet that contains too much fat, cholesterol, sodium, or sugar, or too little fiber using the basic food guide. These are perhaps the greatest shortcomings of the basic food group approach.

The three menus presented in Tables 2-8, 2-9, and 2-10 illustrate this last point. All three of the menus provide the minimum number of recommended servings from each food group, yet the menus are not "equal" nutritionally. Analyses provided below each menu show how closely the basic-food-group choices correspond to the standards set in the "Dietary Guidelines." First, the menus vary in calories from 975 to 2,040. Menus 1 and 2

TABLE 2-8
Menu 1: 975 calories*

	Food Group						
	Breads and Cereals	Vegetables and Fruits: Vitamin A-Rich	Vegetables and Fruits: Vitamin C-Rich	Vegetables and Fruits: Other	Milk and Milk Products	Meats and Alternates	Miscel-laneous
Breakfast							
Orange juice, 6 oz			1				
Cornflakes, 1 c	1						
Whole-wheat toast, 2 slices	2						
Skim milk, 1 c					1		
Lunch							
Tuna (in water), 3 oz						1	
Saltine crackers, 4 pieces	1						
Skim milk, 1 c					1		
Apple, 1				1			
Dinner							
Baked chicken (no skin), 3 oz						1	
Boiled potato, 1 med.				1			
Spinach, ½ c		1					
Total number of servings	4	4			2	2	0

Relationship to Recommendations of the "Dietary Guidelines"

	% Of Calories from Protein:Fat:Carbohydrate	Nutrient Adequacy	Cholesterol, mg	Sodium, mg	Dietary Fiber, g	Sucrose, % of total calories
Recommended	15:30:55	RDA levels	300 or less	3,000	20–30	15% or less
Menu Analysis	32:12:56	4 nutrients below 80% of RDAs	150	1,820	10	5%

*Assumes no salt, butter, or margarine is added at the table.

(Tables 2-8 and 2-9) provide less than 80 percent of the RDAs for four and two essential nutrients, respectively, and both are low in dietary fiber. Menu 2, the one that contains 2,040 calories, is high in fat and cholesterol. Menus 1 and 3 (Tables 2-8 and 2-10) contain the desired levels of cholesterol. Menu 3 provides 1,200 calories, and as the analysis shows, is compatible with the "Guidelines" recommendations.

Attempts are being made to modify the basic food groups so that selections from each group add up to a diet that is adequate as well as balanced in terms of protein, carbohydrate, fat, vitamins, minerals, cholesterol, so-

TABLE 2-9
Menu 2: 2,040 calories*

	Food Group						
	Breads and Cereals	Vegetables and Fruits: Vitamin A-Rich	Vegetables and Fruits: Vitamin C-Rich	Vegetables and Fruits: Other	Milk and Milk Products	Meats and Alternates	Miscellaneous
Breakfast							
Blueberry muffin, 1	1						
Granola, 1 oz	1						
Whole milk, 1 c					1		
Lunch							
Hot roast beef sandwich, 1	2					1	
Gravy, ¼ c							1
Mashed potatoes, ½ c				1			
Orange, 1			1				
Dinner							
Fried chicken, 3 oz						1	
French fries, ½ c				1			
Winter squash, ½ c		1					
Ice cream, 2 c					1		
Total number of servings	4	4			2	2	1

Relationship to Recommendations of the "Dietary Guidelines"

	% Of Calories from Protein:Fat:Carbohydrate	Nutrient Adequacy	Cholesterol, mg	Sodium, mg	Dietary Fiber, g	Sucrose, % of total calories
Recommended	15:30:55	RDA levels	300 or less	3,000	20–30	15% or less
Menu Analysis	14:42:44	2 nutrients below 80% of RDAs	374	1,900	10	7%

*Assumes no salt, butter, or margarine is added at the table.

dium, fiber, and sugar content. It's difficult to accomplish this without making the recommendations overwhelmingly complicated, but improvements are being made.

adequate diet: One that supplies approximately the RDAs for essential nutrients and enough calories to meet the person's need for energy.

Modifying the Basic Food Group Message

The first "basic food group" approach—the Basic Seven Food Groups (Figure 2-6)—was developed to provide an **adequate diet**; that is, a diet that would prevent deficiencies of proteins, vitamin C, niacin, and other essen-

TABLE 2-10

Menu 3: 1,200 calories*

	Food Group						
	Breads and Cereals	Vegetables and Fruits: Vitamin A-Rich	Vegetables and Fruits: Vitamin C-Rich	Vegetables and Fruits: Other	Milk and Milk Products	Meats and Alternates	Miscel-laneous
Breakfast							
Cantaloupe, ¼			1				
Bran Buds®, 1 oz	1						
Skim milk, 1 c					1		
Lunch							
Turkey, 3 oz						1	
Whole-wheat bread, 2 slices	2						
Low-fat yogurt, 1 c					1		
Plum, 1				1			
Dinner							
Spinach salad, 1½ c		1					
Italian dressing, 2 T							
Round steak, 3 oz						1	
Asparagus, ½ c		1					
Whole-wheat roll, 1	1						
Total number of servings	4	4			2	2	0

Relationship to Recommendations of the "Dietary Guidelines"

	% Of Calories from Protein:Fat:Carbohydrate	Nutrient Adequacy	Cholesterol, mg	Sodium, mg	Dietary Fiber, g	Sucrose, % of total calories
Recommended	15:30:55	RDA levels	300 or less	3,000	20–30	15% or less
Menu Analysis	29:31:40	0 nutrients below 80% of RDAs	148	1,790	24	7%

*Assumes no salt, butter, or margarine is added at the table.

tial nutrients. Today we know that although the food-group approach is sufficient for helping people select an adequate diet, it may not be sufficient for selecting a "balanced" diet. Many food-group-approach diets contain too much fat, sodium, alcohol, and other substances and too little fiber. Messages printed in the basic-food-group guides are now being modified to highlight low-fat milk, cheese, yogurt, and meats; whole-grain breads and cereals and other high-fiber foods; and low-salt–low-sugar products.

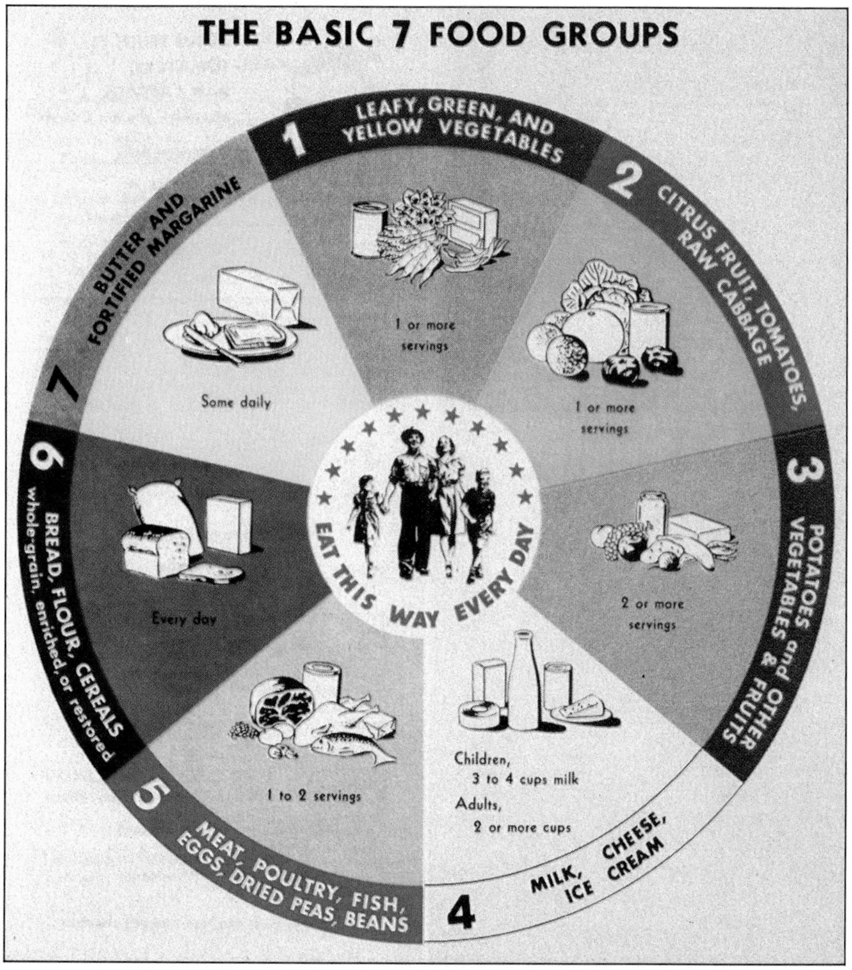

The Basic Seven Food Groups were developed by the U.S. Department of Agriculture in 1946 to help people select adequate diets. The food group guide currently in use, and presented in this book, helps people to select a *balanced* adequate diet.

TABLE 2-11

The eleven principles of nutrition

1. Food is a basic need of humans.
2. Foods provide nutrients needed for life and health.
3. Some nutrients must be provided by the diet.
4. Most health problems related to nutrition originate within cells.
5. Poor nutrition can result from either inadequate or excessive levels of nutrient intake.
6. Malnutrition may be directly related or unrelated to dietary intake.
7. Some groups of people are at greater risk of becoming inadequately nourished than others.
8. Malnutrition can contribute to the development of certain chronic diseases.
9. In addition to nutrients, foods contain other substances that may affect health.
10. Humans have adaptive mechanisms for managing fluctuations in dietary intake.
11. Balance and variety characterize a healthy diet.

In Holland, the basic food guide has been revised to make it easier to choose an adequate, balanced diet. Foods are subdivided into first- and second-preference groups based on the amount of fat, sugar, and fiber they contain.[3] In the U.S., people are being urged to choose foods that are low in fat, cholesterol, and sugar and high in fiber and to moderate their alcohol intake. We are advised to rely less on the "miscellaneous" group for calories and more on additional servings from the breads and cereals group and the vegetables and fruits group. As shown in the following table, these are the foods that U.S. adults are most likely to be consuming in low amounts.[21]

	Number of Servings Daily	
Food Group	Present Average	Recommended Minimum
Breads and cereals	2.8	4
Vegetables and fruits	2.4	4
Milk and milk products	1.9	2
Meats and meat alternates	1.9	2
Miscellaneous (fats and sweets)	1.3	—

The food groups and the advice that goes along with them will continue to change as more is learned about the relationships between diet and health.

■ ■ ■

COMING UP IN CHAPTER 3

Having discussed the broad, basic principles of the science of nutrition (Table 2-11), we are now ready to begin our discussions of specific nutrients. Chapter 3 introduces the "energy nutrients" and describes how the body obtains energy from them. It also addresses nutrition, physical performance, and energy balance.

■ ■ ■

REVIEW QUESTIONS

1. Give an example of a harmful, and of a beneficial effect of specific food additives.
2. List the steps in the progression of a nutrient-deficiency disease.
3. How do adaptive mechanisms provide a buffer against the development of malnutrition?
4. What groups of people are considered to be most vulnerable to the effects of malnutrition? Why are they more vulnerable than other groups of people?
5. Cite three causes of secondary malnutrition.
6. Describe the general role nutrition plays in sustaining cell health.
7. List six factors that influence the amount of essential nutrients needed by humans.

8. Cite five factors that influence the nutrient composition of specific foods.
9. List the 11 principles of human nutrition.
10. List the seven recommendations from "The Dietary Guidelines for Americans."

Answers

1. See the discussion of Principle 9.
2. See Figure 2-3.
3. See the discussion of Principle 10.
4. See the discussion of Principle 7.
5. See the discussion of Principle 6.
6. Refer to the discussion of Principle 4.
7. See the discussion of Principle 3.
8. See the discussion of Principle 2.
9. Refer to Table 2-11.
10. See the discussion of Principle 11.

■ ■ ■

PUTTING NUTRITION KNOWLEDGE TO WORK

1. How does your diet rate for variety? A wide variety of foods is needed for a balanced diet. Americans tend to consume 17 to 22 different food items per day. Write down the foods you ate yesterday (or refer to the exercise you did in Box 2-7). Count the number of different foods you ate. Exclude from the count minor ingredients such as parsley or garlic in spaghetti sauce. Is your diet highly varied (more than 25 different foods) or not very varied (less than 14 different foods)?
2. Think about how much and how frequently you ate when you were growing rapidly in your early teens. How do they compare with your eating pattern now? How do periods of intensive physical training affect your food intake? Are there other factors that influence how much or how often you eat? If yes, what are they?
3. Refer to the RDA tables given on the inside cover of this book. What is the RDA for protein, vitamin C, and calcium for a person of your age and gender? What are they for a 73-year-old man?
4. Can you get all the essential nutrients you need from a "totally" fortified breakfast cereal? Compare the list of nutrients shown on the nutrition label of a fortified breakfast cereal with the list of essential nutrients in Table 2-2. Which essential nutrients are not listed on the cereal label? Does eating a serving of the cereal provide you with 100% of all the essential nutrients?
5. Are you familiar with the menu of a fast-food restaurant that is open for three meals a day? If so, try to select one day of meals that would meet the minimum number of servings from the basic food groups. Try this exercise again, selecting only foods that are neither fried nor salted.

6. Do you know a person from a different country? Ask him or her about the country's traditional foods and meals. Compare and contrast them with your family's traditions.
7. Imagine that you went to a fairly fancy restaurant and, with confidence that it would be delicious, ordered the soup of the day. After enjoying the soup, you ask the waiter what it was, and he replies, "Our chef's favorite, bone marrow soup." What would be your reaction? Would you order the soup again? Why or why not?

■ ■ ■

NOTES

1. *Nutrition Monitoring in the United States*, DHHS Publication No. (PHS) 86-1255 (Hyattsville, Md., July 1986).

2. Food and Nutrition Board, National Research Council, *Recommended Dietary Allowances*, 9th ed. (Washington, D.C.: National Academy of Sciences, 1980).

3. W. Mertz, The essential trace elements, *Science* 213 (1981): 1332–1338.

4. S. T. Omaye, Safety of megavitamin therapy, in *Nutritional Toxicological Aspects of Food Safety*, ed. M. Friedman (New York: Plenum Press, 1904), 169–203.

5. R. E. Hodges, Vitamin C, in *Human Nutrition, a Comprehensive Treatise, Nutrition and the Adult*, eds. R. B. Alfin-Slater and D. Kritchevsky (New York: Plenum Press, 1980), 73–96.

6. T. Moore, *Vitamin A* (New York: Elsevier Publishing Co., 1957).

7. L. Schoeff, Vitamin A, *American Journal of Medical Technology* 49 (1983): 447–452.

8. D. S. Goodman, Vitamin A and retinoids in health and disease, *New England Journal of Medicine* 310 (1984): 1023–1031.

9. *Vital Statistics of the United States 1980, Vol. II: Mortality, Part A*, DHHS Publication No. (PHS) 85-1101 (Hyattsville, Md.: National Center for Health Statistics, 1985).

10. H. S. Mosher, F. A. Fuhrman, et al., Tarichatoxin-tetrodotoxin: A potent neurotoxin, *Science* 144 (1964): 1100–1102.

11. Researchers warn of potato peel toxins, *Nutrition Week*, 3 April 1988: 3.

12. J. M. Kinsbury, *Poisonous Plants of the United States and Canada* (Englewood Cliffs, N.J.: Prentice Hall, Inc., 1964), 6.

13. O. Michelsen, N. G. Yang, and R. S. Goodhart, Naturally occurring toxic foods, in *Modern Nutrition in Health and Disease*, eds. R. S. Goodhart and M. E. Shils (Philadelphia: Lea and Febiger, 1973), 412–433.

14. C. L. Comar and J. C. Thompson, Jr., Radioactivity in foods, in *Modern Nutrition in Health and Disease*, eds. R. S. Goodhart and M. E. Shils (Philadelphia: Lea and Febiger, 1973), 442–454.

15. E. S. Josephson, A historical review of food irradiation, *Journal of Food Science* 5 (1983): 161–189.

16. T. K. Murray, Nutrition aspects of food irradiation, in *Recent Advances in Food Irradiation* (Amsterdam: Elsevier Biomedical Press, 1983).

17. S. Thompson, Food irradiation overview, *Association of Food and Drug Officials Quarterly Bulletin*, October 1984.

18. A. Rogan and G. Glaros, Food irradiation: The process and implications for dietitians, *Journal of American Dietetic Association* 88 (1988): 833–838.

19. Rules and Regulations, *Federal Register*, April 18, 1988.

20. B. Caballero, Food additives in the pediatric diet, *Clinical Nutrition* 4 (1985): 200–206.

21. J. A. T. Pennington, Dietary patterns and practices, *Clinical Nutrition* 5 (1986): 17–26.

CHAPTER 3

FOOD, ENERGY, AND ENERGY BALANCE

Energy is neither created nor destroyed. It can, however, change from one form to another.

—First Law of Thermodynamics

Energy is a basic requirement for life. Every time you blink, think, speak, read, move, or breathe, you use energy. Energy makes the processes of **digestion**, **absorption**, and nutrient utilization possible. It allows us to grow, to develop, to heal, and to resist disease. The energy needed for these and many other body functions comes from only three food components: carbohydrates, proteins, and fats. Collectively, these are known as the "energy nutrients," and they are totally responsible for the caloric value of foods.

digestion: The process by which ingested food is prepared for use by the body. It occurs in the digestive system and involves several mechanical processes and thousands of chemical reactions.

absorption: The process by which nutrients and other substances are transported from the gastrointestinal tract into the body proper.

calorie: A unit of measure for energy. The nutrition "calorie" refers to the kilocalorie (kcal), the amount of energy needed to raise the temperature of a kilogram of water from 15°C to 16°C.

THE CALORIE: A UNIT FOR MEASURING FOOD ENERGY

Just as the foot is a measure of length and the pound is a measure of weight, the **calorie*** is a measure of energy. The caloric value of a food represents how much energy it will supply to the body. Technically speaking, a calorie is *the amount of energy needed to raise the temperature of one kilogram of water* (slightly more than 4 cups) *from 15°C to 16°C* (59°F to 61°F).

In many countries the unit of measure for the energy value of foods is the joule. One calorie equals approximately 4.2 joules. Although it has been strongly urged by the international scientific community that joules be used by all countries as the measure of food energy, the change has not yet been broadly adopted.

Although calories are often thought of as the "fattening" component of food, they are not an *ingredient* of food, as are nutrients. They are units that

*Although this text uses the common term for the amount of energy in food, *calorie*, the "calories" are actually kilocalories (kcal) or Calories (spelled with a capital *C*).

TABLE 3-1
Caloric value of the energy nutrients and alcohol

	Calories per Gram
Carbohydrate	4
Protein	4
Fat	9
Alcohol	7

represent the amount of energy stored in carbohydrates, proteins, and fats. Stored within each gram of carbohydrate and protein is approximately 4 calories' worth of energy. That's equivalent to 112 calories per *ounce* of carbohydrate or protein. (Reminder: there are approximately 28 grams in an ounce.) Fats contain the highest level of stored energy, about 9 calories per gram or 252 calories per ounce. The caloric value of a slice of bread, for example, comes from the 13 grams of carbohydrate, the 2.2 grams of protein, and the 0.8 gram of fat it contains:

$$\begin{aligned} \text{13 grams carbohydrate} \times \text{4 calories per gram} &= 52 \text{ calories} \\ \text{2.2 grams protein} \times \text{4 calories per gram} &= 8.8 \\ \text{0.8 gram fat} \times \text{9 calories per gram} &= \underline{7.2} \\ \text{Total energy value} &= 68.0 \text{ calories} \end{aligned}$$

Alcohol, although not considered an essential nutrient, also supplies energy because of its carbohydratelike chemical structure. Alcohol provides 7 calories per gram. Table 3-1 summarizes these caloric values.

Not all of food's weight is accounted for by its carbohydrate, protein, and fat content. Foods also contain water and other substances such as minerals that add to their weight. An ounce of lean sirloin steak does not contain 28 grams of protein, for example; it contains 16.4 grams of water, 9 grams of protein, and 2.2 grams of fat, plus trace amounts of some minerals.

Measuring the Caloric Value of Foods

The energy value of food is measured in laboratories with an instrument called a bomb calorimeter (Figure 3-1). A known amount of a food is burned in a sealed container that is surrounded by a kilogram of water. The food in the container is ignited with the help of oxygen and heats the water as it burns. The increase in the temperature of the surrounding water is noted, and a caloric value is assigned based on the increase. For example, if a slice of cheese was burned in a bomb calorimeter and raised the temperature of the kilogram of water from 59°F to 185°F, it would indicate that the slice of cheese contained 63 calories. The slice of cheese would release enough heat to make about 4 cups of slightly cool water too hot to touch.

The energy contained in carbohydrates, proteins, and fats is completely released when foods are burned in a bomb calorimeter. The body, however, absorbs less than 100% of the carbohydrate, protein, and fat content of food. Consequently, the measured caloric values of foods must be adjusted to

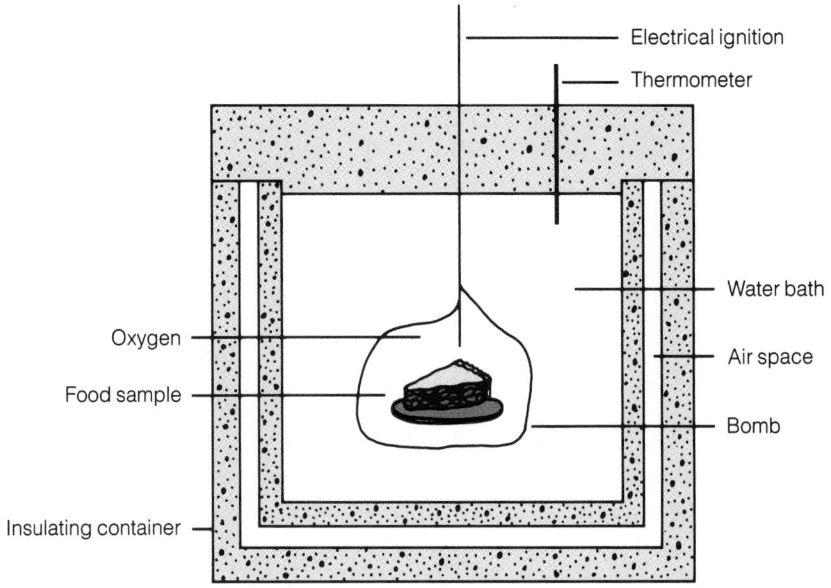

FIGURE 3-1
Determining the caloric value of foods in a bomb calorimeter.

account for the percentages of the energy nutrients that are absorbed by the body. The human body absorbs approximately 99% of carbohydrates, 92% of proteins, and 95% of fats that are consumed.

Characteristics of Energy Nutrients

Soon after the energy nutrients were discovered in the late 1800s, it was recognized that protein is more than a source of energy; that its primary function is as the source of material for construction and repair of body tissues. Because only protein can perform these essential functions, the body "spares" protein from use as an energy source if carbohydrates and fats are available. When the supply of carbohydrates and fats is limited, protein is used to form energy, which makes less protein available for tissue formation and repair. So, protein can only be used for these unique functions if enough carbohydrate and fat is available to meet the body's energy needs.

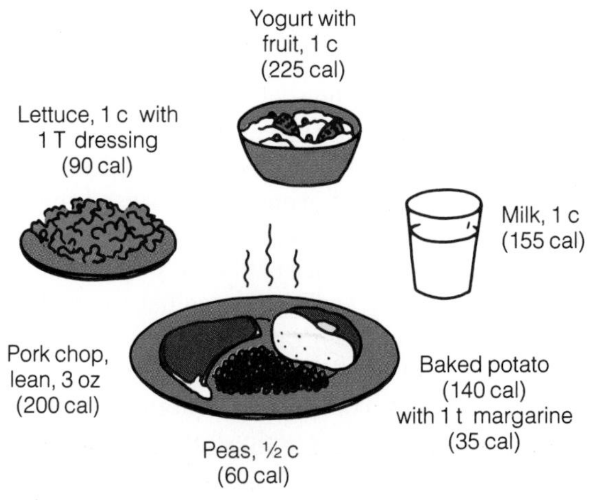

Foods are the body's source of energy. The energy value of food is measured in calories.

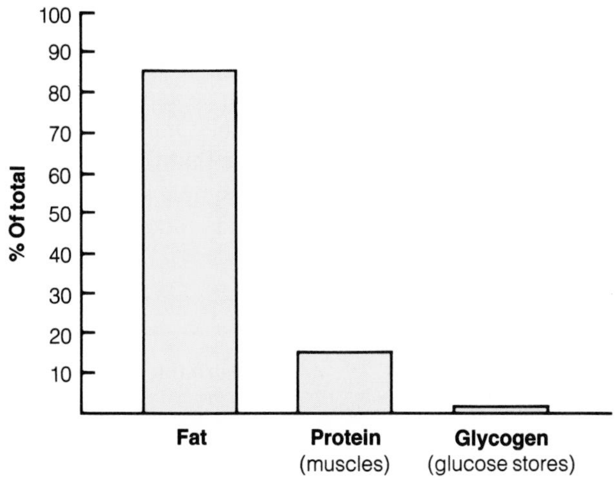

FIGURE 3-2
Body energy reserves in healthy humans.

Of the energy nutrients, carbohydrates can be converted into energy most readily, and unlike protein and fat, carbohydrate can be directly used as a source of fuel by all cells in the body.

The first law of thermodynamics states that energy can be neither created nor destroyed, but that it can change form. The energy stored in the carbohydrates, proteins, and fats we consume can be used for physical movement, digestion, and so on, or it can be changed into a storage form of energy. If the foods we consume supply more energy than we need at the time, most of the excess is converted to fat and stored for later use. When our food intake supplies less energy than we need, stored fat is used to make up the deficit.

Carbohydrate is also stored in muscles and the liver in the form of glycogen, although the glycogen energy stores are much smaller than the fat stores. Glycogen energy stores are usually limited to about 1800 calories, whereas fat stores typically exceed 100,000 calories in normal-weight adults. Figure 3-2 shows the percentages of body energy reserves contributed by fat, protein, and glycogen in normal-weight, healthy adults.

Carbohydrates, proteins, and fats occur in substantially greater amounts in food than do vitamins and minerals, reflecting our larger need for them (Figure 3-3). Only rarely are the energy nutrients the sole nutrients provided by foods. With the exception of sugar and alcohol, foods that supply the energy nutrients also add vitamins, minerals, water, and other substances to our diet.

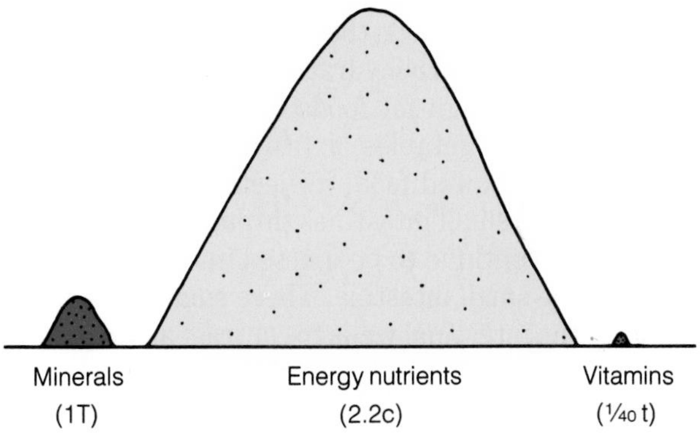

FIGURE 3-3
Comparison of the volume of energy nutrients, minerals, and vitamins needed daily. This is based on a 2,400-calorie diet that provides 55% of its calories from carbohydrates, 30% from fat, and 15% from protein. The U.S. RDAs were used to calculate the amounts of minerals and vitamins.

DIGESTION AND ABSORPTION OF ENERGY NUTRIENTS

Before carbohydrates, proteins, and fats can be used for energy, they must become part of the body proper. That is, they must be broken down into their component parts, which are substances that the body can absorb. The absorbable forms of carbohydrates are the simple sugars, such as glucose. Proteins are largely absorbed as amino acids, and fats as fatty acids and glycerol:

Energy Nutrient	Absorbable Form
Carbohydrates	simple sugars
Proteins	amino acids
Fats	fatty acids and glycerol

A good deal of "processing" is generally required to convert the energy nutrients consumed in food to their absorbable forms. This task is accomplished by digestion.

The processes involved in digesting a meal take perhaps a day or two to complete, and when they are completed, big pieces of food have been broken into microscopic particles. The vast majority of the processes of digestion occur in the **gastrointestinal tract** of the digestive system (Figure 3-4). The digestive tract is about 25 to 30 feet in length and is like a long, irregularly shaped tube. Digestion is accomplished by both mechanical processes and chemical processes.

gastrointestinal tract: The portion of the digestive system that consists of the stomach and intestines. Although the mouth and esophagus are parts of the digestive system and are involved in digestion, the vast majority of digestive processes occur in the stomach and intestines. (The gastrointestinal tract is sometimes referred to as the *gut*.)

Mechanical Processes of Digestion

The muscles of the digestive tract conduct mechanical—physical—processes that help to break down food into absorbable forms. Chewing and the mixing and movement of food along the digestive tract are the major mechanical processes of digestion.

After food is chewed it is swallowed and passes down the esophagus to the stomach. Muscles that act as valves at the entrance and exit of the stomach ensure that the food stays there until it's liquified and ready for the digestive processes of the small intestine. Solid foods tend to stay in the stomach for over an hour, whereas most liquids pass through it in about twenty minutes (Figure 3-5). Foods that are high in fat stay in the stomach longer than high-protein or carbohydrate-rich foods. This is why you feel "full" longer after you eat high-fat foods (such as a hamburger or potato chips) than after you eat vegetables or fruits. When the stomach has finished its work on the swallowed food, it ejects one to two teaspoons of its liquified contents into the small intestines through the muscular valve at its end. Stomach contents continue to be ejected in this fashion until they are totally released into the small intestine. These small pulses of liquified food stimulate muscles in the intestinal walls to contract and relax, thereby caus-

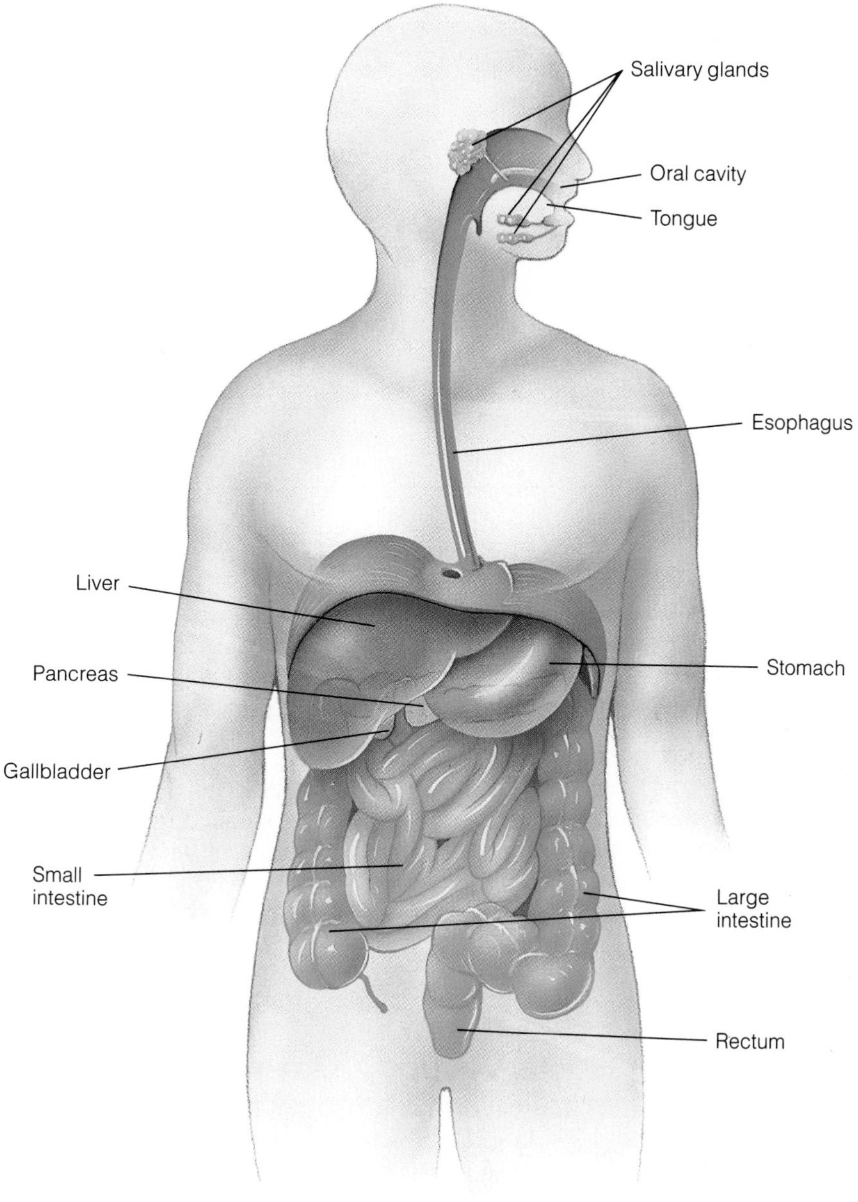

FIGURE 3-4
The digestive system.

ing mixing and movement of the food being digested. Diets that contain a lot of "bulk"—what is more commonly referred to these days as *fiber*—tend to increase the size of the bulge of digesting food in the intestines. Bigger food bulges stimulate a higher level of intestinal muscle activity than do smaller food bulges. Thus, high-fiber meals pass through the digestive system somewhat more quickly than low-fiber meals.

Chemical Processes of Digestion

The chemical processes of digestion begin before food is eaten. Simply thinking about food makes digestive juices start flowing, as the exercise

FIGURE 3-5

The amount of time solids and liquids remain in the stomach.

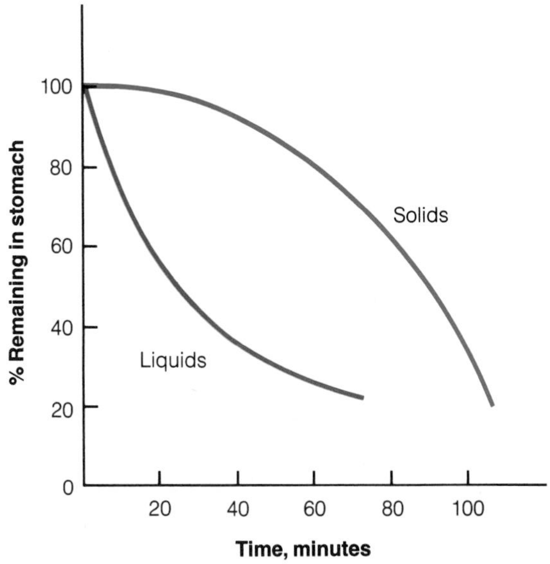

enzymes: Complex protein substances that increase the rate of chemical reactions without being permanently changed themselves in the process; sometimes referred to as *catalysts*. The body contains hundreds of enzymes. They are found in particularly high amounts in the gastrointestinal tract. They are specific in their action, each acting only upon a particular chemical substance. The suffix *-ase* is common for enzyme names; amyl*ase* and sucr*ase* are examples. The suffix *-in* is also common—as in tryps*in* and peps*in*.

described in Box 3-1 demonstrates. After food is consumed, **enzymes** break down carbohydrates, proteins, and fats into absorbable forms. Vitamins and minerals are not broken down before they are absorbed; they are simply released from the foods that hold them during digestion.

Digestive Enzymes Several quarts of digestive juices are produced by the digestive tract each day. The major components of the digestive juices are enzymes manufactured by the salivary glands, stomach, pancreas, and small intestine. All together, nearly a hundred different enzymes participate in the digestion of food.

Enzymes used in digestion are complex protein substances that speed up the chemical breakdown of food. Enzymes may increase the rate of the

BOX 3-1

COMMUNICATING WITH YOUR DIGESTIVE SYSTEM

The brain has a direct communication line with the stomach. This exercise will demonstrate this for you.

Take a deep breath, clear your head, and relax. . . . Now, think about these foods:

- lemon juice, dripping on your tongue
- a golden brown, succulent roast turkey that you can smell roasting in the oven
- a piping-hot pizza smothered with melted cheese
- a peach so sweet the juices drip down your chin when you bite into it

If your mouth is watering and you have become aware of your stomach, the "call" went through. The digestive juices have begun to flow in anticipation of eating. If you want to get over the feeling, think about something far removed from food, such as sports, the news, or your homework.

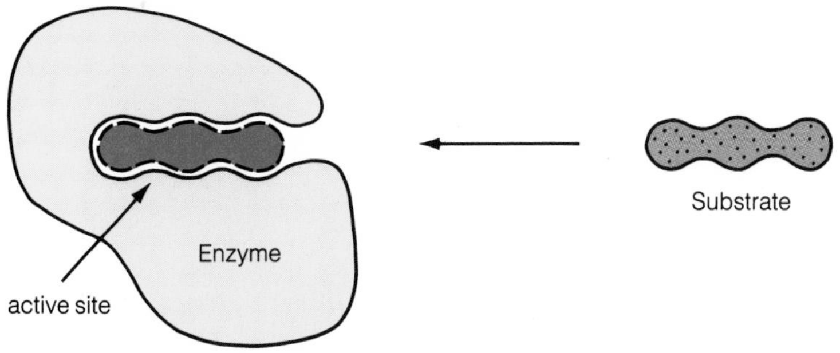

FIGURE 3-6
Simplified representation of an enzyme and its substrate. The substrate must have the proper structure to bind to and be acted on by the enzyme. Note how much larger the enzyme is than the substrate.

chemical reactions by a factor of a million or more. One enzyme that has been studied causes chemical reactions between two substances to occur up to 600,000 times per second. Without enzymes, food would be broken down so slowly that people would starve to death. Even the lack of a single enzyme can cause major digestive problems. People who do not produce lactase, the enzyme that breaks down lactose ("milk sugar") develop cramps, gas, and diarrhea when they consume lactose in milk or milk products. These problems are due to the presence of undigested lactose in the gut.

Features of enzymes:
complex protein substances
speed up chemical reactions
reusable
specific in action

A remarkable feature of enzymes is that they are not changed by the chemical reactions they effect. This makes them reusable. In spite of the fact that they operate in the midst of chemical reactions that change the structure of carbohydrates, proteins, and fats, the enzymes themselves remain intact.

Many enzymes surround food particles during digestion, but each enzyme acts only on one specific type of particle, or **substrate**. The enzyme that speeds up the chemical breakdown of sucrose (table sugar), for example, has no effect on any other substrate. Each enzyme has a uniquely shaped "active site" that enables the enzyme to "recognize" the substrate it acts upon. Only a substrate that fits perfectly into an enzyme's active site will be affected by that enzyme. The relationship between an enzyme's active site and a substrate's shape is shown in Figure 3.6. It is said that a substrate must fit an enzyme's active site like a piece in a puzzle or a key in a lock in order to work.

substrate: The substance acted upon by enzymes. Food particles are the *substrate* of digestive enzymes.

Carbohydrates, proteins, and fat each have a set of their own digestive enzymes. We will discuss the major enzymes involved in digestion of carbohydrates, proteins, and fats in the next chapters. Additional information about digestion appears in appendix C.

Digestion is completed when carbohydrates, proteins, and fats are reduced to substances that can be absorbed. Once absorbed, they become part of the body proper and can be used to produce energy.

Absorption

Absorption is the process by which the end products of digestion are taken into the **lymphatic system** (Figure 3-7) and the blood system for eventual distribution to all cells of the body. Most absorption takes place in the small intestine. It has a lining that is very well suited for maximal absorption of nutrients.

lymphatic system: A network of vessels that absorb some of the products of digestion and transport them to the heart, where they are mixed with the substances contained in blood.

The lining of the small intestine has the appearance of velvet. As Figure 3-8 shows, the surface is lined with closely packed, fingerlike projections

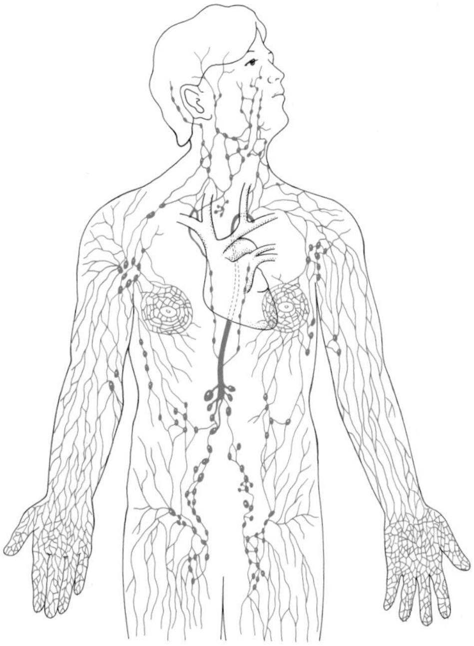

■
FIGURE 3-7
The lymphatic system.

that greatly increase the surface area available for absorption. These fingerlike projections are called *villi*, and each is infiltrated with tiny lymph and blood vessels (Figure 3-9). Absorption occurs when nutrients pass through the cells that line the villi and into the lymph and blood vessels. The break-down products of fat digestion are largely absorbed into lymph vessels, whereas carbohydrates and proteins enter the blood vessels. Particles that cannot be absorbed are not considered nutrients; a substance is a nutrient only if it can be absorbed and used by the body.

Transport of Nutrients to Cells

Cells are the body components that need the absorbed nutrients. How do they get their nutrient supply? Here is a description of the supply line.

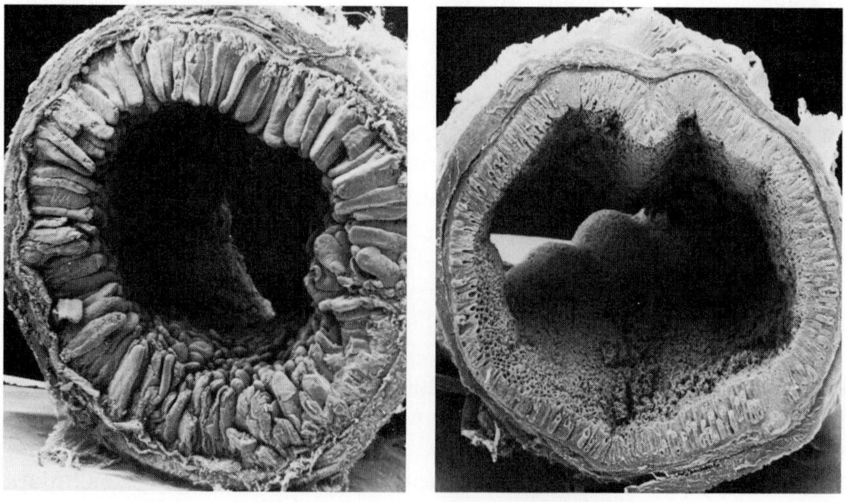

■
FIGURE 3-8
Scanning electron micrographs of cross sections of (*a*) the small intestine and (*b*) the colon (large intestine) of a rat. Note the high density of villi in (a) and the absence of villi and the relative flatness of the lining of the colon in (b).

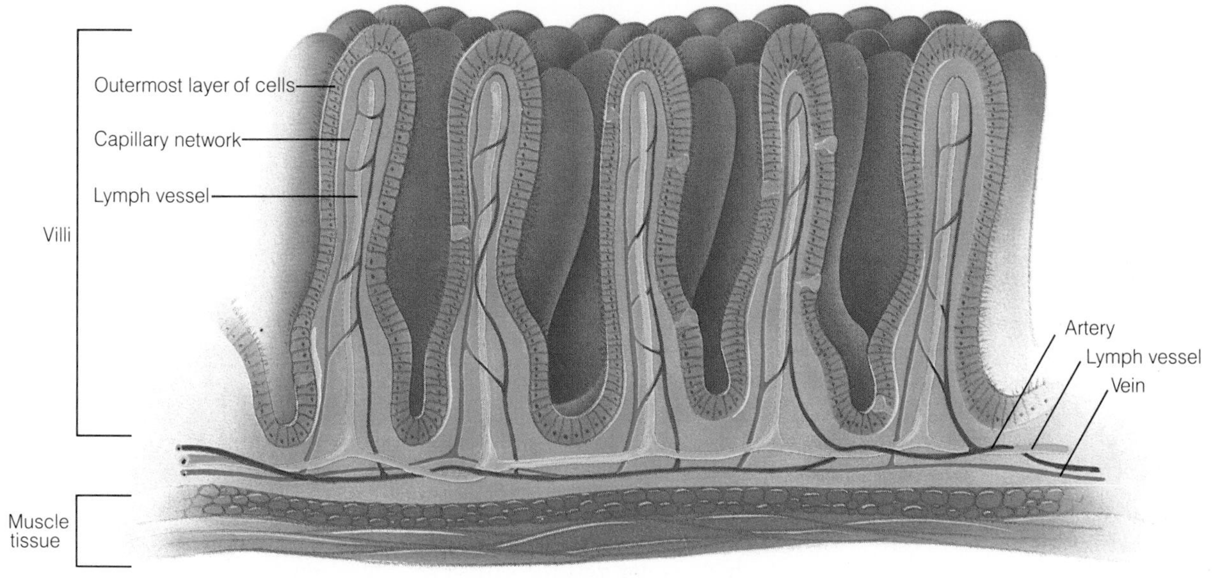

FIGURE 3-9
Structure of a villus, showing blood and lymph vessels.

Nutrients transported by the lymph vessels enter the blood stream shortly after being absorbed. The small vessels of the lymph system that transport absorbed nutrients combine into one large vessel (the thoracic duct) that empties directly into the heart. In the heart the nutrients in lymph are mixed with blood, which is then pumped into the circulatory system and on to the liver. Nutrients absorbed into blood vessels follow a different route. They are directly transported by the portal vein to the liver.

The liver is the largest organ in the body. It weighs slightly more than three pounds in adults and occupies a good deal of the space in the lower chest and stomach areas. The blood the liver receives after a meal is nutrient-dense, and it's the liver's job to process the nutrients and to bring blood nutrient levels back toward normal. If the blood glucose level is high, the liver lowers it by converting glucose to glycogen or fat. The liver can remove amino acids from blood and convert them to fat or glucose. These and many other functions of the liver make it the "central processing plant" for absorbed nutrients. (An expanded description of the processes of absorption is provided in appendix D at the back of this book.)

Blood leaving the liver distributes the energy nutrients to nerve, muscle, bone, and all other cells via the circulatory system. While in transit, the body has opportunities to adjust the level of energy nutrients in the blood by increasing or decreasing their uptake by cells. This fine tuning of blood levels of glucose, fatty acids, glycerol, and amino acids is largely controlled by hormones.

Hormones and Energy Formation

Hormones are chemical compounds that regulate all sorts of chemical processes in the body. Some hormones have profound effects on energy formation, since they help the body adjust to changes in energy needs due to

hormones: Chemical substances produced by specific glands in the body that affect the functions of particular cells.

thyroxine: A hormone secreted by the thyroid gland that increases the rate at which energy is formed in the body. Thyroxine plays a major role in stimulating energy formation during times of growth. Adults who produce too little or too much thyroxine have trouble maintaining a constant body weight because of disruptions in energy metabolism.

epinephrine: (also called *adrenalin*) A chemical messenger derived from an amino acid, it increases blood pressure, the force of the contractions of the heart, and the pulse rate. It is the "fight or flight" chemical that surges into the blood stream in times of stress.

insulin: A hormone secreted by the pancreas that acts to lower blood glucose levels. Insulin helps to transport glucose into cells and to return blood glucose levels to normal after a meal. Inadequate secretion, or a lack of cell sensitivity to the presence of insulin, results in inadequate cell supply of glucose and overutilization of fatty acids for energy. Inadequate "clearing" of blood glucose due to depressed insulin activity leads to an elevation in blood glucose level and diabetes.

glucagon: A hormone secreted by the pancreas that acts to raise blood glucose levels. Glucagon stimulates the breakdown of glycogen and the release of glucose by the liver, thereby increasing blood glucose levels. It helps to maintain normal blood glucose levels between meals and during periods of fasting.

metabolism: The chemical changes that take place within the body.

anabolism: The constructive, or build-up, phase of metabolism; also called *synthesis*. The formation of muscle tissue is an example of an anabolic process. Anabolic processes generally require energy in addition to "building" materials.

growth, pregnancy, illness, physical activity, and fasting. The extra energy needed for growth, for example, is supplied by the direct effect of **thyroxine** (an iodine-containing hormone produced by the thyroid gland) and other hormones that influence the rate at which energy is formed. **Epinephrine**, often referred to as *adrenaline*, can be released rapidly when a person is faced with a "fight or flight" situation. The surge of epinephrine released when a person is threatened allows the body to form energy quickly and increases the person's ability to respond physically to the event.

The hormone **insulin** affects energy formation by increasing the amount of glucose that enters cells. Without the action of insulin, glucose accumulates in the blood, and energy formation from glucose within cells is dramatically decreased. (The disease that develops when blood glucose levels are high is diabetes. More information about the role of insulin in regulating blood glucose levels and in the development of diabetes is given in Chapter 5.)

The hormone that acts to increase blood glucose level is **glucagon.** One of glucagon's major roles is to increase blood glucose level between meals when the body is not getting a fresh supply of glucose from food. It accomplishes this by converting glycogen stored in cells to glucose and, to a lesser extent, by stimulating the conversion of amino acids into glucose. Blood glucose levels and the body's supply of glucose for energy formation are maintained within a normal range by the balancing act performed by insulin and glucagon.

Energy Metabolism

In the end, the amount of energy a person needs from food is the amount of energy required by his or her body's cells to support **metabolism**—the chemical reactions that take place within the body. Some of the reactions serve to build up—synthesize—chemical substances, whereas others serve to break them down. The process of building up chemical substances is called **anabolism.** Reactions that lead to the formation of glycogen from glucose, tissue proteins from amino acids, and storage fat from fatty acids and glycerol are anabolic reactions. They generally require energy.

The other type of chemical reactions, those that are involved in breaking down chemical substances, are referred to as **catabolism.** Catabolic reactions include the breakdown of the energy nutrients for energy formation. All of the body's energy is formed by catabolic reactions.

Where's the Energy in the Energy Nutrients? The sources of energy in the energy nutrients are the **chemical bonds** that hold **molecules** together. Molecules of glucose, amino acids, and fatty acids are linked together by a sharing of energy between adjacent atoms. These energy links are called *chemical bonds*. Energy within chemical bonds is generated by the sharing of electrons of atoms that are next to one another in a molecule (Figure 3-10). When these bonds are broken—almost always with the help of enzymes—energy is released. Figure 3-11 shows chemical bonds of glucose that release energy when they are broken. The released energy is partly captured by adenosine diphosphate (ADP), an amazing molecule that

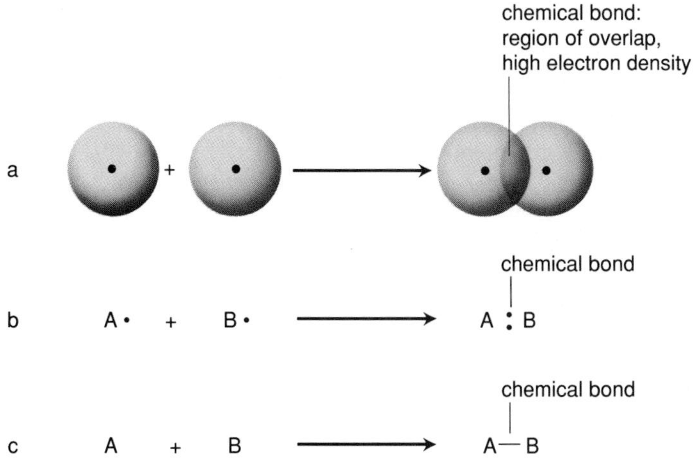

FIGURE 3-10
Schematic representations of a chemical bond. Chemical bonds formed by the sharing of electrons by adjacent atoms in a molecule can be illustrated in several ways. Option c is used most often in this book.

has the ability to capture and store large amounts of energy. The addition of energy to ADP converts it to adenosine triphosphate (ATP). When energy is needed by a cell, ATP releases its trapped energy, making it available for the cell's use. The transfer of energy changes ATP back to ADP, and it is then ready to trap energy again. Thus, ATP functions like a rechargeable battery.

ADP doesn't capture all of the energy that is released when chemical bonds are broken. Some of the energy escapes into the cell in the form of heat. This energy, too, serves a useful purpose; it helps keep the body warm.

Each energy nutrient fulfils the body's energy needs by giving up energy stored in its chemical bonds to ADP. However, the chemical reactions that convert carbohydrates, proteins, and fats into energy differ, and the extent to which each type is used to form energy varies depending on whether the body is at rest or is physically active. Moreover, we can modify the extent to which carbohydrates, proteins, and fats are used to form energy and actually improve energy production for physical activity. More information about how the body obtains energy from food and how the body's ability to produce energy can be increased are discussed in the next section.

catabolism: The break-down phase of metabolism. The release of energy from the energy nutrients is an example of a catabolic process. (Memory aid: Just as a *Cat*erpillar tractor can break down buildings, a *cata*bolic reaction breaks down molecules.

chemical bonds: Energy in the form of electrons that hold atoms within a molecule together (see Figure 3-10).

molecules: Chemical substances formed from the union of two or more atoms. For example, oxygen and hydrogen atoms bond together to form H_2O molecules (water).

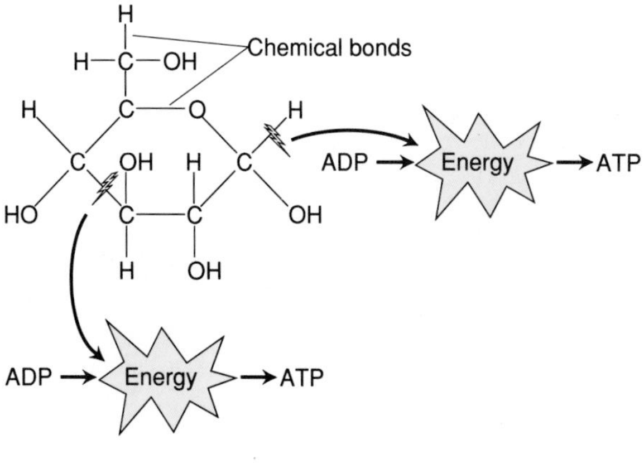

FIGURE 3-11
Structure of glucose showing chemical bonds that yield energy when broken.

FOOD, ENERGY FORMATION, AND PHYSICAL PERFORMANCE

It's the final lap of the 200-yard free-style swim. The top three contenders are neck-and-neck, and it looks as though it will be a very close finish. Each swimmer knows there are just a few seconds left in the race. They are reaching deep inside themselves to find that last burst of energy that will bring them in first.

All of a sudden, Jones in the outside lane pulls out in front. Her struggling competitors are left in her wake. It's Jones by a length!

Why did Jones win the race? Talent and the will to win no doubt were important. But an effective training program that increased her ability to sustain a strong stroke and to perform a final, vigorous "kick" in the last few seconds probably helped. Our ability to produce energy can be improved with the right training diet and conditioning program. To understand how this works, we first need to take a look at how the body forms energy during exercise.

glycolysis: The lysis (splitting) of glucose to yield energy. Glucose, which has 6 carbon atoms, is split by a series of enzymes into two smaller molecules having 3 carbons each. The process releases energy that is then trapped by ADP. Unlike energy formation from fatty acids and certain types of amino acids, glycolysis does not require oxygen; it is anaerobic.

citric acid cycle: A complex series of chemical reactions that lead to the formation of energy from fatty acids, certain amino acids, and glucose fragments. The citric acid cycle requires oxygen; it is aerobic. Also called the *Kreb's cycle* and the *tricarboxylic acid cycle*.

The Two Major Pathways of Energy Formation

Nearly all of the energy our muscles use is formed by the chemical reactions of **glycolysis** and the **citric acid cycle**. These chemical pathways—sets of chemical reactions—continually produce energy in the form of ATP. However, the extent to which each pathway is used primarily depends on the intensity of the muscular work that is being performed. When we slam on the car brakes, steal second base, spike a volleyball, or perform other energy-intense activities, the glycolysis pathway of energy formation is used. Glycolysis provides quick energy for intensive muscular work. Other times, a steady supply of energy is needed for such activities as jogging, bicycling, lawn mowing, and so on—activities that are low to moderate in intensity (Table 3-2). For these activities, we need a constant supply of energy. The citric acid cycle provides us with that kind of energy.

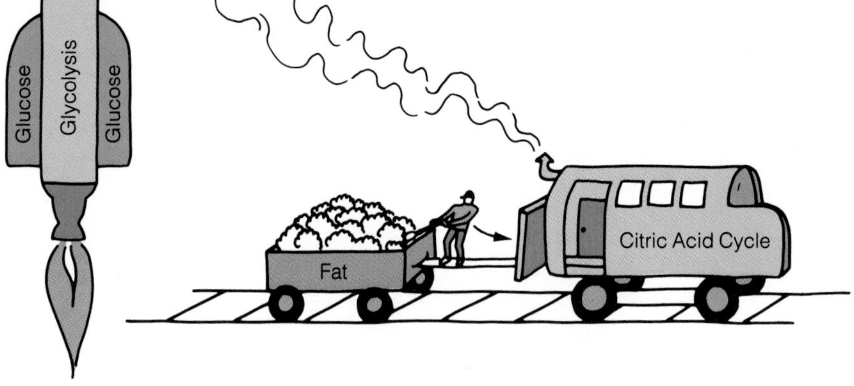

Glycolysis produces bursts of energy, whereas the citric acid cycle provides a constant supply of energy.

TABLE 3-2

Examples of activities fueled by glycolysis and the citric acid cycle

Glycolysis	Citric Acid Cycle
sprinting	long-distance running
high jump	long-distance swimming
golf swing	jogging
weight-lifting	walking
push-ups	hiking/backpacking
pull-ups	bicycling (level)
"kicks"	ice skating
"full-court press"	basketball
tennis serve	tennis volley
wrestling	reading
diving	waiting

As you can see in Figure 3-12, glucose and fatty acids are the body's primary sources of energy. The figure also points out the relative importance of each energy nutrient for different intensities of activity and their involvement in the two pathways of energy formation. We'll discuss how you can "tune up" your body to use the two pathways to their full extent after we take a closer look at glycolysis and the citric acid cycle.

Glycolysis

The vast majority of the energy formed by glycolysis comes from glucose. Glycolysis can produce energy quickly because it is **anaerobic**—it does not require oxygen. Cells, the site of energy formation, cannot be supplied with oxygen fast enough during intense exercise to support the rapid formation of energy. Glycolysis does not produce a great deal of energy—only 2 ATPs per molecule of glucose—but it can produce energy very fast when needed.

anaerobic: "Without oxygen"; the pathway of energy formation that does not require oxygen is glycolysis.

The glucose used to fuel glycolysis is derived from three sources in addition to blood glucose: glycogen (a stored form of glucose), glycerol (a small

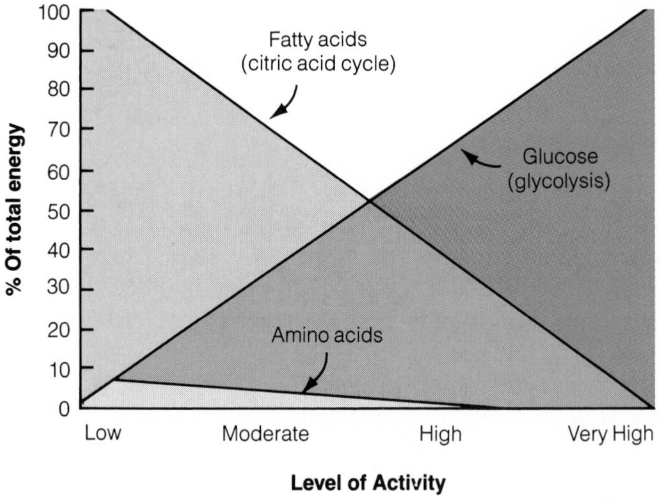

FIGURE 3-12
The sources of energy for varying levels of physical activity.

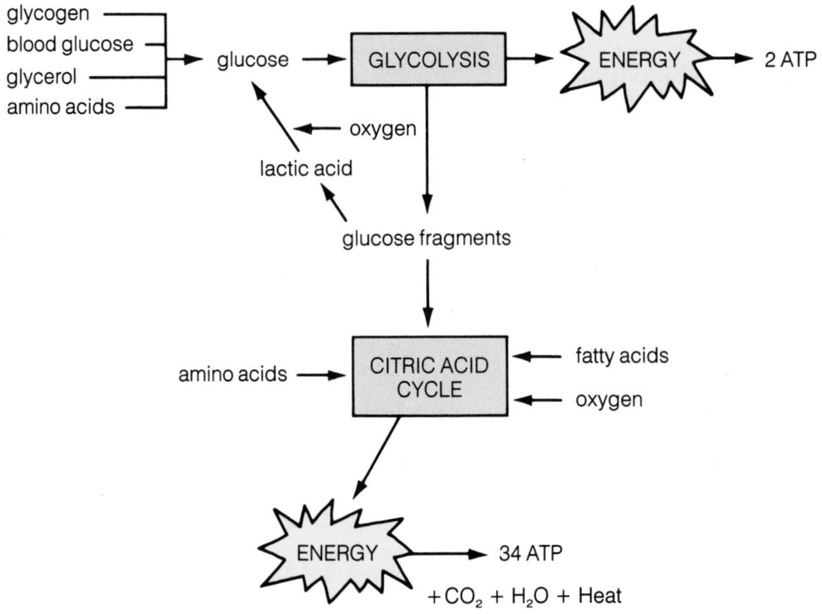

■ **FIGURE 3-13**
Energy formation by glycolysis and the citric acid cycle.

fraction of stored fat molecules), and several amino acids. Of these, glycogen is by far the most important source of glucose for glycolysis. Most adults have about a 1000-calorie store of glycogen in the muscles. (In addition, about 800 calories' worth of glycogen is stored in the liver, but liver glycogen cannot be used to supply glucose to muscles.) Physical activity that is very intense or that requires repeated bursts of energy can be sustained only as long as the body glycogen stores hold out. However, glycogen stores can be increased to above-average levels through "glycogen loading" (Box 3-2).

Glycolysis does not completely capture all of the energy that is available in the chemical bonds of glucose. At the end of glycolysis, glucose fragments remain that are generally used up completely in the citric acid cycle (Figure 3-13). We say *generally*, because sometimes they are not completely used up. Glucose fragments are formed at a higher rate than they can be used in the citric acid cycle if exercise is too strenuous. (You know you've overdone glycolysis when your body tells you about it the next day. Box 3-3 explains why you get stiff muscles from too much strenuous exercise.)

The Citric Acid Cycle

The citric acid cycle uses three types of fuel: glucose fragments produced by glycolysis, fatty acids, and certain amino acids. Fatty acids drawn from the body's stores of fat serve as the largest source of fuel. Considering that normal-weight adult bodies contain over 100,000 calories' worth of fat stores, most people are not likely to run short of fuel for the citric acid cycle as they may for glycolysis.[6]

aerobic: "With oxygen"; the pathway of energy formation that requires oxygen is the citric acid cycle.

The citric acid cycle requires oxygen; it is the **aerobic** pathway of energy formation. It is the body's high-volume energy producer, yielding 17 times more ATP per molecule of fuel than glycolysis. Nearly all of the energy we use at rest and most of the energy that supports low-to-moderate levels of

GLYCOGEN LOADING

Since glycogen is the primary source of glucose for glycolysis, and glycolysis provides the energy for strenuous activity, it has been reasoned that you could increase your endurance by increasing your stores of glycogen. That reasoning turns out to be true. You can approximately double your glycogen stores and substantially increase your endurance level for strenuous activities with a moderately high carbohydrate diet and physical training.[1,2]

During training, a diet that provides about 65% of total calories as carbohydrate leads to a much higher level of glycogen stores than does a diet that is "average" or low in carbohydrates.[3] Table 1 shows the difference diet composition makes to glycogen stores and endurance.

It should be emphasized that dietary carbohydrates increase glycogen stores above normal levels only when combined with a training program. During training, glycogen stores accumulate only in the muscles that are exercised. This fact was demonstrated quite clearly by a study in which a subject was given a high-carbohydrate diet and then exercised only one leg on a stationary bicycle. The muscles in the leg that had done the work increased glycogen stores, whereas the muscles in the other leg did not.[3] So, glycogen stores will increase on a carbohydrate-rich diet only in the muscles that are used during the training program. This is one reason coaches don't emphasize weight lifting for long-distance runners. Athletes are generally coached to exercise and develop the muscles they use most in their particular events.

It was formerly thought that the best way to increase glycogen stores was first to deplete them with exercise and a low-carbohydrate diet, and then to eat a very high carbohydrate diet for several days

continued

TABLE 1
Effect of diet on muscle glycogen stores during training

Carbohydrate Level of Diet for Previous 3 Days	Muscle Glycogen, grams per 100 grams of muscle	Time to Exhaustion
Low	0.6 g	60 minutes
Average	1.8 g	115 minutes
High (60%–70% of total calories)	3.5 g	170 minutes

New ideas in glycogen loading call for tapering off exercise and increasing carbohydrate intake during the week prior to the event. This regimen is only recommended for athletes who participate in strenuous events that last longer than 80 minutes.

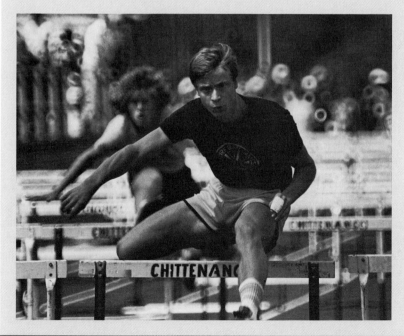

before an event. This method of glycogen loading works, but it produces many undesirable side effects. So much glycogen may be stored by this approach that muscles become stiff from the excess glycogen. People who are "superloading" with glycogen feel heavy and tired. Muscle tissues may be lost by overloading them with glycogen, and chest pains and depression may also occur.[4] For these reasons and others, this traditional approach to glycogen loading is no longer recommended. It has been replaced with a safer method that effectively increases glycogen stores and endurance. (The regimen is recommended only for athletes who participate in strenuous events that last over 80 minutes.) This method calls for tapering-off exercise and increasing carbohydrate intake during the week prior to the event. The diet should provide 60% to 70% of total calories as carbohydrates, rather than the usual level of around 50%.[4,5] The food sources of the carbohydrates should be mainly breads, pastas, rice, cereal, and starchy vegetables (such as potatoes and squash), rather than sweets or sweetened beverages. An example of a diet that provides 68% of total calories as carbohydrate is given in Table 2.

The new approach to glycogen loading can increase glycogen stores safely while allowing for the selection of a balanced variety of foods. Because diets that supply 60% to 70% of total calories as carbohydrate tend to be low in animal products (which, except for skim milk, are poor sources of carbohydrates), the diet may be low in iron, zinc, and vitamin B_{12}. These nutrients are primarily supplied by meats. The menu in Table 2, for example, is a bit low in zinc; it provides 88% of the adult male RDA. It provides adequate amounts of the other nutrients with RDAs, however. Care should be taken to eat a variety of foods while following a moderately high carbohydrate diet.

TABLE 2

A high-carbohydrate diet

Carbohydrates provide 68% of the 2,420 calories in this day's menus, protein provides 11%, and fats provide 21%. Grams of carbohydrate are shown in parentheses.

Breakfast	Dinner
orange juice, 1 c (25)	Spanish rice, 1 c (41)
oatmeal, 1 c (24)	baked potato 1 (35)
brown sugar, 1 T (13)	corn, ½ c (15)
skim milk, 1 c (12)	apple crisp, ½ c (43)
banana, 1 (25)	iced tea, 2 c (0)
Snack	**Snack**
granola, ½ c (29)	cornflakes, 1 c (20)
apple juice, 1 c (30)	canned peaches, ½ c (22)
	skim milk, 1 c (12)
Lunch	
lettuce salad, 2 c (10)	
salad dressing, 2 T (4)	
macaroni and cheese, 1 c (40)	
crackers, 4 squares (8)	
sliced tomato, ½ (3)	
skim milk, 1 c (12)	

physical activity is formed by the citric acid cycle. As you read these words, for example, the citric acid cycle is meeting your energy needs by converting fatty acids from your last meal, your hip, arm, or other fat-storage sites into energy.

The reactions of the citric acid cycle release energy stored in the fatty acids, glucose fragments, and amino acids that enter it. At the completion of one turn of the cycle, these molecules have been totally converted to the end products of ATP, carbon dioxide, water, and heat. An overview of the differ-

BOX 3-3

MUSCLE FEEDBACK

You know when you have overdone strenuous activity, because stiff muscles tell you about it the next day. Muscles become "stiff" after heavy exercise when too much of the exercise was fueled by glycolysis. When this occurs, more glucose fragments are produced than the body can convert into energy by the citric acid cycle. The body deals with excessive levels of glucose fragments by converting them to lactic acid. Lactic acid can be converted to glucose, but oxygen is required to do that. When the body is short on oxygen (as is frequently the case when you overexert yourself), not enough oxygen is available to convert lactic acid to glucose. The result is that lactic acid accumulates in the muscles and makes them feel stiff.

The lactic acid buildup eventually disappears as oxygen becomes available to convert it to glucose. The process of clearing lactic acid from muscles can take a day or two, depending on how much has accumulated. Lactic acid buildup can generally be prevented during strenuous activity by taking occasional breaks that are at least half as long as the period of intense exercise. The breaks give the muscles a chance to replenish their oxygen supply.

Some "Sunday athletes" have stiff muscles on Monday morning due to lactic acid buildup.

ences between the citric acid cycle and glycolysis is given in Table 3-3. Additional information about energy metabolism appears in appendix E, and chapters 5, 6, and 7 provide more information about the metabolism of individual energy nutrients.

Most people have sufficient fat stores to support the citric acid cycle for a long time. Nonetheless, some people's bodies convert fatty acids to energy more readily than others'. The reason has nothing to do with the availability of fat. It has to do with the amount of oxygen a person can deliver to his or

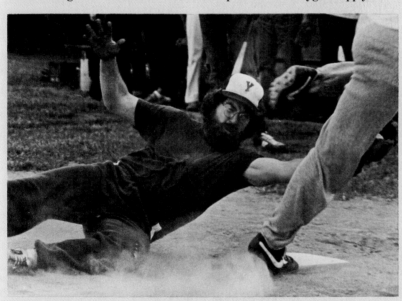

TABLE 3-3
Comparison of glycolysis and the citric acid cycle

	Glycolysis	Citric Acid Cycle
Fuel	glucose	fatty acids, glucose fragments, and amino acids
Is oxygen required?	no (anaerobic)	yes (aerobic)
Energy produced per molecule of fuel	2 ATPs	34 ATPs
Type of physical activity supported	intense, brief periods of activity ("quick" energy)	low- to moderate-intensity, extended-time activities ("ongoing" energy)
By-products of energy formation	glucose fragments	CO_2, H_2O, heat

her muscle cells. The citric acid cycle can increase energy production only to the level that it can be supplied with oxygen. When we reach the point where we are breathing in oxygen as fast as we can, we are at **maximal oxygen consumption** (VO_2 max.). That's the highest amount of oxygen we can make available to cells for the citric acid cycle.

maximal oxygen consumption: The largest potential amount of oxygen available to cells for use in the citric acid cycle of energy formation; also referred to as *VO_2 max*.

The citric acid cycle produces most of the energy for exercising muscles until a person exceeds 50% of maximal oxygen consumption. Beyond that point, most of the energy is formed by glycolysis. (Look back to Figure 3-12 for help in visualizing the shift in energy formation from the citric acid cycle to glycolysis as exercise intensity increases.) Energy formation continues to be generated primarily by glycolysis as long as oxygen consumption exceeds 50% of the maximum. When cells have used up their supply of oxygen, additional energy needs of muscles must be met by glycolysis. When we run short of oxygen for the citric acid cycle and are also low on glycogen (for glycolysis), we feel exhausted; we take a break or call it a day.

It is possible to increase the body's ability to deliver oxygen to cells and to use fatty acids as a source of energy with conditioning programs that emphasize aerobic fitness.

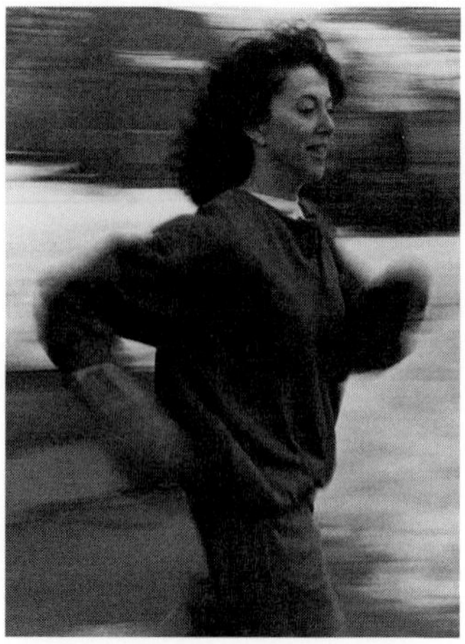

Aerobic fitness programs have been shown to strengthen the heart, lungs, and muscles.

Aerobic Fitness Programs

The goal of aerobic fitness programs is to increase the maximal oxygen consumption level. Increased maximal oxygen consumption means a person can deliver more oxygen to muscle cells and thereby increase the amount of energy produced from fatty acids by the citric acid cycle. Aerobic fitness programs increase maximal oxygen consumption by expanding the network of blood vessels that infiltrate muscle tissues. The programs also condition the heart to deliver a larger amount of blood with each beat. Consequently, more blood and more oxygen are delivered to the muscles. Aerobic fitness training is commonly recommended for athletes who undertake low- to

TABLE 3-4

Age-predicted maximum heart rate adjusted for two levels of aerobic fitness

		Level of Fitness	
Age, years	**Maximum Heart Rate**	"Beginner" (60% of maximum)	"Experienced" (80% of maximum)
15	205	123	164
18	202	121	162
20	200	120	160
22	198	119	158
24	196	118	157
30	190	114	152
40	180	108	144
50	170	102	136
60	160	96	128

moderate-intensity endurance events, as well as for dieters and people who have had heart attacks. It's wise to have a doctor's approval for participating in an aerobic program, because it may be too strenuous for some people with heart disease, kidney disease, or other health problems.

Components of an Aerobic Fitness Program Most programs for improving aerobic fitness emphasize exercises that maintain the heart rate at a particular level for 20 to 30 minutes. The desired heart rate is usually calculated as 60% of the maximum heart rate for beginners, and as 70% to 85% of the maximum for people who are physically fit. Maximum heart rate is the highest number of beats per minute that does not overly strain the heart. It is frequently estimated as 220 minus a person's age in years. Estimates of 60% and 80% of maximum heart rates for people of various ages are given in Table 3-4. People in aerobic exercise programs are advised to monitor their heart rate occasionally to see if it is close to the target rate. You can monitor your heart rate by taking your own pulse. Box 3-4 explains how to do this.

Estimate of maximum heart rate:
220 − age in years

Achieving aerobic fitness usually requires 20 to 30 minutes of moderate exercise 3 to 5 times per week.[4] As people become aerobically fit, their heart rates decrease because they become more efficient at delivering blood

BOX 3-4

HOW TO TAKE YOUR PULSE

It is possible for you to measure your pulse quite easily. Gently place a fingertip in the hollow below your jaw on one side of your neck. If you have been exercising, it is generally quite easy to feel the pulses as blood passes through a major vessel in your neck. Count the pulses for 10 seconds and multiply that number by 6. This gives you your heart rate in beats per minute.

(and therefore oxygen) to their muscles. As a matter of fact, how fast the heart beats at rest and during exercise is an indication of aerobic fitness. Many seasoned long-distance runners have resting heart rates at least 20 beats per minute slower than people who are not aerobically fit. Aerobic fitness also has a beneficial effect on blood cholesterol levels.[7]

A number of issues pertaining to nutrition, physical performance, and sports are addressed in Box 3-5.

ENERGY BALANCE

energy balance: The amount of energy consumed in foods equals the amount used by the body.

negative energy balance: Energy intake is less than energy output; results in use of the body's energy stores.

positive energy balance: Energy intake exceeds energy output; the excess energy is stored in the body as fat.

Every person needs a certain amount of energy to fuel day-to-day body functions and activities. If we consume the same amount of energy from food as we need to support metabolic reactions, we are in **energy balance**. If we consume less than that amount, we are in **negative energy balance**. In that case, the body relies on its stores of fat for energy, and as these stores are used, we lose weight. On the other hand, if we consume more energy from foods than we need, we have a surplus and are in **positive energy balance**. The excess energy is largely stored as fat, which adds to our size and weight. The level of energy "input" required to achieve energy balance can be estimated by measuring the body's energy output for three types of activities: basal metabolism, physical activity, and thermogenesis. Basal metabolism accounts for the largest amount of the energy needs of most people.

Basal Metabolism

basal metabolism: Energy used to support the body's ongoing metabolic processes while the body is in a state of complete physical, digestive, and emotional rest. Basal metabolism represents the energy the body expends to keep the heart beating, the lungs working, body temperature normal, and the energy spent in a variety of other ongoing processes.

Every second, thousands of energy-requiring reactions occur in the body that support life and health. These reactions occur automatically and require no conscious effort, and all together, they constitute our **basal metabolism**. Examples of basal metabolic processes include:

- the beating of the heart
- breathing
- maintenance of body temperature
- the repair and replacement of cells and cell components
- the delivery of nutrients to, and the removal of waste products from cells
- growth

All of the processes involved in basal metabolism act to maintain *homeostasis*, the delicate balance of fluids, nutrients, and other substances that make up the body's internal environment. Each chemical reaction that is part of basal metabolism ultimately contributes to the maintenance of this constant set of conditions under which the body functions best. The basal metabolic processes do not act independently of each other; they are carefully orchestrated so that a constant, favorable internal environment is maintained.

Variation in Basal Metabolism The amount of energy required for basal metabolic processes varies among the organs and tissues of the body and among individuals. The brain and liver, for example, make up only

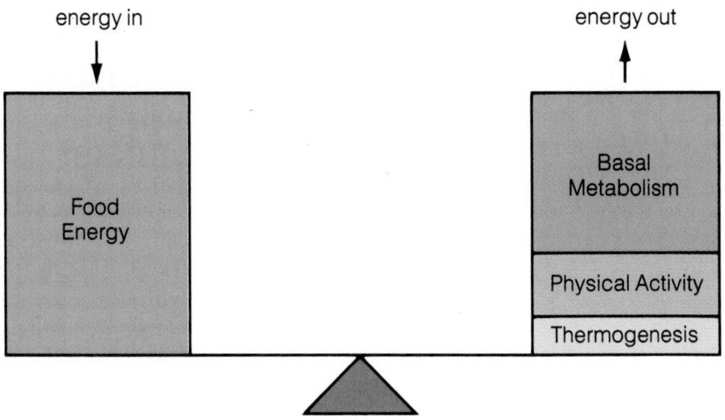

Energy balance exists when the amount of energy we derive from foods equals the amount of energy our bodies use.

about 4 percent of the weight of an adult, but together they consume over 45 percent of the energy used for basal metabolism. Metabolically, they are very active tissues. (See Table 3-5.) Because muscle tissue is metabolically more active at rest than is fat, muscles use more energy for basal metabolism than fat. Consequently, a muscular person requires more energy for basal metabolism than does a person of the same weight who has less muscle.

Growth processes consume a lot of basal metabolic energy. More energy is needed to support processes that build up tissues than is needed to maintain tissues. Young infants have especially high energy requirements for basal metabolism due to their rapid growth. Growth is not considered in calculations of adult energy needs.

The major factors affecting basal metabolic energy need are body composition and growth.

Basal Metabolic Rate A person's **basal metabolic rate** (BMR) is the amount of energy needed to support basal metabolic processes during a twenty-four-hour period. Basal metabolic rate is generally determined in a laboratory setting by carefully measuring a person's oxygen uptake while he or she is at complete physical, digestive, and emotional rest. The measurement is usually taken in the morning before a person has eaten, exercised, or become involved in daily events. The amount of oxygen a person consumes is directly proportional to the amount of energy used by his or her basal metabolic processes. (Resting metabolic rate (RMR), which is measured when a person is resting quietly at various times during the day, can

basal metabolic rate (BMR): The amount of energy used for basal metabolic processes over a 24-hour period.

TABLE 3-5
Consumption of basal metabolic energy by organs and tissues in adults

Organ/Tissue	Basal Metabolic Energy Used, % of total
Liver	27%
Brain	19%
Skeletal muscles	18%
Kidneys	10%
Heart	7%
All others	19%

HOT TOPICS IN SPORTS NUTRITION

PREGAME MEALS

Since the days of ancient Rome, it has been thought that eating meat before a strenuous physical contest confers stamina and strength. A recent study found that more than a third of health and physical education teachers believe that protein is the primary source of energy for muscles.[8] The image of meat as a muscle-building and strengthening food extends across amateur and professional sport teams. You can get an idea of the emphasis placed on meat by glancing at the grocery list for the training camp of a professional team; see Table 1.

From the standpoint of health and performance, however, the only advantage of eating steak before a game is the ceremonial or psychological meaning attached to it. Although a steak meal may give an athlete an emotional boost before an event, what the body needs are foods that are low in fat and high in carbohydrates. Carbohydrates are the most readily digested of the energy nutrients and they spend the least amount of time in the stomach. Steak and other high-fat foods take longer to digest and may still be in the stomach at game time.

Pregame meals should be eaten three to four hours before an event and should include such foods as cereal, breads, potatoes, fruit, and juices. These "light" foods are much less likely to cause stomach upsets and cramping during and after an athletic contest than a steak-type meal. Athletes feel and perform better on high-carbohydrate pregame meals.[4]

TABLE 1

A sampling of the New England Patriots' training camp grocery list*

Food	Amount
Fresh fruits	6,000 lb
Eggs	6,000 lb
Sirloin steak	1,200 lb
Prime rib	950 lb
Sausage	700 lb
Round steak	625 lb
Bacon	600 lb
Fish	400 lb
Milk	2,700 gal
Fruit juices	1,240 gal

*The training camp is about two-weeks long and involves approximately 100 athletes and coaches.

EATING BETWEEN EVENTS

For events such as swim meets, play offs, and track and field meets, athletes have to participate in several competitions in a day. To keep going, they need to eat between events. Carbohydrates are once again the food of choice. Crackers, fruit, cereals, breads, and juices are examples of food that "go down easily" and help keep the energy level up between events. Candy, soft drinks, and other concentrated sources of sugar may actually interfere with performance.

WHAT ABOUT SPORT DRINKS?

The best sport drink yet discovered is water. For most athletic events, it is all that is needed. Physical performance is improved if athletes remain hydrated—maintain normal levels of body water—during exercise. Once the body starts to run low on water, fatigue and weakness set in and performance suffers. Water should be consumed before, during, and after exercise. Particular care should be taken to drink enough water when exercise is performed in warm weather.

Do commercial sport drinks offer any advantage over water? For most events, no, because the body generally has no need for the nutrients provided by the sport drinks. Athletes usually begin events with enough sodium, potassium, and other **electrolytes** to see them through to the end of the event. The nutrient that most likely needs replacing is water and not electrolytes.[9]

Some sport drinks contain excessively high levels of electrolytes that may interfere with performance. When high levels of electrolytes enter the stomach and intestines, they draw water away from the blood and into the digestive tract. Thus, drinks that claim to replace electrolytes lost during exercise may be ineffective in replacing them and may cause a loss of body water. Sport drinks that

electrolytes: Chemical substances that form charged particles and conduct an electrical current when in solution. The chief electrolytes in body fluids are sodium, potassium, and chloride.

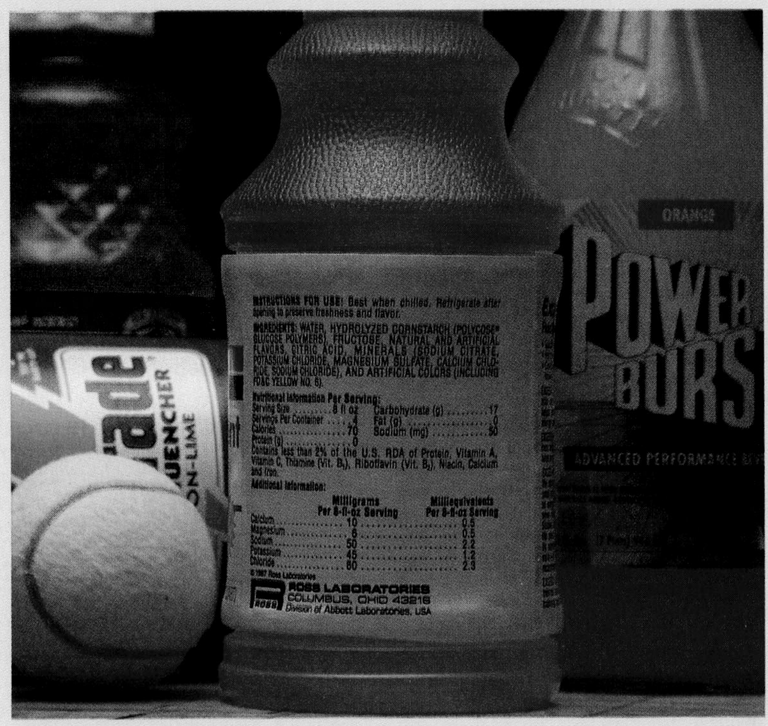

Sport drinks containing no more than 0.2% sodium and potassium by volume may benefit athletes who perform strenuous exercises in very warm environments or over a period of several hours.

contain weak concentrations of sodium, potassium, and certain other electrolytes are more effective than highly concentrated ones in replacing electrolytes lost in sweat during exercise. Sport drinks that contain no more than 0.2% sodium and potassium by volume may benefit athletes who perform strenuous exercise in hot weather and those who are physically active for several hours or more, such as marathon runners.[10]

Soft drinks and sport drinks that are high in sugars such as glucose and sucrose appear to be particularly ineffective in improving energy levels during exercise. These high-sugar beverages stay in the stomach longer than low-sugar beverages do, and the sugar tends to cause a surge in insulin release upon absorption. (The hormone insulin lowers glucose levels.) The insulin surge can lead to a drop in blood glucose levels and to decreased energy production from glycolysis.[4,5] In addition, most soft drinks don't even "quench" thirst, because they contain too much sugar for their water content. Rather than providing the body with water and energy, they may increase the need for water and lead to early fatigue.[4] The bottom line is that heavily sweetened sport drinks should be avoided during an event.

PROTEIN AND PERFORMANCE: IS THERE A MATCH?

Since muscles contain a lot of protein, if you eat a high-protein diet, you'll build muscle, right? Wrong. Here's why.

The body needs a certain amount of protein when muscle cells are forming and when the cells are increasing in size. How much protein is eaten in excess of the required levels in no way affects the number of muscle cells or the size of the muscle cells. The protein content of the typical U.S. diet far exceeds the level required to form and develop muscle cells.[11] The only way to increase muscle size (short of the very dangerous use of steroid hormones) is to exercise them on a regular basis. Exercise programs that emphasize muscle development increase the size and strength of muscle cells, but not their number. Body-building exercises work because they make muscle cells larger, and therefore muscles become stronger.

continued

High-protein diets and protein supplements may have a negative effect on performance. Many high-protein foods such as meat and dairy products tend to be high in fat and low in glycogen-forming carbohydrates. Eating a high-protein meal before an event increases the body's requirement for water, which increases the risk of dehydration during the event.[4] It is very clear that high-protein diets and supplements should not be given a second thought by athletes. An adequate diet that provides ample amounts of carbohydrates for glycogen stores and a weight-training program provide the biggest pay-off for muscle strengthening.

CAFFEINE AND PERFORMANCE

Caffeine affects the body in many ways, one of which is increasing the level of fatty acids in the blood. When blood levels of fatty acids go up, more fatty acids are available for use by muscles for energy formation. Caffeine has been found to increase the amount of fatty acids used by muscles during exercise when provided at levels of about 350 milligrams (the amount in two or three cups of coffee). Endurance appears to be somewhat improved by the action of caffeine.[13,14]

However, there's a down side to caffeine intake that has led to its not being recommended for use by athletes. Caffeine increases both heart rate and water loss. Additionally, it makes some people feel

TABLE 2

Dietary practices of Olympic athletes

Ellington Darden, a professor of nutrition, asked former Olympic athletes if they ate any special foods or took vitamin pills or other supplements as part of their training programs. The athletes' responses illustrate the wide spectrum of nutrition beliefs of accomplished athletes. (These statements are not meant to be taken as advice.)

Kathy Hammond (400-meter run):	"I take no vitamin or mineral pills other than iron. However, I avoid greasy foods in the meal preceding the race."
Leonard Hilton (3-mile run):	"I'm a strong believer in additional vitamin C, E, and B-complex tablets each day."
Jim Ryan (1500-meter and 1-mile run):	"I eat no special foods and take no supplements."
Frank Shorter (marathon):	"Three days prior to a marathon, I try to load up on carbohydrates. I gain several pounds, which I consider to be an advantage as I have more energy."
George Frenn (hammer throw):	"I used to take vitamins by injection and eat many health foods, but not anymore. I think they are all a bunch of hooey."
Ray Seales (boxing):	"I don't eat any bread or starch. It makes me soft inside. I eat a lot of meat and green vegetables, and I also take a vitamin–mineral supplement."

edgy and anxious. The use of high levels of caffeine by athletes has been banned by the International Olympics Committee.[15]

PERFORMANCE AIDS

Do any of these help athletes improve their performance?

wheat germ oil	royal jelly
bee pollen	B-complex vitamins
enzyme supplements	vitamin C
honey	carnitine
vitamin E	

The promoters of these and similar types of products would like athletes to think so, and many athletes believe in them. Table 2 presents the thoughts of some Olympic athletes on the subject. The less frequently heard voice of the experts would say these "performance aids" are a waste of time and money. None of these products has been shown to improve physical performance. If they offer anything, it's a psychological boost. An athlete's belief that a particular supplement or dietary aids will improve his or her performance may, in fact, improve it. (It's the placebo effect.)

"MAKING" WEIGHT

Wrestlers tend to take their weight very seriously. They often want to stay in the lowest possible weight class. Some wrestlers go to great lengths to remain in a particular weight class, even though they have outgrown it. They may fast, "sweat off" weight, make themselves vomit after eating, and suffer through other types of temporary torture to lose weight before a weigh-in. Are these heroic efforts worth it? Hardly.

Wrestlers, like other athletes involved in intense exercise, perform better if they have a good supply of glycogen and a normal amount of body water. Fasting before a weigh-in dramatically reduces glycogen stores, and withholding fluids puts the wrestler at risk of becoming dehydrated. Trying to stay within a particular weight class too long may also stunt or delay a young wrestler's growth.

A current trend in wrestling coaching is a positive one: a movement away from the goal of "making" a weight class to the goal of "growing into" one. Eliminating some of the lowest weight classes for young wrestlers and adding higher weight classes is contributing to meeting this goal.

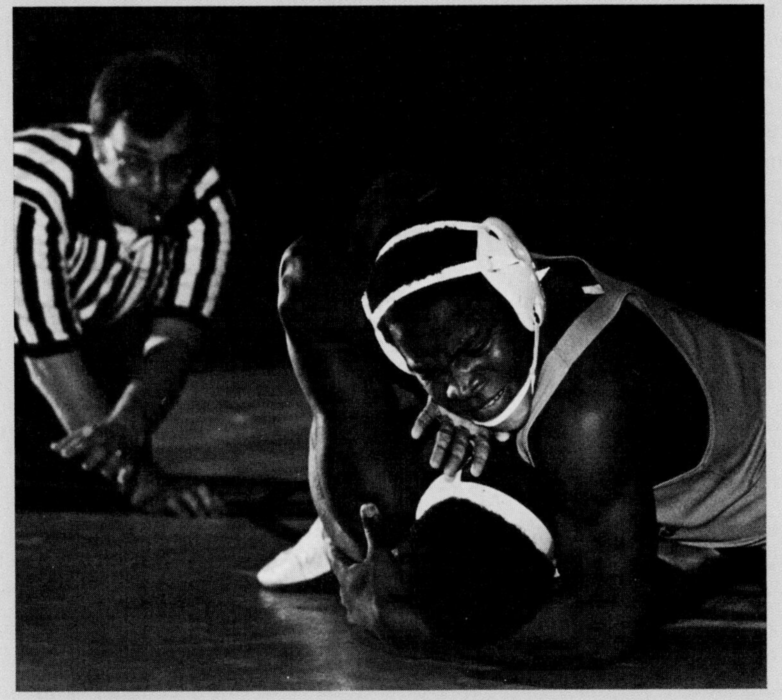

Wrestlers, like other athletes involved in intense exercise, perform better if they have a good supply of glycogen and a normal amount of body water.

also be used to determine the energy costs of basal metabolic processes. It is not significantly different from BMR if measured three to four hours after a meal.)

The laboratory tests required to determine BMR are expensive to conduct and thus not widely used. In practical settings, it is common to use a formula or a rule of thumb to estimate basal metabolic rate. A method for estimating the number of calories you use for BMR, physical activity, and thermogenesis is explained later in the chapter.

Physical Activity

Physical movement is a remarkable process controlled by messages sent from the central nervous system to the muscles. The messages signal the muscles to perform the chemical reactions required to stimulate muscle cells to contract and relax in a coordinated fashion. Energy is required for physical movement for the same reason it is required for basal metabolism: to fuel energy-requiring chemical reactions. Our energy requirement for physical movement is perhaps easier to understand than our energy needs for basal metabolism. We generally move by choice and sometimes we are powerfully aware of how much energy it takes to perform a particular physical activity. On the other hand, we don't get such powerful signals about basal metabolism. Yet, most of us spend more energy on basal metabolism than on physical activity. For example, the energy cost of supporting a physically "inactive" lifestyle is about 30% of the number of calories needed for basal metabolism. An "average" level of activity requires roughly 50%, and an exceptionally high level of physical activity requires about 75% of the number of calories needed for basal metabolism.

Factors that Influence the Caloric Cost of Exercise

Not everyone of the same weight requires the same number of calories to perform a particular exercise. Caloric requirements are affected by a person's physical fitness level. People who are physically fit use calories for muscular work more efficiently than those who are not. Interestingly enough, space flight also affects the caloric cost of exercise, since it's harder to work without the help of gravity (see Box 3-6).

It used to be thought that age and gender affect the caloric cost of exercise, but these factors are no longer considered important. More important than age or gender is a person's body composition and level of fitness.[16]

Estimating the Caloric Cost of Physical Activity

The caloric cost of physical activity can be measured quite accurately by laboratory methods (Box 3-7), or it can be estimated. Noting a person's usual activity level and keeping track of the type and duration of physical activities the person undertakes in a day or week and assigning caloric costs to each can give a reasonably good estimate. This approach is explained in "Putting Nutrition Knowledge to Work" at the end of the chapter. You will use this method to estimate the number of calories you expend in physical activity.

BOX 3-6

PEOPLE USE MORE CALORIES IN SPACE

Gravity, and the lack of it, make important differences in energy output. Astronauts consume an average of 3,000 calories per day from a nutritious assortment of foods on long-term space flights (over 2 weeks in duration), but yet they lose muscle, bone mass, and weight during the flights. The nine *Skylab* astronauts lost an average of six pounds.[17] It appears that body movement requires more energy in near-zero gravity than it does under the influence of the earth's gravity—there's no downward-pulling force out there. Both Soviet and U.S. space travelers are being provided with high-calorie, nutrient-dense rations in an attempt to help prevent the muscle, bone, and weight loss that occurs during space flight.

The efforts to increase the astronauts' calorie intake include making freeze-dried, low-moisture, and irradiated foods more palatable. Astronauts tend not to want to eat all of the food rationed for them. (One even took along a ham and cheese sandwich from home.) During the *Salyut-6* missions, the Soviets customized the astronauts' menus on a personal basis and delivered fresh fruits, vegetables, and condiments by an unmanned resupply spacecraft. These astronauts were able to "pack in" an average of 3,150 calories per day. It is anticipated that future spaceflights will have an automated collection system for data on food intake; a "nutritionist-in-a-computer" will be on board.[17]

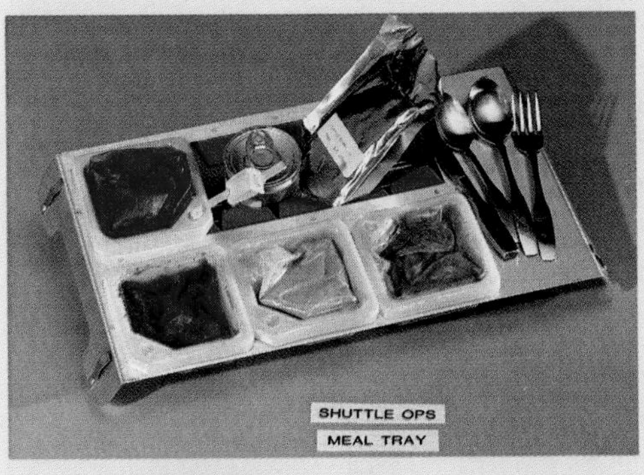

A typical meal prepared by NASA for use aboard the space shuttle. This meal consists of cream of mushroom soup, mixed vegetables, smoked turkey, and strawberries.

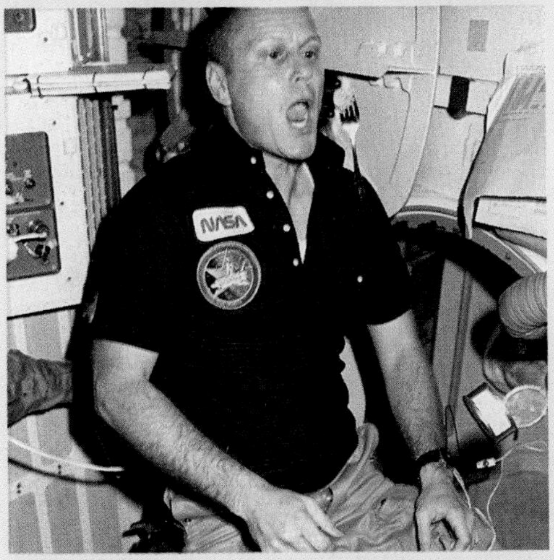

Mealtime in near-zero gravity.

BOX 3-7

LABORATORY ASSESSMENT OF ENERGY OUTPUT DURING EXERCISE

The man shown in the photograph is running on a treadmill. His nose is plugged, and all of his breathing is done through the tube held in his mouth. For at least 12 hours before the test, he has neither eaten nor performed heavy physical exercise. The number of calories the man is expending by jogging is being determined by measuring the amount of oxygen he consumes.

Oxygen consumption during exercise is calculated by subtracting the total amount of oxygen exhaled from the amount inhaled through the tube. About 20 calories are used for every gallon of oxygen consumed. If this man was running at a pace that would take him a mile in 6 minutes, he would use about 5 gallons of oxygen for energy formation, or a total of 100 calories.

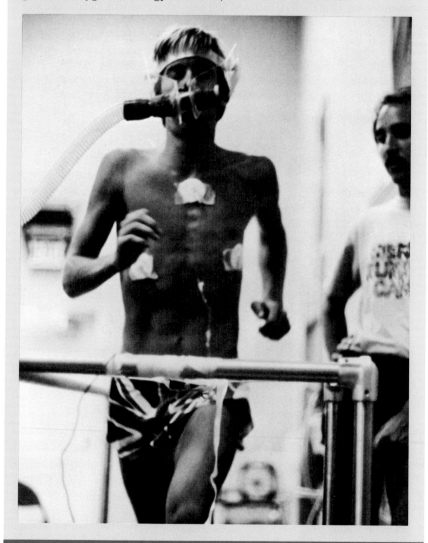

TABLE 3-6

Peanuts per physical activity (PPA) scores for four physical events at two body weights

	120-Pound Person			160-Pound Person		
		PPA Score*			PPA Score*	
Physical Event	Calories Expended	Number	Cups	Calories Expended	Number	Cups
Boston Marathon (26-mile run)	2,500	454	3 c + 1 T	3,400	620	4⅓
U.S. Open (3 hours of tennis)	1,500	282	1¾	2,060	375	2½
10K run	575	105	¾	770	140	1
Aerobic dancing (½ hour, vigorous)	260	47	⅓	340	62	⅖

*These calculations are for shelled peanuts. Thirty peanuts weigh about an ounce and provide 165 calories. There are about 150 peanuts in a cup.

To illustrate the relationship between energy input from food and energy output for physical activity, Table 3-6 tells the number of peanuts it would take to provide energy to fuel four physical events. That is, the table gives "peanuts per physical activity scores." Figures are given for two levels of body weight.

Thermogenesis

The third use of energy is **thermogenesis**—the energy expended by the body in digesting food and absorbing and processing nutrients. People actually heat up a bit after they eat. The heat is a by-product of the intense level of metabolic activity that accompanies digestion and absorption. Although it used to be thought that the amount of energy used for thermogenesis was too small to make a real difference in a person's total caloric need, it now appears that that thinking is wrong.[18] It is suspected that individual differences in thermogenesis may help explain the development and maintenance of underweight and obesity.[18,19]

A number of studies have found that some underweight people burn more calories than would be expected after a meal. The level of heat produced is high enough to make some individuals feel warm an hour or so after eating a large meal. Some obese people, on the other hand, have been found to burn fewer calories for thermogenesis than expected and may have lower calorie requirements as a result.

The rule of thumb used for calculating calorie output for thermogenesis is based on the *average* calorie cost of digesting food and absorbing and processing the energy nutrients; individual differences in diet composition and response to food are not considered. Because of this, we must not put too much stock in it. The rule of thumb is that the calories needed for thermogenesis can be estimated as 10% of the caloric requirement for basal metabolism and physical activity.

One of the exercises in "Putting Nutrition Knowledge to Work" will help you estimate your total calorie need.

thermogenesis: (*thermo* = "heat," *genesis* = "production") The rise in metabolic rate that occurs as a result of eating. It represents the energy the body expends in digesting foods and absorbing and processing nutrients. The elevation in metabolism due to thermogenesis is greatest two hours after a meal and lasts for 3 to 4 hours. Also referred to as *dietary thermogenesis* and *specific dynamic action.*

COMING UP IN CHAPTER 4

The topics of food, energy, and energy balance encompass many issues of concern to human nutrition. The subjects are central components of knowledge about the science and lead logically to the important topics of the regulation of food intake, obesity, underweight and starvation, and eating disorders. These topics are discussed in chapter 4.

REVIEW QUESTIONS

1. How many calories are there in a slice of cheese pizza that contains 18 grams of carbohydrate, 8 grams of protein, and 5.5 grams of fat?
2. Explain how a bomb calorimeter is used to determine the caloric content of food.
3. Which energy nutrients can be used to form body fat?
4. What is a villus? What are its major roles in absorption?
5. Cite three characteristics of enzymes.
6. Which is usually larger, an enzyme or its substrate?
7. Cite three differences between glycolysis and the citric acid cycle.
8. What is the estimated maximum heart rate of a 20-year old?
9. What are the four sources of glucose for glycolysis?
10. What is the main fuel used by the citric acid cycle?
11. What are the major health benefits of aerobic fitness?
12. Define metabolism. State the difference between anabolism and catabolism.
13. Name three hormones and tell how each affects energy metabolism.
14. What does the word *thermogenesis* mean to you?

Answers

1. 153.5 calories.
2. See Figure 3-1 and the text discussion of the bomb calorimeter.
3. They all can.
4. A villus and its roles are discussed in the section on absorption of nutrients.
5. See the subsection on digestive enzymes.
6. Enzymes are usually bigger than their substrates.
7. See Table 3-3.
8. Maximum heart rate = 220 − age in years.
9. Refer to Figure 3-13.
10. Hint: fatty acids.
11. See the discussion of aerobic fitness programs.
12. The answers lie in margin definitions.

13. The information is in the section on hormones and energy formation.
14. Does it agree with the definition given in the chapter?

PUTTING NUTRITION KNOWLEDGE TO WORK

1. Calculate your own total calorie need by following these steps.

Step 1. Determine your BMR calories by the rule-of-thumb method. If you are a male, multiply your body weight in pounds by 11. If you are a female, multiply your body weight in pounds by 10. This is roughly the number of calories you need for basal metabolism each day.

Step 2. Estimate the energy requirements for your usual physical activity.

a. Select the category that best describes your level of physical activity in Table 3-7. Multiply your BMR calories calculated in Step 1 by the % of BMR calories for your activity level.

> *Example:* Assume a person's BMR is 1,500 calories per day and that the person is physically inactive. The BMR of 1,500 calories would be multiplied by 0.30 (for 30%) to estimate calories used to support physical activity: 1,500 calories × 0.30 = 450 calories.

This figure is the estimate of your total caloric expenditure for physical activity unless you also exercise. If you exercise, go to b (below). If not, proceed to c.

b. If you exercise regularly or participate in an athletic program, you need to include those activities in calculating your energy expenditure for physical activity. To do this, write down each activity you perform and the amount of time you spend doing it. Include only the amount of time you spend moving or straining and not the time you are relaxing or taking a break. Then, look up the caloric cost of each activity in Table 3-8. Calculate the energy cost of each activity by multiplying the time you spend on it and the caloric cost of the activity per pound by your weight in pounds. Add the exercise calories to the calories for your activity level to estimate your total activity calories.

TABLE 3-7
Energy expenditure for usual level of activity

Activity Level	% Of BMR Calories
Inactive: Sitting most of the day; less than two hours of moving about slowly or standing.	30
Average activity: Sitting most of the day; walking or standing two to four hours, but no strenuous activity.	50
Active: Physically active four or more hours each day; little sitting or standing; some physically strenuous activities.	75

Example: Assume a person weighs 150 pounds and plays tennis at moderate intensity a half-hour every day.

3.4 calories/pound/hour	×	0.5 hours	=	1.7 calories/pound
1.7 calories/pound	×	150 pounds	=	255 calories

Thus, 450 for activity level + 255 for exercise/sports = 705 total usual activity calories.

Step 3. Estimate the caloric cost of thermogenesis. The caloric cost of thermogenesis is calculated as 10% of the BMR calories plus the physical activity calories.

a. Add your BMR calories to your total activity calories.

b. Multiply that number by 0.10 (or 10%) to get the calories needed for thermogenesis.

c. Add the numbers you got in a and b. The sum is the number of calories you need each day for energy balance and weight maintenance.

Example: (a) 1,500 BMR calories
+ 705 total usual activity calories
2,205
(b) 2,205 calories for BMR + usual activity
× 0.10
221 calories for thermogenesis
(c) 2,205
+ 221
2,426 total calorie need

2. These exercises utilize the "Total Calorie Need" software program.
   a. Calculate your total calorie need using the instructions provided in the software program. The program uses a more complex but more accurate system for determining total calorie need than the method just given in number 1. Compare the results of your computer run with the total calorie need level you calculated. (You will be asked to recall the results of this computer run. Record your total calorie need from the run.)

   b. Assume you are in good physical condition and made it on the sculling (or rowing) team. Training sessions run from 7:00 to 9:00 AM Monday through Friday. You actually row for 60 minutes each session. Use the TCN program to determine how this additional activity would increase your total calorie need.

   c. Joyce needs to lose 20 pounds and has decided to do it by increasing her activity level. She is 20 years old, 5′5″ tall, and weighs 145 pounds. She is usually not physically active. The most exercise she gets is walking to class at about 4 mph for 20 minutes 5 days a week. She has decided to swim at a moderate pace (20 yards/minute) for 30 minutes 5 days a week. Use the TCN program to answer these questions:
      1) What is Joyce's daily caloric need before she starts the swimming program?

TABLE 3-8

Average energy output per pound of body weight for selected types of exercise*

Exercise	Intensity	Calories/lb/hr
Walking	3 mph (20 min/mi)	1.6
	3½ mph (17 min/mi)	1.8
	4 mph (15 min/mi)	2.7
	4½ mph (13 min/mi)	2.9
Jogging	5 mph (12 min/mi)	4.1
	5½ mph (11 min/mi)	4.5
	6 mph (10 min/mi)	4.9
	6½ mph (9 min/mi)	5.2
	7 mph (8½ min/mi)	5.6
	7½ mph (8 min/mi)	6.0
Running	8 mph (7½ min/mi)	6.3
	8½ mph (7 min/mi)	6.7
	9 mph (6⅔ min/mi)	7.1
	9½ mph (6⅓ min/mi)	7.4
	10 mph (6 min/mi)	7.8
	11 mph (5½ min/mi)	8.5
	12 mph (5 min/mi)	9.5
Rebound trampoline	50–60 steps/min	4.1
Cycling (stationary)	mild effort	2.9
	moderate effort	3.4
	vigorous effort	4.3
Cycling (level)	6 mph (10 min/mi)	1.5
	8 mph (7½ min/mi)	1.8
	10 mph (6 min/mi)	2.0
	12 mph (5 min/mi)	2.8
	15 mph (4 min/mi)	3.9
	20 mph (3 min/mi)	5.7
Skating		2.9
Calisthenics	moderate	2.4
	vigorous	2.9
Rope skipping	moderate	4.8
Bench stepping	12″ high, 24 steps/min	3.2

Exercise	Intensity	Calories/lb/hr
Weight lifting		2.9
Wrestling		6.2
Handball	moderate	4.8
	vigorous	6.2
Swimming	resting strokes	1.4
	20 yd/min (mod.)	2.9
	40 yd/min (vig.)	4.8
Rowing	(sculling or machine)	4.8
Down-hill skiing		3.8
Cross-country skiing (level)	4 mph (15 min/mi)	4.3
	6 mph (10 min/mi)	5.7
	8 mph (7½ min/mi)	6.7
	10 mph (6 min/mi)	7.6
Aerobic dancing	moderate	3.4
	vigorous	4.3
Raquetball/squash	moderate	4.3
	vigorous	4.8
Tennis	moderate	3.4
	vigorous	4.3
Volleyball	moderate	3.4
	vigorous	3.8
Basketball	moderate	3.8
	vigorous	4.8
Football	moderate	3.8
	vigorous	4.3
Baseball/golf/woodcutting/horseback riding/badminton/canoeing		2.4
Soccer/hill climbing/fencing/judo/snow shoeing		5.3
Bowling/archery/pool		1.2

*Values calculated from *Guidelines for Graded Exercise Testing and Exercise Prescription*, 2nd ed. American College of Sports Medicine, Lea & Febiger, 1984.

2) What will it be after she starts the swimming program?
3) Approximately how many weeks will it take Joyce to lose 20 pounds if she swims according to her schedule?

4) What if Joyce keeps on swimming and also decreases her daily caloric intake by 200 calories per day. About how many weeks would it then take her to lose 20 pounds?
5) One year later, Joyce weighs 125 pounds and is on the swim team. She swims vigorously (40 yards/minute) for 60 minutes 5 times a week. How many calories does she need each day to maintain her weight?

NOTES

1. J. Bergstrom and L. Hermanson, et al., Diet—muscle glycogen and physical performance, *Acta Physiologica Scandinavica* 71 (1967):140–150.
2. E. H. Christensen and O. I. Hansen, Arbeitsfahigkiet und ernahrung, *Skandinavisches Archiv for Physiologie* 81 (1939):1–12.
3. E. Hultman, J. Bergstrom, and A. E. Roch-Norlund, Glycogen storage in human skeletal muscle, *Acta Medica Scandinavica* 182 (1967):109.
4. D. Elliot and L. Goldberg, Nutrition and exercise, *Medical Clinics of North America* 69 (1985):71–81.
5. W. J. Evans and U. A. Hupnes, Dietary carbohydrates and endurance exercise, *American Journal of Clinical Nutrition* 41 (1985):1146–1154.
6. G. A. Bray, Autonomic and endocrine factors in the regulation of energy balance, *Federation Proceedings* 45 (1986):1404–1410.
7. P. Hespel, Changes in plasma lipids and apoproteins associated with physical training in middle-aged sedentary men, *American Heart Journal* 115 (1988): 786–792.
8. C. A. Pratt and J. L. Walberg, Nutrition knowledge and concerns of health and physical education teachers, *Journal of the American Dietetic Association* 88 (1988):840–841.
9. D. Henderson, Nutrition and the athlete, *FDA Consumer*, May 1987:1 18–21.
10. K. M. Wiche, Quenching the athlete's thirst, *Physician Sports Medicine* 14 (1986):228.
11. B. Torun, N. S. Scrimshaw, and J. R. Young, Effect of isometric exercises on body potassium and dietary protein requirements of young men, *American Journal of Clinical Nutrition* 30 (1977):1983–1993.
12. E. Darden, Olympic athletes view vitamins and victories, *Journal of Home Economics* 65 (1973):8–11.
13. H. Sasaki, Effect of sucrose and caffeine ingestion on performances of prolonged strenuous running, *International Journal of Sports Medicine* 8 (1987) :261–265.
14. J. L. Ivy, D. L. Costill, and W. J. Fink, et al., Influence of caffeine and carbohydrate feedings on endurance performance, *Medical Science Sports* 11 (1979):6–11.
15. J. L. Slavin, Caffeine and sports performance, *Physician and Sports Medicine* 13 (1985):191–193.
16. J. J. Cunningham, A reanalysis of the factors influencing basal metabolic rate in normal adults, *American Journal of Clinical Nutrition* 33 (1980):2372–2374.
17. P. L. Altman and J. M. Talbot, Nutrition and metabolism during space flight, *Journal of Nutrition* 117 (1987):421–427.
18. J. Himns-Hagen, Thermogenesis in brown adipose tissue as an energy buffer, *New England Journal of Medicine* 311 (1984):1549–1555.
19. K. R. Segal, and B. Guten, et al., Thermic effect of food at rest, during exercise, and after exercise, *Journal of Clinical Investigation* 76 (1985):1107–1112.

CHAPTER 4

FOOD INTAKE, BODY WEIGHT, AND HEALTH

One of the very nicest things about life is the way we must regularly stop whatever we are doing and devote our attention to eating.
—Luciano Pavarotti in *Pavarotti: My Own Story*

Food is a source of pleasure as well as a necessity of life; it provides feelings of comfort and security and sensual pleasure as well as relief from hunger. The pleasure and relief provided by food are strong incentives for eating. This "eating reward system" serves to ensure that the body has a chance to get the energy and nutrients it needs to stay alive and well.

The foremost need of the body is energy, the calories supplied by food. But how does the body attempt to match energy intake with its need for energy? How do people know when and how much to eat? As you will read in this chapter, humans experience much stronger signals to eat than not to eat. There are no innate human systems that keep us from eating too much and guide us to select the foods we need. Nonetheless, humans are born with several traits that foster energy balance. We will examine these normal traits and discuss how they can be overridden.

NORMAL EATING SIGNALS

Healthy humans are born with two primary mechanisms that influence when and how much is eaten. The "when" to eat is signaled by the physical sensations of **hunger**, and the "how much" by **satiety**. Hunger and satiety act to roughly balance energy intake with need. About every four hours during the day, the body gives signals that it's time to eat by creating hunger pangs and symptoms such as weakness and loss of attention span that are relieved by eating. We know we have had enough to eat when we feel full and have lost interest in eating more. (If we continue to eat beyond this point, we get the painful feeling of "overfulness.") It takes the body about twenty minutes after starting a meal to send the satiety signals. This is why it's easier to overeat if you eat fast than if you eat slowly. This twenty-

hunger: Unpleasant physical sensation resulting from the lack of food; may be accompanied by weakness, an overwhelming desire to eat, and "hunger pangs" in the lower part of the chest that coincide with powerful contractions of the stomach.

satiety: (sə tī′ə tē) Being full to the point of satisfaction; occurs when a person no longer feels a need for food and loses interest in eating.

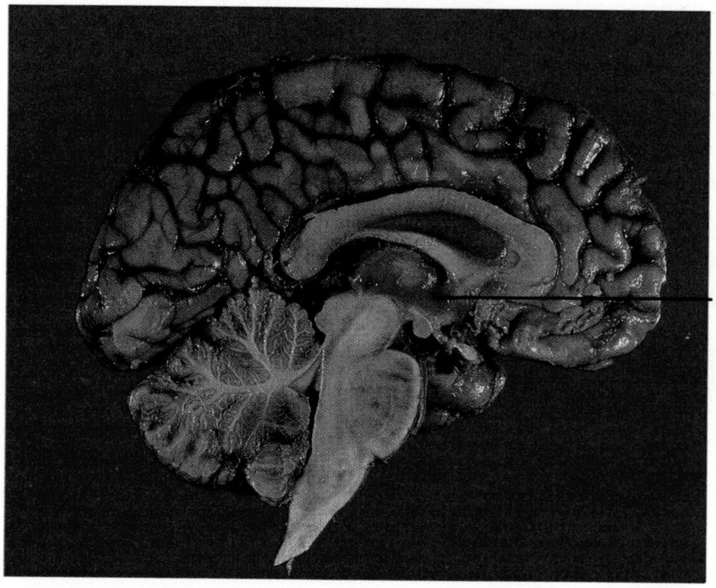

FIGURE 4-1
Cross section of the brain, showing the area of the hypothalamus.

minute time lag also explains why snacking before a meal may decrease a person's interest in eating the meal.

People who eat when they are hungry and stop as soon as they start to feel full tend not to have problems managing their weight. But, as you can tell by taking a quick look around a roomful of people, hunger and satiety are not the only factors that influence how much people eat.

People eat for many reasons that may not be related to the body's need for food. People eat because the clock says it's time for a meal, because their favorite foods are around for the taking, because they are bored or stressed, and for other reasons. A major motivation for eating that may or may not be related to hunger is **appetite**. Unlike hunger and satiety, appetite cues are learned, not inborn.

appetite: The desire to eat; a pleasant sensation that is aroused by thoughts of the taste and enjoyment of food.

Appetite is a desire for food and the pleasure that eating provides. It is cued by psychological signals that have developed out of a person's experiences with food and eating. Appetite is not accompanied by hunger pangs or the sensation of weakness that occurs when a person is hungry, but hunger and appetite usually go together. People tend to be more receptive to appetite signals when they are hungry than when they are not.

The Role of the Hypothalamus in Regulating Food Intake

Hunger, satiety, and appetite have been studied intensively in the hope of discovering the cause of obesity. This line of research quickly centered on the hypothalamus. The hypothalamus is a small, distinct area of the brain located almost directly in the center of the skull (Figure 4-1). It is involved in the regulation of thirst, energy metabolism, and body temperature, and the chemicals it produces affect mood. The hypothalamus also serves as the body's "control center" for regulating food intake. It responds to chemical messages sent by various tissues throughout the body by signaling hunger, appetite, or satiety.

Scientists have long been able to manipulate the feeding behavior of laboratory animals by surgically damaging particular portions of the hypothalamus. If a portion on one side of the hypothalamus is damaged, animals will overeat and gorge themselves if their favorite foods are available. These animals experience exaggerated sensations of hunger and appetite and do not experience normal feelings of satiety. They quickly gain weight and continue to gain. Damage to an area on the other side of the hypothalamus, however, causes the animals to decrease their food intake and to lose weight. They act as if they are "full" all the time and show little desire to eat. Similarly, damage to the human hypothalamus resulting from accidents or tumors has been found to affect the eating behavior of humans.[1]

Results from these and other studies prompted the suggestion that under- and overeating may be due to faulty input from the body's tissues or to abnormal functioning of the hypothalamus. This suggestion has been exceedingly difficult to confirm in human studies because human hypothalami are not available for study. Nonetheless, the results of animal research indicate that the hypothalamus (and possibly other parts of the brain and body) may play a role in the development of weight problems in humans.

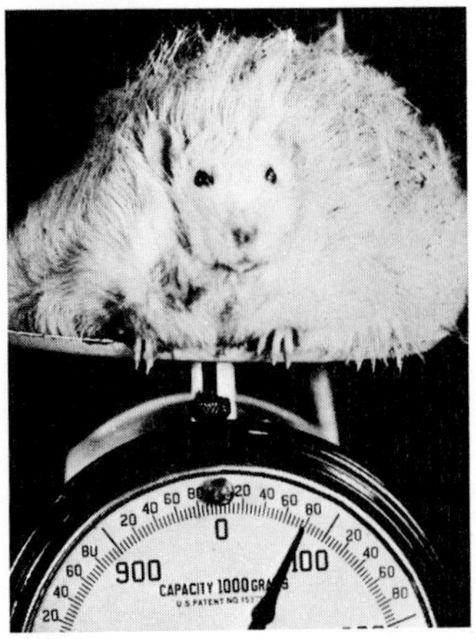

Hypothalamic overeating. This young rat weighs 1,080 grams, more than 3 times the normal weight for its species.

BODY WEIGHT

Optimal Body Weight

Most Americans know how much they weigh and what they would like to weigh for cosmetic reasons. A better basis for identifying optimal body weight is the weight that would be most healthy for the person. Very strong hints about optimal body weights for good health have been provided by life insurance companies.

Life insurance companies have been active in collecting data that relate weight to health since 1919. As a matter of fact, much of the information available on the topic comes from their studies. Working jointly, life insurance companies have collected data on 25 million adults over the age of 25 in the U.S. and Canada. They have published a table that lists weights of females and males at specific heights that correlate with longer-than-average

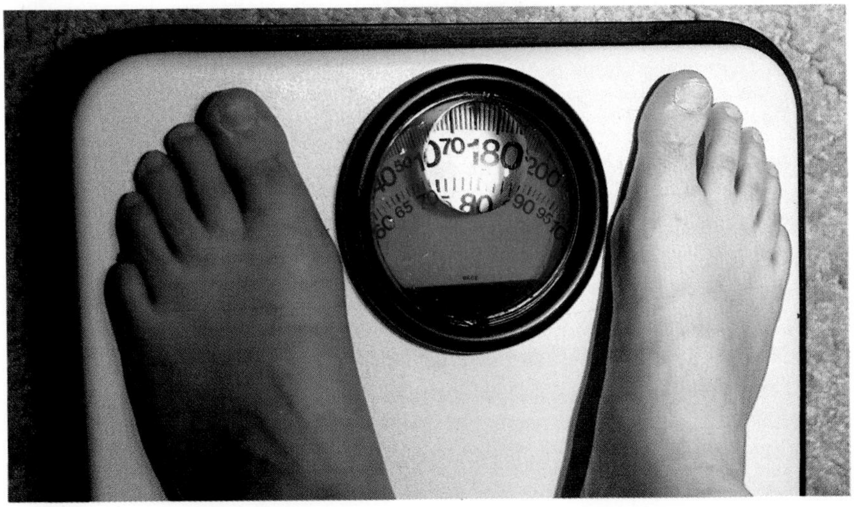

Weight control is important for good health.

TABLE 4-1

Standard body weights based on life insurance data*

Height		Standard Body Weight, pounds	
		Women	Men
4 feet	9 inches	94–106	
4	10	97–109	
4	11	100–112	
5	0	103–115	
5	1	106–118	111–122
5	2	109–122	114–126
5	3	112–126	117–129
5	4	116–131	120–132
5	5	120–135	123–136
5	6	124–139	127–140
5	7	128–143	131–145
5	8	132–147	135–149
5	9	136–151	139–153
5	10	140–155	143–158
5	11	144–159	147–163
6	0		151–168
6	1		155–173
6	2		160–178
6	3		165–183

*Weight of insured persons in the United States and Canada associated with the longest life expectancy. Values listed are for persons with medium frame and aged 25 years and over. Heights and weights are measured without shoes or other clothing.[6]

life expectancy. The information in Table 4-1 was first published in 1959 by the Metropolitan Life Insurance Company and is still considered the weight for height table of choice by many scientists.

As a general guide, people are considered *underweight* if their weight for height is less than 90 percent of the midpoint of their standard weight range. *Normal* weights are considered to be those that are between 90% and 110% of the midpoint of the standard range. People with weights for heights that place them between 110% and 120% of the midpoint of their ranges are considered *overweight*; and those whose weights exceed 120%, *obese*. These guides are summarized in Table 4-2. Box 4-1 explains how you can determine your weight status category.

Although the Metropolitan Life Insurance Company table is widely used to estimate desirable weight, evidence is accumulating that suggests people who weigh slightly below the midpoint of their standard weight range tend to live longer.[2,3] Up until recently, body weights for people in the U.S. have been increasing. In 1863, for example, men who were 5′10″ tall averaged 147 pounds. By 1980, that figure had increased to 175 pounds (Figure 4-2).[4,5] The trend toward higher body weights for height now appears to be declining for women, but not for men. The most recently published (1983) Metropolitan weight-for-height tables showed that, on average, women over the age of 30 weigh a few pounds less for their height than in 1959.[6]

BOX 4-1

HOW TO IDENTIFY YOUR WEIGHT STATUS GROUP

Step 1: Using Table 4-1, identify the standard weight range for a person of your gender and height.

Step 2: Find the middle value (number) of the standard weight range:
a. Subtract the lowest number of the range from the highest number.
b. Divide the difference by 2.
c. Add the lowest number of the range to the number you got in b.

Step 3: Divide your weight in pounds (measured without clothing) by the middle value of your standard weight range.

Step 4: Convert the result of Step 3 to a percentage figure by multiplying it by 100.

Step 5: Refer to Table 4-2 to learn your weight status category.

TABLE 4-2
Categories of weight status corresponding to the life insurance table of standard body weights

Weight Status	Difference from Standard Weight
Underweight	less than 90%
Normal weight	90% to 110%
Overweight	110%–120%
Obese	more than 120%

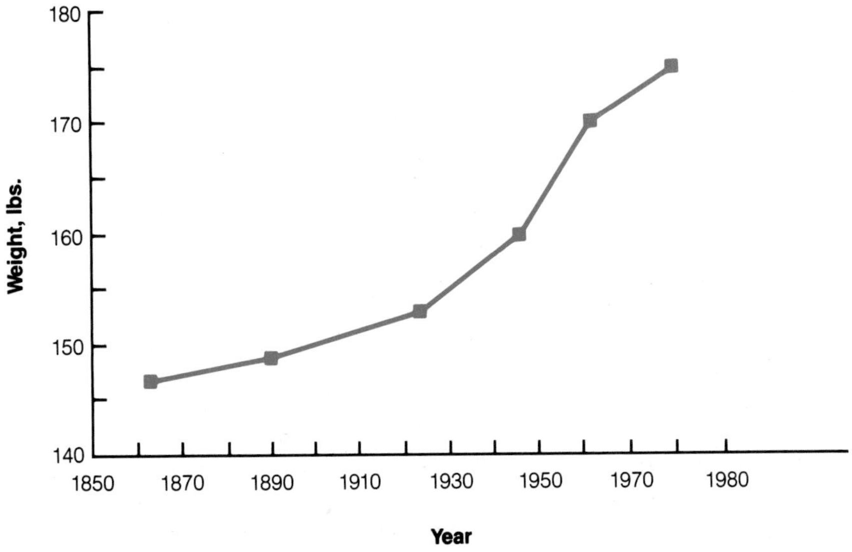

FIGURE 4-2
Increases in average body weight of 30–35-year-old 5′10″ tall males since 1860.[4,5]

Body Fat Content

A person's body weight doesn't tell the whole story about health risks related to body size. It makes a difference to health if fat stores account for too little or too much of body weight.

"Body fat is where it's at" is the gist of many articles about body weight. That's because health risks attributed to weight are probably really related to body fat content. Body fat content is a much more reliable indicator of fitness and health than is body weight alone. Consider a body builder, a wrestler, and a football player as examples. Many of them weigh in as overweight for their height, but they aren't. Their muscular physiques register more pounds on the scale than does fat. So, although the table will indicate they are overweight, they may have less body fat than the amount that poses a risk to health. The opposite situation also exists. People may be classified as normal weight by the table but actually be undermuscled and overly fat. The secretary or lawyer who sits most of the day and gets very little exercise may not look overweight. But, underneath the fitted suit may be a body that contains too much fat. A much more accurate way to determine whether a person is underweight or overweight is to measure body fat content.

Males and females naturally vary in levels of body fat considered normal. For males, it's about 15% of body weight, and for females it is 25%.[7] Body fat content tends to increase with age up to about 50 years for both males and females, and then it starts to decline. The age-related increase in body fat stores for females is shown in Figure 4-3.

Levels of body fat considered to be too low and too high have been defined. The least amounts of body fat compatible with health are approximately 3% for men and 10% to 12% for women.[7] The body maintains these

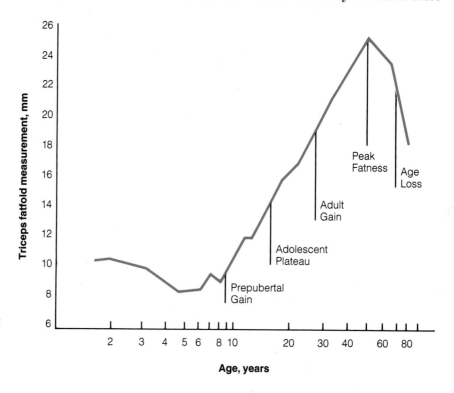

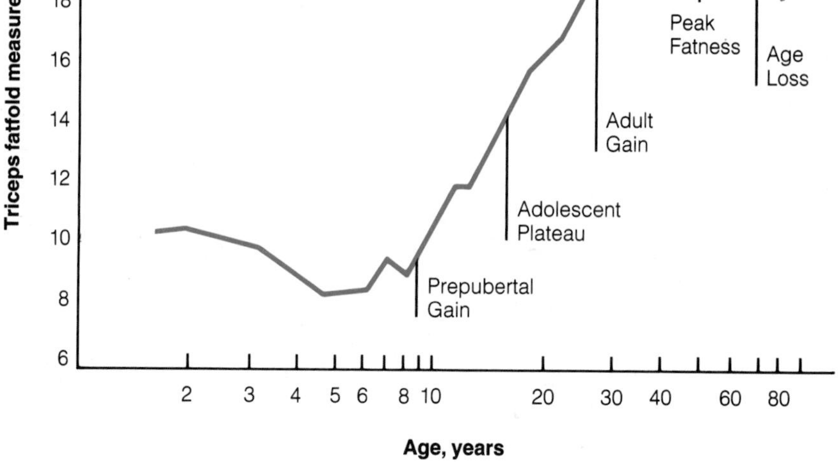

FIGURE 4-3
Changes in female body fat content with age. Body fat was estimated by measures of triceps fatfold thickness in the Ten-State Nutrition Survey.

Overly fat people who store excess body fat primarily in the chest and stomach areas are at higher risk for diabetes, heart disease, and other health problems than are people who store excess fat in the arms and legs.

TABLE 4-3
Percentage body fat content and health

	Minimum Level Compatible with Health	Underfat	Normal Body Fat Content	Overfat
Women	10%–12%	less than 20%	20%–30%	more than 30%
Men	3%	less than 12%	12%–20%	more than 20%

minimal levels tenaciously; this body fat is not used as an energy source, even if a person is starving. Men who have between 3% and 12% body fat and women with 10% to 20% body fat are considered *underfat*. The cutoff points for *overfat* are body fat content of over 20% in men and over 30% in women (Table 4-3).

Where overly fat people store body fat has recently been observed to be related to health. People who store most of their fat around their middles are at higher risk for developing hypertension, diabetes, elevated levels of blood cholesterol, and heart disease than are people who store fat in the arms, thighs, and buttocks.[8]

Assessing Body Fat Content Whether a person has too little or too much body fat can be roughly determined by the "eyeball test," which entails simply looking at the amount of fat stored in the arm, legs, and stomach areas of the body. Another means of estimating fat stores is the "pinch an inch test." People who can pinch more than an inch thickness of fat stores above their navel or at the back of their upper arm may be overly fat. These tests give only a quick "guestimate" of whether a person has too little or too much fat. They do not indicate *how much* of a person's body weight is fat. Much more sophisticated approaches are used for learning this. Three commonly used methods are skinfold thickness measurements, electrical impedence, and underwater weighing.

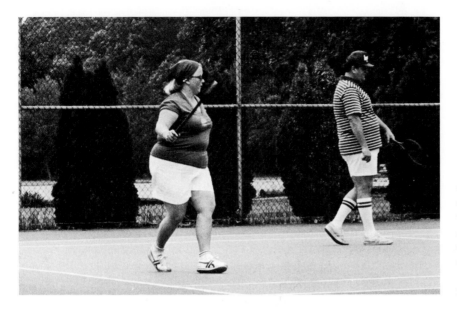

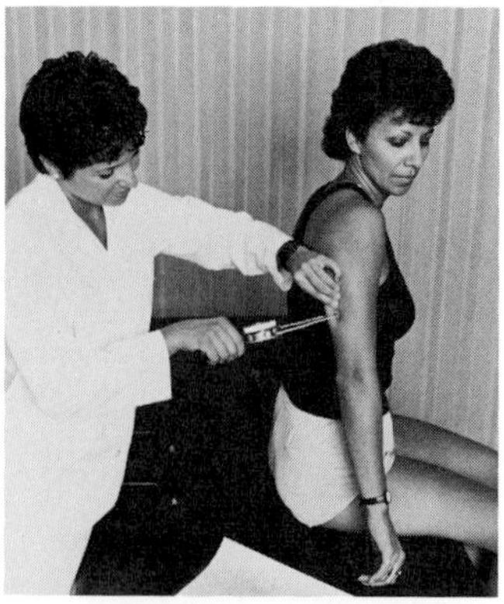

Skinfold calipers are commonly used to estimate body fat content.

1. Skinfold Thickness Measurements

   You can estimate how much fat is present in a person's body by measuring the thickness of the layer of fat below the skin with an instrument called a skinfold caliper. The body sites measured include the back of the arm, the shoulder blade, and an area above the navel. The measurement is "plugged into" an equation that yields an estimate of body fatness. Skinfold thickness measurements by skilled individuals come very close to accurately assessing a person's body fat composition. Measurements taken by amateurs are likely to be incorrect.

2. Electrical Impedence

   A relatively new method for estimating body fat composition is measurement of electrical impedence. Because fat is a poor conductor of electricity and water and muscles are good conductors, you can estimate how much fat a person has by measuring how quickly electrical current is conducted through the body. In electrical impedence measuring, a low voltage transmits an electrical current from a person's ankle to the wrist. (The person hardly feels it.) Although less accurate than underwater weighing estimates, this method enjoys widespread use in fitness centers.

3. Underwater Weighing

   The most accurate method for estimating body fat content is underwater weighing. It has the disadvantage of requiring expensive equipment that is not easily moved from place to place. A person is first weighed on "dry land" and then when totally under water. Because fat is more buoyant than muscle, the less a person weighs underwater compared to their weight out of the water, the greater is their fat content. Perhaps you have noticed the difference body composition makes to how much a person seems to weigh in water. Muscular people do not float very well, and they must put a good deal of energy into swimming in order to keep their head above water. People with more body fat float more easily and need not work so hard to keep from going under.

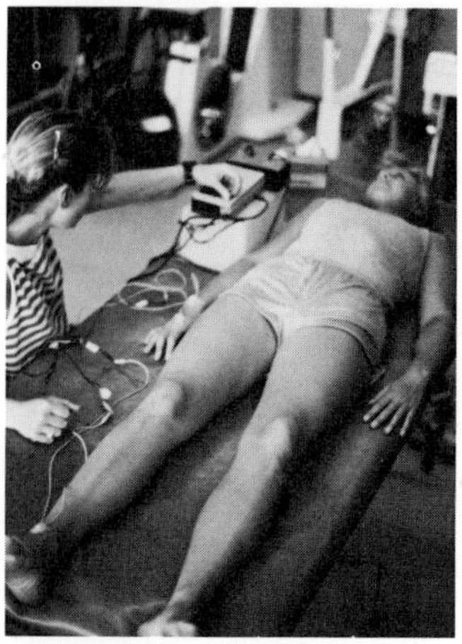

Electrical impedence measurement of body fat content.

As has been discussed, too little as well as too much body fat affects health. Obesity is a crucial health issue in the U.S. In other countries, especially those where there is much poverty, underfat and its consequences are major public health concerns.

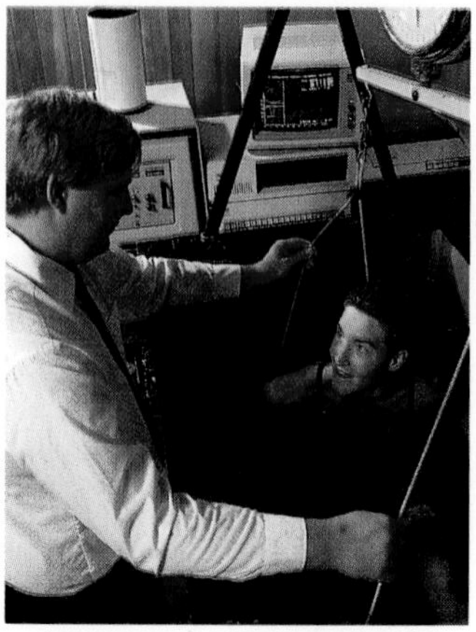

Hydrostatic (underwater) weighing.

■ ■ ■

OBESITY: A LEADING FORM OF MALNUTRITION IN THE UNITED STATES

Perhaps no area within the field of human nutrition is more intensively researched and discussed than the subject of obesity. In spite of all the research and discussion, it remains a disorder for which there is no clearly known cause or reliable treatment. This major public health problem is one of the most complex and misunderstood disorders of our time. Approximately 22% of men and 24% of women in the U.S. are obese.[5]

Interest in solving the mysteries surrounding the cause and cure of obesity is intense because the condition poses serious threats to health. Although it is the direct cause of death for only one disorder (Box 4-2), obesity is associated with a wide range of conditions; see Table 4-4. The increased risk of developing heart disease, diabetes, certain types of cancer, hyper-

BOX 4-2

PICKWICKIAN SYNDROME

For the most part, obesity is indirectly associated with the development or aggravation of diseases and disorders. One disorder, however, is directly caused by obesity. The disorder is called Pickwickian syndrome, after Samuel Pickwick, the obese title character in a novel by Charles Dickens. Pickwickian syndrome occurs among grossly obese people and is characterized by difficulty in breathing, especially when the person is lying down. The weight of the chest exerts more pressure on the lungs than can be "lifted" during the process of inhaling. The lack of oxygen that results can lead to death by suffocation.[2] Fortunately, the condition is alleviated when the person loses weight.

TABLE 4-4

The mismatch between obesity and health[2]

Problems associated with Obesity			
shortened life span	hypertension	infertility	accidents
heart disease	depression	complications during pregnancy	complications from surgery
diabetes	high blood cholesterol levels	injury to weight-bearing joints	gout
certain types of cancer	gallbladder disease	varicose veins	skin disorders

tension, and other disorders may contribute to shortened life span and decreased quality of life for people who are obese.[2]

A consequence of obesity that has perhaps the greatest impact on quality of life stems from people's attitudes about it. Obesity is a visible disorder, against which many Americans hold strong biases. Biases against obesity translate subtly or overtly into job discrimination, social isolation, ridicule, and rejection. The consequences of obesity are much better understood than its causes. The scientific literature does, however, offer several theories about its causes.

Causes of Obesity

The difficulty of identifying the root causes of obesity clearly indicates how complicated it is. We know that whatever causes behaviors or conditions that produce obesity results in a positive energy balance—caloric intakes that exceed the body's need for calories. What is not known with any certainty is why some people develop eating habits or other conditions that lead to a positive energy balance and why these habits and conditions are so difficult to modify.

Two theories about the causes of obesity have contributed to our knowledge: the "nature" theory and the "nurture" theory (Table 4-5). The nature

■
TABLE 4-5
Causes of obesity

The Nature Theory	The Nurture Theory
Obesity is linked to genetic traits inherited from parents. There appear to be "natural" differences in individual rates of thermogenesis. Some animals are genetically obese, so perhaps some humans are, too. Each person has a biologically determined weight.	Obesity is related to: overeating habits formed in childhood psychological factors routine availability of highly preferred foods physical inactivity increased fat cell numbers due to overeating

theory attempts to explain obesity by genetic (inborn) traits. The nurture theory examines the roles of environmental factors such as early childhood food experiences and exercise in obesity development. Neither theory adequately explains why people become obese; it appears that "nature" and "nurture" each play a role.

The Nature Theory Are some people born with a tendency to become obese? Evidence supporting this notion has been found in studies of obesity in families and twins.

Obesity tends to run in families. One well-known study published in 1965 found that 80% of the children raised in families where both parents were obese were obese themselves. If one parent was obese, 40% of the children were also obese. However, if neither parent was obese, only 14% of the children were.[9] These results do not provide conclusive evidence that obesity is inherited. It is frequently argued that children adopt the eating and exercise patterns of their parents. Families have a lot more in common than their genes.

To sort out the effects of upbringing and genetic traits on obesity development, scientists have studied twins adopted at birth. In general, twins raised by adoptive parents tend to have body builds similar to those of their biological parents.[10] When twins are adopted by different sets of parents at birth and reared apart, they tend to resemble each other in height and weight.[11] Not every study has found these results, however. Adopted children have also been found to have body weights that more closely resemble those of the children and parents in their adoptive families than their biological siblings and parents.[12]

Inborn differences in thermogenesis—the energy expended for digestion, absorption, and processing of nutrients—may also be related to obesity. People whose thermogenesis "thermostats" are set on low use fewer calories for these processes than others. The difference in caloric need may be great enough to lower total caloric requirement and make it easier for some people to gain weight on a modest caloric intake than others who have a higher rate of thermogenesis.[13]

The genetic links to obesity uncovered in twins studies and the finding of individual differences in thermogenesis strongly support a genetic component to obesity, but they do not explain all cases of obesity. Only 4 out of 10 obese children become obese adults; most obese adults were of normal weight as children and infants.[14] The overall incidence of obesity is on the rise in the U.S., and the cause of this increase is clearly not genetic.[15] Although genetic traits may be related to obesity in childhood and adulthood, they are not the only cause.

The Nurture Theory Two important factors associated with the development of obesity appear not to be related to genetic traits: eating habits and physical activity habits. Children learn to eat to satisfy hunger as well as for reasons unrelated to the need for food. Instead of eating to cure hunger pangs, they may learn to eat to relieve boredom, to escape a stressful situation, or to please their parents. Consider parents who insist that children "clean their plates" or who reward good behavior with cookies, candy, or other high-calorie treats. The child's natural eating cue—hunger— may become obscured by other eating signals. Eating habits that develop during childhood can be very difficult to change.

The types of food available to a person may influence whether the person eats too much and becomes obese.[16] Most children and adults in the U.S. live in environments where much more appetizing food is available to them than they need. The opportunity to overeat is generally no farther away than the refrigerator, a vending machine, the corner grocery, or the dining table. The nearly continuous access to highly preferred foods has been cited as one reason people in the U.S. become obese.[4] This notion has found strong support in animal research.

Until recently, it was widely thought that obesity is a condition of humans. It had long been observed, for example, that laboratory rats and other animals would not overeat or become obese if given free access to large amounts of standard laboratory foods. Such observations led to the conclusion that humans lack the inborn mechanisms of other animals that control how much is eaten when a surplus of food is available. Several discoveries from feeding experiments have struck down this assumption. We now know that the type of food offered to laboratory rats and humans makes a big difference in how much is eaten.[17]

Rats and humans share strong preferences for many of the same types of foods. If given free access to cookies, peanut butter, marshmallows, chocolate bars, and sugared cereals, rats will ignore their standard laboratory food and become obese from eating too much of these "highly preferred" foods. If returned to a diet of only the standard foods, the rats will stop overeating and eventually return to normal weight.[17] See Figure 4-4.

A strain of rats that are genetically obese has been discovered and is widely used in feeding and obesity research. These "Zucker" rats overeat and become obese even on the most monotonous diet. When offered "highly preferred" foods, the rats become enormously obese, even more so than they do on a monotonous diet. The combination of the genetic tendency toward obesity and access to favorite foods produces the most extreme degrees of obesity in these rats.[4]

The results of human-feeding experiments correspond to some extent to those of the rat studies. When normal-weight and obese human volunteers

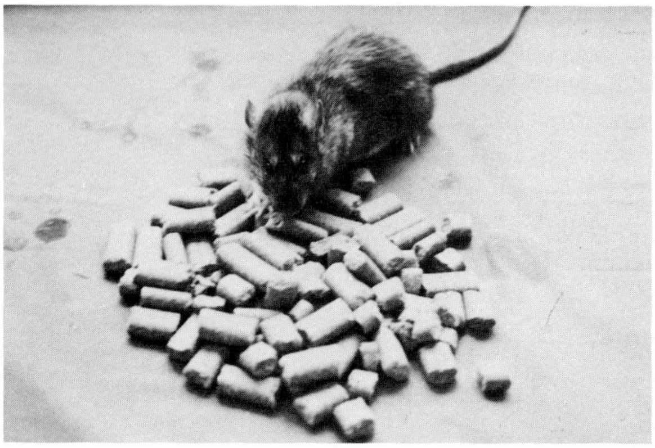

(a)

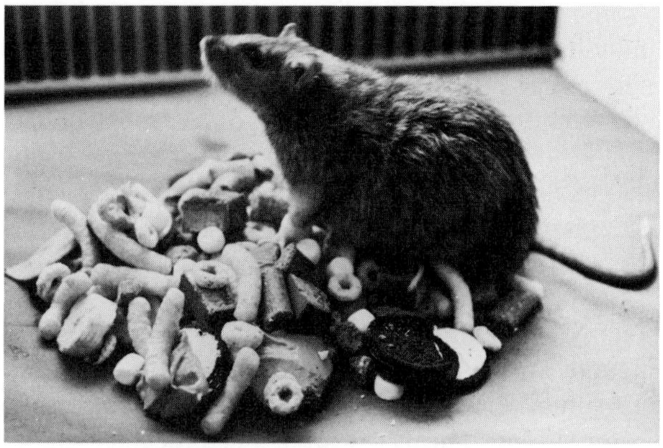

(b)

■ FIGURE 4-4

Normal rats *(a)* remain lean on a standard rat diet, and *(b)* become obese if they are provided with unlimited access to human snack-food items.

are given a monotonous but nutritionally adequate liquid diet (analogous to the standard laboratory rat food), normal-weight subjects will eat enough to maintain their weight. Obese subjects, on the other hand, eat less and lose weight rapidly.[18] In other experiments, both normal-weight and obese humans have tended to gain weight if offered unlimited amounts of "highly preferred" foods.[19] The similarities in the results of animal and human feeding experiments have helped to explain why some people with no family history of obesity become obese while people who have a genetic tendency toward obesity remain obese. They have led Theodore Van Itallie, a leading obesity researcher, to conclude:

> There may not be anything basically wrong with most obese people. The problem simply may lie in the fact that human beings have had to learn how to store fat in order to survive. When it becomes easy rather than difficult to obtain extra calories from the environment, obesity is the natural outcome—perhaps *thin* people are the ones who are abnormal.[20]

Physical Activity Patterns and Obesity Physical inactivity has been directly related to the development of obesity in children and adults.[21,22] For some people, a very low level of physical activity may be a primary reason for obesity, whereas a high level of physical activity may explain why others are not obese. One study showed that Japanese migrating to Hawaii and California gained between 13 and 19 pounds in only a few years. They did not gain the weight because of a high-calorie diet; they actually ate fewer calories in the U.S. than they had in Japan. The difference was their activity level; they became less active as they adjusted to U.S. lifestyles.[23]

A number of surveys have shown that certain groups of people with relatively high caloric intakes are less likely than people with lower calorie intakes to be obese. These are people who are physically active. Thus, obesity is not a result of caloric intake alone. Some obese people don't eat any more than normal-weight people; they are simply much less physically active.

Maintenance of Obesity

Whatever the cause of obesity—nature, nurture, or a combination of the two—it is a condition that is very hard to change once established. The tenacity demonstrated by the human body in maintaining obesity once established has led scientists to look for body mechanisms that act to maintain the obese state. So far, two major body mechanisms that may promote the maintenance of obesity have been uncovered. The first has to do with the number of fat cells obese people produce, and the second with the body's "idea" of its ideal weight—the "set-point" theory of obesity maintenance.

Fat Cells and Obesity Observations that obese people tend to have more fat cells than normal-weight people once led many people to believe that the number of fat cells a person forms during childhood and adolescence is responsible for the maintenance of obesity. It was assumed that fat cells, like nerve or muscle cells, increase in number only during growth periods. If a person overate during childhood, it was reasoned, he or she would form an excess number of fat cells. This high level of fat cells would tend to make and keep the person obese.

It now appears that humans can add fat cells throughout life.[24] When a person's existing fat cells reach the maximum size (by becoming stuffed with storage fat), the body produces new cells to handle the need for additional fat storage. The presence of a higher number of fat cells appears to make it difficult to lose weight. It has been suggested that the body may trigger eating signals when the amount of fat stored in the fat cells begins to decrease.[25]

Set-Point Theory The set-point theory of obesity holds that each person is "programmed" to weigh a certain amount or to contain a particular level of body fat. If you weigh less or more than this predetermined amount or have a lower or higher level of fat, your body will automatically make adjustments in food intake or in the amount of energy expended for basal metabolism or thermogenesis so that you get back to your "set point." According to this theory, people become obese because they have high set points.[26]

Scientific evidence that supports the set-point theory is limited. However, the theory offers an attractive explanation for why most people regain lost weight. Many people who manage to reduce their body weight and keep it at the lower level report that they have to "diet" constantly; if they eat enough to satisfy their desire for food, they regain the weight. Why people tend to "defend" a particular body weight is not at all clear. It is clear, however, that a strong tendency exists for people to maintain a particular weight and that this tendency is not easily modified.

Most examinations of the possible causes of obesity lead to the same conclusion: it is easier to prevent obesity from developing than to try to undo it once it has been established. Preventing obesity is viewed as the most effective way to "cure" the problem.

Preventing Obesity

The surest route to the prevention of obesity is the early establishment of healthy eating and exercise patterns. Children are less likely to overeat if they are not encouraged (or forced) to clean their plates, not encouraged to eat when they are not hungry, and not rewarded with food. Small children know when they feel hungry, and they should not be encouraged to eat when they are not hungry or to continue eating when they have had enough. Parents, however, need to control what foods are available to their children. Children appear to be much better judges of *when* and *how much* they

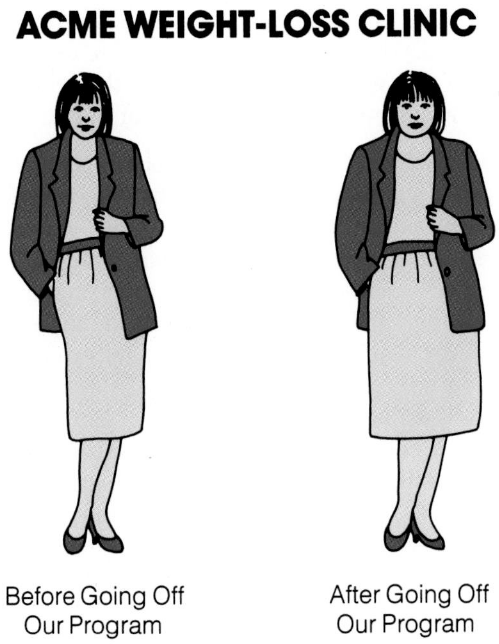
ACME WEIGHT-LOSS CLINIC
Before Going Off Our Program
After Going Off Our Program

If the advertisements for weight loss programs were completely truthful, they would include photographs of their clients before and after they *went off* the program.

should eat than they are of *what* they should eat. Children are not born knowing how to select a balanced diet; they have to learn that.[27]

The chances of children becoming obese are decreased if they are physically active. Children who spend most of their free time watching television, for example, are more likely to be obese than children who play actively during their free time.[28] Children who enjoy sports and other forms of physical activity may be more likely to engage in exercise in their adult years, too.

Children's attitudes toward eating and physical activity are influenced by their parents' behaviors. This makes the prevention of obesity a family affair. The "do as I say, not as I do" approach rarely works. Establishing good habits in children sometimes must begin with correcting the poor habits of adults.

Approaches to the Treatment of Obesity

There are hundreds of approaches to weight loss, and the vast majority of them do not work. Overall, only 5% to 20% of the people who enter weight-loss programs lose weight and maintain the loss for a year.[29] Programs that claim better results almost uniformly calculate their success rates on the number of people who *lose some* weight, rather than the number who *maintain* their loss. Any approach to weight loss that includes a reduction in caloric intake can produce weight loss. The real test of a weight-loss program is its success in helping people *stay* at their lower weights. *No weight-loss program can be considered successful unless it leads to a permanent loss in body fat.*

Some popular approaches to weight loss are discussed in Box 4-3. The method of choice, however, is one that changes a person's eating and exercise behaviors permanently. It is not reasonable to expect to reach a point where weight maintenance requires no effort. The effort can be easier if new and improved behaviors became a way of life, however.

BOX 4-3

SOME POPULAR APPROACHES TO WEIGHT LOSS THAT DON'T WORK

A number of popular schemes and "last-ditch" approaches to weight loss are described in this box. As you read about each one, ask yourself these questions:

Does the approach help to improve eating behaviors?

Are only modest changes in eating behavior recommended?

Is exercise a part of the plan?

If the answer to one or more of these questions is no, the approach lacks at least one key ingredient for weight-loss maintenance.

WEIGHT-LOSS DIETS

Bookstore shelves are loaded with books offering help with weight loss. Let's take a look:

Fit for Life
Fit or Fat
Win the Food Fight
Life Extension
The Doctor's Quick Weight Loss Diet
Dr. Atkin's Diet Revolution
The Last Chance Diet
The Cambridge Diet

The reason for the great number of diet books on the market is that there are a lot of people who want to lose weight. They want to lose it quickly, painlessly, and once and for all! It hasn't seemed to occur to many people that none of the diets works very well in the long run. Many people are so anxious about their weight that they are much more interested in getting it off quickly than in keeping it off. Admittedly, most of the diets that become popular do help people lose weight. (As a nation, we lose millions of pounds every year on these diets.) The problem is that the weight is not lost for very long—only until it's "found" again.

Popular weight-loss diets typically have several features that give them market appeal.

A Gimmick Some gimmick distinguishes the diet from the ones that preceded it. It is often advertised as the unique element of the diet and the element that makes it work, which explains why others have failed. Gimmicks that have been used in the past include the grapefruit gimmick (grapefruit "burns up fat"), the high-carbohydrate gimmick (it improves your mood so you're happier and won't eat so much), the high-protein gimmick (it spares your muscles while using up your fat), and the doctor gimmick (the book was written by a doctor, so it must be good).

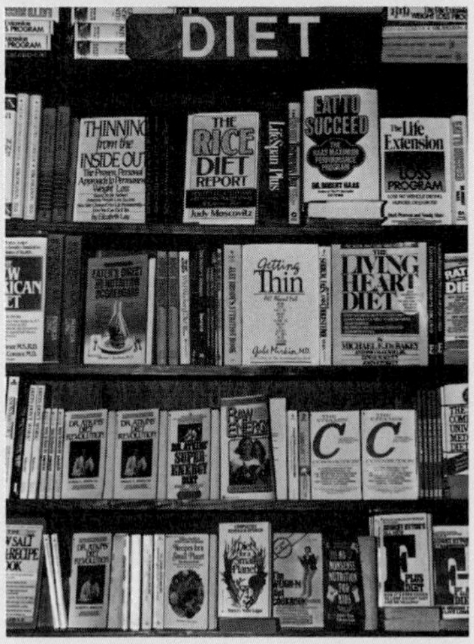

Bookstores offer a wide selection of "diet" books.

Quick Results Can you imagine a weight-loss book selling if it promised "slow" results?

Easy to Use Popular diets that offer black-and-white advice, that are easy to follow, and that allow the dieter few choices have appeal.

Calorie Cutback All of the popular diets have the feature of being low in calories. Although this feature may be overshadowed by the diet's gimmick, it is the real reason people will lose weight if they follow the diet.

FASTING

The most extreme type of weight-loss diet is fasting. A fast is either a total fast, in which case only water is allowed, or a partial fast, which allows several hundred calories a day. Either type should be undertaken only in a hospital with close medical supervision.

Obese people can, and have, lost a tremendous amount of weight by fasting. It appears to be worth the effort and expense when it is used to get a person's weight down so that required surgery can be performed. People who have lost large amounts of weight by fasting have reported that it was easier for them to get employment and to increase their earnings after their fasts.[30] Although there may be benefits, fasting has some of the same problems that plague other approaches. They are the problems of weight regain, the loss of muscle mass, and an inadequate intake of nutrients.

Fasting does not correct the underlying causes of a person's obe-

continued

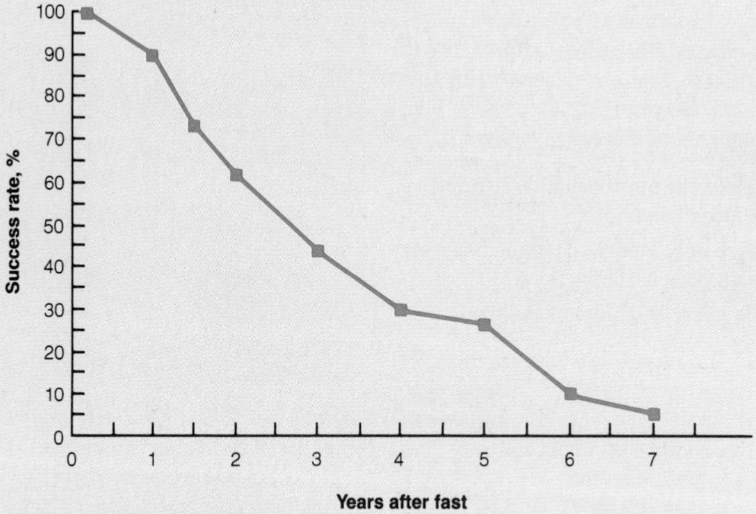

FIGURE 1
Percentage of 121 obese patients who maintained weight loss after a two-month fast.[30]

sity and it is not effective in preventing a rebound in body weight. Most people who lose weight by fasting regain it all in 2 to 3 years. Within 7 years, about 94% of people who lost weight during a two-month fast weighed as much or more than they did before the fast (Figure 1).[30]

ORGANIZED WEIGHT-LOSS PROGRAMS

Group approaches to weight loss are widely available in the U.S. and Europe. Programs such as Overeaters Anonymous,™ TOPS™ (Take Off Pounds Sensibly), and Weight Watchers™ offer reasonably balanced, low-calorie diets as well as group support and encouragement for weight loss. Some group programs are beginning to incorporate exercise and help in bringing about behavioral changes. The primary criticism of the programs is the lack of scientific data that show they help people maintain their weight loss.

DRUGS

Several types of pills that suppress appetite are sold over the counter, most of them containing the chemical phenylpropanolamine (PPA). They may be effective in helping people lose weight for a few months, but then they lose their effectiveness. Potential side effects of appetite-suppressing drugs include nervousness, irritability, and insomnia.

SURGERY AND OTHER DRASTIC MEASURES

These "weight-loss approaches of last resort" include jaw wiring, stomach balloons, and surgery.

Jaw Wiring Jaw wiring entails the partial closing of a person's jaw with wire so the mouth cannot open very wide; the opening is large enough to allow the person to drink with a straw (which means that high-calorie drinks such as milkshakes can be consumed). People whose jaws have been wired have trouble speaking, sneezing, coughing, yawning, and maintaining good oral hygiene. Because they are at risk of choking, people with wired jaws are generally given pliers and taught how to undo them if they start to choke. The opportunity to go off their liquid diets is as close as the pliers.

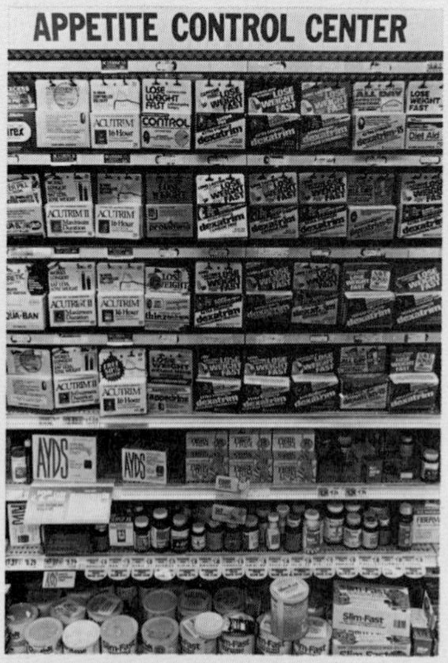

Appetite suppressants are not a long-term solution to obesity.

Stomach Balloons Stomach balloons are actually latex tubes that are inserted into a person's stomach to reduce the amount of food the stomach can hold. The long-term effectiveness of this method is not well-studied, but it appears that stomach balloons decrease food intake, at least temporarily.[31] This procedure is not expected to increase in popularity, because the balloons sometimes burst and the fragments may obstruct the intestines.

Surgery *Lipectomy* is a type of surgery used to help people "spot reduce." Also called *liposuction*, the procedure involves vacuuming

FIGURE 2

Diagram of stomach "stapling" surgery. The stomach is surgically closed near the top so that food will bypass the main part of the stomach and go directly to the small intestine which has been connected to the part of the stomach above the staples. Digestive juices from the stomach and uppermost part of the small intestine are routed to the food as shown.

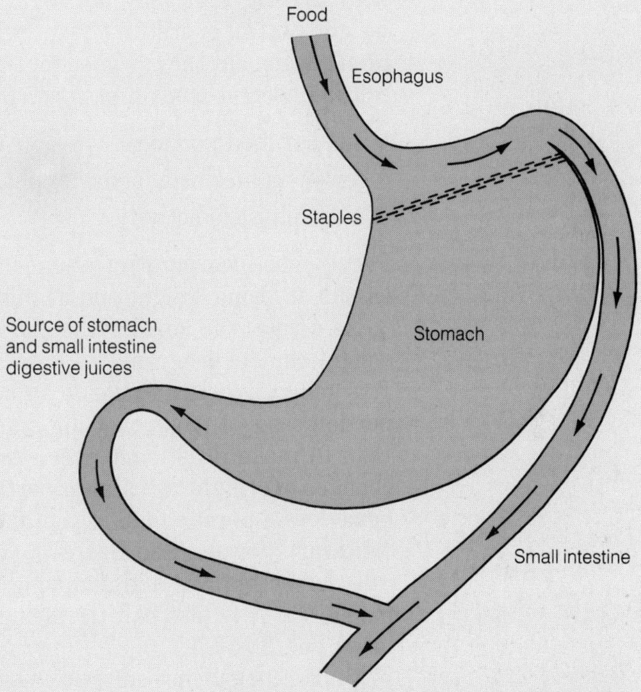

out fat cells that have accumulated under the skin around the thighs, stomach, buttocks, or other parts of the body. It appears to keep people shapely only if they do not gain weight. If they overeat, fat will again accumulate in the fat cells that remain after a lipectomy, and new fat cells may eventually form. Lipectomies are expensive, and they are not recommended for weight control; they are simply intended to reshape parts of a person's figure.

In the past, a surgical procedure that reduced the length of the small intestine was performed for weight loss. It led to many digestion and absorption complications and is no longer performed. The current, most common surgical approach for weight loss is the procedure called "stomach stapling," or "gastric bypass."

Stomach stapling is usually reserved for the highest risk, most stubborn cases of obesity. Obese people who suffer from poorly controlled diabetes or severe joint problems, for example, may elect this operation as a final shot at improving their condition with weight loss.

The purpose of stomach stapling is to reduce the size of the stomach. By stapling closed about 90% of the stomach (Figure 2), people are able to eat only a tablespoonful or two at a time. If this amount is exceeded, they get sick to their stomachs. Many people who have had this surgery can no longer tolerate certain foods such as meats, milks, breads, sweets, and fried foods. Their diets tend to be highly inadequate.[32]

Food intake is drastically reduced by stomach stapling, and weight loss tends to be rapid during the first few months. By stretching the stomach with more food as time goes on, a person can eat larger amounts of food and slow the rate of weight loss. One study reported food intake to increase from an average of 745 calories per day three months after surgery to 1,089 calories after a year.[33] Weight loss tends to plateau after a year, and most people regain some of the weight that was lost.[34] Two years after surgery, however, people still tend to weigh less than their presurgery weight.[35] Some people have had the procedure repeated when the stomach stretched to the point where weight gain resumed.

Surgery and other drastic measures of weight loss may be particularly attractive to obese people who have repeatedly experienced failure with other weight-loss approaches. Stomach stapling, jaw wiring, or stomach balloons may be viewed as the only way for them to lose weight. According to Dr. Philip White, formerly the staff nutritionist of the American Medical Association, this situation makes for a good deal of abuse. Dr. White has noted that these radical approaches keep obesity specialists busy treating over ten million patients and billing at a level of one to two billion dollars annually.

THE SENSIBLE APPROACH TO WEIGHT CONTROL

Although the idea may not seem very exciting, the sensible approach to weight control is still the best. Sensible diets are like sensible shoes; they aren't flashy but they're good for you in the long run. The basic elements of a sensible weight-control program include:

- smaller food portions
- fewer high-calorie foods, emphasis on nutrient-dense foods
- more physical activity

People who incorporate these elements into new habits are the most successful at losing weight and keeping it off.[24,36]

As a rule, the smaller the changes in personal behavior required by a weight-control program, the greater the chances the program will succeed. It is generally much easier to adjust to modest changes—such as reducing portion sizes of foods or using stairs instead of elevators when possible—than to make drastic changes. Weight-loss programs that require major changes overnight are almost certain to fail. The closer the changes are to behaviors a person finds acceptable and can "live with," the greater their "sticking" power. (See Box 4-4). The sensible approach to weight control calls for acceptable and enduring changes in eating and physical activity habits. (It may also call for facing the truth about the calorie content of foods; see Box 4-5.)

Unlike the quick results promised by many weight-loss programs, a sensible diet is planned around the gradual loss in weight of a pound or two a week. Diets that produce a higher rate of weight loss are generally so different from a person's usual diet that they are totally abandoned after weight loss is achieved. Resumption of the person's old habits makes the person regain the lost weight.

BOX 4-4

BEHAVIOR CHANGES FOR LIFETIME WEIGHT CONTROL

Eat smaller portions and don't take second helpings.

Stop eating before you feel overly full.

Increase your intake of vegetables and fruits.

Limit the availability of high-calorie snacks and desserts.

Roast, broil, and steam foods rather than frying them.

Select lean cuts of meat and low-fat dairy products.

Go easy on butter, margarine, sauces, and gravies.

Eat slowly; give your stomach a chance to notify your brain about how much you've eaten.

Walk more.

Make a habit of using stairs whenever possible.

Make time to enjoy participating in your favorite sport more often.

If you watch TV, do floor exercises while watching.

BOX 4-5

FOODS THAT REALLY DO HAVE CALORIES

- cookie pieces
- food "sampled" during meal preparation
- food that doesn't taste very good
- candy, popcorn, and soft drinks eaten in a movie theatre
- foods eaten while discussing weight-control diets
- foods you grab and eat on the run
- alcohol-containing drinks
- foods eaten along with grapefruit or a diet soda
- foods eaten directly from their storage container
- foods you eat when you're not thinking about eating

Eating to Lose Weight

The weight-loss pattern of most people on calorie-restricted diets is not smooth. Even though the calorie content of the diet stays the same, a person may lose three pounds in one week, no pounds the next, and two pounds the week after. Several conditions are thought to contribute to the plateaus and valleys in the rate of weight loss. Weight usually comes off more quickly at the beginning of a weight-control diet than later on. The initial losses are generally greater due to losses in body water in the first few days. If caloric reductions are maintained, most of the weight lost after the first week or so is from fat stores. Exercising as part of a weight-control program may lead to the addition of lean muscle mass, which weighs more (per volume) than fat does. Slight changes in BMR and thermogenesis may also contribute to variations in the amount of weight lost over time.

Because of these conditions, it is difficult to predict precisely the rate at which an individual will lose weight on a calorie-restricted diet. It can be roughly estimated, however, by the rule of thumb that a one-pound loss in body weight corresponds to a 3,500-calorie deficit, on average.

1 pound weight loss per week = roughly −3,500 calories, or −500 calories per day on average. Individual variations in the rate and timing of weight loss are associated with calorie deficits.

You can estimate how many calories are needed to produce an average weight loss of a pound a week by subtracting 500 calories from your usual daily calorie intake level. If you were to cut back by 750 calories per day, you'd lose an average of about a pound and a half per week. Since calories expended by increased physical activity also count toward the calorie deficit, a person could, for example, increase energy expenditure by 200 calories per day and reduce intake by only 550 calories and still achieve the pound-and-a-half per week weight loss.

An example of a sensible weight-loss diet is presented in Table 4-6. The menus shown average 1,379 calories per day if the snacks are included and 1,262 calories if they are not. You'll notice that the menus provide a wide assortment of common foods that contribute to a balanced diet. For a person with a usual daily intake of about 1,900 calories, adherence to this seven-day diet would lead to about a pound of weight loss per week on average. For some people who are tall or physically active, this diet would be too low in calories. Portion sizes would have to be increased to ensure a gradual weight loss.

Reducing caloric intake to below 1,200 calories per day is not advised, because it's too difficult to get the nutrients you need from food at such low

TABLE 4-6

A seven-day low-calorie diet (average calories: 1,262 without snacks; 1,379 with snacks)

	Day 1	Day 2	Day 3	Day 4	Day 5	Day 6	Day 7
Meal 1	orange juice, 6 oz (85 cal) Cheerios®, 1 c (97) whole-wheat toast, 1 slice (65) margarine, 1 t (35) skim milk, 1 c (90)	cantaloupe, ¼ (50) bran flakes, 1 c (127) English muffin, 1 (138) margarine, 1 t (35) skim milk, 1 c (90)	peanut butter, 2 T (190) whole wheat toast, 2 slices (130) orange, 1 (80) skim milk, 1 c (90)	orange juice, 6 oz (85) bran muffin, 1 (100) margarine, 1 t (35) skim milk, 1 c (90)	orange juice, 6 oz (85) cornflakes, 1 c (95) whole-wheat toast, 1 slice (65) margarine, 1 t (35) skim milk, 1 c (90)	pineapple juice, 6 oz (105) low-fat yogurt, 1 c (145) graham cracker, 1 (55)	orange juice, 6 oz (85) poached egg, 1 (80) whole-wheat toast, 1 slice (65) margarine, 1 t (35) skim milk, 1 c (90)
Meal 2	hamburger (lean) 3 oz (190) bun, 1 (112) tomato, ½ (13) skim milk, 1 c (90)	bean soup, 1 c (170) crackers, 4 (50) ham, 1½ oz (96) rye bread, 1 slice (65) mustard, 1 t (4) skim milk, 1 c (90)	chef's salad, 2 c (285) (includes 1 oz each of ham, turkey, and cheese, 1½ c lettuce, ½ egg) salad dressing, 2 T (130) skim milk, 1 c (90)	vegetable-beef soup, 1 c (80) turkey, 3 oz (150) mayonnaise, 1 t (30) white bread, 2 slices (140) skim milk, 1 c (90)	low-fat cottage cheese, ½ c (81) peaches, ½ c (75) grapes, 10 (35) roll, 1 (112) margarine, 1 t (35) iced tea, 1 c (0)	hamburger (lean), 3 oz (190) bun, 1 (112) catsup, 1 T (15) cole slaw, ½ c (59) skim milk, 1 c (90)	chicken salad, 1 c (254) whole-wheat crackers, 4 (64) pineapple, ½ c (95) skim milk, 1 c (90)
Meal 3	baked chicken (no skin), 3 oz (164) peas, ½ c (60) macaroni, ½ c (98) margarine, 1 t (35) skim milk, 1 c (90)	chow mein, 1 c (95) rice, ½ c (113) fortune cookie, 1 (43) tea, 1 c (0)	baked fish, 3 oz (16) sweet potatoes, ½ c (117) green beans, ½ c (15) skim milk, 1 c (90)	spaghetti, ½ c (95) tomato sauce, ½ c (43) meat balls, 2 (159) corn, ½ c (70) roll, 1 (112) margarine, 1 t (35) tea, 1 c (0)	lettuce, 1 c (6) French dressing, 1 T (65) beef (lean), 3 oz (220) peas, ½ c (55) roll, 1 (112) margarine, 1 t (35) skim milk, 1 c (90)	tomato soup, 1 c (90) macaroni and cheese, ½ c (215) spinach (cooked), ½ c (20) beets, ½ c (30) margarine, 1 t (35) skim milk, 1 c (90)	pork (lean), 3 oz (201) noodles, ½ c (95) broccoli, ½ c (20) margarine, 1 t (35) tea, 1 c (0)
Calories without snack:	**1,224**	**1,166**	**1,380**	**1,314**	**1,291**	**1,251**	**1,209**
Snack	banana (100)	peanuts, 1 oz (165)	Fudgesicle®, 1 (91)	low-fat yogurt, 1 c (145)	apple, 1 (80)	sherbet, ½ c (134)	pear, 1 (100)
Calories with snack:	**1,324**	**1,331**	**1,471**	**1,459**	**1,371**	**1,385**	**1,309**

levels of calories, and the diets likely represent too dramatic a change to be maintained.

Can you stay on your sensible diet when you eat out? Yes, if you are armed with some knowledge. As the examples in Box 4-6 show, "diet plates" bear scrutiny. They tend to include foods not thought of as fattening, rather than foods that are actually low in calories. Steak or lean hamburger and cottage cheese, two foods that are relatively high in calories, are often featured on diet plates, and potatoes and bread, two lower-calorie foods, typically are not because they are commonly thought to be "fattening." Not all "diet plates" qualify for a sensible weight-loss diet.

Physical Activity

Weight-control efforts that include a physical activity program offer several bonuses. Exercise burns off calories, which contributes to weight loss and weight control (if it is continued). Muscular bodies use more calories for basal metabolism than do fatter bodies. Regular exercise improves circulation, stamina, and in many cases, a person's alertness and feeling of well being. It may also decrease appetite. Obese people who get involved in exercise tend to have less appetite and to eat less than those who do not exercise.[37,38]

■ ■ ■
UNDERWEIGHT

Because obesity is so common in the U.S. and many other developed countries, it is sometimes given far more attention than the opposite problem, underweight. Worldwide, however, underweight is much more common than obesity. It represents one of the most serious threats to the health of the world's population, especially for children. Although children require adequate calories and nutrients for growth and health, the body's first need is for energy. Without enough energy, children fail to grow and they become susceptible to a host of diseases.

Globally, the most common cause of underweight is the lack of food. Underweight is prevalent in countries where periods of food shortage and starvation are a fact of life. Underweight only occasionally results from a lack of food in the U.S. It is most commonly caused by child neglect, illnesses such as cancer and thyroid disease, bizarre diets, and eating disorders.

Health problems that stem from being underweight are related to the body's inadequate supply of energy for vital functions such as growth, disease resistance, and recovery from illness. Underweight children tend to be short in stature and susceptible to infectious diseases. They are less able to fight off diseases such as measles, tuberculosis, and chicken pox and it takes them longer to recover from disease. Underweight children tend to be irritable and to show little interest in their surroundings.

Because their food intake is low and generally lacking in variety, children who are underweight are more likely than normal-weight children to develop deficiency diseases. Deficiencies of vitamin A, protein, zinc, and iron are commonly associated with underweight. Of these, a calorie deficiency

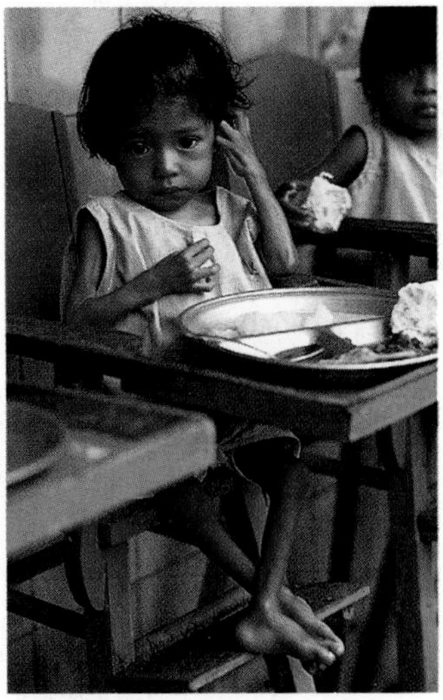

This little Guatemalan girl suffers from marasmus, progressive emaciation due to a dietary deficiency of calories.

BOX 4-6

HOW "DIET" ARE DIET PLATES?

No doubt you have seen "diet plates" listed on restaurant menus. Just how low in calories are they in comparison with other restaurant meals?

Let's consider two types of "diet" meals and a popular fast-food meal. The meals are shown here.

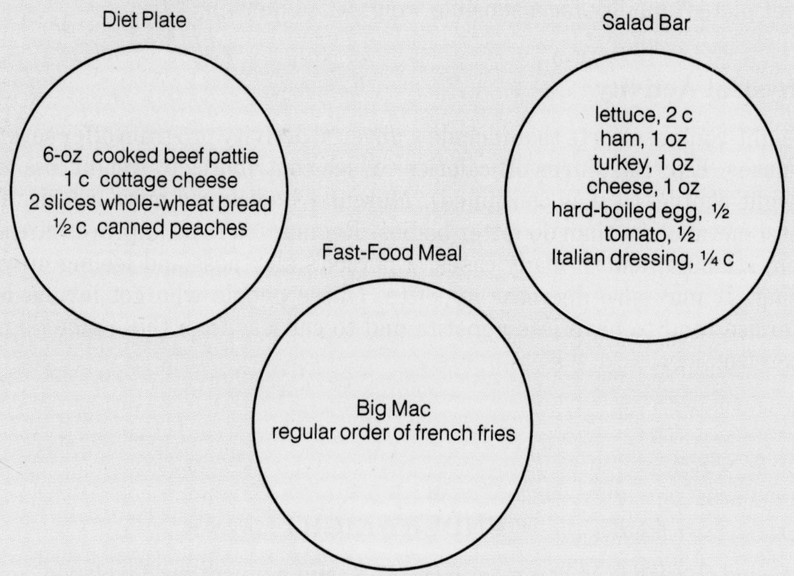

Which meal provides the fewest calories? The diet plate weighs in at about 940 calories, very close to the 980 calories in the fast-food meal. Neither of these is very "diet" for a person interested in low-calorie meals. The salad-bar meal shown has the fewest calories, approximately 630. Most of the calories in the salad-bar meal are in the salad dressing. If you doubled the amount of salad dressing (from 2 ounces to 4 ounces), you would increase the calorie content of the meal to 970—right up there with the "diet plate."

makes the most difference in a child's appearance. Children who primarily lack calories may come to look like "skin and bones" and be uncomfortable most of the time. This condition is called *marasmus*. Children who are deficient in protein—children with kwashiorkor—may actually look normal weight or even fat. They appear fat because their bodies have accumulated a great deal of water as a result of the protein deficiency.

The Causes of Underweight

More is known about causes of underweight than about the causes of obesity. Although underweight can be rooted in psychological causes or stem from disease, its most common cause is simply a shortage of food. The cure for the majority of cases of underweight is food. But that solution is seldom easily achieved. Between people and food is a complex series of economic,

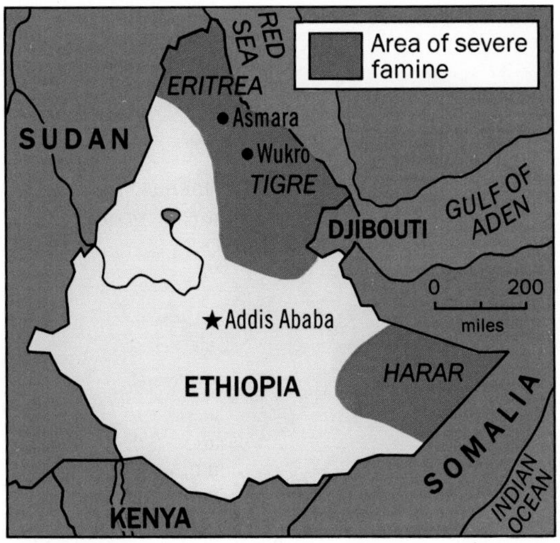

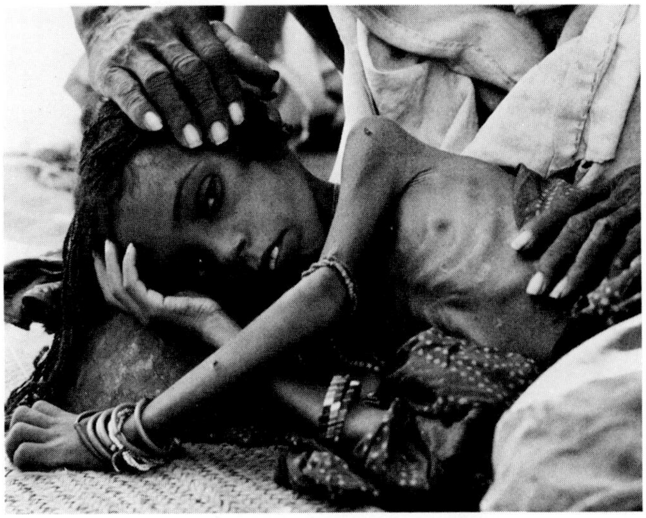

(Left) Area of the famine in Ethiopia in 1987. *(Right)* This girl and her family walked 30 days to escape the Ethiopian army.

political, and social barriers. The complexities of solving food availability problems are the primary reason that millions of people continue to starve.

Starvation and underweight in today's world appear to be more the result of human errors than natural causes such as floods and droughts.[39] Many countries produce food surpluses, and millions of tons of grain spoil each year waiting to be sold while millions of people go hungry. Humans starve when they are unable to produce enough to support themselves and they do not receive food from other people for some reason. The famine in northern Ethiopia can serve to illustrate factors that can affect food availability and lead to mass starvation.

Drought is often regarded as the primary cause of the Ethiopian famine that reached severe levels in the mid 1980s. Drought did play a role, but the dry conditions were not due solely to a lack of rain. The drought conditions were exacerbated by the desertification of the land caused by overgrazing of animals on the poor soil available for farming. Without the grasslands, areas became deserts after a series of dry years, and then they could support neither animals nor plants.

Ongoing political battles in this part of Africa intensified the starvation situation. People in control of the emergency food supplies denied their enemies food or allowed them to receive inadequate amounts of food aid. Other starving people were relocated to areas where the chances of successful farming were no better than where they had been.[39] The famine in this part of Africa is likely to last as long as the political battles and poor farming practices continue, regardless of the rainfall. (Interestingly, it was some rock musicians and the proceeds from their benefit concert and the sale of their record "We Are the World" that made a substantial contribution to improving food availability in Ethiopia for a time.)

Physical Effects of Starvation

As explained in chapter 1, the biological systems of humans developed during times when "feast and famine" was the way of life. Consequently, humans have adaptive mechanisms that help them adjust biologically to temporary food deprivation. If the deprivation extends beyond a certain point,

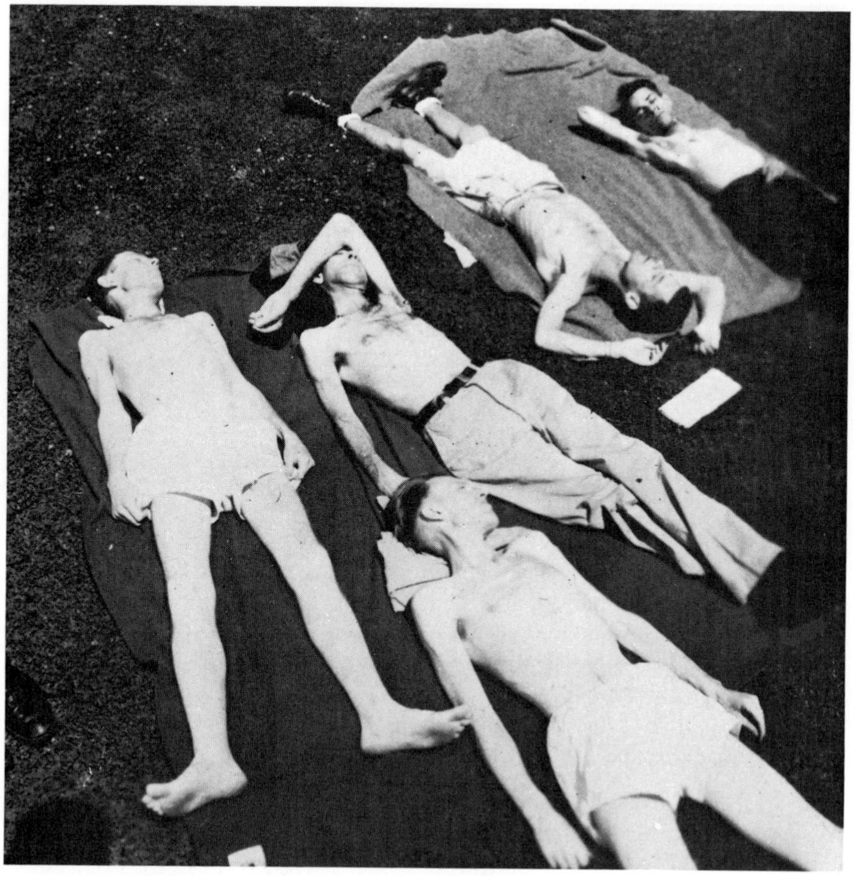

Semistarved volunteer subjects rest in the sun during an experiment undertaken in 1944–1945. Volunteers were conscientious objectors of World War II.

however, human adaptive mechanisms are not sufficient to maintain survival. Healthy adults can survive the longest without food, and children and those who are ill or in poor nutritional health are most vulnerable. Survival during periods of starvation extracts both biological and psychological costs. As you will see, the effects of starvation on the human body are profound.

A Starvation Experiment

The most complete description of the effects of starvation on the human body comes from studies on 32 normal-weight men who were conscientious objectors to World War II.[40] In order to learn how to treat the starving survivors of concentration camps in Europe, these men volunteered to live for a year in a laboratory where they would submit to semistarvation and periodic examinations. During the first six months, the men received about 50% of the calories needed to maintain their weight; the second six months they received enough calories to regain the weight they had lost. During the six months of semistarvation, the men lost an average of 50 pounds. They became emaciated and lost a substantial amount of body fat and muscle tissue. Their hearts shrank because their bodies used heart-muscle protein as a source of energy. Their heart rates declined by almost half, and their basal metabolic rates decreased by an average of 30%. The declines in heart rate and basal metabolism caused a chilling effect; the volunteers constantly

BOX 4-7

DESCRIPTION OF A STARVATION EXPERIENCE

Samuel Legg was a volunteer in the starvation studies conducted during 1944–45 at the University of Minnesota. His description of the experience paints a vivid picture of starvation. The following is a portion of a talk Legg gave about his experiences in the starvation study.

"In November 1944, I went out to Minnesota to take part in a nutrition experiment. Actually it was an attempt to determine the minimum basis on which large populations can be brought back from a starving situation. . . .

"We got every kind of psychological test it is possible to devise. In these tests we were asked what seemed to be stupid questions, personal inventories, intelligence tests, and power tests to determine our mental ability. We had all of them and took them over and over again. They probably were fairly valuable, because one of the increasingly important aspects of starvation, we found, was our psychological outlook when we were normal and . . . when we weren't, which produced some extremely interesting results. . . .

"The psychological aspects of starvation are unbelievable. We went there because we were concerned about people abroad and wanted to do what we could to help those less fortunate than ourselves, and I think we lost that feeling after about two months. At the end of five months of starvation our attitude was 'to heck with the people abroad; I am hungry.' That was all that was important. The only important thing left was whether I was ever going to get food. I was only interested in myself.

"We had to keep answering questions, and our whole attitude was introspective. We lost our semblance of humanity and became similar to beasts. I remember seeing a guy on a corner in Minneapolis and I got mad at him because he could go and have something to eat. A couple of days later I saw a kid on a bicycle. My first thought was 'how could anybody get that much energy?' Then I thought 'he is probably going home to supper. I hate him.' That is one of the most awful things I know.

"When the war ended we were on the way back—[that is] on the first month of rehabilitation. We were sitting at the supper table when the news came. The end of the war meant a lot to us, of course. We talked about it for as long as twenty seconds, and then the discussion was about what we were going to eat tomorrow. News like that, which was so important, meant a lot to us, and to think that for only twenty seconds we talked about it and that was all. . . .

"What does all that mean? It comes to this. If you are going to bring people back [from starvation], you must send them tremendous amounts of food. Quality of food is not as important as quantity."

complained of being cold, and they needed three or four blankets at night in the heat of July. This experience with feeling cold led the men to voice concern for people in the cold climates of Europe who were short on fuel and food during the war.

During the semistarvation period the men experienced unremitting hunger, rapid and dramatic mood swings, sleeplessness, depression, irritability, and a nagging sense of being old. They reported thinking and dreaming of little else but food and eating (Table 4-7). Samuel Legg, one of the subjects in the study, brought the realities of starvation closer to home in a speech, parts of which appear in Box 4-7.

TABLE 4-7

Effects of semistarvation

Physical Effects	Psychological Effects
weight loss	intense preoccupation with food
use of body's fat and protein tissues to meet energy needs	poor ability to concentrate
	confusion
decreased basal metabolic rate	irritability
decreased physical activity	sense of being old
decreased heart rate	sleep disturbances
intolerance to cold	depression

■ ■ ■

EATING DISORDERS

Starvation and periods of feast and famine are not always imposed upon people; sometimes people impose these conditions upon themselves. This is the case with the eating disorders that exist in developed countries where a high priority is placed on being slim.

anorexia nervosa: (*an*, "not"; *orexis*, "appetite"; *nervosa*, "assumed to have psychological origins") A condition in which a person *appears* to have no appetite. People with anorexia nervosa do have appetite, but they don't eat in response to it because they have a pathological fear of gaining weight.

bulimia: (literally, "ox hunger"; also referred to as *bulimia nervosa*) Condition characterized by alternating episodes of dieting and binging on food.

Twenty years ago, few nutrition textbooks devoted more than a paragraph to the subject of eating disorders. Although these disorders were known to have serious effects on health, they were considered rare and of passing interest. This cannot be said today. **Anorexia nervosa** and **bulimia**,* the two major eating disorders, are becoming increasingly common in the U.S.[41] The current estimate is that 1 in 200 teenage girls have anorexia nervosa, and that 1 in 20 adolescent and young adult females experience bulimia.[41,42]

Anorexia nervosa and bulimia have "condition" similarities and "people" similarities (Table 4-8). Both appear to result from deeply rooted psychological disruptions, although physical conditions have not been ruled out as contributing factors. They are conditions that develop during the teen or

■

TABLE 4-8

Similarities between anorexia nervosa and bulimia

Condition-Related Similarities	People-Related Similarities
long-term	females
teenagers and young adults are at high risk	middle- to upper-income families
	obsession with body appearance
serious potential health consequences	feel "fat" whether or not they are
	preoccupied with food, eating, and dieting
	frequently depressed
	low self-esteem

*The official name for bulimia became *bulimia nervosa* in 1987. In this book we refer to the condition as *bulimia*.

early adult years, and they are primarily disorders of females from middle- and upper-class families.[43] Females are 9 times more likely to develop an eating disorder than males,[44] a situation that may be related to the greater pressure placed on females to be thin in certain societies.[45] Among females, professional dance students, college students majoring in dietetics, and women in careers that emphasize body size are at especially high risk for developing anorexia nervosa or bulimia.[46,47]

Characteristically, people with either anorexia nervosa or bulimia are obsessed with the appearance of their bodies and are preoccupied by thoughts of food, eating, and dieting.[44] No matter what their size, they tend to consider themselves as "fat."[43] In most cases this represents a very distorted body image. Anorexia nervosa and bulimia occur most frequently in people who have a history of depression and low self-esteem.[43]

Anorexia Nervosa: Beyond Slimness

People with anorexia nervosa are much more likely to be dangerously thin than are people with bulimia. They act as if they do not recognize that the bodies they see in their mirrors are starving. To them, the mirror shows a body that is overweight. In order to lose weight, a person with anorexia will follow a strict, very low calorie diet and exercise at nearly every opportunity. Most are very knowledgeable about the caloric values of foods and

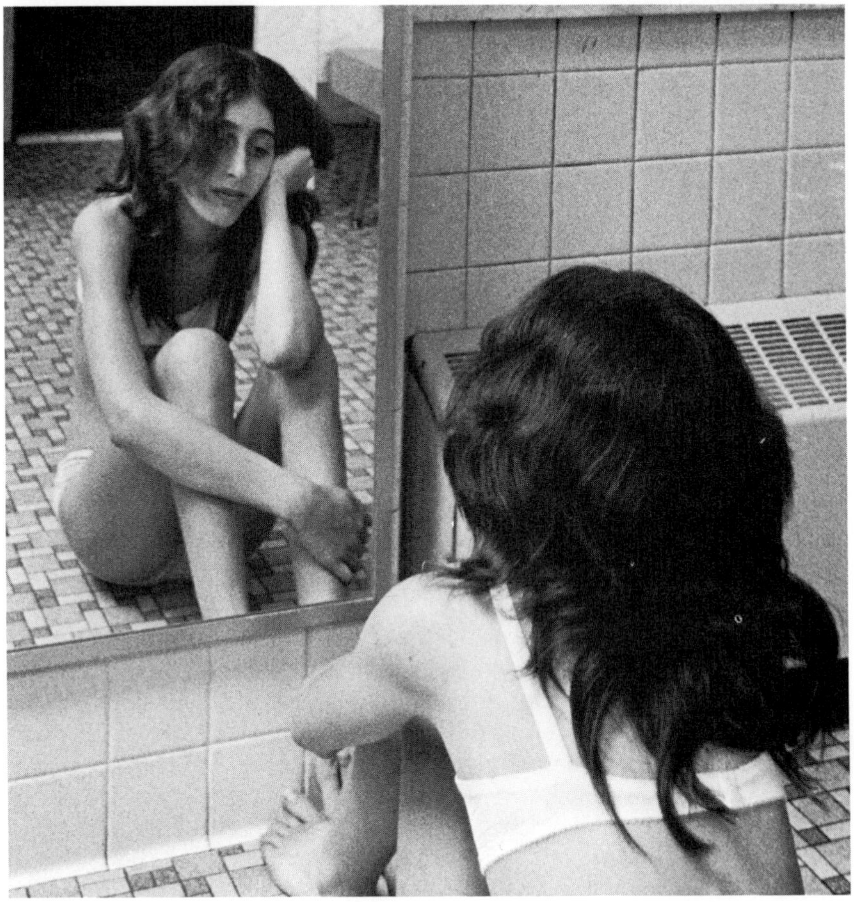

This person with anorexia nervosa looks starved to us, but she thinks that she is too fat.

BOX 4-8

ANOREXIA NERVOSA: A CASE HISTORY

Mary was raised by her grandmother and parents on a prosperous ranch on the outskirts of a small town. Her grandmother had a domineering personality and was very influential in directing Mary's development. Although Mary got along very well with her parents, she felt that her father ignored her and that her mother could have protected her from the grandmother's demands.

Mary showed no signs of an eating disorder until her fourteenth year. She had gained some weight that year and was heavier than many of her classmates. Weighing 120 pounds, she occasionally was teased by classmates for being "chubby." Mary's response was to withdraw from her friends and to stay away from social events. She made it her full-time job to excel in schoolwork—and to lose weight.

As time went on, Mary ate less and less. Within 5 months, her weight had dropped from 120 pounds to 85 pounds. She exercised every chance she got. When seen by a doctor 10 months after she started to lose weight, Mary weighed 72 pounds and looked nearly starved to death. Although she felt tired all the time and depressed, she continued to maintain her rigorous diet and exercise program. Mary was referred to a psychologist and was diagnosed as having anorexia nervosa.

During psychological counseling, Mary revealed that she deeply resented the lack of attention she got from her parents. She felt she had little control over her life and that she could not live up to her grandmother's high expectations. One of the few things Mary had absolute control over was her weight. There was nothing the grandmother could do about that!

After several episodes of gaining and losing weight during adolescence, Mary stabilized her weight at a near-normal level. Spending more time with her parents and gaining independence from her grandmother's demands helped her recover from anorexia nervosa.[43]

carefully avoid high-calorie foods and sweets. They also may avoid foods high in carbohydrates, such as breads and pastas.[48]

One of the hallmarks of people with anorexia nervosa is their steadfast refusal to eat when offered food. Although preoccupied with eating, people with anorexia will deny that they are hungry when presented with food. This persistent refusal to eat is the symptom that causes the most concern, frustration, and rage among their parents and friends.[43]

Females with anorexia nervosa are generally described as "perfect" children by their parents. In school, they tend to be well-liked, to achieve good grades, and to be obedient, respectful, and athletic, as well as stubborn.[43] It is not uncommon for their parents to have unreasonably high expectations for their performance and to be domineering in their control over their children's lives.[43] (Box 4-8 presents a case history that highlights this characteristic.) Rather than fostering self-confidence and independence, the parents of anorexics may be unduly critical of the child's performance and decisions. Although people with anorexia nervosa may feel helpless in controlling large parts of their lives, they assume firm control in one area—their weight.[43]

A questionnaire has been developed for identifying possible cases of anorexia.[46] Some of the responses that people who are at risk of developing an eating disorder tend to give include the following:

- Prefer to eat alone
- Prepare food for others but don't eat it myself
- Am terrified about being overweight
- Am preoccupied with thoughts of food and weight
- Binge occasionally
- Know calorie content of foods
- Feel "stuffed" after meals
- Weigh myself frequently
- Wake up early in the morning
- Think about burning up calories while exercising
- Take a long time to eat meals
- Eat "diet" foods
- Feel that food controls my life
- Am constipated frequently
- Regret eating sweets or "fattening" foods
- Feel an impulse to vomit after eating

Physical Consequences and Treatment The primary physical effects of anorexia nervosa are the same as those experienced during starvation. Heart rate, basal metabolism, and body temperature decrease; muscle tissue is used as a source of body energy; depression settles in, and a preoccupation with food and eating takes over. Growth and sexual maturation come to a halt, as do normal feelings of sexuality.[43,49] If the weight loss that accompanies anorexia nervosa is not reversed, the most devastating consequence of the disorder occurs; approximately 6% of the people with anorexia nervosa starve to death.[50]

Psychotherapy that focuses on correcting disturbed family interactions and building a person's self-esteem and confidence is the cornerstone of the treatment of anorexia nervosa. If these problems are resolved, normal nutrition and weight gain will often follow.[43] About half of people with anorexia recover completely with treatment; the other half continue to live with the disorder well into their adult years.[50] The earlier anorexia nervosa is discovered and treated, the more likely it is that the condition will improve.[51]

Bulimia: The Binge–Purge Eating Disorder

Unlike people with anorexia nervosa, people with bulimia are often of normal weight or slightly overweight, and the signs of bulimia often do not appear until people are in their 20s or 30s. Instead of dieting constantly, people with bulimia tend to interrupt their usual eating pattern by **binging**—eating a large amount of food in a short period of time. The foods chosen for binges are often high-calorie foods such as ice cream, candy, potato chips, cookies, and other desserts. Table 4-9 presents the list a 26-

binge: Consumption of excessive quantities of food in a short period of time.

TABLE 4-9

Three days' food intake by a person with bulimia (Foods listed in the colored boxes were purged.)

Day 1	Day 2	Day 3
	Breakfast	
whole-wheat toast, 1 slice margarine, 1 t low-cal jam, 1 t strawberries, 3 pear, 1 skim milk, 1 c orange juice, 1 c coffee, 1 c diet soda, 1 can	bread, 1 loaf butter, ⅓ c jelly, ⅔ c milk, ? amount orange juice, ? amount coffee, 1 c	bread, 1 loaf butter, ⅓ c cookies, 1 bag apple, 1 coffee, 1 c
	Lunch	
minestrone soup, 1 c crackers, 2 turkey and Swiss cheese sandwich with tomatoes, lettuce, and mayonnaise apple, 1	Chinese food, lots donut holes, 12 soft drinks, ? amount cookies, ? amount	cookies, 1 bag M and M's, 1 bag donut holes, ? amount milk, ? amount yogurt, ? amount
	Dinner	
	ice cream, ? amount cookies, ? amount candy bars, ? amount soft drinks, ? amount McDonalds food, ? amount shakes, ? amount	Girl Scout cookies, ? amount milk, ? amount soft drink, ? amount ice cream, ? amount candy bars, ? amount
	Snacks	
Butterfinger® candy bar, 1 $100,000 Dollar® bar, 1 M and M's®, 1 bag cookies, 1 bag ice cream, ½ gal marshmallows, ? amount toast, ? amount milk, ? amount soft drink, ? amount orange juice, ? amount	apple, 1 water	mixed vegetables, ? amount orange juice, ? amount

year-old woman attending a bulimia clinic submitted as the record of what she ate in a three-day period. Notice that she failed to record the amounts of all the foods she ate during binges; it is likely that she didn't give a lot of attention to the amount she was eating. Bulimics appear to be unable to control their binges once they start. Although the binges are often a source of pleasure, they are usually followed by overwhelming feelings of guilt.

Food binges by bulimics are generally followed by attempts to rid the body of the food that was consumed so that the "terrible" consequence of weight gain can be avoided. To do this, they **purge** themselves of the food they have eaten by self-induced vomiting, taking laxatives or diuretics, and subsequent fasting. Of these, only self-induced vomiting successfully rids the body of calories, and it is the most common method employed.[52] Laxatives and diuretics may help with weight loss, but the loss is from water. Approximately 78% of bulimics vomit daily, some of them many times each day.[53] Common characteristics of people with bulimia include:

purge: Self-induced vomiting or laxative use intended to prevent weight gain.

- Binge and purge regularly (By definition, a bulimic person binges and purges at least twice a week for a period of three months or longer.)
- Use vomiting, laxatives, or diuretics to help prevent weight gain
- Binge primarily on high-calorie, sweet-tasting foods
- Have no control over eating once a binge has begun
- Enjoy the binges but feel depressed afterwards
- Alternate periods of binging with periods of fasting[55]

Box 4-9 presents excerpts from the case histories of four bulimics.

Physical Consequences and Treatment Frequent vomiting causes erosion of tooth enamel and enlargement of salivary glands. Without enamel, the teeth are smaller and they decay easily. Salivary glands are forced to work overtime to produce enough fluids to resupply those lost by vomiting. As a result, the glands may enlarge. The large amounts of fluid that are lost from the stomach can produce another problem: mineral deficiencies. Stomach fluids contain a variety of minerals required for the normal functioning of the stomach during digestion. If not replaced, a deficiency of minerals such as chloride and sodium may develop. The excessive use of laxatives, diuretics, and diet pills also causes health problems for people with bulimia. Laxatives, especially in the large doses taken by some people with bulimia may lead to a dependence on them for normal bowel function. Diuretics are powerful drugs that can affect blood pressure and mineral balance. Diet pills lose their effect with time, but they continue to produce unhealthy side effects as long as they are taken.

Evidence that bulimia may be related to pre-existing physical conditions is accumulating. It is suggested that bulimia may be related to metabolic changes that lead to overeating. The metabolic changes may be initiated by feast and famine cycles.[56] Recent evidence indicates that people with bulimia have trouble knowing when they are full. A chemical substance that contributes to signaling "I'm full" may be produced in abnormally low amounts in people with this eating disorder.[57]

The primary approach to treating bulimia is the formation of good eating habits around regular meals and a nutrient-dense, well-balanced diet.[56] Group and individual psychotherapy to improve a person's self-esteem and

BOX 4-9

BULIMIA: CASE HISTORY NOTES

These notes highlight behaviors of several adolescent females with bulimia. The notes and the cases are real, but the names are not. These represent extreme examples of behaviors that accompany this condition.[54]

Sarah

Sarah, a 16-year-old suffering from bulimia for several years, reported eating foods that totaled over 30,000 calories in a day by binging and purging.

Jane

Jane, a 17-year-old who had "flunked" treatment in two reputable clinics for eating disorders was being treated in a psychiatric institution. She sometimes binged and purged 10 to 20 times per day and she was very thin. She had to be watched by two attendants at all times to prevent the practice and to allow her extremely irritated throat and stomach to heal. Between bouts of binging and purging, Jane would semistarve herself; she had anorexia nervosa as well as bulimia.

Sandra

Sandra used laxatives to help rid her body of the food she consumed during binges. Within a year, she needed 30 to 50 laxative pills (daily) to produce malabsorption. Due to her dependence on laxatives, she had lost all normal bowel function.

Joan

Joan's bulimia had come to be very expensive. The fast foods, candy, and ice cream she routinely binged on cost an average of $70 a day. She stole money from the cash register of the restaurant where she worked part-time to cover the food purchases.

confidence and to modify attitudes about food, eating, and body image are also important components of treatment.[43]

Eating disorder clinics have sprung up across the country, many of them associated with hospitals. Services for people with eating disorders are also generally available through health maintenance organizations, college student health services, and other professional health-care providers.

Anorexia Nervosa–Bulimia Combination

About 30% to 50% of people with anorexia nervosa also show signs of bulimia, occasionally breaking their semistarvation dietary pattern with binges and purges.[42] Generally, these people are severely underweight and experience great difficulty in attempting to change their eating behaviors.

TABLE 4-10
Summary of eating disorders

Anorexia Nervosa	Bulimia	Anorexia Nervosa and Bulimia
1 in 200 adolescent females	1 in 20 adolescent and young adult females	30%–50% of people with anorexia nervosa
very underweight	normal weight or slightly overweight	underweight
very physically active	recurrent episodes of food binges followed by purges	periodic interruption of very low calorie diets with binging and purging
very low food intake	preference for sweets and high-calorie foods for binges	existence of both is more serious than existence of just one
carbohydrate "phobia"	enlarged salivary glands	
avoidance of high-calorie foods	tooth erosion	
starvation effects on health	dental decay	
cessation of growth		
cessation of sexual maturation		
absence of sexual feelings		
may binge and purge on occasion		

They are at the highest risk of developing serious health problems and of dying from the conditions.[46] Table 4-10 summarizes the characteristics of the eating disorders we have discussed.

Prevention of Eating Disorders

Family environment seems to have the greatest influence on the development of eating disorders. Children who are reared in homes where perfection is expected, where independence and self-confidence are not encouraged, and where body weight and dieting are overemphasized are more likely to develop an eating disorder than are children reared under different circumstances.[43] Eating disorders appear to be more common in the U.S. than in other countries,[58] very likely because the culture values thinness. Although this attitude appears to be changing slowly, the prevailing view of a "perfect body" is still one that is unhealthfully thin. Shifting public opinion from "thin is in" to "healthy and fit are in" will help to bring society's expectations about desirable body weights into a healthful, realistic range.

COMING UP IN PART TWO

The nine chapters in Part Two present the nutrients: carbohydrates, proteins, fats, vitamins, minerals, and water. Knowledge of these nutrients is an essential component of the science, and many contemporary issues in nutrition relate to the effects of particular nutrients on health and disease.

The organization of the material presented is consistent throughout the chapters in Part Two. Information on the functions, categories, food sources, recommended dietary intake levels, and the consequences of deficient and excessive intakes is presented for each nutrient. The first three chapters in Part Two focus on the energy nutrients, beginning with carbohydrates, our leading source of food energy.

REVIEW QUESTIONS

1. What are three differences between hunger and appetite?
2. What percentages of body fat are considered too high and too low for adult males and females?
3. What are three methods for estimating percent body fat? Which method is the most accurate?
4. What did you learn in this chapter about the consequences of starvation on the human body?
5. In what ways are anorexia nervosa and bulimia similar? How are they different?

ANSWERS

1. See the Normal Eating Signals section.
2. The answer can be found in Table 4-3.
3. See the Assessing Body Fat Content subsection.
4. Table 4-7 summarizes the consequences.
5. These are broad questions. The answers are discussed in the Eating Disorders section and summarized in Tables 4-8 and 4-10.

PUTTING NUTRITION KNOWLEDGE TO WORK

1. Describe how you feel when you are hungry. How long does the feeling last once you start eating? How do you know when you have eaten enough?
2. The next time you are in a group of more than 25 adults, look around and count how many of the people appear to be overweight and how many appear underweight. Compare your observation with the textbook statement that one in four or five adults is overweight and one in twenty is underweight.
3. Use the common features of weight-loss diets discussed in Box 4-3 to design a fad diet. Then, develop one that is based on the sensible approach to weight control. In what ways are the two diets similar, and how are they different?
4. You have read about the nature and nurture theories of obesity development. Based on your readings, which do you think has the stronger influence on the development of obesity? (There is no right or wrong answer to this question, but it's instructive to ponder the question.)
5. Enough food is produced by the countries of the world to meet the caloric requirements of every person on earth, yet huge numbers of the world's people die of starvation each year. Cite five distinct barriers that preclude access to the world food supply by populations who are in need of food. Suggest at least one reason for each of the barriers.

NOTES

1. J. R. Vasselli, M. P. Cleary, and T. B. Van Itallie, Modern concepts of obesity, *Nutrition Review* 41 (1983):361–373.
2. Consensus Development Conference Statement on Health Implications of Obesity (Bethesda, Md.: National Institutes of Health), February 11–13, 1985.
3. A. P. Simopoulos and T. B. Van Itallie, Body weight, health, and longevity, *Annals of Internal Medicine* 100 (1984): 285–295.
4. T. B. Van Itallie, Obesity: The American disease, *Food Technology*, December 1979, 43–47.
5. T. B. Van Itallie, Paper presented at the Fourth International Congress on Obesity. New York, October 3–5, 1983.
6. 1983 Metropolitan height and weight tables, Metropolitan Life Foundation *Statistical Bulletin* 64 (1983):2–9.
7. D. Elliot and L. Goldberg, Nutrition and exercise, *Medical Clinics of North America* 69 (1985): 71–81.
8. L. Lapidus, C. Bengstonn, et al., Distribution of adipose tissue and risk of cardiovascular disease and death: A 12-year follow-up of participants in the population study of women in Gothenburg, Sweden, *British Medical Journal* 289 (1984):1257–1261.
9. J. Mayer, Genetic factors in human obesity, *Annals of the New York Academy of Sciences* 131 (1965):412–421.
10. A. J. Stunkard, T. I. A. Sorensen, et al., An adoption study of human obesity, *New England Journal of Medicine* 314 (1986):193–198.
11. J. Shields, *Monozygotic Twins Brought up Apart and Together* (London: Oxford University Press, 1962).
12. S. M. Garn, Effect of parental fitness levels on the fitness of biological and adoptive children, *Ecology of Food and Nutrition* 6 (1977):91–93.
13. J. Himns-Hagen, Thermogenesis in brown adipose tissue as an energy buffer, *New England Journal of Medicine* 31.1 (1984):1549–1555.
14. A. P. Simopoulos, Obesity and body weight standards, *Annual Review of Public Health* 7 (1986):481–492.
15. *Nutrition Monitoring in the United States*, Human Nutrition Information Service, DHHS publication no. (PHS) 86-1255 (Hyattsville, Md.: National Center for Health Statistics, 1986).
16. S. Schachter, Some extraordinary facts about obese humans and rats, *American Psychologist* 26 (1971):129.
17. A. Scalfani and O. Springer, Dietary obesity in adult rats: Similarities to hypothalamic and human obesity syndrome, *Physiology and Behavior* 17 (1976):461.
18. R. G. Campbell, S. A. Hasim, and T. B. Van Itallie, Studies of food intake regulation in man: Responses to variations in nutritive density in lean and obese subjects, *New England Journal of Medicine* 285 (1971):1402.
19. K. P. Porikos, G. Booth, and T. B. Van Itallie, Effect of covert nutritive dilution on the spontaneous food intake of obese individuals: A pilot study, *American Journal of Clinical Nutrition* 30 (1977):1638.
20. T. B. Van Itallie, Obesity: the American disease, *Food Technology*, December 1979, 45.
21. J. Mayer, Obesity Diagnosis, *Postgraduate Medicine* 25 (1959):469.
22. J. R. Vasselli, M. P. Cleary, and T. B. Van Itallie, Modern concepts of obesity, *Nutrition Reviews* 41 (1983):361–373.
23. M. G. Marmot, S. L. Syme, et al., Epidemiologic studies of coronary heart disease and stroke in Japanese men living in Japan, Hawaii, and California: Prevalence of coronary and hypertensive heart disease and associated risk factors, *American Journal of Epidemiology* 102 (1975):514–525.
24. K. O. Brownell, Public health approaches to obesity and its management, *Annual Review of Public Health* 7 (1986):521–533.
25. G. A. Bray, Metabolic response to positive energy balance, in *Controversies in obesity*, ed. B. C. Hansen (New York: Praeger Publishers, 1983), 3–14.

26. N. J. Rothwell and M. J. Stock, Regulation of energy balance, *Annual Review of Nutrition* 1 (1981):235–256.

27. M. Story and J. E. Brown, Do young children instinctively know what to eat? The studies of Clara Davis revisited, *New England Journal of Medicine* 316 (1987):103–106.

28. W. H. Dietz and S. L. Gortmaker, Do we fatten our children at the television set? Obesity and television viewing in children and adolescents, *Pediatrics* 75 (1985):807–812.

29. A. Palgi, B. R. Bistrian, and G. L. Blackburn, Two to seven year maintenance of weight loss, *Clinical Research* (abstract) 32 (1984):632A.

30. D. Johnson and E. J. Drenick, Therapeutic fasting and morbid obesity, *Archives of Internal Medicine* 137 (1977):1381–1382.

31. A. Geliebter, S. Westreich, and D. Gage, Gastric distention by balloon and test-meal intake in obese and lean subjects, *American Journal of Clinical Nutrition* 48 (1988):592–594.

32. E. K. Brown, E. A. Settle, and A. M. Van Rij, Food intake patterns of gastric bypass patients, *Journal of the American Dietetic Association* 80 (1982):437–444.

33. J. L. Raymond, C. A. Schipke, et al., Changes in body composition and dietary intake after gastric partitioning for morbid obesity, *Surgery* 99 (1986):15–19.

34. W. Pories, The effectiveness of gastric bypass over gastric partition in morbid obesity, *Annals Surgery*, October 1982, :389–397.

35. T. Andersen, O. G. Backov, et al., Randomized trial of diet and gastroplasty compared with diet alone in morbid obesity, *New England Journal of Medicine* 310 (1984):352–356.

36. R. W. Jeffery, A. R. Folsom, et al., Prevalence of overweight and weight loss behavior in a metropolitan adult population, *American Journal of Public Health* 74 (1984):349–352.

37. R. Woo, The effect of increasing physical activity on voluntary food intake and energy balance, *International Journal of Obesity* 9 (1985):155–160.

38. B. E. Dickson-Parnell and A. Zeichner, Effects of a short-term program on caloric consumption, *Health Psychology* 4 (1985):437–438.

39. A. H. Ehrlich and P. R. Ehrlich, Why do people starve? *The Amicus Journal*, Spring 1987, 42–49.

40. A. Keys, Human starvation and its consequences, *Journal of the American Dietetic Association* 22 (1946):582–587.

41. *Facts about anorexia nervosa*, Office of Research Reporting, National Institute of Child Health and Human Development (Bethesda, Md.: National Institutes of Health, 1983).

42. C. Johnson, C. Lewis, and J. Hagman, The syndrome of bulimia: Review and synthesis, *Psychiatric Clinics of North America* 7 (1984):267–273.

43. H. Brunch, Anorexia nervosa: A review, in *Ross Timesaver* 18 (1976): 29–34.

44. A. Hall, J. W. Delahunt, and P. M. Ellis, Anorexia nervosa in the male: Clinical features and follow-up on nine patients, *Journal of Psychiatric Research* 19 (1985):315–321.

45. D. M. Zuckerman, A. Colby, et al., The prevalence of bulimia among college students, *American Journal of Public Health* 76 (1986):1135–1137.

46. D. M. Garner and P. E. Garfinkel, The eating attitudes test: An index of the symptoms of anorexia nervosa, *Psychological Medical* 9 (1979):273–279.

47. S. Crockett and J. M. Littrell, Comparison of eating patterns between diabetic and other college students, *Journal of Nutrition Education* 17 (1985):47–49.

48. A. Drewnowski, K. A. Halmi, et al., Taste and eating disorders, *American Journal of Clinical Nutrition* 46 (1987):442–450.

49. J. L. Treasure, P. A. Gordon, et al., Cystic ovaries: A phase of anorexia nervosa, *Lancet* ii (1985):1379–1382.

50. D. M. Schwartz and M. G. Thompson, Do Anorectics Get Well? Current Research and Future Needs, *American Journal of Psychiatry* 138 (March 1981):319–323.

51. A. H. Crisp, Psychopathology of weight-related amenorrhoea, in *Advances in Gynaecological Endocrinology*, ed. H. S. Jacobs (London: Royal College of Obstetricians and Gynaecologists, 1978), 111–117.
52. J. H. Lacey and E. Gibson, Controlling weight by purgation and vomiting: A comparative study of bulimics, *Journal of Psychiatric Research* 19 (1985):337–341.
53. R. L. Pyle, J. E. Mitchell, and E. D. Eckert, Bulimia: A report of thirty-four cases, *Journal of Clinical Psychiatry* 42 (1981):60–64.
54. M. Story, Personal communication, 1987.
55. *Diagnostic and Statistical Manual for Mental Disorders*, 3rd ed. (OSM III-R) (Washington, D.C.: American Psychiatric Association, 1987), 65–69.
56. K. Healy, R. M. Contry, and N. Walsh, The prevalence of binge-eating and bulimia in 1063 college students, *Journal of Psychiatric Research* 19 (1985):161–166.
57. T. D. Geracioti and R. A. Liddle, Impaired cholecystokinin secretion in bulimia nervosa, *New England Journal of Medicine* 319 (1988):683–688.
58. S. Dalvit-McPhillips, A dietary approach to bulimia treatment, *Physiology and Behavior* 33 (1984):769–775.

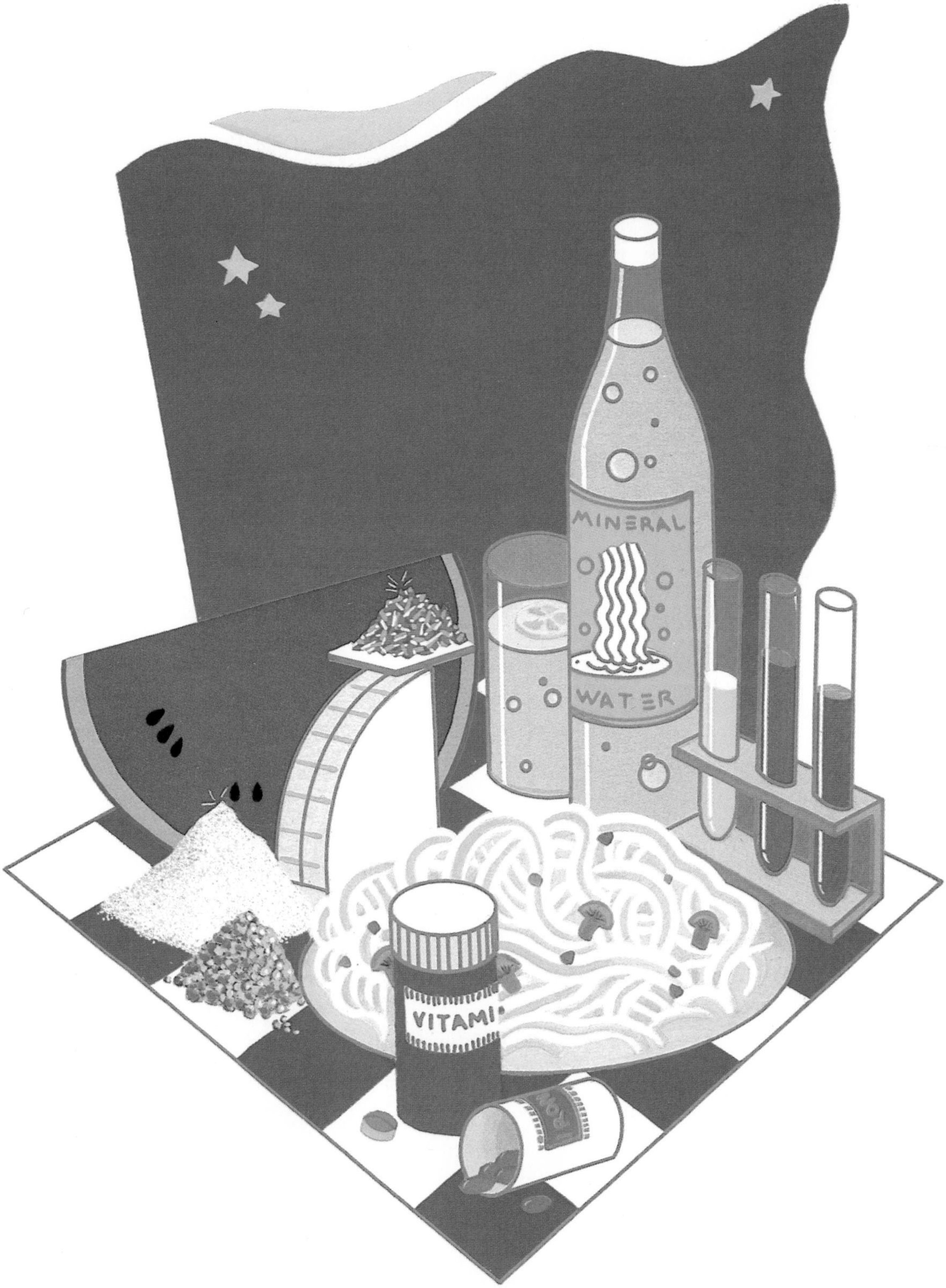
MINERAL
WATER
VITAMI

PART TWO

THE NUTRIENTS

CHAPTER 5

CARBOHYDRATES

Carbohydrates are the leading source of energy for most of the world's people. Foods rich in carbohydrates such as rice, beans, millet, cassava, pasta, and breads are staples of most human diets. In the U.S. and some other economically developed countries, however, carbohydrates take a back seat to foods that are rich in protein and fat.

Carbohydrates are composed of three elements: carbon, hydrogen, and oxygen. They are produced in plants from carbon dioxide, water, sunlight, and chlorophyll through the process of photosynthesis. Plants supply all but a small fraction of our total carbohydrate intake; most animal products are poor sources of carbohydrates.

HOW THE BODY USES CARBOHYDRATES

Carbohydrates serve one major function in the body: they provide energy. Unlike protein and fat, carbohydrates can be converted to energy by every cell in the body. The cells of the central nervous system, certain cells in the kidneys, and red blood cells must have a constant supply of carbohydrates for energy formation. Under normal circumstances, the brain alone uses 4 to 5 ounces of carbohydrate in the form of glucose for energy formation every day. (That's about 500 calories' worth of carbohydrate.) Of particular importance to people living on low-protein diets is the fact that carbohydrates, like fats, spare protein for use in building and maintaining organs, muscles, bones, and other protein-containing tissues. If energy needs are met by foods rich in carbohydrates, then the small amount of protein in the diet need not be used for energy formation.

Categories of Carbohydrates

Carbohydrates are a diverse group of substances. They range from simple sugars to complex, indigestible dietary fibers. They are usually grouped into two basic classes, the simple sugars and the complex carbohydrates. Except for dietary fibers, all of the complex carbohydrates are comprised of chains of simple sugars. Alcohol is a close chemical relative of carbohydrates

TABLE 5-1
Simple sugars and complex carbohydrates

Monosaccharides	Disaccharides	Polysaccharides
Glucose	Sucrose: glucose + fructose	Starch and glycogen: chains of maltose
Fructose	Lactose: glucose + galactose	
Galactose	Maltose: glucose + glucose	Dietary fiber: chains of undigestible carbohydrates and carbohydratelike substances

and is classed along with them. Rarely a "natural" ingredient of foods, most alcohol is ingested as a component of beverages such as beer and wine.

Simple sugars consist of molecules called **monosaccharides** and **disaccharides**. Complex carbohydrates that contain three or more saccharide units are referred to as **polysaccharides**. Two minor categories of carbohydrates are **alcohol sugars** and **alcohol**. Each type of carbohydrate has a particular chemical structure that determines how it is digested and used by the body. Tables 5-1 and 5-2 summarize some basic information about carbohydrates.

■ ■ ■
THE SIMPLE SUGARS

There are three major monosaccharides: glucose ("blood sugar"), fructose ("fruit sugar"), and galactose. The body converts nearly all of the fructose and galactose consumed to glucose soon after they are absorbed. Once converted to glucose, monosaccharides are available for energy formation.

A disaccharide consists of two monosaccharide molecules. Sucrose ("table sugar") and honey are formed from the monosaccharides glucose and

monosaccharide: (*mono* = "one," *saccharide* = "sugar") A carbohydrate whose chemical structure contains one sugar molecule. Monosaccharides are the basic chemical units from which all sugars are built.

disaccharide: (*di* = "two") A sugar consisting of two monosaccharide molecules.

polysaccharides: (*poly* = "many") Complex carbohydrates (starches, dietary fibers, and glycogen) consisting of three or more monosaccharides or monosaccharidelike substances.

alcohol sugars: Monosaccharides whose chemical structures contain an alcohol group.

alcohol: A chemical substance primarily derived from carbohydrates.

© 1989 H. L. Schwadron **"Just pull my sweet tooth."**

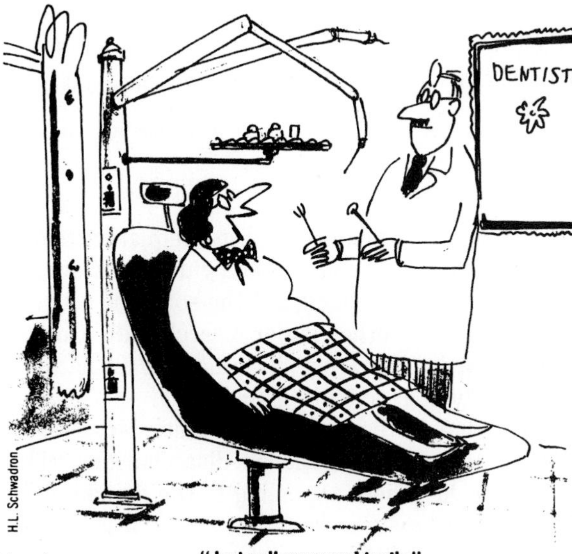

(note: oligo- = *"few")*

TABLE 5-2

Categories of carbohydrates and their primary food sources

Carbohydrate Type	Common Name(s)	Primary Food Source
Monosaccharides		
glucose	dextrose, blood sugar	sweeteners, fruits
fructose	levulose, fruit sugar	high-fructose corn syrup, honey, fruits
galactose	—	Rarely found free in food; it is a component of lactose
Disaccharides	oligosaccharides	
sucrose	table sugar	beet and cane sugar, other sweeteners, fruit
lactose	milk sugar	milk and milk products
maltose	malt sugar	germinating grains
Polysaccharides, Plant Sources	complex carbohydrates	
starches	dextrins	wheat, corn, other grains, beans, potatoes
dietary fiber	roughage, bulk	grains, beans, nuts, vegetables, fruits
Polysaccharide, Animal Sources		
glycogen	—	muscle meat, liver (trace amounts only)
Alcohol Sugars		
mannitol		fruits, vegetables
sorbitol		fruts, vegetables
xylitol		fruits, vegetables
Alcohol	ethanol	alcoholic beverages

fructose. Both table sugar and honey consist of equal parts of glucose and fructose. Lactose ("milk sugar") consists of a glucose molecule and a galactose molecule. Milk and milk products are the sole food sources of lactose. Maltose ("malt sugar") is the other major disaccharide. Comprised of two molecules of glucose, it is the rarest disaccharide. In nature, maltose is found almost exclusively in germinating grains.

Most simple sugars have a distinctly sweet taste. Fructose is the sweetest, followed by glucose, galactose, and the disaccharides.[1] The sweetness of the simple sugars makes them appealing to the human palate. (Box 5-1 explains something candy makers have known for a long time about the chemistry of sweetness.)

BOX 5-1

HOW SWEET IT IS

Ever wonder why the liquid in a chocolate-covered cherry is so extremely sweet? It's because, like honey, it contains an *invert sugar*, a disaccharide that has been chemically rearranged into monosaccharides. Here's how a chocolate-covered cherry is made. Sucrose is mixed with a small amount of enzymes and an acid. A cherry is added, and the whole thing is dipped in chocolate. Confined within the hardened chocolate covering, the enzymes and acid break down the sucrose into fructose and glucose. The chemical reactions produce a syrup that is actually sweeter than sucrose.

Humans, like most mammals, are born with a preference for sweet tastes. Even before birth, a fetus reacts positively (moves toward the source of sweetness) if a sucrose solution is injected into the womb, and withdraws from bitter and sour-tasting fluids. After birth, infants will select sweet-tasting fluids over solutions with other tastes. The preference for sweet solutions may decline with age, but a preference for a sweet taste is a lifelong human trait.[2]

Dietary Sources of Sugar

More than one hundred sweet substances are correctly described as sugars. Sucrose, or table sugar, is the most common. It is manufactured by a process that converts the juice of sugar cane or sugar beets first to molasses, then to brown sugar, then to "raw" sugar, and finally to pure white sucrose crystals. Per capita consumption of sucrose in the U.S. is approximately 5.4 ounces per day, which amounts to about 123 pounds per year.[3]

Most of the sugar in the U.S. diet is added to foods during processing. Of the total amount of sugar produced, 65% is used by the food and beverage industry in the manufacture of soft drinks, beer, wine, bakery products, cereals, candy, and processed foods.[4] A 12-ounce cola, for example, contains about 10 teaspoons of sugar. Standard-size servings of some presweetened cereals contain 4 teaspoons of added sugar. Added sugars can make up as much as 45% of the total calories in a breakfast cereal (Table 5-3). Sometimes you can get a rough estimate of the sugar content of a breakfast cereal by noting the shelf on which it is displayed in the grocery store. The cereals on the lower shelves—at about eye level for six-year-old shoppers—often are the sweetest.

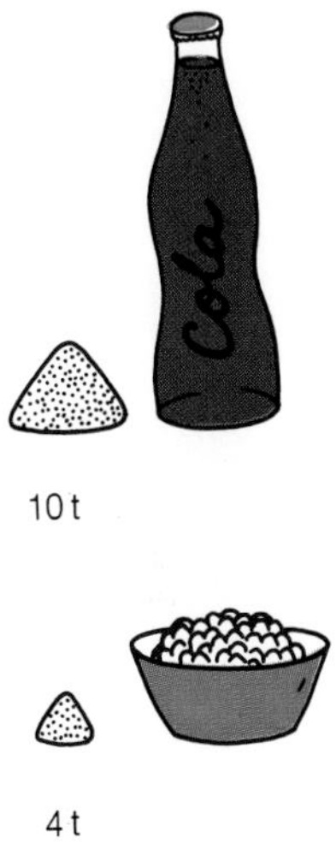

The amount of sucrose in a 12-ounce cola soft drink and the amount in one cup of a presweetened cereal.

Do you know what levulose, dextrose, and sorghum are? They are three simple sugars. If you read nutrition information labels on food packages, you have probably noticed them. A wide array of simple sugars are added to foods, and many have names that make them difficult to recognize as sugars. Table 5-4 lists some of them. As an example, consider this food ingredient label:

> INGREDIENTS: *Bleached flour*, sugar, *vegetable shortening*, dextrose, *water*, high-fructose corn syrup, *carob, whey blend, cornstarch, salt, sodium bicarbonate, lecithin, artificial flavorings and colors.*

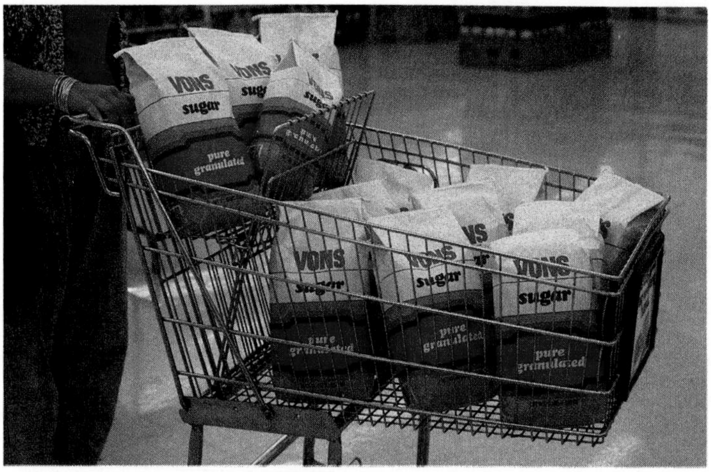

The average amount of sugar consumed annually by each person living in the United States—123 pounds.

TABLE 5-3

Sucrose and calories in one-ounce servings (approximately 1 cup) of selected breakfast cereals

Cereal	Sucrose: Amount, g*	Sucrose: % Of Total Calories	Total Calories*
Raisin bran	9	45	80
Frosted Flakes®	11	40	110
Ice Cream Cones®	11	37	120
All Bran®	5	29	70
Frosted MiniWheats®	6	24	100
Bran Flakes®	5	22	90
Life®	6	20	120
100% Natural®	6	17	140
Grape-Nuts®	3	11	110
Product 19®	3	11	110
Special K®	3	11	110
Wheaties®	3	11	110
Wheat Chex®	2	8	100
Cornflakes	2	7	110
Cheerios®	1	4	110
Shredded wheat	0	0	110

*According to nutrition statements on packaging, 1987.

TABLE 5-4

Names of sugars added to foods

Brown sugar	Fructose	Mannitol	Sorbitol
Confectioner's sugar	Glucose	Mable syrup	Sorghum syrup
Corn syrup	Lactose	Molasses	Sucrose
Dextrose	Levulose	Powdered sugar	Sugar
High-fructose corn syrup	Maltose	Raw sugar	Xylitol
Honey	Maltodextrin		

This product contains three added sugars: sugar, dextrose, and high-fructose corn syrup. Ingredients are listed on labels in the order of greatest weight. Since these sugars are listed second, fourth, and sixth in the list, the product probably contains a good deal of sugar.

High-fructose corn syrup is a relative newcomer to the sweetener scene. Food companies have known about its remarkable sweetening powers for some time, but it hasn't been widely used in foods because it was costly to process. New technology has made it inexpensive to manufacture, and it is taking over a good portion of the sweetener market. Made from cornstarch, high-fructose corn syrup can contain up to 90% fructose, which makes it a very sweet fluid. High-fructose corn syrup is used in candy, soft drinks, bakery products, and cereals and in "sucrose-free" seltzers. A close look at the labels of these seltzers reveals that they are indeed sucrose-free, but they are by no means sugar-free. Many are loaded with fructose, which contains 4 calories per gram just as the other sugars do.

Our inborn preference for a sweet taste and the wide availability of sugary foods can put us at odds with what we think we ought to be eating. Although they please the taste buds, sweet foods are generally thought of as being "bad for you." Some writers and others who tend to draw (and publicize) unfounded conclusions have gone so far as to suggest that excessive sugar intake is the root of hyperactivity, mental illness, and violent and criminal behavior. On top of these problems, it has been claimed that sugar depletes nutrients from our bodies. None of these purported relationships is scientifically sound. One relationship between sugar and health that is beyond question, however, is the one between sugar intake and tooth decay.[5]

Sugars and Tooth Decay

The suspicion that diet may be related to tooth decay was expressed as long ago as 350 B.C., when Aristotle posed the question, "Why do figs when they are soft and sweet, produce damage to the teeth?"[6]

Tooth decay is the leading dental health problem in the world. It has been bothersome to humankind for thousands of years, but it did not become a widespread problem until late in the seventeenth century when great quantities of sucrose began to be imported from the New World.[7,8] Sugar consumption is so closely linked to the development of tooth decay that periods of sugar shortage, such as those that occurred during World Wars I and II, corresponded to decreased rates of tooth decay in the U.S. and Europe (Figure 5-1).[7]

The Development of Tooth Decay Tooth decay—or *dental caries*—is caused by bacteria that live on our teeth. Bacteria enter the mouth along with food, and some of them adhere to the teeth. If allowed to stay there, they multiply and form a sticky material called dental **plaque**. Bacteria living in plaque readily use simple sugars as a food source. They multiply rapidly in the presence of mono- and disaccharides. If not disturbed by toothbrushes or mouth rinses, areas of plaque will spread over the surface of teeth and lead to the development of tooth decay.

plaque: A soft, white, sticky material that forms on the surface of teeth and contains a dense collection of bacteria.

Bacteria in plaque excrete acids as waste products, and these acids are the real culprits in tooth decay. They dissolve the mineral compounds in the enamel and dentin components of teeth (Figure 5-2). This allows bacteria to

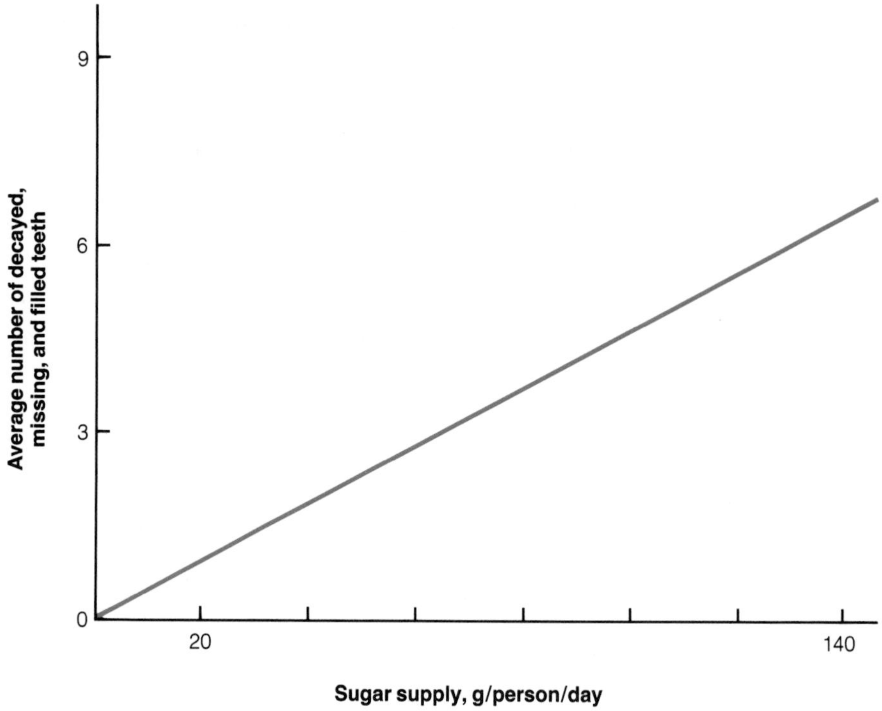

FIGURE 5-1
The relationship between dental problems and the availability of sugar, based upon data collected in 47 countries.

invade the pulp, the soft, inner part of teeth where blood vessels and nerves are located. When this happens, one of the most intense pains ever felt occurs—a toothache.

The accumulation of plaque on teeth also contributes to the development of gingivitis and periodontal disease. Gingivitis is a condition that produces inflamed gums, and periodontal disease reduces the mineral content of teeth. Both are associated with the loss of teeth.

Other Factors and Tooth Decay Fluoride, an essential nutrient, helps to protect teeth from tooth decay. Teeth that contain sufficient fluoride are less susceptible to the eroding influence of bacterial acids. Fluoride is thus a very important factor in the prevention of tooth decay. We'll discuss fluoride in chapter 12.

Certain foods can inhibit the development of tooth decay. Bacteria that cause tooth decay cannot use proteins and fats as food. Consequently, bacteria on teeth decrease in numbers when high-fat or high-protein meals are consumed. Examples of foods that promote and inhibit tooth decay are shown in Table 5-5. Foods that inhibit tooth decay are low in sugar and other carbohydrates.

Whether people who consume foods that promote tooth decay actually develop decayed teeth depends on a number of factors. One of the most important factors is whether sugars are consumed with meals or between meals. Consuming sugary foods and sweetened beverages between meals is more hazardous to dental health than consuming them with meals.[9,10] People who drink coffee or tea sweetened with sugar throughout the day tend to have more decayed teeth than people who drink sweetened beverages only with meals.[10] Candy, cookies, crackers, and syrups eaten between

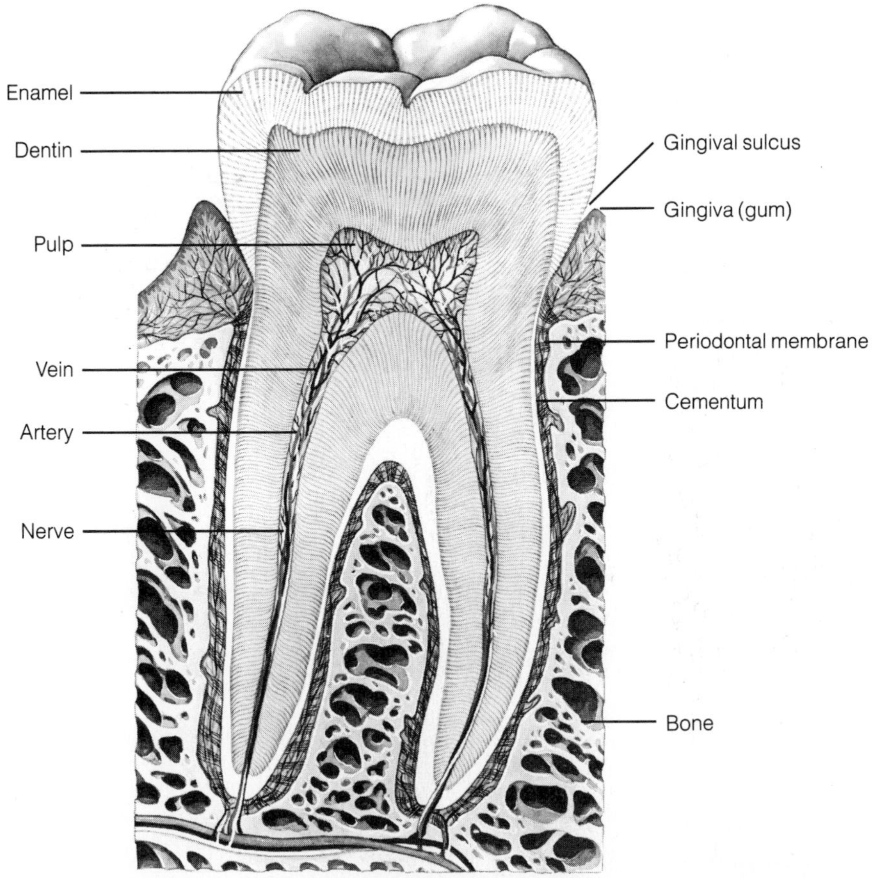

(a)

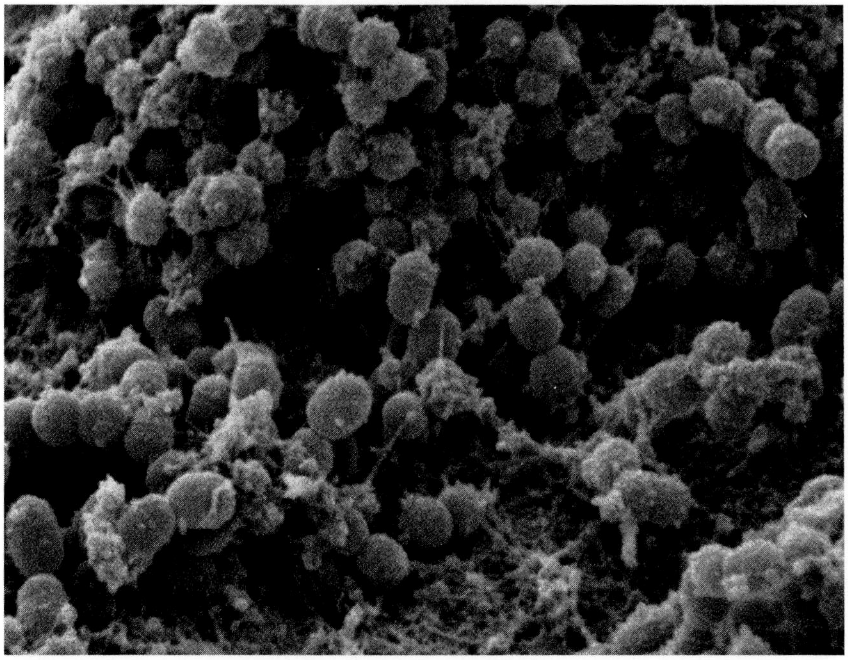

(b)

FIGURE 5-2
(a) Cross section of a healthy tooth. (b) Bacterial plaque on a tooth surface. Acids secreted by the bacteria dissolve mineral compounds in the enamel and dentin.

Chewing gums sweetened with alcohol sugars do not promote tooth decay.

TABLE 5-5

Foods and tooth decay[12]

Foods that Promote Tooth Decay	Foods that Inhibit Tooth Decay
sugar	milk
fruit drinks	cheese
soft drinks	eggs
candy	meat
crackers	nuts
milk chocolate	peanut butter
cookies	fats and oils
cereals	club soda
chocolate milk	coffee
chewing gum	tea
raisins	artificial sweeteners
jelly	sugar-free gum
jam	ice cream
syrups	puddings
pastries	yogurt

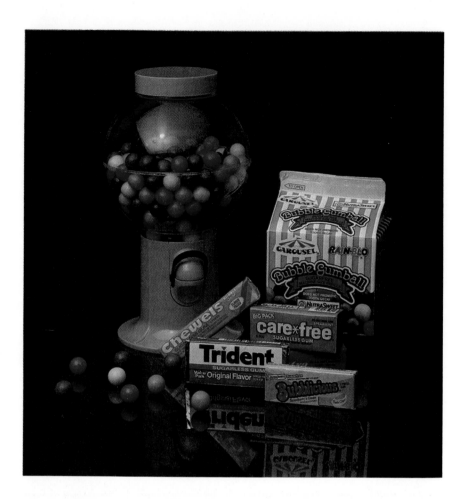

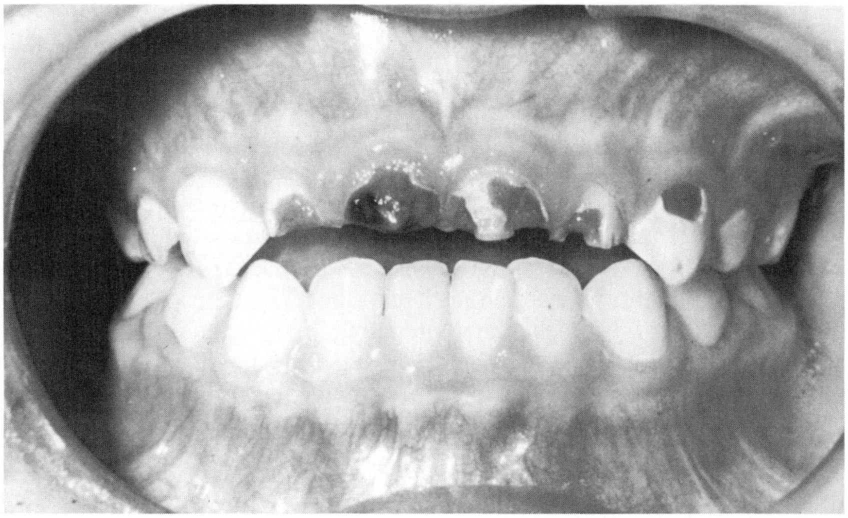

FIGURE 5-3
Nursing-bottle caries of a 25-month-old bottle-fed child. Although rare, this pattern of tooth decay has also been observed in very young children who are regularly breast-fed at bedtime and fall asleep with milk in their mouths.

meals are much more likely to promote decay than when the same foods are mixed with a meal.[9] Chewing as few as two sticks of sugar-containing gum a day also significantly increases tooth decay.[11]

Sugars that are consumed with a meal have less opportunity to stick to teeth, because they are generally wiped off and diluted by other, less sugary foods. Sugary between-meal snacks are not as likely to be cleaned from the teeth or diluted, so they tend to give mouth bacteria a bigger dose of sugar. It takes less than five minutes of sugar exposure for acid production by bacteria to increase, and acid production generally continues for thirty minutes after sugary snacks are eaten.[12] This is sometimes referred to as an *acid bath.*

The tooth-decay-promoting effect of exposing the teeth to sugars between meals is vividly demonstrated by a condition known as nursing-bottle caries (Figure 5-3). Infants and young children who routinely fall asleep while sucking a bottle of fruit drink, sugar water, or other sugary fluid often develop tooth decay. After the child falls asleep, the sugary fluid may continue to drip into the mouth. Due to the pressure in the mouth, a pool of the fluid accumulates between the tongue and the front teeth. As shown in the photo, the teeth that tend to become decayed first are the front, upper ones. Children with nursing bottle caries suffer a good deal of pain and some have been known to lose all of their baby teeth before the age of five.[13]

Trends Tooth decay, although still one of the most serious health problems of our time, is on the decline in the U.S., Sweden, Scotland, the Netherlands, England, New Zealand, and other countries.[14] Decreased rates of tooth decay are strongly associated with declining consumption of sugary foods between meals and the increased availability of fluoridated drinking water and mouth rinses.[8] Switzerland has instituted a national education program that has helped to reduce tooth decay in that country. A "happy tooth" emblem is displayed on labels of foods that have been found to be safe for teeth (Figure 5-4). As a result of this program, a majority of candies sold in Switzerland now contain sweeteners that do not promote tooth decay, and studies show that less candy is being eaten between meals.[12]

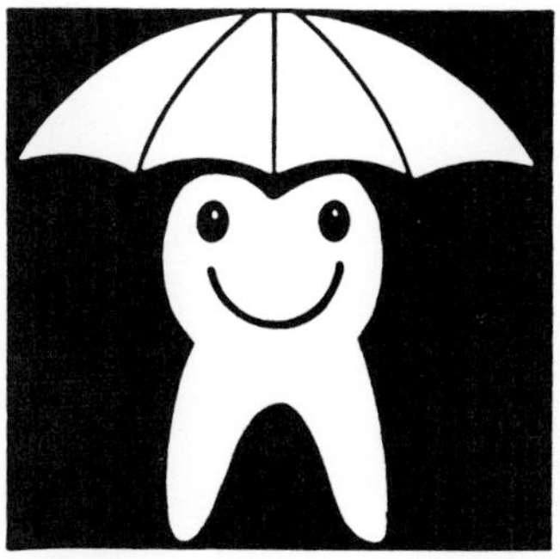

FIGURE 5-4
This symbol is placed on food packages in Switzerland to indicate products that are safe for teeth.

The opposite trend is observed in some economically developing countries. Soft drinks, candy, and sugary snacks are now widely available throughout most of the developing world. Unfortunately, fluoridated water and other tooth-decay-preventive measures are not so common in these countries. The combination of increased sugary snack consumption and inadequate fluoride intakes adds up to a rising incidence of tooth decay.[7]

A growing body of expert opinion indicates that many people in the U.S. would benefit from lower sugar intakes. The reason is not only that sugars promote tooth decay, however. It is also because sugars and most sugary foods provide "empty calories." Such foods take up space in a diet that would be better occupied by fresh fruits, vegetables, grains, and other nutrient-dense foods. Foods that are high in sugar tend to be high in fat as well. In general, fat intake increases in direct proportion to sugar intake.[15] Cutting down on sugar may well be paralleled by a bonus reduction in fat intake.

ARTIFICIAL SWEETENERS

Many chemicals other than simple sugars impart a sweet taste to foods. Of the hundreds identified so far, saccharin and aspartame (also known as Nutrasweet™) are used commercially. Saccharin is a complex, noncarbohydrate substance with no caloric value; it cannot be broken down by the body to yield energy. Since aspartame is a protein, it contains four calories per gram. (You'll read more about aspartame in chapter 6.) Most aspartame-sweetened products contain few calories, however, because very little aspartame is needed to sweeten a product. Gram for gram, saccharin and aspartame are several hundred times as sweet as sucrose.[16] They are at the top of the list when the relative sweetening power of all sweet substances now used are compared (Figure 5-5).[1]

Concerns about a possible relationship between saccharin intake and cancer have led to decreased use of saccharin in foods. Aspartame is now the most common artificial sweetener. It is found in soft drinks, gelatins, whipped toppings, jellies, fruit drink mixes, cereals, puddings, and some medications. Because aspartame breaks down when it is heated and loses its sweetening power, it is not used in cooked food products.[17] Many other

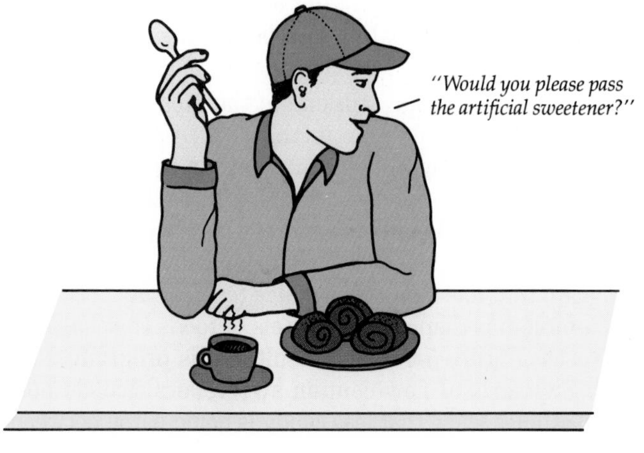
"Would you please pass
the artificial sweetener?"

SACCHARIN

ASPARTAME

XYLITOL

FRUCTOSE

HIGH-FRUCTOSE CORN SYRUP

GLUCOSE

SUCROSE

SORBITOL

MALTOSE

LACTOSE

FIGURE 5-5
Relative sweetness of sweeteners.

artificial sweeteners are being developed and will be introduced onto the market in years to come. It is likely that products one hundred times sweeter than aspartame will be developed.

Artificially sweetened products are often touted as beneficial for dieters because they help a person cut down on caloric intake. In fact, artificially sweetened products *may not* help people control their weight. Two studies have shown that people who use them regularly tend to gain *more* weight over time than people who do not.[18,20]

ALCOHOL SUGARS AND ALCOHOLS

Alcohol sugars and alcohols are chemically similar to the simple sugars, in that they are formed when simple sugars ferment. They are converted to alcohol by enzymes such as those found in yeast.

TABLE 5-6

Alcohol content and caloric value of selected alcohol-containing beverages

Alcohol-Containing Beverage	Amount	Ethanol, g	Calories
Beer			
regular	12 oz	16	150
light	12 oz	13	95
Liquor (86-proof; gin, rum, vodka, whiskey, etc.)	1½ oz	16	105
Wine			
sweet	3½ oz	15	200
dry red	3½ oz	10	110
dry white	3½ oz	10	115
Cordials and liqueurs (80-proof)	1½ oz	17	145

Alcohol sugars occur naturally in very small amounts in foods such as fruits, and they are used as sweetening agents for chewing gums and "dietetic" candies. Their use in so-called dietetic candies is a bit misleading. They contain 4 calories per gram just as the other carbohydrates do, and thus they do not necessarily lower the caloric value of a food product.

The alcohol sugars have a sweet taste. Xylitol is by far the sweetest among them and is the sweetest of all the real sugars.[1] Mannitol and sorbitol, the other two major alcohol sugars, are about half as sweet as xylitol.[19] The extensive use of the alcohol sugars as sweetening agents is limited by their tendency to cause diarrhea and other side effects.[20]

One negative feature of the simple sugars that is not shared by the alcohol sugars is a tendency to promote tooth decay. Bacteria that cause tooth decay do not feed on the alcohol sugars.[7] Thus, chewing gums sweetened with alcohol sugars may pose less risk of tooth decay than regular chewing gums.

Alcohol enters our diets through alcohol-containing beverages such as beer, wine, and whiskey (Table 5-6). These beverages mainly add calories to our dietary intake; alcohol is nutrient-free except for the energy provided in the form of alcohol. Annual per capita consumption of alcohol-containing beverages in the U.S. for persons over the age of 14 years is 14 cases of beer, 12 fifths of wine, and 12 fifths of distilled spirits. This is an increase of 34% since 1960 (Figure 5-6). However, about 80% of the alcohol consumed in the U.S. is by the 30% of adults who consume it regularly.[21]

Alcohol is used by the body as an energy source, but it is not first converted to glucose as the other carbohydrates are. It is converted to fatty acids and enters the citric acid cycle along with other fatty acids. (The citric acid cycle was discussed in chapter 3, pages 78 to 82.) This is why alcohol provides 7 calories per gram instead of the 4 calories that other carbohy-

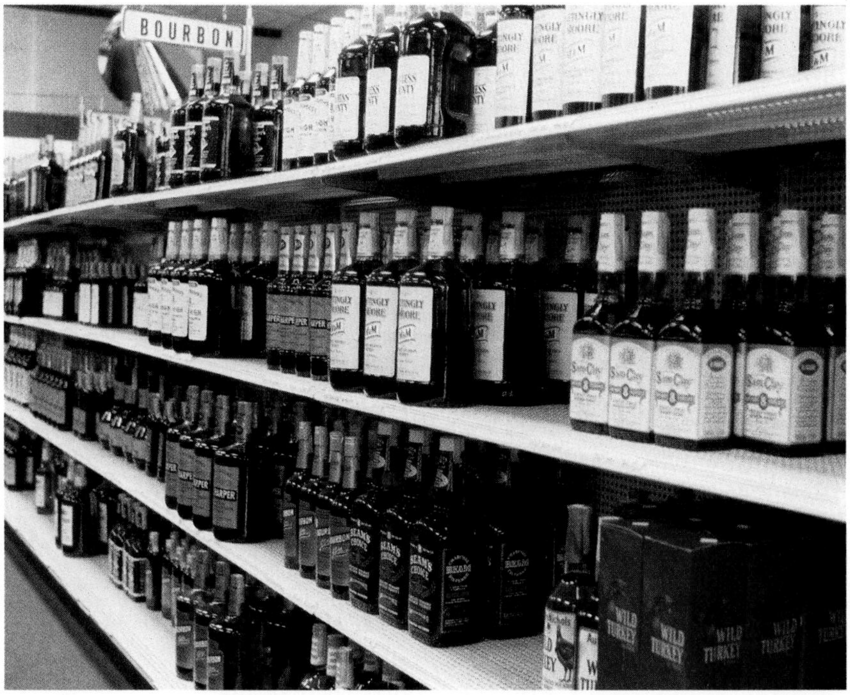

Annual per capita consumption of alcoholic beverages by persons over the age of 14 in the U.S. is 14 cases of beer, 12 fifths of wine, and 12 fifths of distilled spirits. It is believed that 80% of this amount is consumed by 30% of the adult population.

drates do. Alcohol that is consumed in excess of our need for energy is converted to fat and stored. People who drink too much alcohol continue to feel the intoxicating effects until it has been used to form energy or has been stored as fat. A potentially fatal condition can result from high intakes of alcohol in a short period of time, when the body cannot convert it to energy or fat fast enough to keep the toxic effects of high blood-alcohol levels from impairing body functions.

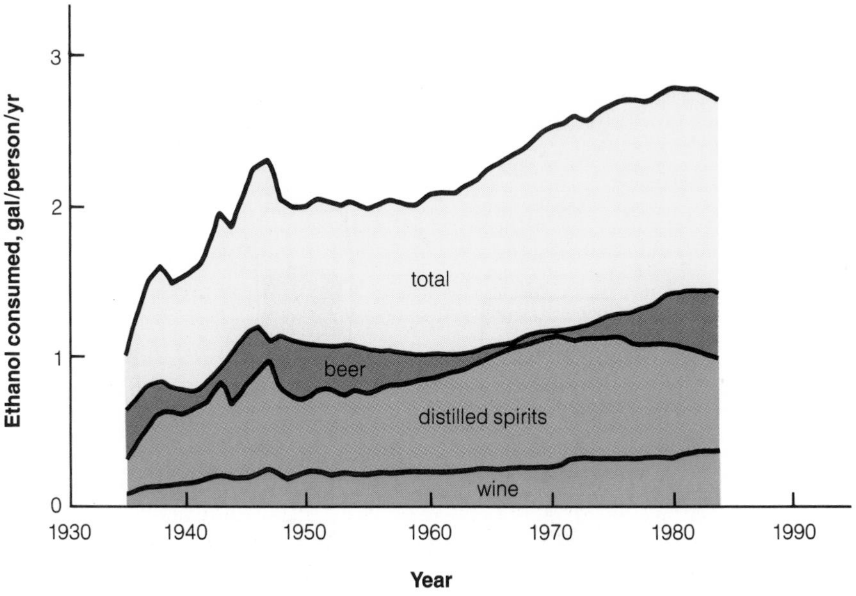

FIGURE 5-6
Estimated U.S. consumption of ethanol from various types of beverages. Data through 1969 are for persons 15 years and over; data from 1970 through 1983 are for persons 14 years and over.

Alcohol-containing beverages consumed in moderation by nonpregnant adults appear to cause no harm, and they may slightly decrease the risk of heart disease.[22] A moderate amount of alcohol is considered one to two standard-size drinks per day. Heavy drinking (usually defined as 6 or more drinks per day) puts people at high risk of developing a variety of social, economic, and health problems. Among the health problems that are common in heavy drinkers are malnutrition, hypoglycemia, ulcers, heart disease, hypertension, certain types of cancer, and cirrhosis of the liver.[23,24] Cirrhosis of the liver is the eighth-leading cause of death in the U.S., and over 90% of the cases are associated with heavy drinking.[21,25] Excessive drinking also increases a person's chances of becoming involved in an accident.

Alcohol, because it provides only calories, does not contribute to our intake of proteins, vitamins, or minerals. You will never find alcohol legitimately recommended as a component of a balanced diet. You will, however, often see the advice that it be consumed in moderation, if at all, and that it be avoided entirely if one is pregnant.

THE COMPLEX CARBOHYDRATES

starch: A polysaccharide produced by plants from glucose; the plant storage form of glucose.

dietary fiber: Polysaccharides and carbohydratelike substances that, because of their chemical structure, cannot be digested by enzymes in the human digestive tract.

The polysaccharides that make up complex carbohydrates consist of plant **starches**, most types of **dietary fiber**, and glycogen. None of these has the sweet taste of the simple sugars. With the exception of the dietary fibers,

These foods are among the best sources of dietary fiber.

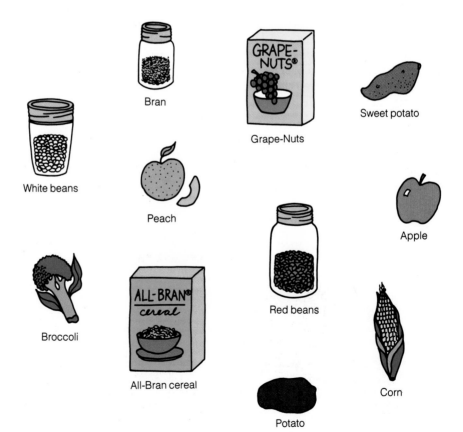

BOX 5-2

CRUNCHINESS AND FIBER VALUE

Not all fruits and vegetables that look fibrous and are crunchy to chew are rich in fiber. Lettuce, for example, looks and feels like it ought to be a high-fiber food, but it is not. Raw carrots have no more fiber value than cooked carrots. Cooking can remove the crunchiness, but it has no effect on the fiber value of foods.

Foods such as dried beans, potatoes, and corn conceal their fiber content very well. Although they are not crunchy and they do not look fibrous, they are among the best sources of fiber.

The bottom line is that you can't tell a plant's fiber content by its looks or its crunchiness. Tables on the dietary fiber content of foods reveal the hidden truths.

complex carbohydrates consist of maltose units linked together in various patterns. Dietary fibers are the most complex of the carbohydrates. Made from many different carbohydrate and carbohydratelike substances, they all have one property in common: they cannot be broken down by human digestive enzymes.

Dietary Fiber

Dietary fibers are found only in plants and come in two basic types. One type is the fibrous components of plant cells, particularly plant cell walls. The other type is nonfibrous components of plant cells that are primarily found inside the cell. (Box 5-2 explains that not all crunchy foods are good sources of fiber.) Fibrous sources of dietary fiber, such as seeds and the bran that covers wheat, rice, rye, and some other whole grains, do not dissolve in water. However, they do "hold" water and will swell up when combined with water. This type of fiber is referred to as **insoluble fiber**. Nonfibrous dietary fibers form a gel-like solution when they are combined with water. Because they form a solution with water, they are known as the **soluble fibers**. Our primary sources of the soluble fibers are the pulp of fruits, vegetables, oat bran, and dried beans. You can see the difference in the water solubility of the two types of fiber in Figure 5-7.

insoluble fiber: Dietary fiber that is not soluble in water. This type of fiber "holds" water and is found in the fibrous components of plant cell walls. Most whole grains and seeds are good dietary sources of insoluble fiber.

soluble fiber: Dietary fiber that dissolves in water and results in the production of a gel. Soluble fibers are mainly found in the pulp part of fruits and vegetables. Oat bran and pectin, a substance found in fruits and used to make jelly "gel," are examples of soluble fibers.

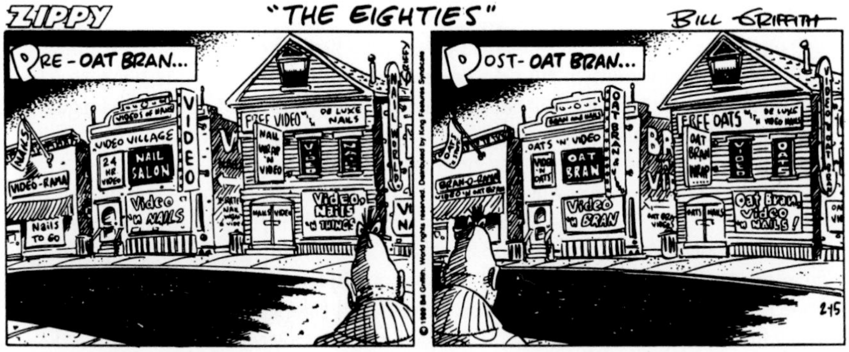

By permission of Bill Griffith and King Features Syndicate, Inc.

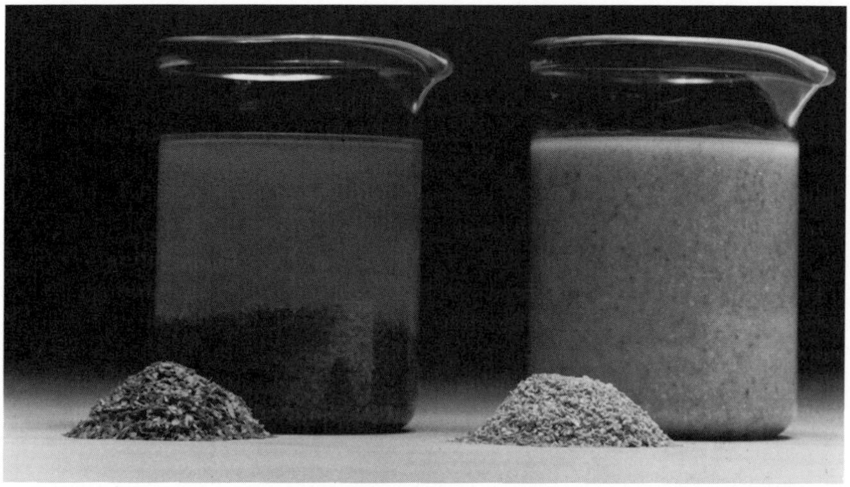

FIGURE 5-7
Water-solubility of fibrous and nonfibrous dietary fibers. Nonfibrous dietary fiber dissolves in water to produce a gel.

The Special Effects of Dietary Fiber Even though dietary fibers are not directly absorbed into the body proper, they have a number of effects on digestion and absorption. The type of effect varies according to what type of dietary fiber is present. Cellulose, a fibrous component of cell walls, facilitates the movement of food through the digestive tract. Gel-forming, nonfibrous fibers such as the pectins in fruit have the opposite effect. They slow down the passage of food through the intestinal tract.[26] Fibrous forms of dietary fiber such as wheat bran tend to bind with certain minerals during digestion and decrease their absorption.[27] Some types of gel-forming fibers appear to decrease glucose and cholesterol absorption, a feature that has contributed to the recent growth in popularity of oat bran, guar, and fibers found in some dried beans.[26,28]

Average dietary fiber intake for U.S. adults is 13 grams per day.[29] An intake of 25 to 35 grams per day is regarded as desirable.[30] Food sources of dietary fiber are shown in Table 5-7. Most of the fiber-containing foods listed there are good sources of a variety of nutrients and are relatively low in calories. (If you are thinking about adding more fiber to your diet, read Box 5-3.)

BOX 5-3

A NOTE OF CAUTION

Some newcomers to increased-fiber diets experience diarrhea, cramping, bloating, and gas for the first several days (or more). This is because it takes the intestines and their bacterial colonies a while to adjust to the larger supply of fiber. Thus, fiber should be increased gradually. Increased fiber intakes should also be accompanied by increased consumption of fluids. If diarrhea and the other symptoms continue beyond a few days, there is likely too much fiber in the diet. The amount of dietary fiber needed to promote peak intestinal performance varies substantially among individuals. Some people develop diarrhea on relatively small amounts, whereas others need a lot of fiber to prevent constipation. It has been noted that the optimal level of dietary fiber intake is the level that produces neither diarrhea nor constipation.

TABLE 5-7
Food sources of dietary fiber

Food	Amount	Dietary Fiber, g*
Grains		
All Bran®	¾ c	11.2
Grape-Nuts®	¾ c	5.9
shredded wheat	1 biscuit	2.7
oatmeal	¾ c	2.1
cornflakes	¾ c	2.1
whole-wheat bread	1 slice	2.0
bran	1 T	1.8
Rice Krispies®	¾ c	0.9
white bread	1 slice	0.6
Fruits[1]		
banana	6″ long	4.0
pear (with skin)	1 med.	3.8
strawberries	10 large	3.3
apple (with skin)	1 med.	3.2
peach (with skin)	1 med.	2.3
grapefruit, canned	½ c	0.5
Legumes[2]		
kidney or navy beans	⅓ c	6.2
peas	½ c	5.7
peanuts	3 T	2.5
peanut butter	2 T	2.3
Nuts		
Brazil nuts	¼ c	2.7
Vegetables		
corn, canned	½ c	4.7
potato (with skin)	1 med. (2¼″)	3.5
broccoli	½ c	3.4
carrots, boiled	½ c	2.8
green beans	½ c	2.7
brussels sprouts	½ c	2.0
cauliflower	½ c	1.4
tomato, fresh	1 small	1.4
potato chips	1 oz	0.9
lettuce, iceberg	½ c	0.8

*Recommended adult intake is 25–35 grams per day.
[1]You may wonder that prunes are not among the top sources of dietary fiber. The distinct effect of prunes on the intestinal tract is not primarily due to their fiber content; it is due to the natural laxative they contain.
[2]Legumes: Seed pods that will split into two distinct halves. Examples include beans (such as kidney, pinto, black, and red), peas, chick-peas, lentils, and peanuts.

■ ■ ■

HOW THE BODY DIGESTS AND ABSORBS CARBOHYDRATES

Carbohydrates are the most rapidly digested and absorbed energy nutrient. See Figure 5-8. They need only to be broken down into their monosaccharide building blocks to be absorbed. When we consume monosaccharides such as glucose and fructose in fruit, no digestive processes are required to make them absorbable. Disaccharides simply need to be broken in two by digestive enzymes for absorption. Polysaccharides, such as starch, contain many monosaccharide units that must be separated by enzymes, so they take a bit longer to be absorbed.

The digestion of carbohydrates begins in the mouth with the action of salivary amylase on polysaccharides. The longer polysaccharides stay in the mouth, the more they are broken down into *dextrins*, short chains of maltose units. Since foods don't stay in the mouth very long, only a very small amount of digestion occurs there. Salivary amylase is inactivated when it mixes with stomach acids, putting a temporary halt to carbohydrate digestion. It resumes when foods enter the small intestines from the stomach.

Polysaccharides and dextrins entering the small intestine are broken down into disaccharides by the action of pancreatic amylase and intestinal amylase. These newly generated disaccharides and those such as lactose and sucrose that are consumed in foods are then reduced to monosaccharides by other enzymes. Each enzyme that acts on the disaccharides is named after the disaccharide it acts upon: sucrase acts on sucrose; lactase, on lactose; and maltase, on maltose.

Most of the breakdown of the disaccharides occurs on the surface of the small-intestine lining. That is where the largest amounts of the disaccharide-splitting enzymes are located. Once carbohydrates are in the form of glucose, fructose, or galactose, they can be absorbed. Nearly 100% of the carbohydrates we consume are absorbed, the exception being the dietary fibers. For the most part, dietary fibers exit the body in the same form that they entered, but they do provide a little bit of energy. Here's why. Al-

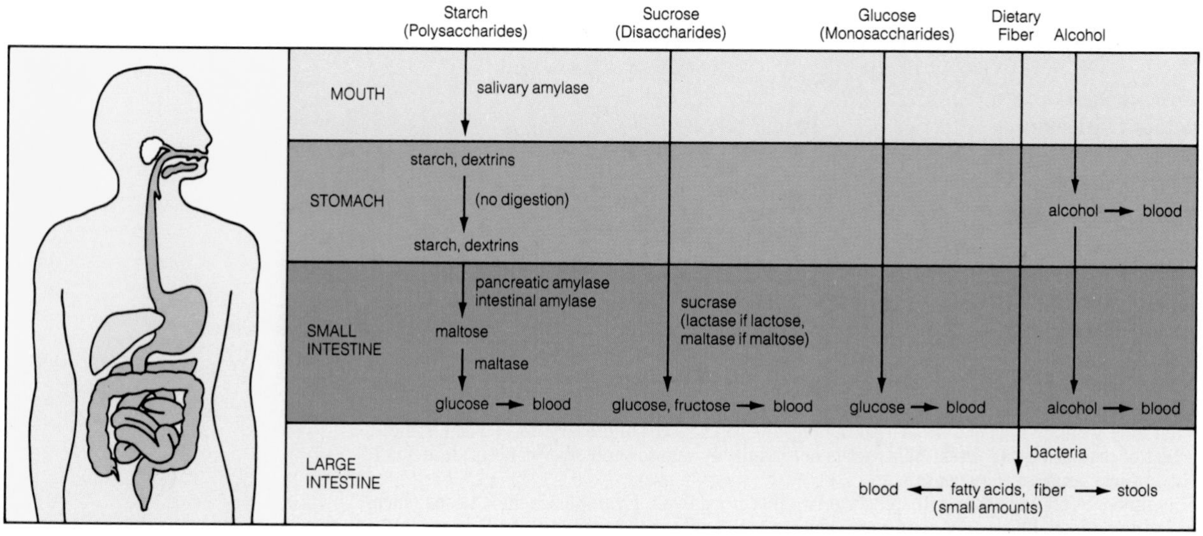

■ **FIGURE 5-8**
Overview of the digestion and absorption of carbohydrates and carbohydratelike substances.

though humans do not produce the types of enzymes needed to break down dietary fiber, certain bacteria that dwell in the large intestine do. Bacteria that consume dietary fibers as food do not break them down completely. They excrete fatty acids and gases as the end products of dietary fiber consumption. The gas produced by the bacteria sometimes causes discomfort after a meal containing a lot of dietary fiber has been consumed. Some of the fatty acids produced by the bacteria are absorbed by the large intestines. The large intestine is not set up to absorb fats very well, so only a small proportion of the fatty acids formed by bacteria from dietary fiber is absorbed.

Carbohydrate digestion doesn't always go as programmed. Problems can occur when particular carbohydrate-digesting enzymes are not available. One of the most common disruptions in human digestion results from the absence of lactase, an enzyme that breaks down the lactose in milk and milk products.

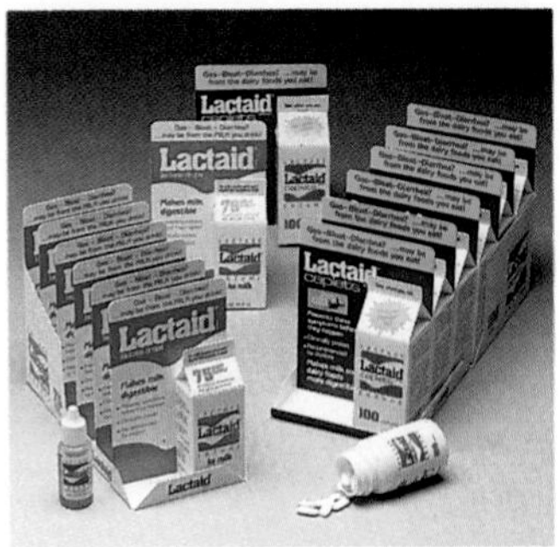

FIGURE 5-9
Milk treated with lactase is available in many large grocery stores, and lactase can be purchased in pharmacies and some grocery stores. Adding lactase drops to milk breaks down the lactose in about 24 hours, making the milk suitable for people who are lactose-intolerant. Lactase tablets can be taken with meals in which lactose is consumed.

Lactose Intolerance

The proportion of people who genetically lack the enzyme lactase beyond the age of 5 or 6 is remarkably high among Asians (85%–95%), Africans (50%–99%), native Americans (85%–95%), and American blacks (70%–75%). Lactase deficiency is less common among Caucasians but still affects a significant proportion. Reports that lactase activity is lost with aging have not been confirmed.[5]

Symptoms of lactose intolerance occur 15 minutes to several hours after an individual consumes more lactose than can be digested. The reaction can be very painful, and some people with a severe intolerance report that lactose makes them feel as though a total intestinal revolt is occurring. Symptoms of lactose intolerance include bloating, diarrhea, gas, and cramps, all of which are related to the effects of undigested lactose. Free lactose in the large intestines is a favorite food of the bacteria residents. Unfortunately, they don't completely break down lactose, either. When they consume lactose, they excrete fatty acids, gases, and other substances. Some of the fatty acids are absorbed by the large intestine, but the gas accumulates and causes cramps and diarrhea.[31]

Not all of the side effects associated with lactose intolerance are considered undesirable—at least not by one researcher. This researcher states, "Although we think of lactose intolerance as a source of distressing symptoms, some degree of incomplete absorption of carbohydrates is not only common, but also desirable. In our constipated society, it may be the ingestion of milk and other sources of poorly absorbed carbohydrates that keeps us regular."[31]

Most lactase-deficient individuals can consume small amounts of milk and milk products because they do produce some lactase. Many can tolerate aged cheese and cultured-milk products such as yogurt because the lactose is partially broken down during processing. Lactase-treated milk and lactase drops and tablets are commercially available and are becoming popular (Figure 5-9). Lactase-treated milk tastes a little different from regular milk; it's sweeter, because the lactose has been converted to glucose and galactose, which are sweeter-tasting than lactose. It is important that people with lactose intolerance consume foods that contain adequate amounts of calcium, such as lactase-treated milk. Studies have shown that they are at risk of consuming too little calcium and are more likely than people who are not lactose-intolerant to develop osteoporosis.[32]

Absorption of Monosaccharides

Glucose, fructose, and galactose are absorbed into the blood stream after a meal and circulated to the liver, the body's central processing plant for nutrients. The liver contains enzymes that process sugars. These enzymes can:

1. convert fructose and galactose into glucose
2. convert glucose to glycogen or fat for storage
3. use the glucose to meet the liver's energy needs
4. add nitrogen and other elements to glucose to produce the nonessential amino acids that make up body proteins (more on this in chapter 6).

The liver has many opportunities to process the monosaccharides because they continually reenter the liver through the circulatory system. Cells outside the liver that receive glucose from circulating blood can use it for energy, convert it to glycogen or fat, and change it to nonessential amino acids, just as the liver does. Figure 5-10 provides an overview of the major ways in which the monosaccharides are used by the liver and the cells of the body.

The Action of Insulin

Cells function best when they receive a certain level of glucose, and even small decreases in the amount can cause problems. Because of its importance, the level of glucose that enters cells is closely regulated. The hormone insulin regulates glucose entry into cells.

Insulin is a powerful hormone produced by the pancreas that dramatically increases the amount of glucose that can cross cell membranes and therefore enter cells. It does so by interacting with special receiving platforms called *receptors* located on cell membranes. When occupied by insulin, the receptors cause the rate of glucose transport across cell membranes

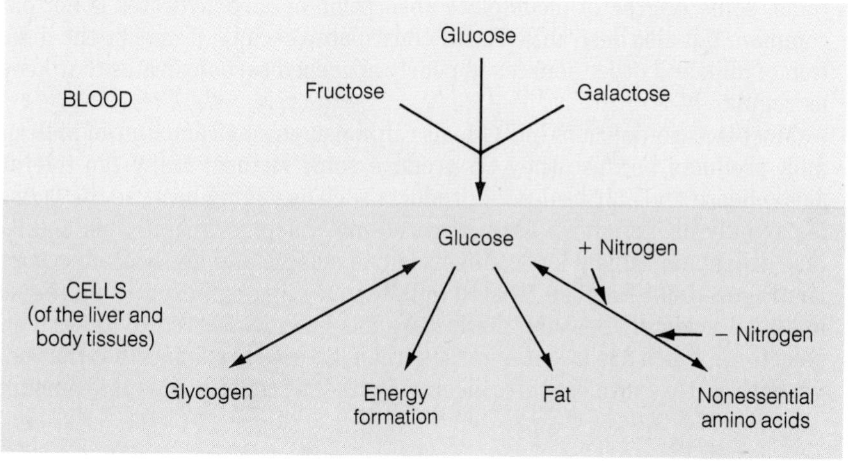

FIGURE 5-10
The major ways the body uses monosaccharides received in foods.

BOX 5-4

EARLY METHODS OF DIABETES DIAGNOSIS

Before the advent of a chemical test to detect glucose in the blood or urine, diabetes was typically diagnosed by tasting the urine of individuals suspected of having the disease. When the taste was sweet, diabetes was diagnosed. Sometimes ants helped out in the laboratory. Because ants are attracted to sweet substances, they were used to identify urine samples that contained glucose.

to increase by 5 to 10 times. Without insulin or its receptors, glucose accumulates in the fluid surrounding cells and in the blood, leaving the cells themselves in a state of semistarvation. The disease associated with this excess glucose accumulation is diabetes mellitus, more commonly referred to as **diabetes**. When excess insulin is secreted, glucose is rapidly taken up by cells. This leaves the fluid surrounding cells and blood with abnormally low amounts of glucose. **Hypoglycemia** is the disorder associated with low blood glucose levels. It is much less common than diabetes.

diabetes: A disorder of carbohydrate metabolism characterized by high blood-glucose levels. It results from the inadequate production of insulin by the body, or more commonly, from abnormal utilization of insulin. Two major types of diabetes are recognized: insulin-dependent and non-insulin-dependent.

hypoglycemia: (*hypo* = "low," *glyc* = "glucose," *emia* = "in the blood") A condition in which blood glucose levels are abnormally low. It can be caused by certain tumors, an excessive level of insulin secretion, or other processes that interfere with the body's utilization of glucose or insulin.

Diabetes

Diabetes is the seventh-leading cause of death in the U.S. and is frequently a contributor to hypertension, kidney disease, blindness, and to death from heart disease.[25,33] Diabetes is a complex, chronic disease for which there is care, but currently no cure. It affects an estimated 11 million people in the U.S.[34]

In diabetics, either the pancreas does not produce enough insulin, or the body does not properly use the insulin that is produced. As a result, excess glucose accumulates around cells and in the blood, and overflows into the urine. (Box 5-4 explains how high levels of glucose in urine were detected in the past.)

Diabetes resulting from an inadequate supply of insulin appears to result from a viral infection that damages the cells of the pancreas that produce insulin.[35] Individuals who develop this type of diabetes seem to be genetically susceptible to the effects of the virus of the pancreas. They are more likely to develop diabetes as a result of the viral infection than are people who are not genetically susceptible. Medications used to treat high blood pressure, arthritis, and some other long-lasting disorders may also contribute to the development of diabetes. The other type of diabetes, the type that is due to poor utilization of existing insulin, is thought to be related to a decreased sensitivity of cell receptors to insulin. Consequently, although insulin is present, it does not function normally in the transport of glucose across cell membranes.[35]

Diabetes resulting from a deficiency of insulin accounts for only about 10% of all cases and is called *insulin-dependent diabetes mellitus*. Diabetes that occurs in the presence of insulin production accounts for 90% of all cases.[36] Because people who have this form of the disease are not insulin-deficient, it is referred to as *non-insulin-dependent diabetes mellitus*. An overview of the two types of diabetes is given in Table 5-8.

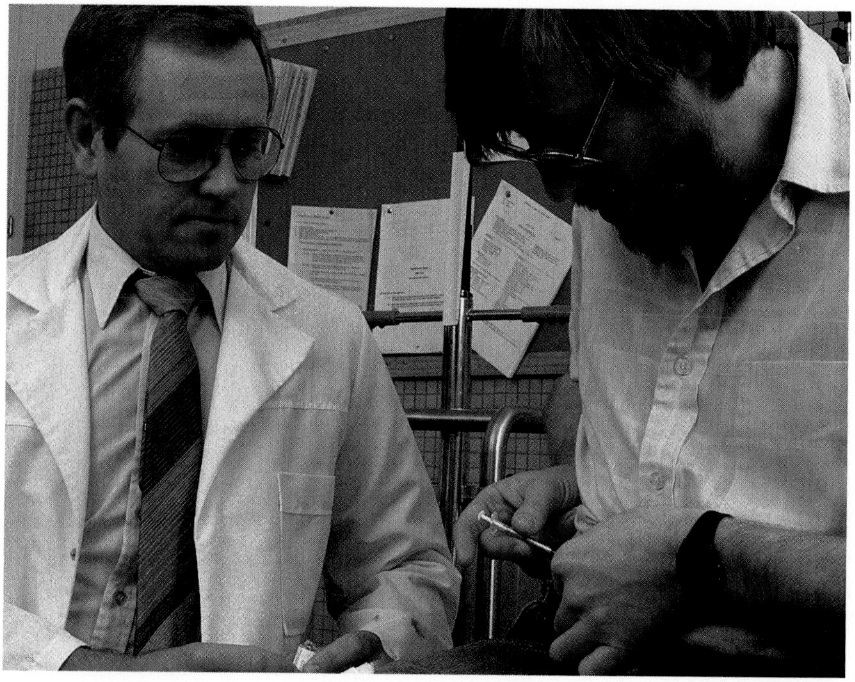

A doctor instructs a diabetic on how to use insulin.

TABLE 5-8
Summary of the two types of diabetes

Characteristic	Insulin-Dependent Diabetes	Non-Insulin-Dependent Diabetes
Insulin deficiency	yes	no
Proportion of total cases	10%	90%
Risk factors	genetic predisposition plus viral infection, long-term use of certain medications	obesity
Treatment	insulin injections, dietary management	weight loss, dietary management

The majority of people with non-insulin-dependent diabetes mellitus are obese adults who have measurable or excessive amounts of insulin.[35] The problem appears to be that they have too few functioning insulin receptors. Overeating, excessive body fat, and low activity levels decrease the concentration of functioning insulin receptors and may contribute to the cause of this common type of diabetes. Receptor numbers tend to increase with starvation, weight loss, and exercise.[35]

The treatment goal for diabetes is the maintenance of normal blood glucose levels. Many of the complications of diabetes, such as poor vision and impaired wound healing, can be prevented, or their onset delayed, if blood glucose values are kept within the normal range. Increasingly, people with diabetes are taking more responsibility for their own treatment by closely monitoring and controlling their blood glucose levels.

For people with insulin-dependent diabetes, blood glucose levels can be maintained within the normal range by insulin injections and dietary management. People with this type of diabetes are taught how to test their blood glucose levels and to adjust their insulin dosages and diets as needed. The keys to blood glucose control among people with non-insulin-dependent diabetes are weight loss, physical activity, and dietary management.

Dietary Management of Diabetes

Current dietary recommendations for the management of diabetes are shown in Table 5-9. It is recommended that 55 to 60 percent of total calories be from carbohydrates (mainly the complex type), 30 percent or less from fat, and the rest from protein (20 percent). Simple sugars do not have to be excluded from the diet. If included, they should be consumed in modest amounts and along with a meal, not separately as a snack. The recommendations call for diets that provide 300 milligrams or less of cholesterol and no more than 3000 milligrams of sodium per day. These recommendations, although intended for persons with diabetes, are very similar to those given in the "U.S. Dietary Guidelines." The diet recommended for persons with diabetes is a model diet for most adults. Many people with controlled diabetes (they maintain normal blood glucose levels) have superb eating habits.

Recommendations for diabetics used to call for a high-fat, high-protein, low-carbohydrate diet. Intake of simple sugars was strongly discouraged. Emerging evidence of the effects of high-fat diets on heart disease, the high prevalence of heart disease among people with diabetes, and research results on the influence of different types of carbohydrates on blood glucose levels have produced a radical change in diet therapy for diabetes.[37] It was previously assumed that all carbohydrates had a similar effect on blood glucose levels. Consequently, it was thought that it did not matter very much which carbohydrates were consumed; that what mattered was the total amount of carbohydrates consumed. All carbohydrates were restricted.[38] A new approach to assessing the influence of dietary carbohydrates on blood glucose level, the glycemic index, has been developed. It is based on the findings that different types of carbohydrates, and even different food sources of carbohydrates, affect blood glucose levels differently. (The influence of various simple sugars and food sources of carbohydrates on blood glucose level is shown in Figure 5-11.) To the surprise of many health professionals and diabetics, foods such as cornflakes and carrots were found to cause greater rises than sucrose or fructose in blood glucose level. The reasons for these results aren't clear. It is clear, however, that different types and sources of carbohydrate affect blood glucose levels differently and that foods with a low glycemic index should be emphasized as preferable sources of carbohydrates for the person with diabetes.[45]

Old beliefs about carbohydrates and diabetic diets have been difficult to topple. Although a low-fat, moderate-protein, high-carbohydrate diet (that may include some simple sugars with meals if desired) is currently recommended, it has been a difficult change for some people to accept because it is so different from traditional thoughts and therapy.[38,39]

TABLE 5-9

American Diabetes Association dietary recommendations for persons with diabetes

Dietary Factor	Recommendation
Calories	Should be prescribed to achieve and maintain a desirable body weight.
Carbohydrate	Should comprise 55 to 60 percent of the calories with the form and amount to be determined by individual eating patterns and blood glucose and lipid responses. Unrefined carbohydrates should be substituted for refined carbohydrates to the extent possible. Modest amounts of sugars may be acceptable as long as metabolic control and desirable body weight are maintained.
Protein	Should follow the Recommended Dietary Allowance (NRC 1980) of 0.8 g/kg body weight for adults, although more may be needed for older persons. Some reduction in protein intake may prevent or delay the onset of the kidney complications of diabetes.
Fat	Should comprise 30 percent or less of total calories, and all components should be reduced proportionately. Replacement of saturated with polyunsaturated fat is desirable to reduce cardiovascular risk.
Cholesterol	Should be restricted to 300 mg/day or less to reduce cardiovascular risk.
Alternative sweeteners	Both nutritive and non-nutritive sweeteners are acceptable in diabetes management.
Sodium	Should be restricted to 1,000 mg/1,000 kcal, not to exceed 3,000 mg/day, to minimize symptoms of hypertension. Severe sodium restriction, however, may be harmful for persons whose diabetes is poorly controlled and for those with postural hypotension (low blood pressure and consequent dizziness when first standing up) or fluid imbalance.
Alcohol	Should be moderate and may need to be restricted entirely by persons with diabetes and insulin-induced hypoglycemia, neuropathy, or poor control of blood sugar, blood lipids, or obesity.
Vitamins and minerals	Should meet recommended levels for good health. Supplements are unnecessary for persons with diabetes except when caloric intake is exceptionally low or the variety of food intake is limited. Calcium supplements may be necessary under special circumstances.

Source: American Diabetes Association Task Force on Nutrition and Exchange Lists. 1987. Nutritional recommendations and principles for individuals with diabetes mellitus: 1986. *Diabetes Care* 10:126–32. Reproduced with permission of the American Diabetes Association, Inc.

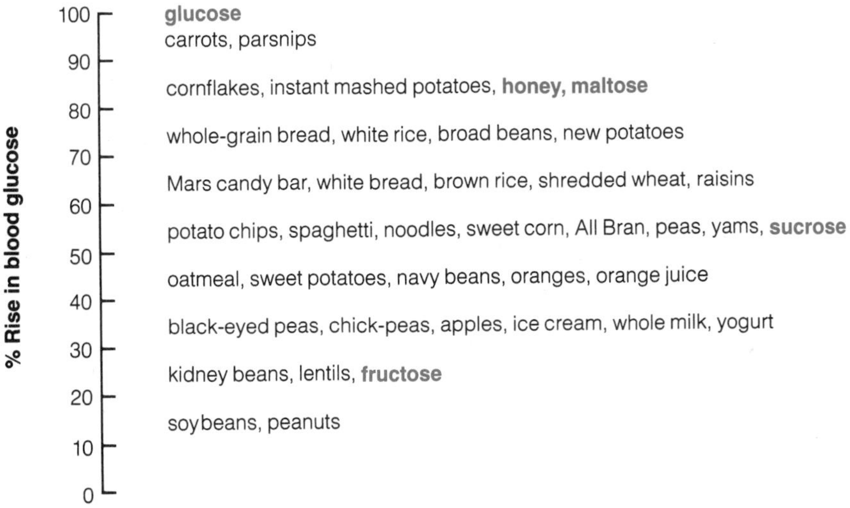

FIGURE 5-11
Glycemic index: A ranking of selected foods on the basis of their effect on blood glucose levels, with glucose serving as the standard (100%). Sugars are in color.

Hypoglycemia

Hypoglycemia is a disorder that gets a lot of attention. Consumers appear to think of it as a common problem, whereas many health professionals dismiss it as rare or "only in a person's head." It has been called the "sugar blues," a "glucose crash," and "low blood sugar"—the condition it actually represents. Hypoglycemia is thought to be a rare disorder because it is not often diagnosed. The true incidence of hypoglycemia is unknown.

Hypoglycemia is most often caused by an excessive availability of insulin in the blood. The oversupply of insulin may be caused by certain tumors or may be due to the release of abnormally high amounts of insulin in response to elevations in blood glucose after a meal or snack. Hypoglycemia also occurs during prolonged starvation, but blood glucose levels become abnormally low only when the condition threatens life.

Hypoglycemia is accompanied by abnormally low blood glucose levels, weakness, and behavioral signs such as nervousness and irritability. Symptoms of hypoglycemia such as weakness and irritability may occur before blood glucose levels become low enough for the diagnosis of hypoglycemia. It appears there is considerable variation in how people respond to low normal blood glucose levels. These symptoms disappear rapidly after food is consumed.[40]

It has been speculated that a high simple-sugar intake stimulates excessive secretion of insulin and may cause hypoglycemia. This notion has not been verified among healthy people in research settings, however.[41] The diagnosis of diet-related hypoglycemia requires that blood glucose levels be low at the same time the symptoms of hypoglycemia are present.[40]

Standard diet therapy for hypoglycemia is five to six well-balanced, small meals per day and avoidance of simple sugars and alcohol.[42]

■ ■ ■

RECOMMENDED INTAKE OF CARBOHYDRATES

Currently, there is no RDA for carbohydrates. Since the body requires energy and it can be produced by any of the energy nutrients, it has been difficult to identify a specific "best" level of carbohydrate intake. The body

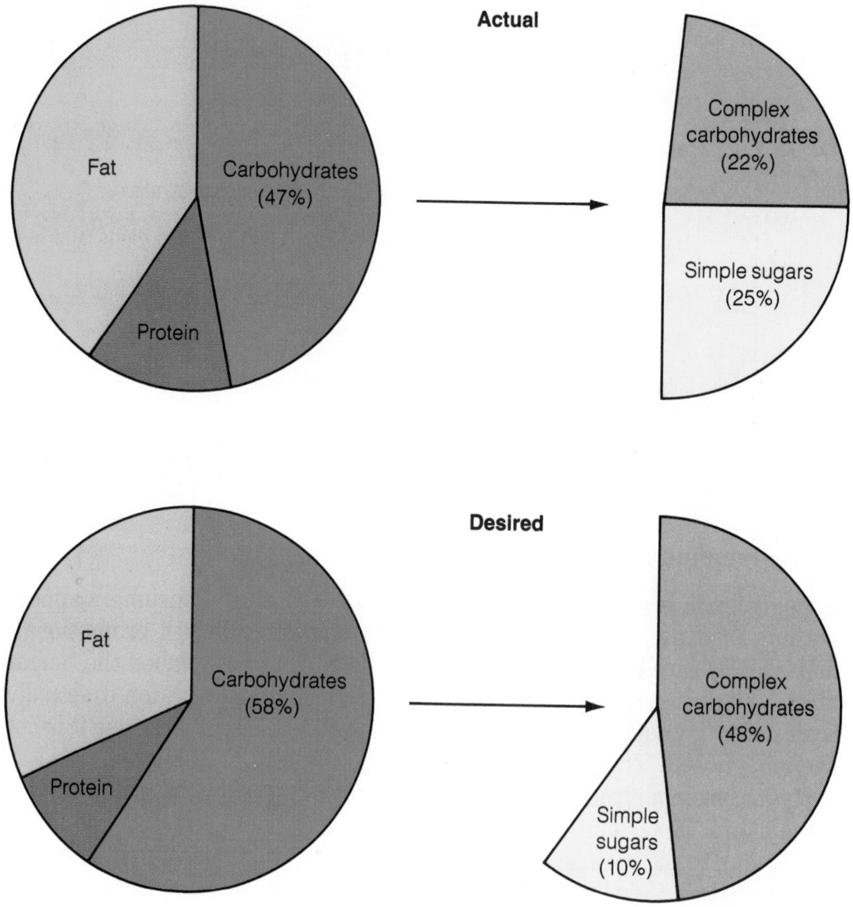

FIGURE 5-12

Actual and desired levels of carbohydrate intake for the U.S. diet.

will spare protein from use as a source of energy when a minimum of about 100 grams (400 calories' worth) of carbohydrates is consumed each day. (The desired level of carbohydrate intake is higher than this amount.) If less than this amount is consumed, the body uses protein and fat for meeting energy needs. The excessive use of proteins and fat for energy formation leads to a buildup of incompletely utilized fatty acids in the body. (The fatty acid fragments are called *ketone bodies*; we will discuss them in the chapter on fats.) When this occurs, people tend to tire easily, get headaches, and become irritable.

Recommendations for diets that promote health indicate that about 58% of the total calories in a person's diet should come from carbohydrates, particularly the complex, "starchy" sources such as potatoes, pasta, breads, and cereals.[23,43] Foods rich in complex carbohydrates are often good sources of dietary fiber, vitamins, and minerals and are not high in calories. Most people in the U.S. are currently getting too few of their calories from complex carbohydrates and too many from simple sugars and fat (Figure 5-12). As pointed out earlier, simple sugars are often a major ingredient of "empty-calorie foods" and if consumed frequently may promote the development of tooth decay. America's high-fat diet has been linked to increased risks of developing heart disease and certain types of cancer.

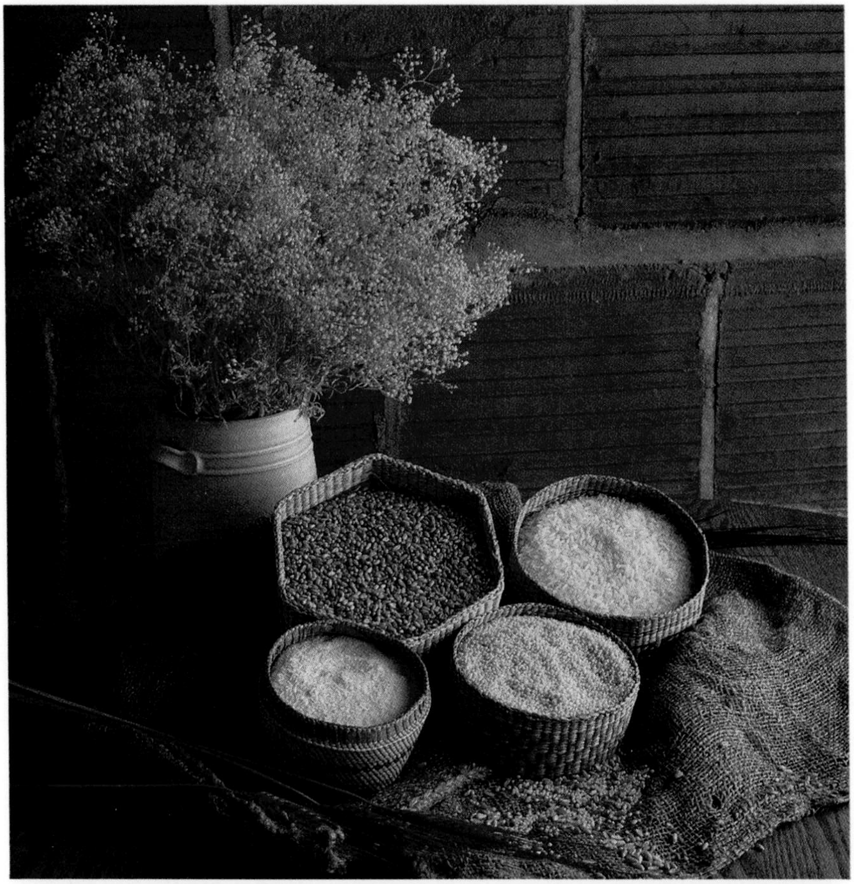

The world's major food sources of carbohydrates (*clockwise from upper right*), rice, cassava flour, millet, and wheat.

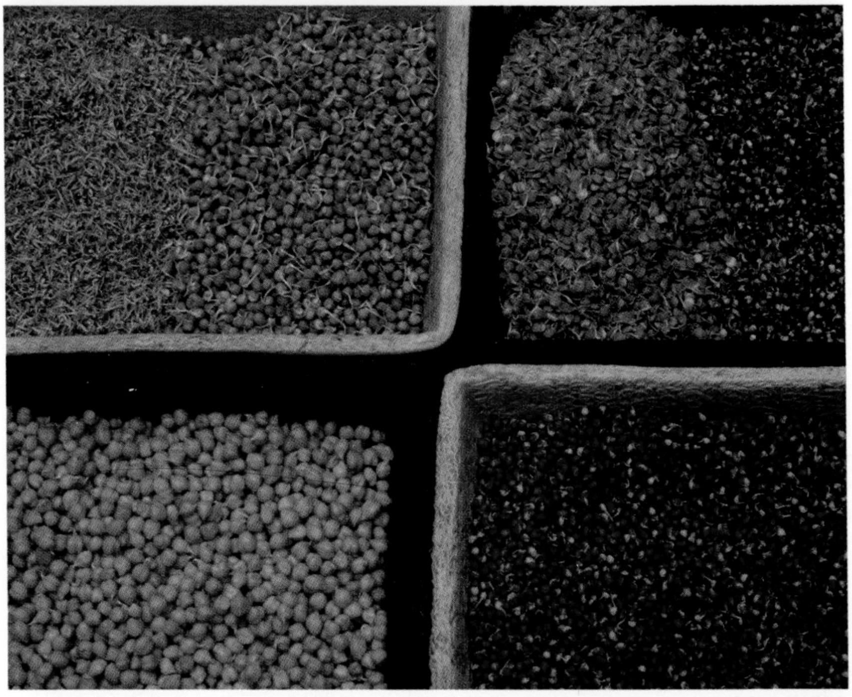

Legumes are good sources of soluble dietary fiber, a complex carbohydrate. This photograph shows chick-peas (also called *garbanzos*), azuki beans, mung beans, lentils, and sprouting alfalfa seeds.

On average, a little over half of our carbohydrate intake comes from simple sugars; they make up about one out of every four calories consumed in our overall diets.[44] The usual carbohydrate intake of people in the U.S. is in sharp contrast to that of most of the rest of the world. In many countries, as much as 80% of a population's average caloric intake comes from complex carbohydrates contained in bulgur, cassava, millet, and rice.

FOOD SOURCES OF CARBOHYDRATES

I never met a carbohydrate I didn't like
—Boynton, 1979

Plants, the original source of carbohydrates in nature, provide far more carbohydrates than animal products. You won't see meats, eggs, fats, or oils listed in the "good food sources of carbohydrates" table (Table 5-10), although you will find milk. Milk is in the table because it contains lactose. But, as you can see from the calorie percentage column of the table, whole milk supplies far fewer of its total calories as carbohydrates than does skim milk. Most cheeses contain very little carbohydrate; the lactose is removed with the fluids that are drained off from cheese during manufacture. All of the grains, legumes, and vegetables listed provide high amounts of complex carbohydrates. They should be the featured sources of carbohydrates in our diets.

TABLE 5-10
Carbohydrate content of common foods

Food	Amount	Carbohydrate Content: Grams	Carbohydrate Content: % Of Total Calories*
Sugars and Sweeteners			
white sugar	1 t	4	100 (100)
honey	1 t	6	100 (100)
maple syrup	1 t	4	100 (100)
corn syrup	1 t	5	100 (100)
Grains and Grain Products			
cornstarch	1 t	3	100 (0)
Apple Jacks®	1 c	26	94 (58)
cornflakes	1 c	15	84 (8)
noodles	½ c	19	84 (3)
white rice	½ c	25	84 (1)
whole-wheat bread	1 slice	12	74 (14)
oatmeal	½ c	12	74 (0)
Cheerios®	1 c	16	73 (5)
Legumes			
lima beans	½ c	17	72 (8)
white beans	½ c	21	71 (8)
kidney beans	½ c	20	67 (8)

TABLE 5-10, *continued*

Food	Amount	Carbohydrate Content: Grams	Carbohydrate Content: % Of Total Calories*
Fruits			
apple	1 med.	20	92 (79)
banana	1 med.	25	93 (85)
pear	1 med.	25	90 (58)
peach	1 med.	10	93 (78)
orange	1 med.	18	90 (76)
Vegetables			
carrots	1 med.	7	93 (61)
baked potato	1 med.	35	89 (4)
corn	½ c	15	86 (19)
broccoli	½ c	4	80 (40)
Beverages			
colas	12 oz	40	100 (95)
fruit drinks	1 c	29	98 (100)
grapefruit juice (sweetened)	6 oz	25	95 (76)
orange juice	6 oz	18	90 (95)
skim milk	1 c	12	53 (100)
whole milk	1 c	11	28 (100)

*Recommended intake is 58% of total calories. The numbers in parentheses represent the percent of total carbohydrate contributed by simple sugars. (Simple sugar content of foods taken from Leveille, G.A., et al., *Nutrients in Foods*; Cambridge, Mass.: The Nutrition Guild, 1983.)

COMING UP IN CHAPTER 6

The spotlight is on proteins in chapter 6. They are a much more diverse group of chemical substances and they perform a wider variety of roles in the body than do carbohydrates. Although they qualify as a category of the energy nutrients, their primary role in the body is in the construction of hundreds of protein substances that are needed for growth and health.

REVIEW QUESTIONS

1. What is the plant storage form of glucose?
2. What is the animal storage form of glucose?
3. Which three elements are found in all carbohydrates?
4. What is the major function of carbohydrates?
5. Why is it said that carbohydrates reserve protein?
6. What are the three monosaccharides?
7. Name the three disaccharides and their monosaccharide components.

8. Which infectious disease is strongly associated with the frequent consumption of simple sugars?
9. What is the most common cause of nursing-bottle caries?
10. Cite three differences between saccharin and aspartame.
11. How many calories per gram do alcohol sugars provide?
12. Does xylitol, mannitol, or sorbitol promote tooth decay?
13. Why does alcohol provide 7 calories per gram, not 4 as the other types of carbohydrates do?
14. With the exception of the dietary fibers, complex carbohydrates consist of ___________ units linked together in different patterns.
15. What are the two major types of dietary fiber?
16. Name two good sources of soluble fiber.
17. Name two good sources of insoluble fiber.
18. The vast majority of carbohydrate digestion takes place in the ______ __________.
19. What are the two primary enzymes involved in the digestion of starches?
20. List three population groups that experience high rates of lactose intolerance.
21. Is it true that people with lactose intolerance cannot digest any amount of lactose?
22. Diagram the major ways the body uses monosaccharides received in foods.
23. What is the major function of insulin?
24. What is the major function of glucagon?
25. What are the two major types of diabetes?
26. Is it true that most people with diabetes have too little insulin?
27. What is the glycemic index? Name three foods with high glycemic indexes and three foods with low glycemic indexes.
28. What is the major cause of hypoglycemia?
29. What percent of total calories should be provided by complex carbohydrates?
30. List five good sources of complex carbohydrates.

Answers

1. Starch.
2. Glycogen.
3. Carbon, hydrogen, and oxygen.
4. To serve as a source of energy.
5. Because protein will be "spared" for use in tissue construction, enzyme formation, and other protein-building activities within the body if carbohydrates are available to meet energy needs. (The protein-sparing effects of fats are discussed in chapter 7.)
6. Glucose, fructose, and galactose.
7. Sucrose (glucose + fructose), lactose (glucose + galactose), and maltose (glucose + glucose).
8. Tooth decay.

9. The practice of giving a child a bottle containing sugary fluids at bedtime.
10. Aspartame is a protein substance, it breaks down when heated, and it supplies 4 calories per gram. Saccharin provides no calories and is not broken down by digestive enzymes.
11. Four.
12. No.
13. Because alcohol is converted to fatty acids, not to glucose.
14. Maltose.
15. Soluble and insoluble.
16. Fruits, vegetables, dried beans, whole oats.
17. Whole grains (excluding oats) and seeds.
18. Small intestines.
19. Amylase and maltase.
20. Asians, Africans, native Americans, American blacks.
21. No; there is wide variation in the severity of lactose intolerance among individuals.
22. See Figure 5-10.
23. To increase the rate of transport of glucose into cells. It lowers blood glucose level.
24. To increase the rate of transport of glucose out of cells—or, to raise blood glucose level. As discussed in chapter 3, glucagon raises blood glucose level, whereas insulin lowers it.
25. Insulin-dependent and non-insulin-dependent diabetes.
26. No; most (90%) cases of diabetes are non-insulin-dependent.
27. See Figure 5-11.
28. An excess supply of insulin in the blood.
29. Approximately 48%.
30. See Table 5-10.

■ ■ ■

PUTTING NUTRITION KNOWLEDGE TO WORK

1. Can you identify the sources of simple and complex carbohydrates from these food labels? Try to identify each product.

   Food Label A INGREDIENTS: Oat flour, sugar, corn syrup, cornstarch, wheat starch, salt, gelatin, sodium phosphate, natural and artificial flavors, artificial colors (and added vitamins and minerals).

   (The label lists 3 complex carbohydrates and 2 simple sugars. The product is a presweetened, fortified breakfast cereal.)

   Food Label B INGREDIENTS: Peanuts, dextrose, corn syrup, hydrogenated vegetable oil (palm oil), and salt.

   (Does this product contain glucose? What is dextrose? The product is peanut butter.)

   Food Label C INGREDIENTS: Sugar, enriched wheat flour, vegetable and animal shortening, cocoa, high-fructose corn syrup, corn flour, leavening, whey, chocolate, salt, lecithin, vanilla.

(Which ingredient is contained in the highest amount in this food product? Sugar. It's a chocolate sandwich cookie that some people dunk in milk.)

Food Label D INGREDIENTS: Meat by-products, water sufficient for processing, fish, poultry by-products, carrots, peas, whole egg, wheat germ meal, vegetable gums, potassium chloride, sodium tripolyphosphate, caramel coloring, DL methionine, choline chloride, vitamin B_1, B_6, E, and D_3 supplements, manganous sulfate, iron sulfate, sodium nitrite, folic acid.

(Any sugar in this food product? Sugars are not added to cat food.)

2. Presweetened breakfast cereals vary little in their caloric content—they tend to contain about 110 calories per ounce. The energy nutrient they contain is nearly 100% carbohydrates. Given this information, about how many grams of carbohydrate would be in one ounce of this type of breakfast cereal?

   (110 calories ÷ 4 calories per gram of carbohydrate = 27.5 grams of carbohydrate.)

3. The nutrition label on a can of light beer states that 12 fluid ounces contain 105 calories, 5.0 grams of carbohydrates, 0.7 grams of protein, and 0.0 grams of fat. How many grams of alcohol does the beverage contain?

   (There are 7 calories per gram of alcohol. The answer is 11.7 grams of alcohol.)

4. How does your diet rate for fiber? How often do you eat these types of food: less than once per week, 1 to 3 times a week, 4 to 6 times a week, or daily?
   a. Whole-grain breads or cereal
   b. Several types of vegetables
   c. Fresh fruit

   (The best answer to these three questions is "daily.")

5. Develop a one-day menu that consists of foods you like that would provide 25 grams of dietary fiber. Make sure you include portion sizes for the menu items. Table 5-7 may help you develop the menus.

6. How sweet is your diet? How often do you consume these things: less than once per week, 1 to 3 times a week, 4 to 6 times a week, or daily?
   a. Regular soft drinks, sweetened fruit drinks, punches or ades
   b. Sweet desserts and snacks such as cakes, pies, cookies, and ice cream
   c. Canned or frozen fruits packed in heavy syrup or fresh fruit with added sugar
   d. Candy
   e. Coffee or tea with added sugar
   f. Jam, jelly, or honey on bread or rolls

   The more often you choose the items listed above, the higher your diet is likely to be in sugars. However, not all of the items listed contribute the same amount of added sugars. You may be getting plenty of sugar if you answered "4 to 6 times a week" or "daily" for several of the categories. This does not mean that you should eliminate these foods from your diet. If need be, you can moderate your intake of sugars by choosing foods that are high in sugar less often, and by eating smaller portions.

NOTES

1. G. E. Inglett, *Symposium: Sweeteners* (Westport, Conn.: AVI Publishing, 1974).
2. H. R. Lieberman, Sugars and behavior, *Clinical Nutrition* 4 (1985): 195–199.
3. *Sugar and sweetener outlook and situation reports*, Economics Research Service (Washington, D.C.: U.S. Department of Agriculture, 1984), 28.
4. Sugar: How sweet it is—and isn't, *FDA Consumer*, February 1980, 21–24.
5. *The Surgeon General's Report on Nutrition and Health*, PHS publication no. 88-50210 (Washington, D.C.: U.S. Department of Health and Human Services, 1988).
6. E. S. Forster, The Works of Aristotle, in *Problemata, UN VII* (London: Oxford University Press, 1927), 931.
7. J. H. Shaw, Diet and dental health, *American Journal of Clinical Nutrition* 41 (1985): 1117–1131.
8. O. H. Leverett, Fluorides and the changing prevalence of dental caries, *Science* 217 (1982): 26–30.
9. A. Ismail, Food cariogenicity in Americans aged from 9 to 29 years assessed in a national cross-sectional study, 1971–74, *Journal of Dental Research* 65 (1986): 1435–1440.
10. A. Ismail, B. A. Burt, and S. A. Eklund, The cariogenicity of soft drinks in the United States, *Journal of the American Dental Association* 109 (1984): 241–245.
11. R. L. Glass, Effects of dental caries incidence of frequent ingestion of small amounts of sugars and stannous EDTA in chewing gums, *Caries Research* 15 (1981): 256–262.
12. C. F. Schachtele and S. K. Harlander, Will the diets of the future be less cariogenic? *Journal of the Canadian Dental Association* 3 (1984): 213–219.
13. Diet and dental health, *Nutrition News* (National Dairy Council) 44 (1981): 1–4.
14. R. L. Glass, The First International Conference on the Declining Prevalence of Dental Caries, *Dental Research* (Supplement) 61 (1982): 1304–1383.
15. A. Wretland, World sugar production and usage in European countries, in *Sugars in Nutrition*, eds. H. L. Sipple and K. W. McNutt (New York: Academic Press, 1974), 81–92.
16. D. H. Jordan Goff, *Journal of Food Science* 49 (1984): 306–307.
17. *Dietary Guidelines for Americans: Sugar*, Home and Garden bulletin no. 232-5 (Washington, D.C.: U.S. Department of Agriculture, 1986).
18. S. D. Stellman and L. Garfinkel, Artificial sweetener use and one-year weight change among women, *Preventive Medicine* 15 (1986): 195–202.
19. C. W. Lecos, Sugar: How sweet it is—and isn't, *FDA Consumer*, February 1980.
20. N. Finer, Sugar substitutes in the treatment of obesity and diabetes mellitus, *Clinical Nutrition* 4 (1985): 207–214.
21. *Prevention '82*, Office of Disease Prevention and Health Promotion, DHHS publication no. (PHS) 82-50157 (Washington, D.C.: U.S. Department of Health and Human Services, 1982).
22. A. L. Klatsky, M. A. Armstrong, and G. D. Friedman, Relations of alcoholic beverage use to subsequent coronary artery disease hospitalization, *American Journal of Cardiology* 58 (1986): 710–714.
23. *Dietary Guidelines for Americans*, 2nd ed., Home and Garden bulletin no. 232 (Washington, D.C.: U.S. Departments of Agriculture and Health and Human Services, 1985).
24. A. B. Eisenstein, Nutritional and metabolic effects of alcohol, *Journal of the American Dietetic Association* 81 (1982): 247–252.
25. *Vital Statistics of the United States, 1980*, vol. II: Mortality, part A, DHHS publication no. (PHS) 85-1101 (Hyattsville, Md.: National Center for Health Statistics, 1985).

26. D. J. A. Jenkins and A. L. Jenkins, Dietary fiber and the glycemic response, *Proceedings of the Society of Experimental Biology and Medicine* 180 (1985): 422–431.
27. J. L. Kelsay, Effects of fiber on mineral and vitamin bioavailability, in *Dietary Fiber in Health and Disease*, eds. D. G. Vahouny and D. Kritchevsky (New York: Plenum Press, 1982), 91–103.
28. R. L. Shorey and P. J. Day, et al., Effect of soybean polysaccharide on plasma lipids, *Journal of the American Dietetic Association* 85 (1985): 1461–1465.
29. E. Lanza and D. Y. Jones, et al., Dietary fiber intake in the U.S. population, *American Journal of Clinical Nutrition* 46 (1987): 790–797.
30. *Diet, Nutrition, and Cancer Prevention: A Guide to Food Choices*, NIH publication no. (DHHS) 85-2711 (Washington, D.C.: U.S. Department of Health and Human Services, 1985).
31. W. J. Ravich and T. M. Bayless, Carbohydrate absorption and malabsorption, *Clinical Gastroenterology* 12 (1983): 335–337.
32. T. M. Smith and J. C. Kolars, et al., Absorption of calcium from milk and yogurt, *American Journal of Clinical Nutrition* 42 (1985): 1197–2000.
33. United Kingdom Prospective Diabetes Study III. Prevalence of hypertension and hypotensive therapy in patients with newly diagnosed diabetes: A multicenter study, *Hypertension* 7 (1985): 8–13.
34. Can strict blood sugar control in diabetes avert or lessen blood vessel damage? *NIH Record 35 (1983): 12.*
35. R. A. Arky, Prevention and therapy of diabetes mellitus, *Nutrition Reviews* 41 (1983): 165–173.
36. J. S. Skyler, C. M. Beatty, and R. B. Goldberg, Managing diabetes: an updated look at diet, *Geriatrics* 39 (1984): 57–68.
37. Nutritional recommendations and principles for individuals with diabetes mellitus, *Diabetes Care* 10 (1986): 126–132.
38. P. A. Carpo, Simple versus complex carbohydrate use in the diabetic diet, *Annual Review of Nutrition*, 1985, 95–114.
39. E. L. Bierman, Diet and diabetes, *American Journal of Clinical Nutrition* 41 (1985): 1113–1116.
40. R. L. Nelson, Hypoglycemia: Fact or fiction? *Mayo Clinic Proceedings* 60 (1985): 844–850.
41. M. J. Hogan and F. J. Service, et al., Oral glucose tolerance test compared with a mixed meal in the diagnosis of reactive hypoglycemia: A caveat on stimulation, *Mayo Clinic Proceedings* 58 (1983): 491–496.
42. *Handbook of Clinical Dietetics*, American Dietetic Association (New Haven: Yale University Press, 1981).
43. *Recommended Dietary Allowances*, 9th ed., Food and Nutrition Board, Na-
tional Research Council (Washington, D.C.: National Academy of Sciences, 1980).
44. S. O. Welsh and R. M. Marston, Review of trends in food use in the United States, 1909 to 1980, *Journal of the American Dietetic Association* 81 (1982): 120–125.
45. D. J. A. Jenkins and T. M. S. Wolever, et al., Low-glycemic-index starchy foods in the diabetic diet, *American Journal of Clinical Nutrition* 46 (1988): 248–254.

CHAPTER

6

PROTEINS

The term *protein* is derived from the Greek word *protos* for "first." The derivation indicates the importance ascribed to this substance when it was first recognized. An essential structural component of all living matter, protein is involved in almost every biological process in the human body, and it makes up more than half the dry weight of most cells. In addition to the carbon, oxygen, and hydrogen found in carbohydrates, all proteins contain nitrogen and some contain sulfur. Proteins come in different shapes and sizes, and each plays a unique role in the body.

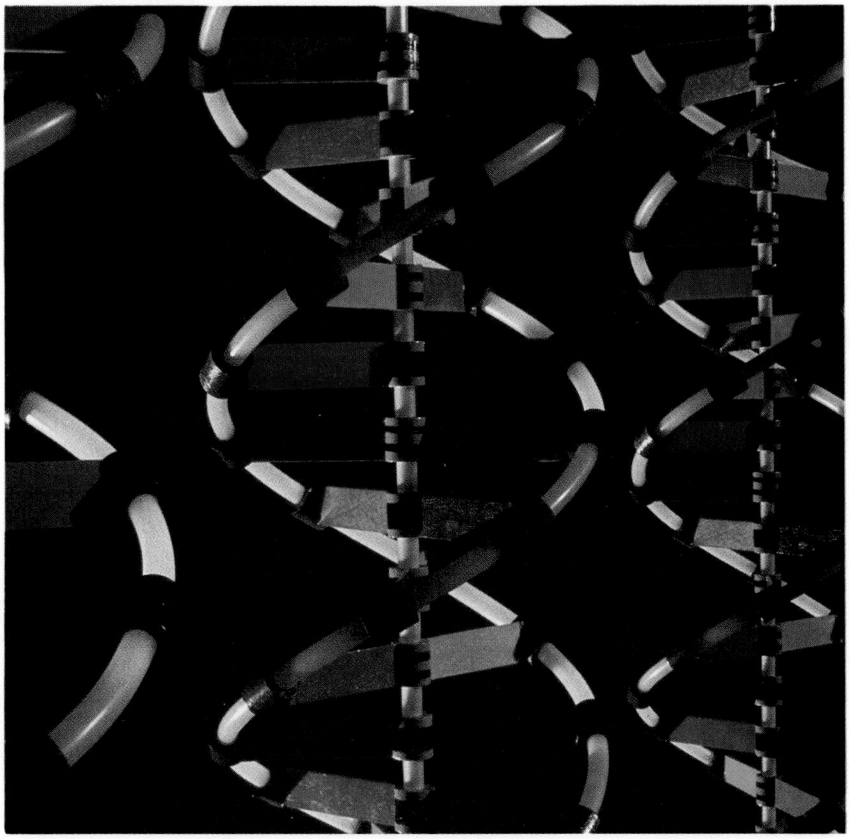

Model of deoxyribonucleic acid (DNA), the amazing genetic material that directs the synthesis of proteins in the body.

HOW THE BODY USES PROTEIN

The primary role of proteins is to provide the building materials for the various components of the body's tissues. Proteins are the basic chemical components of **myosin, actin, collagen, elastin**, and **keratin**—substances in the muscles and connective tissues. They provide the basic building units of **hemoglobin**, enzymes, hormones, **neurotransmitters, antibodies**, and protein "carriers" of certain nutrients in the blood. Proteins are also used in energy formation, but this is not their primary role.

Amino Acids

Proteins are comprised of subunits called *amino acids*. (Amino acids have been described as the "building blocks" of protein.) To better understand the structure and function of proteins, you need to know some things about amino acids.

The "backbone" of a single amino acid is an *amino* group, which contains nitrogen (N), a carbon (C) unit, and an acid group (chemically denoted by *COOH*). In addition, an amino acid contains a "side chain" of varying composition. There are 20 naturally occurring amino acids, and the differences among them are due to what is contained in their side chains. The structures of amino acids vary from that of the simplest, glycine:

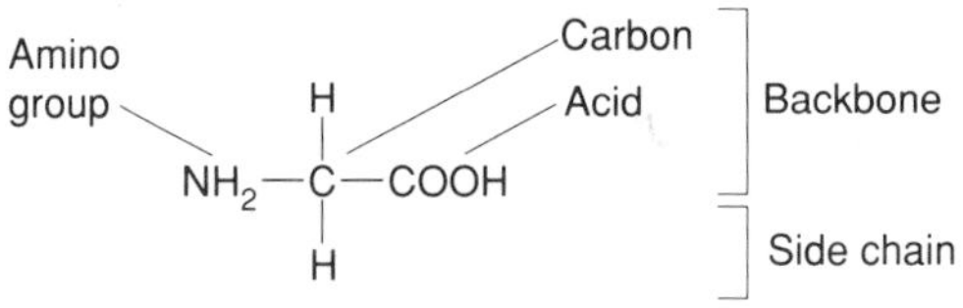

to that of the most complex, tryptophan:

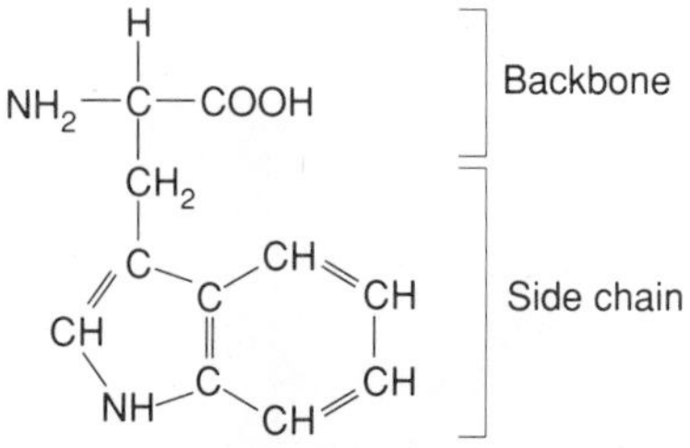

(You may not need to memorize any of the chemical structures shown in this book. Your instructor will advise you as to how important they are in your course. They are included to give you a "picture" of what is being discussed.)

myosin: A protein present in muscle. Myosin comprises about 65% of total muscle protein and is responsible for the elastic property of muscles.

actin: With myosin, the other major protein found in muscle. It combines with myosin when muscles contract.

collagen: Protein found in connective tissue in bones, skin, ligaments, and cartilage. Collagen accounts for about 30% of the total body protein.

elastin: Protein found in elastic connective tissue such as blood vessels and ligaments.

keratins: Proteins in skin, hair, and nails that provide external protection.

hemoglobin: The iron-containing protein in red blood cells.

neurotransmitters: Small molecules most often formed from amino acids that direct cells to perform specific chemical reactions. Epinephrine (adrenalin) and serotonin are two examples.

antibodies: Substances secreted in response to the presence of a foreign protein (antigen). They counteract the harmful effects of bacteria, viruses, and other sources of foreign protein that enter the body.

Calvin and Hobbes by Bill Watterson

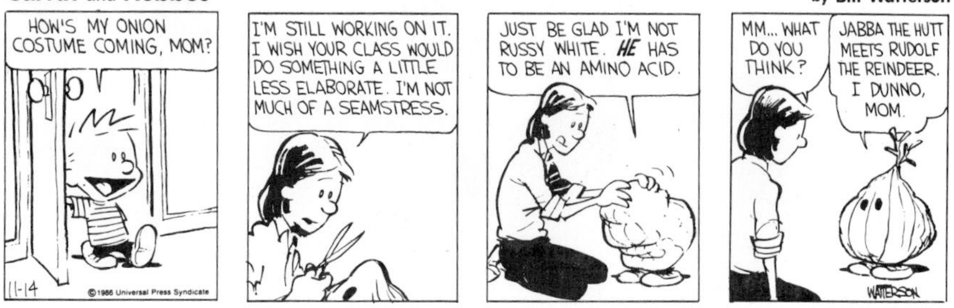

TABLE 6-1
Essential and nonessential amino acids

Essential		Nonessential	
leucine	tryptophan	alanine	glutamine
isoleucine	valine	arginine	glycine
lysine	methionine	asparagine	proline
phenylalanine	histidine	aspartic acid	serine
threonine		cysteine*	tryosine
		glutamic acid	

*Cysteine may be required by infants and may, at some point, be recognized as an essential amino acid.

Classification of Amino Acids Of the 20 naturally occurring amino acids, 9 cannot be manufactured (synthesized) by the body, or cannot be produced in adequate amounts, and therefore must be supplied by the diet. These 9 amino acids are called the **essential amino acids**. The other 11 *can* be manufactured by the body and are referred to as the **nonessential amino acids**. (The essential and nonessential amino acids are listed in Table 6-1.) There are no specific dietary requirements for the nonessential amino acids. Proteins in foods contain both essential and nonessential amino acids.

essential amino acids: Amino acids that cannot be synthesized in adequate amounts by humans and therefore must be obtained from the diet.

The body manufactures the nonessential amino acids from carbohydrates and nitrogen and by chemically rearranging essential and nonessential amino acids. Nonessential amino acids are as important to protein synthesis as the essential amino acids are, but they are seldom given as much attention because the body does not require dietary sources of them. Of the billions of types of proteins that can be made from the 20 amino acids, the body manufactures and uses only several thousand types.

nonessential amino acids: Amino acids that can be readily produced by humans from components of the diet. Because the body can produce them, there are no dietary requirements for them and no deficiency diseases associated with inadequate intakes of them.

Structure of Proteins

Proteins are made up of chains of amino acids connected by so-called peptide bonds that form between a nitrogen atom of one amino acid molecule and the ending carbon atom of another amino acid molecule (Figure 6-1). **Dipeptides** consist of two amino acids, **tripeptides** of three, and **polypeptides** of four or more amino acids held together by peptide bonds. The numbers of amino acids in protein substances that perform specific tasks in the body range from one to several thousand. Neurotransmitters such as epinephrine and serotonin are made from a single amino acid, whereas the polypeptide myosin (a protein found in muscle) is comprised of more than 4,500 amino acids.

dipeptides: Proteins consisting of two amino acids.

tripeptides: Proteins consisting of three amino acids.

polypeptides: Proteins consisting of four or more amino acids. (Most proteins contain at least 50 amino acids.)

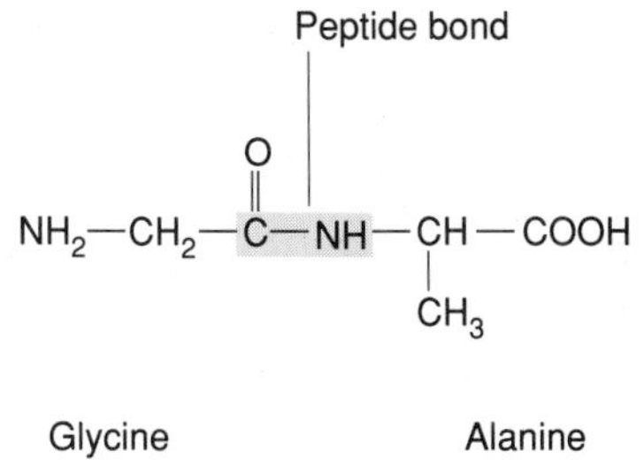

FIGURE 6-1
A peptide bond links two amino acids together.

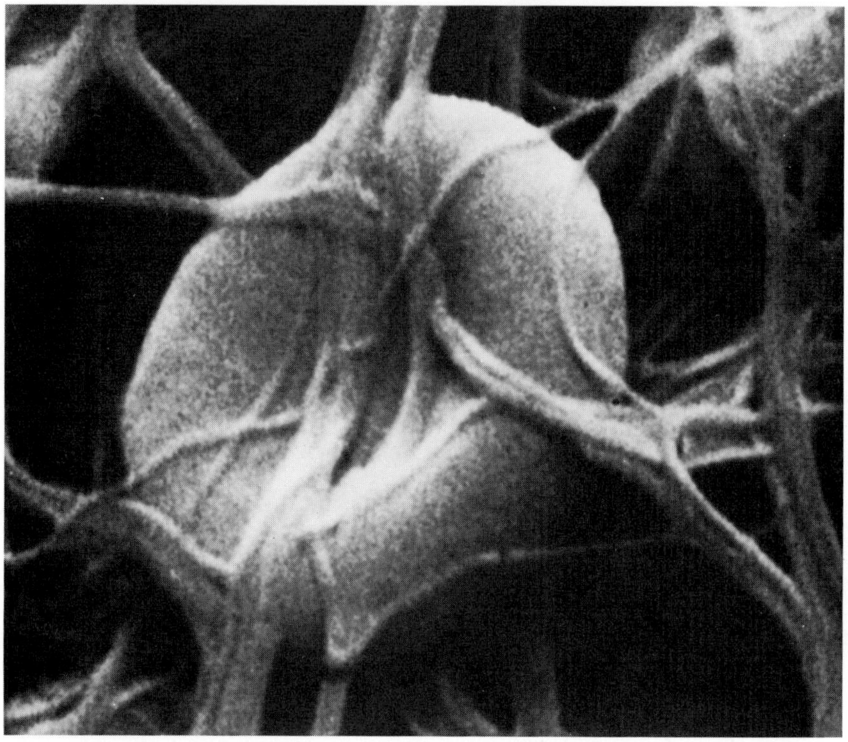

FIGURE 6-2
A red blood cell enmeshed in fibrin.

Classification of Proteins

fibrous proteins: Long, thin strands of polypeptides.

globular proteins: Tightly folded strands of polypeptides.

albumin: One of the most common proteins in blood. It is a relatively small polypeptide that carries certain nutrients in blood and serves as a source of amino acids for cells.

globulins: Polypeptides that constitute a component of blood (e.g., gamma globulin). They help protect the body from infectious diseases.

One way proteins are classified is by their shape. The two basic shapes are **fibrous** and **globular**. Fibrous proteins consist of two parallel strands of amino acids linked by their side chains. Myosin and actin (the muscle proteins) and collagen, elastin, and fibrin (proteins of the connective tissues) are all fibrous proteins. You can see what a fibrous protein looks like in Figure 6-2. The protein shown is fibrin, which aids blood clotting after an injury. Enzymes, hemoglobin, **albumin**, and **globulins** are examples of globular proteins. Globular proteins have irregular, curly, twisted structures. (A drawing of a globular protein, carboxypeptidase, appears in Figure 6-3.) When they are heated or exposed to stomach acid, globular proteins denature—"unfold." Although the term *denature* may sound like something that shouldn't happen to anything we eat, it's actually a helpful

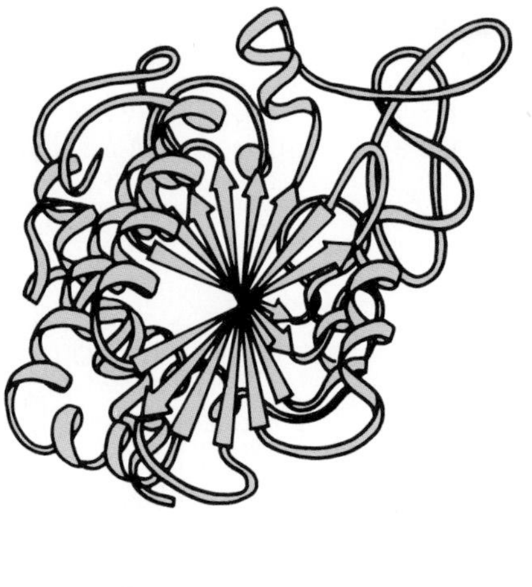

FIGURE 6-3
Structure of carboxypeptidase, a globular protein. Carboxypeptidase is an enzyme that serves in the breakdown of protein.

process. The unfolding of amino acid chains improves their digestibility, because it gives digestive enzymes easier access to the amino acids.

Proteins are also classified by their ability to be used by the body in protein synthesis. This ability depends on their essential amino acid content. How well a dietary protein supports protein synthesis is referred to as its "quality." The quality of dietary sources of protein is an especially important issue in geographic areas where few high-quality protein foods are available and among vegetarians.

PROTEIN QUALITY

The quality of a protein source depends on its content of essential amino acids. **Complete proteins** contain all of the essential amino acids in the amounts needed to support protein synthesis in the body. If any essential amino acid is missing in a protein source, or if any is present in only a relatively low amount, the protein source cannot be used for protein synthesis. Protein sources that lack particular essential amino acids are considered **incomplete proteins**. Proteins found in milk, meat, eggs, and other animal products are complete proteins, whereas proteins in plant sources are incomplete proteins.

complete proteins: Proteins that contain all of the essential amino acids in amounts sufficient to support growth and tissue maintenance.

incomplete proteins: Proteins that are deficient in one or more essential amino acids.

In spite of the fact that not every protein made in the body contains all of the essential amino acids, the lack of just one essential amino acid halts protein production in the body. If it strikes you as inefficient for the body to shut off all protein synthesis for the want of one or two amino acids, consider what would happen if protein synthesis continued. Cells would end up with an imbalanced assortment of protein. That would seriously affect cell functions and homeostasis. Without the needed level of *each* essential amino acid, proteins consumed can only be used to form energy. The body does not store amino acids, so they must be available for the body's use all at once. This means we need to consume a sufficient amount of complete protein consistently throughout our lives.

As we've said, the proteins found in plants are incomplete. However, the essential amino acid composition of plant sources of protein can be made complete by combining them with other sources of protein in a meal.

Complementary Proteins

Which combinations of plant proteins complement each other depends on which essential amino acids are missing from the particular plants or present only in low amounts. The essential amino acid that is missing or found in the lowest amount is referred to as the **limiting amino acid**. The goal of combining plant foods to obtain a complete source of protein is to select foods that complement each other's limiting amino acids; in other words, to select **complementary proteins**. The three most common limiting amino acids in plant foods are lysine, methionine, and tryptophan (Table 6-2). Wheat, rice, nuts, and seeds contain limited amounts of lysine but a good amount of methionine. All of the **legumes** except peanuts contain a high amount of lysine but a low amount of methionine. Thus, combining a grain such as rice with a legume such as dried beans provides a source of complete

limiting amino acid: The essential amino acid with the lowest concentration in a given food.

complementary proteins: Two or more incomplete proteins that produce a complete protein when combined. The limiting amino acid in one food is complemented by the presence of that amino acid in the other food(s).

legumes: Seeds such as peas, various beans, and peanuts that split into two parts.

TABLE 6-2
Limiting amino acid content of plant sources of protein

Plant	Limiting Amino Acid
Wheat, rice, barley, millet	lysine, threonine
Corn	lysine, threonine, tryptophan
Lima, navy, pinto, white, and kidney beans	cystine, methionine
Soybeans	methionine
Sesame and sunflower seeds	lysine
Peanuts	lysine, methionine, threonine
Green peas	methionine

protein. The following are examples of combinations of plant foods that provide complete protein.[1]

- rice and dried beans
- rice and green peas
- bulgur (wheat) and dried beans
- barley and dried beans
- corn and dried beans
- corn and green peas
- corn and lima beans (succotash)
- soybeans and seeds
- peanuts, rice, and dried beans
- seeds and green peas

An example of a dish that contains complementary sources of plant proteins is the Kenyan food isyo (Figure 6-4). Isyo consists mainly of corn and beans, but other plants are added when available.

Several methods are used to assess the protein quality of foods. We will discuss three common methods: amino acid score, biological value, and the protein efficiency ratio.

amino acid score: An estimate of protein quality derived by comparing the amino acid composition of a food with that of a high-quality protein such as egg white or milk or with an established amino acid reference pattern.

Amino Acid Score A food's **amino acid score** is determined by dividing its content of each essential amino acid by the amino acid content of an equal amount of a high-quality source of protein such as egg white or milk. The lowest score for any of the essential amino acids designates the limiting amino acid in the test food and gives a rough estimate of its protein quality. Foods with one or more low scores are considered to be poor-quality sources of protein and must be combined with complementary sources of protein to yield a protein of high quality.

biological value: The percentage of absorbed protein that is retained by the body for use in growth and tissue maintenance.

Biological Value A food's **biological value** represents the percentage of the protein absorbed from it that the body can use for growth and tissue maintenance—rather than for energy production. The biological value of egg white serves as the standard against which other protein sources are judged. Sources of complete protein have high biological values, whereas sources of incomplete proteins have low values. The lower the biological value of a food, the more likely it is that its protein will be used for energy, rather than protein synthesis.

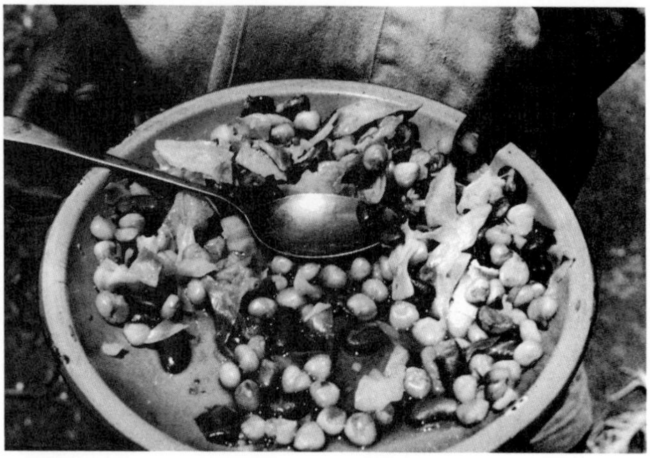

FIGURE 6-4
Isyo is the main source of protein for the Akamba community in Kenya. It consists of well-cooked corn and beans, often mixed with another vegetable such as cabbage.

Assessment of biological value accounts for the incomplete digestion and absorption of some proteins. Thus it provides a more accurate picture of protein utilization than do amino acid scores. Nonetheless, there is a high degree of correspondence between biological values and amino acid scores.

In the mid 1970s, a liquid-protein diet based on the incomplete protein collagen (also known as gelatin) was sold over the counter for weight loss. Despite enthusiastic promotional claims for the product, its safety and effectiveness had not been tested. Because it supplied an incomplete source of protein, muscle mass—including that of the heart—was lost by people who used the diet. Even though many people who used the diet were supervised by their doctors, by early 1978, 58 women who had been on the diet for three months or longer had died. The exact causes of the deaths are not known, but excessive use of the heart muscle as a source of protein may have played a role.[2] Liquid-protein diets are no longer recommended, even if monitored by a physician.

Protein Efficiency Ratio A **protein efficiency ratio** (PER) represents a particular protein's ability to promote growth in laboratory animals. The standard for comparison is the growth produced by the complete protein found in egg white or milk. It is known that gains in muscle mass, bone, and other lean tissues of the body of growing animals decline when only incomplete proteins are consumed, and that the more incomplete the protein is, the greater is the decline in the growth rates. Thus, the protein efficiency ratio is a useful measure of the extent to which different types of food protein promote growth.

protein efficiency ratio: A measure of the growth-promoting effect of dietary protein sources.

Many different dietary patterns can provide humans with sufficient amounts of high-quality protein. Well-planned vegetarian diets are as capable of supplying complete sources of proteins from combinations of plant foods as are the diets of people who consume animal products.

VEGETARIANISM

About 3% of the people in the U.S. practice some form of vegetarianism, and the percentage appears to be increasing.[3] People choose to be vegetarians for health, religious, and philosophical reasons. Vegetarian diets

TABLE 6-3
Comparison of the types of foods consumed by nonvegetarians and vegetarians

	Foods Eaten				
Type of Diet	Beef and Other "Red" Meats	Pork, Poultry, Fish, Seafood	Eggs	Milk, Cheese, and Other Milk Products	Vegetables, Fruits, Grains and Grain Products, Legumes, Nuts, Seeds, Oils, Sugars
Nonvegetarian	X	X	X	X	X
Semivegetarian		X*	X	X	X
Lacto-ovovegetarian			X	X	X
Lactovegetarian				X	X
Vegan					X

*May exclude some types of food in this group.

have been practiced for centuries by some religious groups, bearing testimony to the general safety of well-established vegetarian eating patterns.[1]

The most common categories of vegetarian diets are **semivegetarian** (a relatively new type, which excludes only "red" meats), **lacto-ovovegetarian, lactovegetarian**, and **vegan**. (*Lacto-* refers to milk; *ovo-*, to eggs.) As Table 6-3 shows, these diets become more restrictive as they move from semivegetarian to vegan. Less common vegetarian diets include **macrobiotic** and **fruitarian** regimens. These two types of vegetarian diets exclude many types of foods and are generally inadequate in many nutrients.[1]

semivegetarian diet: Diet that includes some meats in addition to plants, generally excluding "red" meats.

lacto-ovovegetarian diet: Diet that includes plants, milk products, and eggs.

lactovegetarian diet: Diet that includes plants and milk products.

vegan diet: Diet that excludes all animal products.

macrobiotic diet: A vegan diet that is restricted to unprocessed, unrefined foods and foods believed to be endowed with special health properties.

fruitarian: Person whose dietary staples are fruits.

Health Status of Vegetarians

If foods are selected carefully, it is possible to obtain complete nutrition from vegetarian diets.[1] In fact, well-balanced vegetarian diets have some advantages over many omnivorous diets (diets consisting of both plant and animal foods). Vegetarian diets typically contain twice as much dietary fiber, lower levels of saturated fat and cholesterol, and fewer calories than omnivorous diets.[1,4,5] Vegetarians following established dietary practices tend to have lower levels of blood cholesterol and are less likely to be overweight than people who regularly eat meat.[1,5] Furthermore, they are less likely to develop heart disease, diabetes, and cancer of the colon than nonvegetarians.[1,6] Table 6-4 shows the basic groups around which balanced vegetarian diets are built. Vegetarian diets that are nutritionally inadequate generally violate the principle that a wide variety of foods is needed for a healthy diet.

Excessively restrictive or poorly planned vegetarian diets, especially when consumed by people whose needs for protein and other nutrients are high (such as those of children and pregnant women), can compromise health.[7] The example vegetarian diet shown in Table 6-5 was fed to a three-year-old whose mother had put him on a "relatively" macrobiotic diet. The child weighed 35 pounds and was underweight for his height and age. His diet was determined to be low in calories, calcium, iron, vitamin B_{12}, and

TABLE 6-4
Sample vegetarian meal plan for adults

Food Group	Minimum Number of Servings per Day
Protein Foods	2
1½ c cooked dried beans 8 oz tofu 2 c fortified soy milk ½ c nuts 4 T peanut butter 2 c yogurt 2 oz cheese 2 eggs	
Whole Grains	6
1 slice bread (whole-wheat best) 1 muffin ¼ c seeds ½ c cooked cereal ½ c brown rice ½ c pasta	
Vegetables	
Vitamin A–rich ½ c broccoli, brussels sprouts, collards, squash	1
Other ½ c "other" vegetables such as potatoes, green beans, corn, lettuce	2
Fruits	
Vitamin C–rich berries, ¾ c cantaloupe, ¼ orange, 1 grapefruit, ½ orange juice, ½ c	2
Other apple, 1 banana, 1 pear, 1 peach, 1 grapes, ½ c	2
Fats	(depends on caloric need)
margarine, 1 t butter, 1 t oil, 1 t mayonnaise, 2 t cream cheese, 1 T	

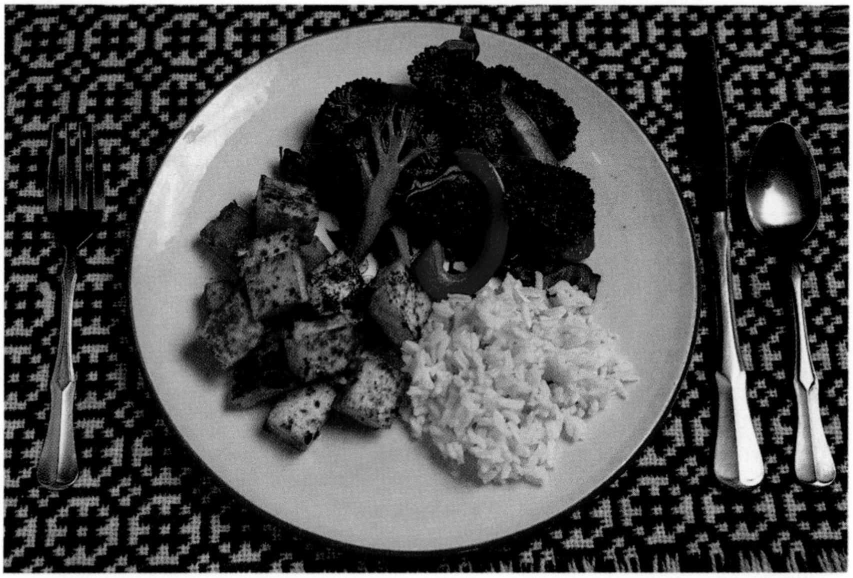

Tofu, broccoli, sweet red peppers, and rice make up this vegetarian meal.

vitamin C and to be high in sucrose. Although low intakes of certain vitamins and minerals would not guarantee that the boy would be deficient in them, his poor diet did put him at risk of developing deficiency diseases and likely caused him to be underweight.

Nutrient Deficiency Risks of Vegetarians

Dietary deficiencies of protein, iron, zinc, calcium, riboflavin, and vitamins B_{12} and D are commonly found among vegetarians consuming an imbalanced assortment of foods.[7] Iron, zinc, and calcium in plants are poorly absorbed due to the presence of substances such as phytates, oxalates, and dietary fiber that can bind these minerals in the intestines.[10] So although these nutrients may be adequate in a vegetarian diet, they are incompletely absorbed. Vegetarian diets that exclude milk or appropriately fortified soy milk may contain inadequate amounts of calcium, riboflavin, and vitamin D. Vitamin B_{12} is found only in appreciable amounts in animal products, and vegetarians who don't eat any type of meat, milk, or eggs are at high risk of becoming deficient in this vitamin.[1] Poor growth and a higher incidence of osteoporosis are common consequences of inadequate vegetarian diets.[7,9]

Nutritional deficiencies may be very common among lifelong vegans. A study of 138 vegans from birth identified deficiencies of vitamin B_{12} in 69%, iron in 63%, vitamin D in 14%, and folic acid in 3%.[10] Among the common vegetarian diets, those of vegans are the most difficult to balance.[1]

DIGESTION AND ABSORPTION OF PROTEINS

Proteins are complex and often large molecules that require many types of enzymes for their digestion. Figure 6-5 presents an overview of protein digestion that highlights the major enzymes involved. Protein digestion begins in the stomach with the action of the enzyme pepsin and hydrochloric acid. Pepsin attacks specific peptide bonds and begins breaking the polypeptides contained in foods into smaller chains of amino acids. Hydrochloric

TABLE 6-5

Three days of food intake for a three-year-old on a "relatively" macrobiotic diet*

Day 1	Day 2	Day 3
Breakfast	Breakfast	Breakfast
brown rice, 1 c	Cream of Wheat, 1 c	Cream of Wheat, 1½ c
sesame seeds, 1 T	milk, 1¼ c	milk, 1 c
maple syrup, 1 T	raisins, 2 T	raisins, 2 T
apple juice, 6 oz	peanuts, 2	apple juice, ¼ c
	yogurt, 2 t	yogurt, ⅓ c
Lunch	Lunch	Lunch
tater tots, 2 T	vegetable soup, 3 T	whole-wheat bread, 2 slices
2% milk, 4 oz		peanut butter, 3 T
applesauce, 1 T		apple juice, 6 oz
graham cracker, ¼, with frosting, ½ t		
celery, ⅕ stalk		
Dinner	Dinner	Dinner
raisins, 1 T	figs, 2	rice, ⅗ c
chocolate chips, 1 T	rice, ½ c	peas, ⅗ c
pecans, 3	peas, ⅙ c	cod, 2 oz
milk, 2 oz	beans, ⅙ c	oil, 1 T
apple juice, 6 oz	onion, ⅓ T	almonds, 3
jelly beans, 2	oil, ⅓ T	jelly beans, 3
rice, ½ c	carrots, ⅙ c	
peas, ½ c	winter squash, ½ T	
carrots, ⅕ c	oil, ⅙ T	
celery, 4 T	soy sauce, ⅒ t	
oil, 1 t	green onions, ½ t	
onion, 1 t	pear, ½	

Food Constituent Analysis

Food Constituent	Average of the 3 Days	Intake Standard/RDA
Calories	1,000	1,300
Protein	27 g	23 g
Fat	29 g	32 g
Carbohydrate	160 g	130 g
Sucrose	36 g	25 g or less
Cholesterol	160 mg	300 mg or less
Calcium	440 mg	800 mg
Iron	6.4 mg	15 mg
Vitamin B_{12}	1.1 mcg	2.0 mcg
Vitamin C	14 mg	45 mg

*This "relatively" macrobiotic diet includes seafoods. This dietary intake was reported by the mother of a three-year-old male. The child was underweight for his height and age.

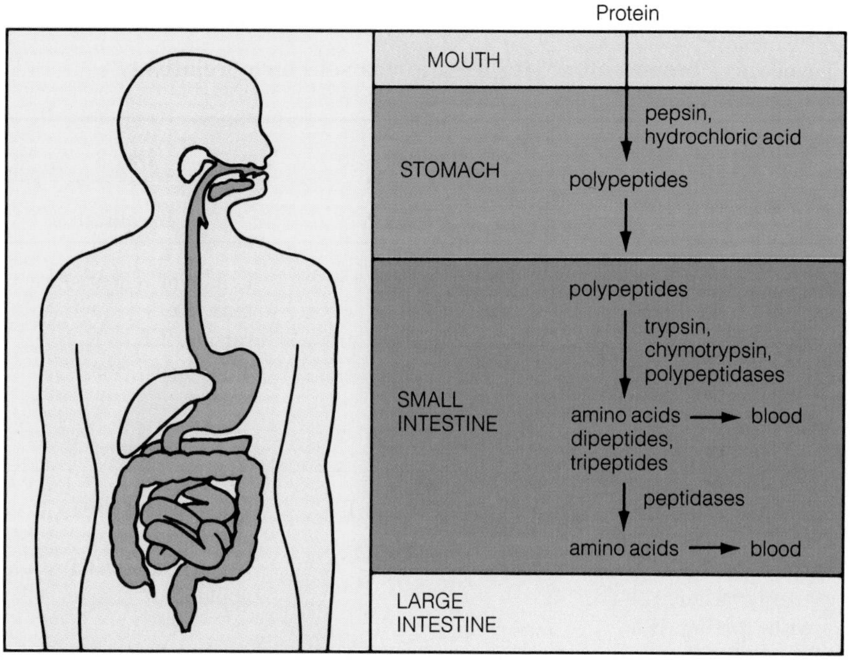

FIGURE 6-5
Overview of the digestion and absorption of protein.

acid denatures (or "uncoils") the proteins, making their peptide bonds more accessible to pepsin and the protein-digesting enzymes in the small intestines.

Trypsin from the pancreas, and chymotrypsin and polypeptidases from the small intestine continue the process of breaking peptide bonds until amino acids and dipeptides remain. Amino acids and dipeptides are absorbed into the cells that line the small intestine. In these cells the dipeptides are broken down to single amino acids by peptidase. The amino acids then pass into the blood stream and are circulated to the liver.

Once amino acids have entered the liver, they can be

- synthesized into proteins
- converted to nonessential amino acids
- converted to glucose or fat
- used for energy production
- released back into the bloodstream

When amino acids are used to form glucose, fat, or energy, the nitrogen component is taken off. The nitrogen may then be used in the formation of nonessential amino acids or converted to urea and excreted in the urine. Free amino acids that leave the liver are taken up by cells throughout the body. Cells use amino acids in the same ways as the liver does. A summary of the ways in which amino acids are used by the body appears in Figure 6-6.

Now let's look at how the cells make proteins.

Cells: The Body's Protein Manufacturing Plants

Amino acids are the raw ingredients that cells use to produce proteins. Each cell is capable of manufacturing the enzymes and other protein substances it needs in order to function. The instructions for how the amino acids are to be linked together to form particular proteins are provided by

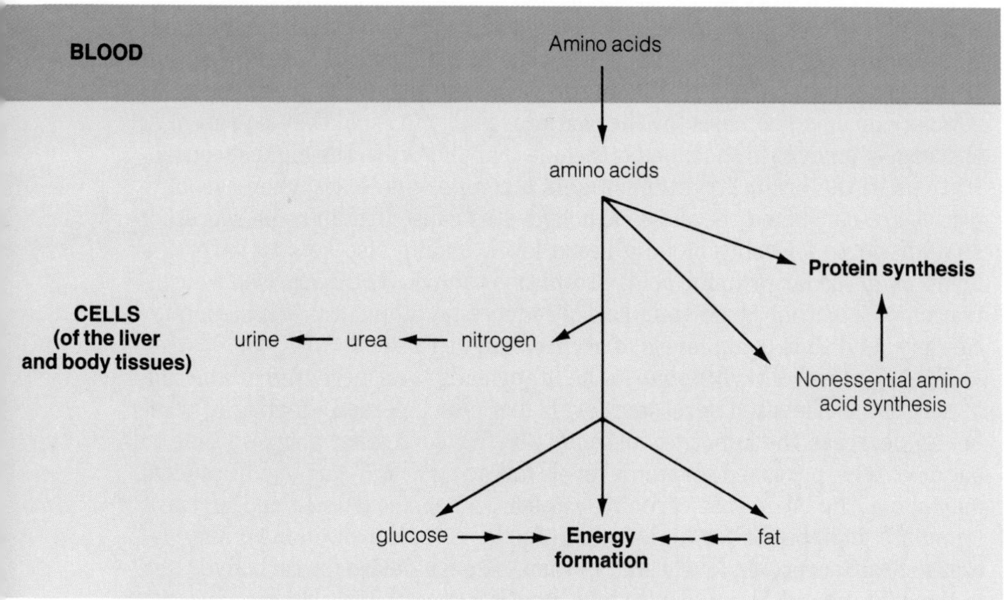

FIGURE 6-6
The major ways the body uses amino acids received in foods.

DNA (deoxyribonucleic acid); that is, DNA dictates the sequence in which amino acids attach to each other. When the process of lining up specific amino acids and binding them together has been completed, the cell has synthesized a new protein. (But remember, protein synthesis occurs only if all of the necessary amino acids are available in the cell.)

Cells also form some very simple substances from amino acids that have profound effects on body processes. One of the simplest types, but the most powerful in terms of their effect on body functions and behavior, are the neurotransmitters.

Amino Acids and Neurotransmitters

Neurotransmitters act as chemical messengers within the body's network of over 100 billion nerve and brain cells. They influence functions such as memory, mood, appetite, and muscular coordination. Known neurotransmitters number around 35, most of which are formed from just one or two amino acids.

Three major neurotransmitters are **serotonin, dopamine**, and **norepinephrine**. Serotonin is derived from the essential amino acid tryptophan, whereas dopamine and norepinephrine are made from the nonessential amino acid tyrosine. The level of activity of each of these neurotransmitters is influenced by diet composition.[11] This fact makes them rather unique, because diet composition doesn't generally affect the production of the body's chemical messengers. This area is a fascinating one, and we'll take a look at one example of the influence of diet on neurotransmitter synthesis and discuss how it may affect our behavior. The neurotransmitter we'll discuss is serotonin, and the behavior, food intake.

The level of serotonin in the brain is influenced by carbohydrate and tryptophan intake.[12] When a high-carbohydrate diet is consumed, tryptophan in the blood is selectively transported into the brain. Why does a high-carbohydrate diet result in the selective increase of tryptophan in the brain?

serotonin: (sir′ə tō′nin) A neurotransmitter formed from the amino acid tryptophan. It is involved in the processes of sleep, pain, appetite, and perception of well-being.

dopamine: (dō′pə mēn′) A neurotransmitter formed from the amino acid tyrosine. It is thought to be involved with emotions, motor functions, and hormone release.

norepinephrine: (nôr′ep′ə nef′rin) A neurotransmitter formed from tyrosine involved in motor function and hormone release.

Tryptophan is a large amino acid that must "compete" with five other large amino acids for carriers to transport them across the "blood–brain barrier." The blood–brain barrier controls the type and amount of substances that cross through the blood vessels to the brain. Although the six amino acids compete on an equal basis for the carriers, the amino acid that is present in the largest amount in the blood is the one that ends up in the highest concentrations in the brain. Tryptophan gets a competitive edge when carbohydrates are consumed, because carbohydrates cause insulin to be secreted. In addition to lowering blood glucose level, insulin also acts to lower the levels of all the large amino acids *except* tryptophan. The decreased concentration of the other large amino acids reduces tryptophan's competition for carriers, and thus brain levels of tryptophan increase.[13]

The high level of tryptophan in the brain leads to an increased production of serotonin. Elevated serotonin levels increase a person's feeling of well-being, decrease the appetite, and may play a role in what people decide to eat next. The increased serotonin levels following a high-carbohydrate meal may signal the brain that carbohydrates have been consumed and, in turn, stimulate an appetite for high-protein foods. A high-protein meal may decrease brain serotonin levels and, in turn, signal a desire for carbohydrates in the next meal.[13] It appears to be a biological possibility that some people crave carbohydrates. There is much more to learn about the effects of diet on behavior, but it is clear that the two are related in some ways.

The Role of Protein in Tissue Maintenance

Protein tissues in the body are constantly maintained through replacement. For instance, about one-half of the total amount of protein in the body's supply of hemoglobin is broken down and replaced every 120 days. Half of the supply of collagen is replaced every 300 days; and half of the muscle tissues, every 150 days. Taste cells and cells that line the small intestine are subjected to a lot of wear and tear; they are replaced more often: taste cells about every seven days, and the cells lining the small intestine about every 3 days. Certain enzymes exist only a few minutes and are recycled continuously.

The breakdown of existing proteins releases their amino acids, and some of those amino acids become available for new protein synthesis. Free amino acids are not stored by the body, and some of them are quickly converted to energy, nonessential amino acids, glucose, or fat. Since they are not stored, the body needs a dependable supply of incoming amino acids to replace those lost during protein tissue turnover.

The protein requirement of adults is actually a reflection of the need for amino acids in replacing proteins. Adults "lose" about 35 grams of protein each day due to the body's tissue maintenance activities. If protein intake is less than this amount or if complete proteins are not consumed, too few amino acids are available to replace those lost.

nitrogen balance: Nitrogen intake minus nitrogen excretion.

Nitrogen Balance A person's protein intake is generally estimated by determining the amount of nitrogen in foods consumed, rather than by analyzing the foods' amino acid content. Since proteins contain a fairly constant proportion of nitrogen, estimates of protein intake based on foods' nitrogen content correspond closely to actual protein intake. The nitrogen component of amino acids that are used for energy formation is excreted,

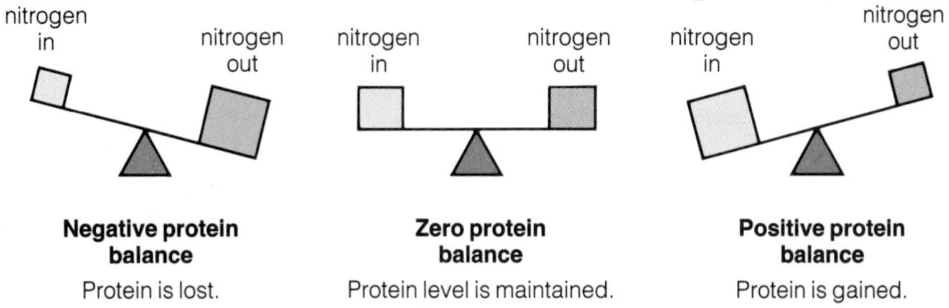

FIGURE 6-7
Schematic representation of nitrogen balance.

primarily in the urine. Thus the amount of nitrogen in the urine will reflect how much of the protein intake was used to form energy rather than to synthesize proteins. If more nitrogen is excreted in the urine than was consumed, the body has lost nitrogen—and therefore protein; the **nitrogen balance** is negative. (See Figure 6-7.) Low-protein and low-calorie diets produce negative nitrogen balances. Over time, a negative nitrogen balance can lead to substantial losses of protein from the liver, muscles, intestinal wall, heart, and other tissues of the body.

A zero nitrogen balance indicates equilibrium between nitrogen intake and output. It shows that protein intake meets or exceeds the protein requirement. If nitrogen excretion is less than intake, a positive nitrogen balance exists. Some of the protein consumed is being used for synthesizing new protein tissue and is thus being retained in the body. With adequate protein and caloric intakes, growth, pregnancy, and recovery from illnesses are accompanied by positive nitrogen balances.

FOOD SOURCES OF PROTEIN

Meat, poultry, fish, and dairy products account for two-thirds of the protein consumed in the U.S. The remaining one-third is supplied by grains, beans, eggs, and other products.[14] Sugars, fats, and oils supply only trace amounts of protein. Table 6-6 presents a list of food sources of protein and the percentages of calories in the foods that are contributed by protein. On the average, there are 8 to 9 grams of protein in a cup of milk, 7 grams of protein in each ounce of lean meat, and 4 grams per ounce of cooked, dried beans.

A new source of protein has entered American diets. Most people don't consume very much of it, but it can drastically change how foods taste. The new source is the sweetener aspartame.

Aspartame—A Protein Sweetener

It has long been known that certain amino acids have an intensely sweet taste and that they held potential for use as low-calorie sweeteners. Developing a protein sweetener that was tasty, inexpensive to produce, and nontoxic absorbed a lot of industry time and money. The product that was finally developed is aspartame—a dipeptide containing the amino acids aspartic acid and phenylalanine. Although it is generally recognized as safe, precautions about the use of aspartame by pregnant women and young children have been issued.[15,16]

■
TABLE 6-6
Food sources of protein

Food	Amount	Protein Content: Grams*	Protein Content: % Of Total Calories Provided by Protein
Animal Products			
shrimp	3 oz	21	84
low-fat cottage cheese	1 c	38	74
chicken (skin removed)	3 oz	20	70
pork chop (lean)	3 oz	20	59
tuna	3 oz	24	56
beef liver	3 oz	20	46
beef steak (lean)	3 oz	24	44
beef roast (lean)	3 oz	25	41
skim milk	1 c	9	40
fish (haddock)	3 oz	19	38
leg of lamb	3 oz	22	37
hamburger (regular)	3 oz	21	34
sausage (pork links)	3 oz	17	28
Swiss cheese	1 oz	8	30
egg	1 med.	6	30
cheddar cheese	1 oz	7	27
low-fat yogurt	1 c	8	27
whole milk	1 c	9	23
hot dog	1	6	15
Legumes and Nuts			
soybeans (cooked)	1 c	20	33
split peas (cooked)	1 c	9	31
lima beans (cooked)	1 c	12	27
dried beans (cooked)	1 c	15	26
peanuts	¼ c	9	17
peanut butter	1 T	4	17
walnuts	¼ c	7	14
almonds	¼ c	7	13
Grains			
corn	1 c	5	29
egg noodles	1 c	7	25
oatmeal		5	15
whole-wheat bread	1 slice	2.5	15
macaroni	1 c	5	13
white bread	1 slice	2.2	13
rice	1 c	4	11

*Adult RDAs are 44 g for women and 56 g for men.

Aspartame is fully absorbed by the body and increases blood levels of aspartic acid and phenylalanine. In laboratory animals, large doses of aspartame have caused decreased synthesis of serotonin by the brain.[17] The effect of aspartame on brain serotonin and possibly other neurotransmitter levels may be related to some of the physical signs reported among humans who have consumed relatively high amounts of it. Depression, headaches, increased appetite, and seizures have been reported among individuals consuming more than five cups of aspartame-sweetened beverages per day.[18,19] These conditions have disappeared when aspartame was removed from the diet.[18] It appears that some people may be sensitive to aspartame and should avoid using it.[20]

Individuals with phenylketonuria (PKU), a rare genetic disorder that causes phenylalanine to accumulate in the blood, must limit the amount of phenylalanine in their diets. If PKU is not managed adequately with a low-phenylalanine diet, mental retardation results. Since aspartame contains phenylalanine, all products containing it must carry a warning label.[1]

RECOMMENDED INTAKE OF PROTEIN

The amount of protein a person requires is affected by the quality of the protein consumed (complete or incomplete), total caloric intake (sufficiency for meeting energy needs), body size, pregnancy, and growth. The amount needed is less when the person consumes complete proteins. For example, people who consume animal products require fewer grams of protein than do vegans. The amount of protein needed in the diet decreases as caloric intakes increase; with sufficient calories from carbohydrates and fat, protein is not needed as an energy source. Growth and pregnancy increase people's needs for protein.

The adult RDA for protein is 44 grams for women and 56 grams for men. With intakes at the RDA levels, approximately 70% of dietary protein is used for tissue maintenance and 30% for energy production. To account for

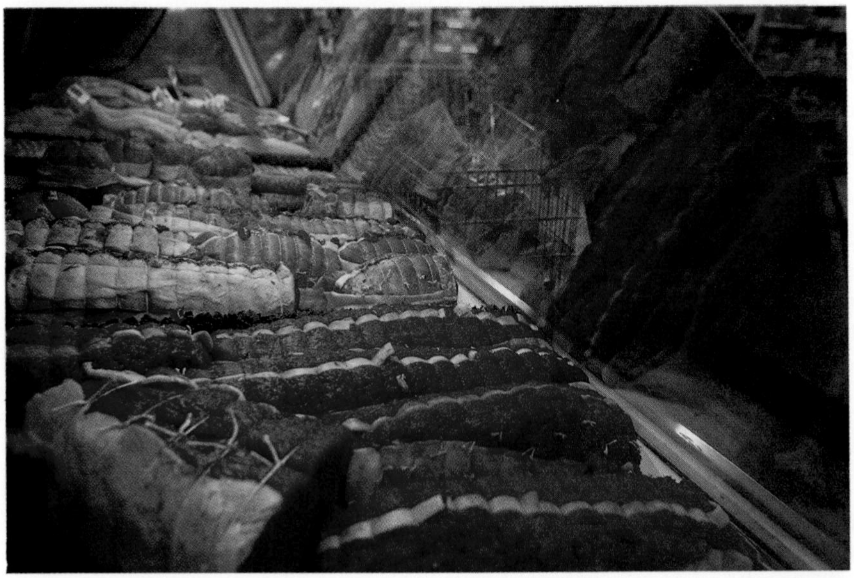

Two-thirds of the protein Americans consume is from animal sources.

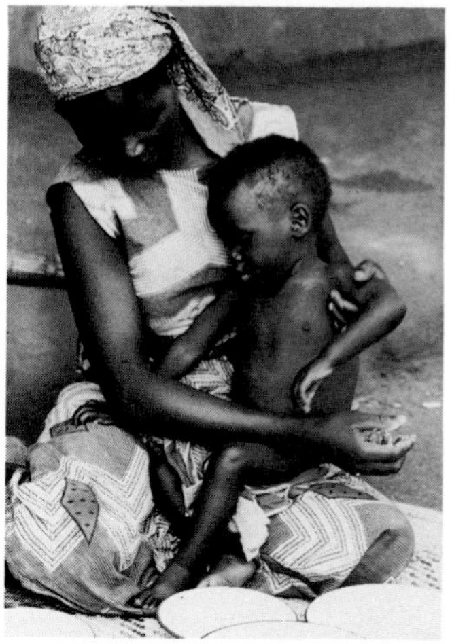

FIGURE 6-8
This two-year-old with kwashiorkor is unable to stand.

the differing protein needs of large and small adults, another recommendation specifies the intake of 0.8 grams of protein per kilogram (2.2 pounds) of body weight. An adult who weighed 210 pounds would have a calculated recommended protein intake of 76 grams, but for a 110-pound person it would be only 40 grams. Both recommended levels assume that people are consuming a mix of animal and plant sources of protein.

The typical U.S. diet is high in protein—a feature not associated with health benefits. The major negative side effect of high-protein diets is that they are generally rich in fat. Most meats and dairy products that are good sources of protein are also loaded with fat. Many people think that lean hamburger is a rich source of protein and not high in fat—after all, it's labeled "lean." But, 48% of the calories in "90% lean" hamburger are fat calories. Low-fat meats and dairy products do help lower the total fat intake, but they may not reduce it as much as consumers hope.

Trends

The percent of calories provided by protein in the typical U.S. diet has remained relatively stable since 1900, but the sources of protein have changed. In the early 1900s about half of the protein consumed came from plant sources and half from animal sources. Now, two-thirds of the protein intake comes from animal products.[14]

Plants contribute a significant proportion of the world's supply of protein. As countries develop economically, however, the proportion of dietary protein obtained from animal products tends to increase. The increased intake of animal sources of protein is accompanied by an increased consumption of fat, and by elevated rates of some of the "diseases of civilization" such as heart disease and cancer.[21]

Protein Deficiency

Protein deficiency can occur by itself or in combination with a deficiency of calories and nutrients. Because food sources of protein generally contain essential nutrients such as iron, zinc, vitamin B_{12}, and niacin, diets that produce protein deficiency usually cause a variety of other deficiencies, too. Protein deficiency leads to a loss of muscle tissue, growth retardation, reduced resistance to disease, weakness, **edema**, and kidney and heart problems.

edema: Condition in which fluid accumulates in the spaces between cells; swelling.

Kwashiorkor is a severe form of protein deficiency in children. It usually develops after a child has been weaned from breast milk and given high-carbohydrate, low-protein foods. As seen in Figure 6-8, children with kwashiorkor may look fat due to edema. They are actually very skinny. Children with protein deficiency are apathetic, irritable, small, and highly vulnerable to infection.[22]

kwashiorkor: (kwä'shē ôr' kôr) A deficiency disease primarily caused by a lack of complete protein in the diet. It usually occurs after children are taken off breast milk and given solid foods that have protein of low biologic value.

COMING UP IN CHAPTER 7

In chapter 7 you'll find out why we need fats in our diet, what they do for us, and why the U.S. diet is getting a bad reputation as an artery clogger.

■ ■ ■

REVIEW QUESTIONS

1. What is the primary function of proteins in the body?
2. Name four body components that consist mainly of protein.
3. What are the basic components of amino acids?
4. What is the major difference between essential and nonessential amino acids?
5. Proteins are made up of chains of amino acids connected by ________ bonds.
6. List three ways proteins are categorized.
7. What's a limiting amino acid?
8. What do limiting amino acids have to do with complementary proteins?
9. Give five examples of complementary proteins from plant protein sources.
10. Would a child grow if given only foods of low biologic value?
11. What does the protein efficiency ratio measure?
12. What are the most common categories of vegetarian diets, and how do they differ?
13. Vegetarian diets can promote health or disease, depending on the variety of foods that they contain. Name three health advantages associated with well-balanced vegetarian diets and three deficiency diseases associated with imbalanced ones.
14. Where does protein digestion begin?
15. Name three enzymes that break peptide bonds.
16. Draw a diagram of the major ways the body uses amino acids received in foods.
17. Name a neurotransmitter, and cite the amino acid from which it is produced.
18. If the amount of nitrogen excretion is less than the amount of nitrogen intake from protein-containing foods, then a person's nitrogen balance is ____________. (positive, negative, or zero)
19. Name two types of food that contain almost no protein.
20. On average, how much protein is supplied by a cup of milk? How much by an ounce of lean meat?
21. List three factors that affect how much protein should be consumed in a diet.
22. The protein-deficiency disease is ____________.

Answers

1. To provide building materials for the various components of body tissues.
2. Pick any four: muscles (myosin and actin), collagen, elastin, keratin, hemoglobin, enzymes, hormones, neurotransmitters, antibodies, protein carriers.
3. An amino (nitrogen-containing group), carbon, acid, and a side chain containing various types of molecules.
4. Essential amino acids are required for body processes but cannot be produced in sufficient amounts by the body. Consequently, essential

amino acids have to be provided in the diet. Nonessential amino acids are also required for body processes. However, they are not a necessary part of our diet because they can be produced in sufficient quantities by the body.

5. Peptide.
6. Essential/nonessential, fibrous/globular, complete/incomplete.
7. The essential amino acid that is missing or found in the lowest amount in a food.
8. You select complementary proteins that together yield a complete protein by combining foods that compensate for each other's limiting amino acids.
9. Refer to Table 6-2.
10. No. Foods containing proteins of low biologic value are incomplete sources of protein. These foods would provide energy but not the assortment of essential amino acids that are needed to support growth.
11. The ability of a particular protein to promote growth in laboratory animals compared to the growth produced by egg white or milk.
12. See Table 6-3.
13. *Health advantages:* reduced risk of heart disease, overweight, diabetes, and certain types of cancer.
    Deficiency diseases: kwashiorkor, iron deficiency, zinc deficiency, vitamin B_{12} deficiency, riboflavin deficiency, vitamin deficiency, folic acid deficiency.
14. In the stomach.
15. Your choices: pepsin, trypsin, chymotrypsin, polypeptidases.
16. See Figure 6-6.
17. The answer can be found in the margin definitions next to the content on amino acids and neurotransmitters.
18. Positive.
19. Fats and oils, sugars and sweeteners, alcohol.
20. 8–9 grams of protein per cup of milk; 7 grams of protein per ounce of lean meat.
21. Select any three: protein quality, total caloric intake (Are enough calories supplied by carbohydrates and fats to spare protein for use in protein synthesis?), growth, and pregnancy.
22. Kwashiorkor.

■ ■ ■

PUTTING NUTRITION KNOWLEDGE TO WORK

1. A friend tells you about a terrific low-calorie, high-protein diet that will make you lose weight like a hamburger on a grill. The diet consists of three eggs, 1 cup of low-fat cottage cheese, 2 ounces of cheddar cheese, and 3 ounces of tuna a day, and you are allowed to drink all the zero-calorie diet soda you want. Use Table 6-6 to calculate the amount of protein in the diet. This diet provides about 800 calories per day. If you followed it, would you be in negative, zero, or positive nitrogen balance? How would most of the protein be used by the body?

(The diet described contains a high proportion of protein and fat calories. It would provide about 94 grams of protein—close to twice the adult female and male RDAs for protein. You would likely be in negative nitrogen balance if you followed this diet, because it would provide too few calories to meet your need for energy. Hence, the protein would primarily be used as a source of fuel to meet the body's energy needs. Only a small portion of the protein would likely be used to build and maintain body tissues.)

2. Assume that the only protein you receive in your diet comes from chicken *or* dried beans. How many ounces of chicken (no skin) would you need to consume to meet your RDA for protein? (See Table 6-6.) How many cups of dried beans (cooked) would be needed? Would meeting your RDA for protein from only dried beans fulfill your requirement for protein?

   (The RDA for protein for men 19–22 years of age is 56 grams, and for females of the same age, it is 44 grams. Since chicken (no skin) has 20 grams of protein per 3 ounces, you would need to consume approximately 8.4 ounces of chicken if male, and 6.6 ounces if female to meet the RDA level. The corresponding figures for the dried beans part of the question are 3.7 cups and 2.9 cups for males and females. Dried beans provide incomplete protein, whereas chicken is a complete protein. This means you could consume dried beans by the gallon and never fulfill your body's need for protein.)

3. About how much protein did you consume yesterday? To get a rough estimate, write down everything you ate and drank yesterday and how much of each food and beverage you consumed. Then use Table 6-6 to estimate the protein content of yesterday's diet.

   (Comments: Did your protein intake come in below, above, or at your RDA for protein? If you generally consume a diet like the one you did yesterday, the estimate may be fairly close to your usual protein intake. If your diet varies a lot from day to day, the estimate may not even come close. In that case, you would have to estimate the protein content of your daily intake for at least a week to get a somewhat accurate picture of your protein intake.)

NOTES

1. Position paper on the vegetarian approach to eating, *Journal of the American Dietetic Association* 77 (1980): 61–68.

2. G. A. Bray, *Obesity: Comparative Methods of Weight Control* (Westport, Ct.: Technomic Publication Co., Inc., 1980).

3. Roper Poll results, in A demographic and social profile of age- and sex-matched vegetarians and nonvegetarians, J. H. Freeland-Graves, S. A. Greninger, and R. K. Young, *Journal of the American Dietetic Association* 86 (1986): 913–918.

4. J. Dwyer, Health implications of vegetarian diets, *Comprehensive Therapy* 9 (1983): 23–28.

5. H. Lithell and A. Bruce, Changes in lipoprotein metabolism during a supplemented fast and an ensuing vegetarian diet period, *Upsala Journal of Medical Science* 90 (1985): 73–83.

6. D. A. Snowdon and R. L. Phillips, Does a vegetarian diet reduce the occurrence of diabetes? *American Journal of Public Health* 75 (1985): 507–512.

7. D. O. Truesdell and P. B. Acosta, Feeding the vegan infant and child, *Journal of the American Dietetic Association* 85 (1985): 837–840.

8. *Recommended Dietary Allowances*, 9th ed., Food and Nutrition Board, National Research Council (Washington, D.C.: National Academy of Sciences, 1980).

9. W. T. van Staveren and J. H. Dhuyvetter, et al., Food consumption and height/weight status of Dutch preschool children on alternative diets, *Journal of the American Dietetic Association* 85 (1985): 1579–1584.

10. I. Chanarin and U. Malkowska, et al., Megaloblastic anemia in vegetarian Hindu community, *Lancet* ii (1985): 1168–1172.

11. W. M. Lovenberg, Biochemical regulation of brain function, *Nutrition Reviews* (Supplement) 44 (1986): 6–11.

12. J. H. Growdon and R. J. Wurtman, Dietary influences on the synthesis of neurotransmitters in the brain, *Nutrition Reviews* 37 (1979): 129–136.

13. R. J. Wurtman, Ways that foods can affect the brain, *Nutrition Reviews* (supplement) 44 (1986): 2–6.

14. S. O. Welsh and R. M. Marston, Review of trends in food use in the United States, 1909–1980, *Journal of the American Dietetic Association* 81 (1982): 120–125.

15. Council on Scientific Affairs, Aspartame: Review of safety issues, *Journal of the American Medical Association* 254 (1985): 400–402.

16. R. J. Wurtman, Neurochemical changes following high-dose aspartame with dietary carbohydrates, *New England Journal of Medicine* 309 (1983): 429–430.

17. H. Yokogoshi and C. H. Roberts, et al., Effects of aspartame and glucose administration on brain and plasma levels of large neutral amino acids and brain 5-hydroxyindoles, *American Journal of Clinical Nutrition* 40 (1984): 1–7.

18. R. J. Wurtman (letter to the editor), *Lancet* ii (1985): 1060; and R. B. Lipton, L. C. Newman, and S. Solomon, Aspartame and headache, *New England Journal of Medicine* 318 (1988): 1200–1201.

19. J. E. Blundell and A. J. Hill, Paradoxical effects of an intense sweetener (aspartame) on appetite, *Lancet* i (1986): 1092–1093.

20. B. Caballero, Food additives in the pediatric diet, *Clinical Nutrition* 4 (1985): 200–206.

21. *The Surgeon General's Report on Nutrition and Health*, PHS publication no. 88-50210 (Washington, D.C.: U.S. Department of Health and Human Services, 1988), 83–138 and 177–248.

22. N. S. Scrimshaw, Nutrition and preventive medicine, in *Public Health and Preventive Medicine*, 12th ed., ed. J. M. Last (Norwalk, Conn.: Appleton-Century-Crofts, 1986), 1515–1542.

CHAPTER 7

FATS

Dietary fat. Body fat. Cholesterol. Blood lipids. Saturated fats. Polyunsaturated fats. Fish oils, corn oil, safflower oil. Sound familiar? Americans have a large "fat" vocabulary. Hardly a week passes that we don't hear something about new research on dietary fat and clogged arteries and a new diet or drug therapy for unclogging them. TV commercials for margarines and oils keep us informed about the various types of vegetable oils that are available and tell us why one type of margarine or oil is better than the others for our hearts. The latest weight-loss book lets us know how we can get rid of that awful, excess body fat. The word *fat* suggests a lot more than "energy nutrient" to most people. In this chapter we'll discuss the functions, categories, and food sources of dietary fats and examine some of the health issues that surround them.

The fats are a group of substances found in food that have one major property in common: they dissolve in fat and not in water. If you have attempted to mix vinegar and oil before pouring it over a salad, you have observed the principle of water solubility and fat solubility first-hand. The

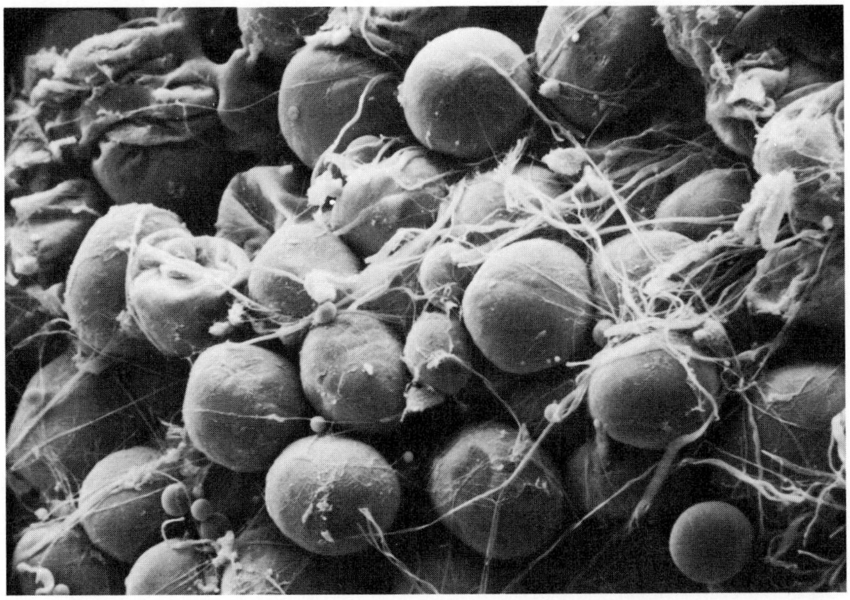

Fat cells: the central energy storehouses of the human body.

vinegar and oil do not mix—dissolve into each other—because their chemical structures make them repel each other. Each will mix only with chemical substances like itself. Fats dissolve in other fats.

lipids: Compounds that are insoluble in water and soluble in fat; commonly referred to as *fats*.

Actually, fats are a subcategory of the fat-soluble substances known as **lipids**. Lipids include all types of fats and oils. Fats are often distinguished from oils by their property of being solid at room temperature. Butter, margarine, lard, shortening, and animal fat are in this group because they don't melt into liquids if left on a shelf. Oils, on the other hand, are liquid at room temperature. The physical difference between fats and oils is due to their chemical structures. In this book we refer to lipids as *fats*, because that is the more common, familiar term.

Like carbohydrates, fats consist of carbon, hydrogen, and oxygen, but they contain more hydrogen and less oxygen than the carbohydrates do. The carbons in fats are usually bound to hydrogen, whereas the carbons in carbohydrates are frequently bound to oxygen. This difference explains why fats deliver more than twice as much energy as carbohydrates. You see, more energy is stored in carbon–hydrogen bonds than in carbon–oxygen bonds. Fats in the diet are compact, concentrated sources of energy.

■ ■ ■

HOW THE BODY USES FAT

A discussion of the functions of fats must address their functions in foods in our diet as well as their functions in our bodies.

Dietary Fat

linoleic acid: The only known essential fatty acid for adults.

essential fatty acid: A fatty acid that is required but cannot be produced by the body; it must be provided in the diet. (See *linoleic acid.*)

Plants and animals produce fat for the same reason that humans do: as an energy reserve. When we consume a fat, we are actually consuming a plant or animal's energy store. In addition to energy, fats in foods also supply fat-soluble nutrients. Fats carry **linoleic acid**—the **essential fatty acid**—and the fat-soluble vitamins A, D, E, and K. Linoleic acid is a component of every cell membrane, and it is needed for normal growth. Thus one reason we need fats in our diet is so that we can get a supply of linoleic acid and the fat-soluble vitamins.

Fats increase the flavor and palatability of foods. Although "pure" fats by themselves are tasteless, they absorb and retain the flavors of substances that surround them. Because fats in meats and other foods exist in different "flavor environments," the characteristic flavors of foods containing fat are due to the flavors that have been incorporated into the fat. This characteristic of fat explains why placing butter next to garlic in the refrigerator would be a mistake.

Fats in foods contribute to the sensation of feeling full (as they should at 9 calories per gram). Fats stay in the stomach longer than do carbohydrates and proteins, and they are absorbed over a longer period of time. Foods containing fat "stick to the ribs."

Dietary fat performs one other important role. Just as do carbohydrates, it spares protein from being used as an energy source. Diets that include some fat help keep dietary protein available for tissue synthesis and maintenance.

The roles of dietary fat are summarized in Table 7-1.

TABLE 7-1
Roles of dietary fat

provide a concentrated source of energy
carry linoleic acid (the essential fatty acid) and the fat-soluble vitamins
increase the flavor and palatability of foods
provide sustained relief from hunger
spare protein from use in energy formation

Body Fat

The body has two sources of fats: those consumed as dietary fat and those produced from carbohydrates and proteins. Although humans eat only a few times a day, they need energy throughout the day. To ensure a constant supply of energy, the body converts consumed carbohydrates and proteins not used to meet immediate needs to a storage form of energy. Although glycogen, the storage form of glucose, makes up some of these stores, most of these stores are converted to fat.

Fat is more than skin-deep in the body; it also surrounds organs such as the kidneys, heart, and pancreas to cushion them and protect them from physical damage when the body takes bumps and blows. Protective fat differs from storage fat in that it is harder and is never completely used to meet energy needs—even during starvation. The primary function of this type of fat is protection of the organs.

Body fat plays an important role in insulating the body; it serves to help the body maintain a constant, normal internal temperature. This role is particularly important to people who live or work in cold climates. People who are noticeably fat are better able than thin people to maintain normal body temperature in cold temperatures. This is a special concern for people who swim in cold waters. The English Channel swimmer pictured in Figure 7-1 is not the lean, visibly muscular type we tend to expect for an athlete, but he is in peak physical condition for swimming the 22 miles in 60-degree water. On the other hand, just as an extra layer of body fat helps keep people warm in cold temperatures, it makes it easier for them to overheat in hot temperatures. An extra layer of insulation makes it take longer for heat to escape from the body and cool the body.

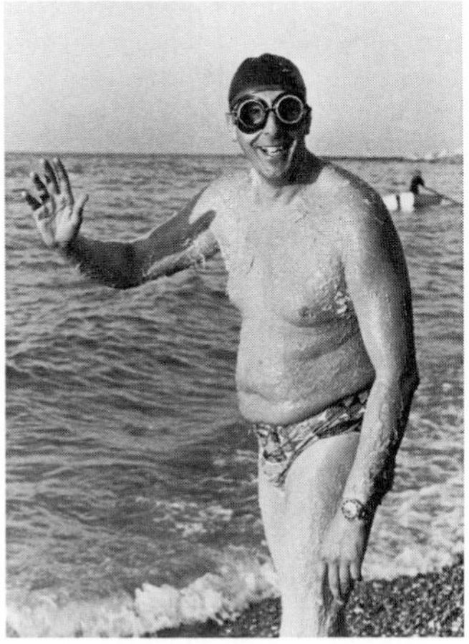

FIGURE 7-1
"King of the Channel," Mike Read of Ipswich, England, as he embarked on his twentieth English Channel swim at the age of thirty-nine.

Another crucial role of body fat is as a component of all cell membranes. The fat component of the membranes plays the leading role in controlling which chemical substances enter and exit cells. The types of fats in cell membranes reflect to some extent the types of fats in the diet.

Fats are also used by the body as a raw material for producing **prostaglandins** and **steroid hormones**. Prostaglandins are hormonelike substances that are involved in many body processes, and the steroid hormones include the sex hormones estrogen and testosterone. More information about the prostaglandins and the steroid hormones is presented when the specific types of fats used in their formation are discussed later in the chapter.

The roles of body fat are summarized in Table 7-2.

prostaglandins: (präs′tə glan′din) Hormonelike substances derived from specific types of fatty acids. Over 90 different types of prostaglandins are found in the human body.

steroid hormones: (stir′oid) Hormones such as estrogen and testosterone that are synthesized from cholesterol.

■
TABLE 7-2
Functions of body fat

source of stored energy
organ cushioning
body insulation
component of cell membranes
raw materials for prostaglandin and steroid hormone synthesis

■ ■ ■

STRUCTURE OF FATS

glycerol: water-soluble, glucoselike component of fats; accounts for about 16% of the weight of a fat molecule.

fatty acids: fat-soluble molecules containing carbon, hydrogen, and an acid group (COOH). When combined with glycerol, they form a fat. Fatty acids come in many forms. They may be short-, medium-, or long-chained; and saturated, monounsaturated, or polyunsaturated.

triglyceride: A fat in which the glycerol molecule has three fatty acids attached to it; also called *triacylglycerol*.

Fats consist of two basic components: glycerol and fatty acids. **Glycerol** is a relatively simple molecule that resembles glucose. **Fatty acids** are generally larger and more complex than glycerol, and there are many types of them. Different types of fatty acids can be attached to glycerol to yield an array of fats. The fatty-acid side chains attached to the glycerol give individual fats unique properties. (In that respect these side chains are similar to the side chains of the amino acids.)

Categories of Fats

Number of Fatty Acids Fats are categorized in a number of ways (Table 7-3). At the basic level, they are grouped according to the number of fatty acids that are attached to glycerol. Each glycerol can have up to three fatty acids attached to it. If three fatty acids are attached, the fat is called a ***tri*glyceride**. A diagram showing the chemical structure of fatty acids and glycerol and how they combine to form a triglyceride is shown in Figure 7-2.

■
TABLE 7-3
Classification of fats and fatty acids

Fats	
By the number of fatty acids attached to glycerol	
glycerol + 1 fatty acid	monoglyceride
glycerol + 2 fatty acids	diglyceride
glycerol + 3 fatty acids	triglyceride
Fatty Acids	
By length of carbon chain	
4 to 6 carbons long	short-chain fatty acid
8 to 10 carbons long	medium-chain fatty acid
12 or more carbons long	long-chain fatty acid
By number of double bonds	
no double bond	saturated fatty acid
1 double bond	monounsaturated fatty acid
2 or more double bonds	polyunsaturated fatty acid

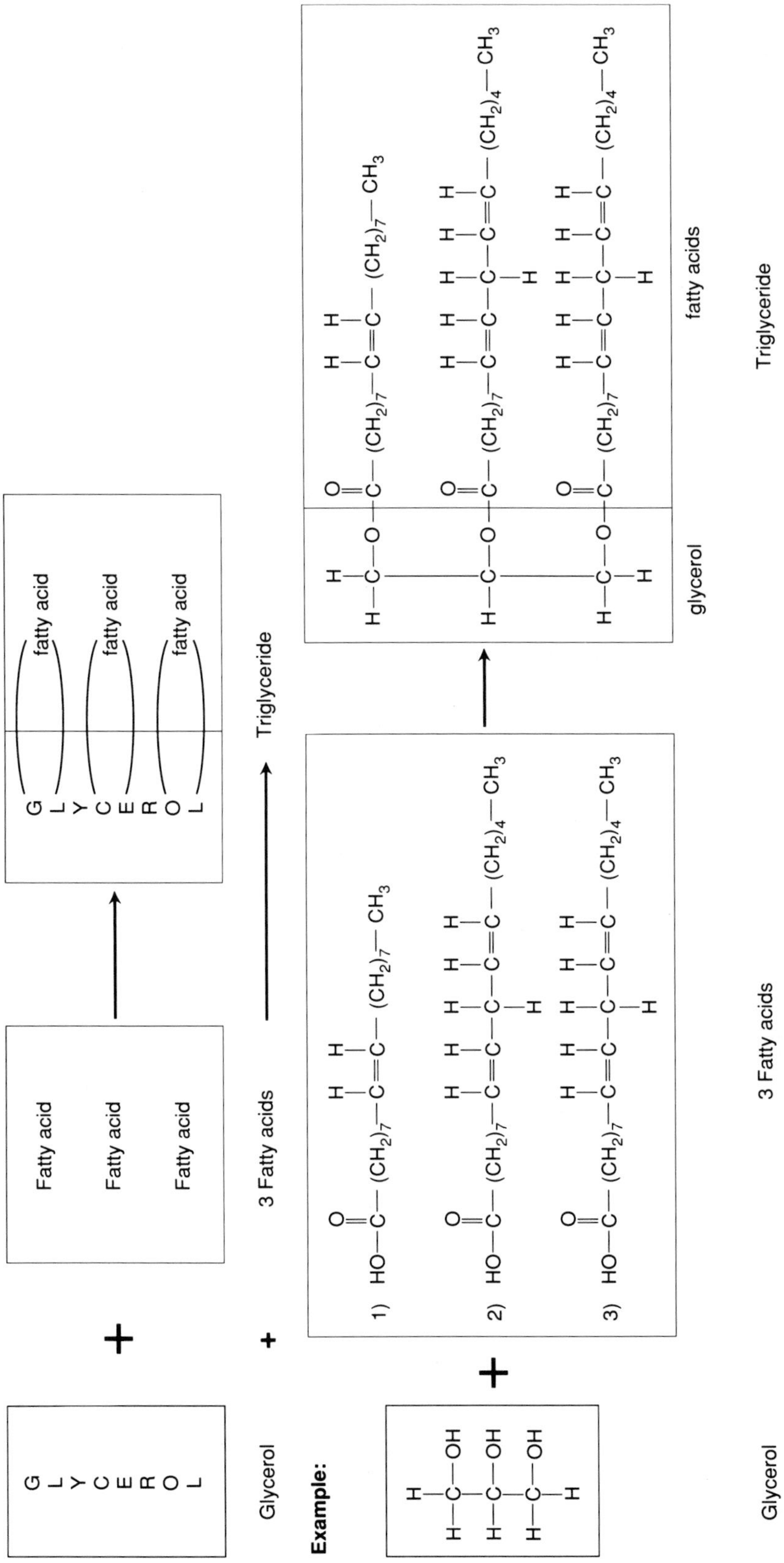

FIGURE 7-2
Formation of a triglyceride from glycerol and three fatty acids.

(Remember, formulas are included only to give you an idea of what the chemical substances are; unless instructed otherwise, do not feel you must memorize them.) Nearly all (98%) dietary fat and body fat is in the form of triglycerides. ***Di*glycerides** consist of two fatty acids attached to glycerol; ***mono*glycerides** consist of one fatty acid attached to glycerol.

diglyceride: A fat in which the glycerol molecule has two fatty acids attached to it; also called *diacylglycerol.*

monoglyceride: A fat in which the glycerol molecule has one fatty acid attached to it; also called *monoacylglycerol.*

Length of Carbon Chain The fatty acids attached to glycerol vary in the length of their carbon chain. Short-chain fatty acids contain 4 to 6 carbons; medium-chain fatty acids contain 8 to 10; and long-chain fatty acids contain 12 or more carbons. Milk, butter, and cheese are rich in short-chain fatty acids, whereas vegetable oils are high in medium- and long-chain fatty acids.

Number of Carbon–Carbon Double Bonds How the carbons in a fatty acid chain are attached to each other determines the properties of the particular fat and thus how the fat is classified. Atoms within molecules attach to each other by sharing their electrons (the negatively charged particles that surround the atoms' nuclei). The movement of electrons around adjacent atoms binds the atoms together. Each carbon atom has 4 electrons to share with adjacent atoms. Carbons can link themselves together by sharing one or two electrons with each other. When each carbon shares one electron, a **single bond** is formed. Two carbons are linked by a **double bond** when they each share two of their electrons (Figure 7-3).

single bond: Bond formed by the sharing of an electron by two adjacent atoms within a molecule.

double bond: Bond formed by the sharing of four electrons between adjacent atoms.

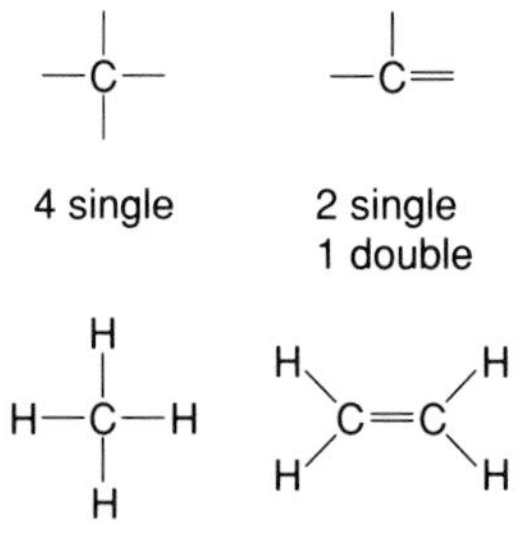

FIGURE 7-3
Single bonds and double bonds. Each bond constitutes a shared electron.

A singly bonded carbon atom within a fatty-acid chain has two electrons available for binding with two atoms of hydrogen. If a carbon atom is doubly bonded, however, it has only one electron available for binding with hydrogen. Consequently, fatty acids containing only single bonds (C—C) have more hydrogens than fatty acids containing at least one double bond (C=C).

Double bonds are weaker than single bonds because there is an imbalance between the positive and negative charges surrounding the carbon atoms. Double bonds are overly charged with negative electrons and are weaker than single bonds. The double bond breaks when an electron gets pulled away by a positively charged atom (such as an oxygen atom) in the molecule's environment. Have you ever smelled butter that has been out on the kitchen shelf for too long or oil that has passed its prime in the deep fat fryer? Both of these strong, irritating odors are caused by the breakdown of some of the double bonds in fatty acids.

SATURATED AND UNSATURATED FATTY ACIDS

Fatty acids that contain only single bonds between carbon atoms (C—C) are called **saturated fatty acids**—meaning they contain the maximum number possible of hydrogen atoms; they are *saturated* with hydrogen atoms. Those containing one or more double bonds (C=C) are called **unsaturated fatty acids**, because they contain fewer than the maximum possible number of hydrogens. Examples of saturated and unsaturated fatty acids are shown in Figure 7-4.

saturated (fatty acid): One that contains only single bonds between adjacent carbons. The carbons are "saturated" with hydrogens; they contain the maximum possible number of hydrogens.

Fats that consist of saturated fatty acids and glycerol are referred to as *saturated fats*, whereas fats composed of one or more unsaturated fatty acid(s) and glycerol are referred to as *unsaturated fats*. Saturated fats are generally solid at room temperature and are most commonly found in animal products. The double bonds in unsaturated fats make them soft or liquid at room temperature. The more double bonds an unsaturated fat has in its fatty acids, the softer—or more liquid—it is at room temperature. Plants are the predominant source of unsaturated fats.

unsaturated (fatty acid): One that contains one or more double bonds between adjacent carbons. The carbons are not saturated with hydrogens; they contain fewer than the maximum possible number of hydrogens.

Unsaturated fatty acids can contain up to six double bonds. If one double bond is present in a fatty acid, it is called a ***mono*unsaturated fatty acid**. If

monounsaturated (fatty acid): One that contains one double bond between carbons.

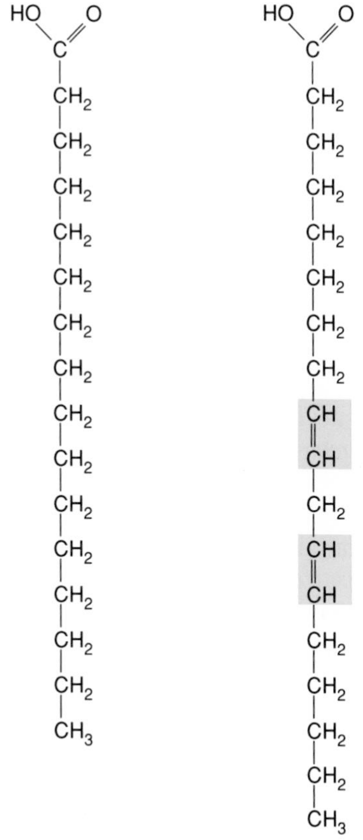

Palmitic acid
a saturated fatty acid

Linoleic acid
an unsaturated fatty acid

FIGURE 7-4

Chemical structure of a saturated fatty acid and an unsaturated fatty acid. The CH=CH groups in the unsaturated fatty acid contain double bonds.

polyunsaturated (fatty acid): One that contains two or more double bonds between carbons.

two to six double bonds are present, the fatty acid is described as ***poly*unsaturated**. Unlike the saturated fatty acids, the body is able to synthesize only a few types of unsaturated fatty acids. An important fatty acid the body cannot produce is linoleic acid, the essential fatty acid. Its chemical structure has two double bonds.

The actions of monounsaturated fatty acids in the body are more similar to those of polyunsaturated fatty acids than those of saturated fatty acids. This is an important point when the effects of the different types of fatty acids on blood cholesterol levels are being considered. We'll return to this issue when we discuss cholesterol later in the chapter.

saturated fat: A fat that contains glycerol and saturated fatty acids.

unsaturated fat: A fat that contains glycerol and one to three unsaturated fatty acids.

Food Sources of Saturated and Unsaturated Fats

Although most food sources of fat contain a mixture of saturated, monounsaturated, and polyunsaturated fatty acids, one type usually predominates. Referring to Table 7-4, you can pick out foods that are high in each type of fatty acid. Cheese, cow's milk, butter, beef, coconut oil, and palm oil contain more saturated fatty acids than unsaturated fatty acids. Coconut oil and palm oil are unique as plant sources of saturated fatty acids. They are sometimes used in coffee lighteners, candy, bakery products, shortening, cooking oil, and other products. Because coconut and palm oils are often the cheapest oils available to the food industry, they are used to reduce production costs of foods manufactured with oil. They are also used by the food industry because their single bonds are less likely to break down and taste bad than are fats that contain unsaturated fatty acids.

Foods that contain more unsaturated fatty acids than saturated ones include human milk, eggs, vegetable oils and margarines (except those made from coconut and palm oil), chicken, turkey, pork, and nuts and seeds.

The Omega Fatty Acids A long-established but rarely used classification system for unsaturated fatty acids has recently come into vogue. It is the system that classifies fatty acids by the distance of the first double bond from the omega end (the $—CH_3$ end) of the fatty acid. (Refer to Figure 7-4 for a look at the omega end of a fatty acid.) The first double bond in linoleic acid (the essential fatty acid) is six carbons from its omega end; this classifies linoleic acid as an *omega-6 fatty acid*. The fatty acids that have made the term *omega* popular, however, are the omega-3 fatty acids found in fish oils. Omega-3 fatty acids have their first double bond three carbons from the omega end, and they contain three to six double bonds. This is an exceptionally high level of unsaturation for fatty acids. The omega-3 fatty acids also appear to have exceptional effects on health. (The discussion of omega-3 fatty acids continues in Box 7-1.)

Hydrogenation: Turning a Liquid Oil into a Solid Fat

hydrogenation: the addition of hydrogen to unsaturated fatty acids; the process converts double bonds to single bonds.

Unsaturated fatty acids such as those in vegetable oils can be partially or completely converted to the saturated and solid form by **hydrogenation**, the addition of hydrogen to the double bonds between carbon atoms (Figure 7-5). The process causes a loss of some of the double bonds in unsaturated fatty acids but has the advantage of making oils spreadable and longer-lasting. Shortenings and margarines are produced from oils in this way. The

TABLE 7-4
Fat profiles of selected foods

Food	Amount	Total Fat, g	P/S*	Percentage Fatty Acid Composition: Saturated	Monounsaturated	Polyunsaturated
Dairy Products						
brick cheese	1 oz	8.4	.04	67	30	3
cheddar cheese	1 oz	9.4	.05	67	30	3
cottage cheese	1 c	9.5	.05	67	30	3
American cheese	1 oz	8.9	.06	67	30	3
whole milk	1 c	8.2		65	31	4
butter	1 T	12.0	.06	65	31	4
Human Milk	1 c	10.8	.24	48	40	12
Egg	1 med.	5.6	.41	37	48	15
Oils and Margarines						
coconut oil	1 T	13.6	.02	92	6	2
corn oil	1 T	13.6	13.6	13	25	62
corn oil margarine	1 T	11.4	1.33	17	61	22
olive oil	1 T	13.5	.61	14	77	9
palm oil	1 T	13.6	.19	52	38	10
peanut oil	1 T	13.5	1.87	18	48	34
soybean oil	1 T	13.6	3.95	15	25	60
soybean oil margarine	1 T	11.4	1.25	22	50	28
sunflower oil	1 T	13.6	6.36	11	21	68
Meats						
hamburger, regular (21% fat)	3 oz	17.6	.08	53	43	4
chicken, roasted (no skin)	3 oz	5.6	1.04	26	46	28
pork chop	3 oz	21.4	.31	39	49	12
turkey, roasted	3 oz	4.6	.88	40	25	35
Nuts and Seeds						
cashews	1 oz	13.2	.85	21	62	17
macadamia nuts	1 oz	20.9	.13	16	82	2
peanuts, dry-roasted	1 oz	14.0	2.32	15	52	33
peanut butter	1 T	8.2	1.79	18	51	32
sunflower seeds (dried)	1 oz	14.1	6.20	11	20	69

*P/S = the ratio of the grams of polyunsaturated fatty acids to the grams of saturated fatty acids. A ratio of 1 or greater is recommended.

■
FIGURE 7-5
Hydrogenation of the double bonds of an unsaturated fatty acid.

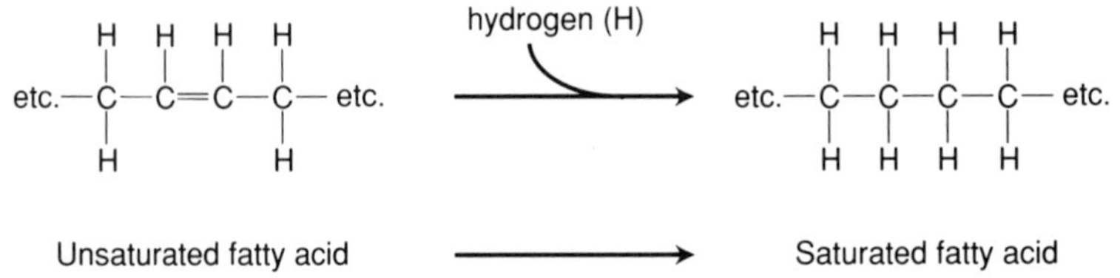

labels on shortenings and margarines often state "made from partially hydrogenated vegetable oil." The harder (more solid) the hydrogenated fat is, the more saturated fatty acids it contains.

You can identify the extent to which hydrogenation reduces the unsaturated fatty acid content of vegetable oils by referring to the Oils and Margarines section of Table 7-4. The table shows that corn and soybean oils contain about 60% polyunsaturated fatty acids, and that margarines made from them contain 40% and 32% less polyunsaturated fatty acids. The saturated fatty acid content of oils is only slightly increased by hydrogenation. The main effect of the hydrogenation of oils is the conversion of polyunsaturated fatty acids to monounsaturated fatty acids.

■ ■ ■

FATLIKE SUBSTANCES

A number of fatlike substances are classified as fats. We will discuss five of them: cholesterol, lipoproteins, phospholipids, waxes, and artificial fats.

Cholesterol

cholesterol: A fat-soluble, colorless liquid found in animals but not in plants. Cholesterol is used by the body to form steroid hormones such as testosterone and estrogen and is a component of animal cell membranes.

So much has been said about the heart disease–promoting effects of high blood **cholesterol** levels that some Americans believe that *all* cholesterol is bad. Actually, a certain amount of cholesterol is required for normal body processes. It is needed for the formation of steroid hormones and it serves as a component of all cell membranes in animals. The steroid hormones

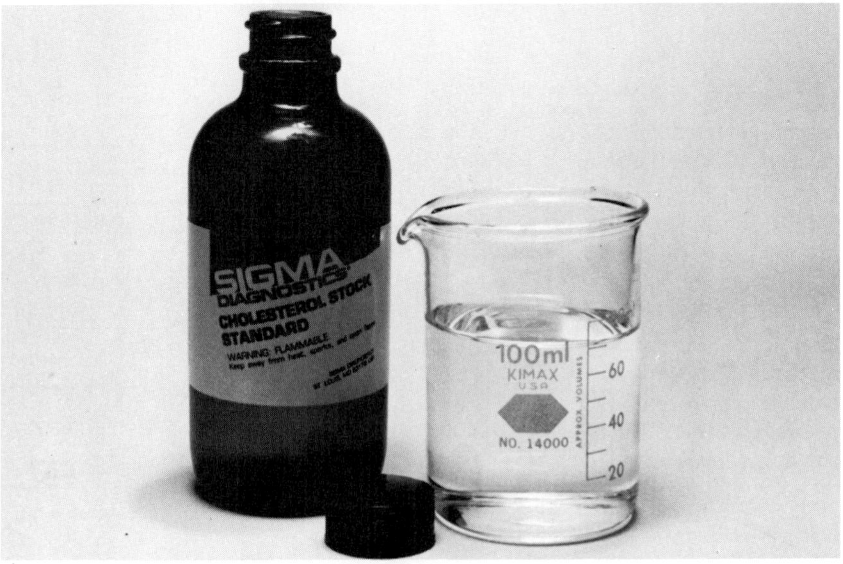

Chemical-grade cholesterol.

BOX 7-1

THE OMEGA-3 FATTY ACIDS

Omega-3 fatty acids and the diets of Eskimos have become hot topics. It has been recognized for many years that Eskimos consuming a traditional diet are at low risk of developing heart disease, high blood pressure, and a number of other diseases common in the U.S. and other economically developed countries.[1,2] It now appears that the Eskimos' protection from these diseases is partially related to the large amount of fish in their diets. Greenland Eskimos, for example, eat about a pound of fish each day.[2] This amount of fish assures a constant source of the omega-3 fatty acids. The typical U.S. diet does not provide nearly as much of the omega-3 fatty acids. This type of polyunsaturated fat is primarily found in fish and seafood (see table) and is contained only in trace amounts in other types of food.[3]

Omega-3 fatty acid content of selected seafoods[3]

Seafood, 3½-oz serving	Omega-3 Fatty Acids, grams
mackerel, Atlantic	2.6
scad	2.1
spiny dogfish	2.0
lake trout	2.0
herring	1.8
tuna	1.5
salmon	1.5
whitefish, lake	1.5
sturgeon	1.5
anchovies	1.4
bluefish	1.2
mullet	1.1
conch	1.0
oysters	0.6
brook trout	0.6
squid	0.6
catfish	0.5
shrimp	0.5
perch	0.4
crab	0.3
pike, walleye	0.3
cod	0.3
flounder	0.2
haddock	0.2
lobster	0.2
scallops	0.2
swordfish	0.2

The effects of omega-3 fatty acids on body processes have been studied extensively, and the research continues. Results so far indicate that they have a profound effect on the synthesis of certain types of prostaglandins, and that this in itself may account for many of the beneficial effects attributed to the omega-3 fatty acids. Prostaglandins are a versatile group of hormonelike substances that have both positive and negative effects on body processes. They induce psoriasis (a skin condition), asthma, and the inflammation that occurs with arthritis. Certain types of prostaglandins promote blood clotting, the buildup of cholesterol plaque within the walls of arteries, and affect blood pressure.[1,4,5,6]

If omega-3 fatty acids are consumed at a level of about 4 grams per day, production of the prostaglandins that promote the formation of cholesterol plaque and increase blood pressure are reduced.[5,6] One study undertaken in the Netherlands reported that as few as two fish meals per week provides protection against heart disease.[2]

Americans are being encouraged to increase their consumption of fish, but not their consumption of concentrated sources of fish oils.[4] Excessive intake of fish oils may slow blood clotting (especially important to people whose blood does not clot normally) and cause toxicities of vitamins A and D (vitamins that are stored in some fish oils) and of environmental contaminants that accumulate in the fat stores of fish and produce fragile cell membranes.[4] The omega-3 fatty acids become part of the lipid layer of cell membranes. This makes the membranes become fragile, because the omega-3 fatty acids contain many more double bonds (which are easily broken down) than do other fatty acids. As with all nutrients, there is an optimal range of intake of the omega-3 fatty acids, but the limits of this optimal range are yet to be defined.

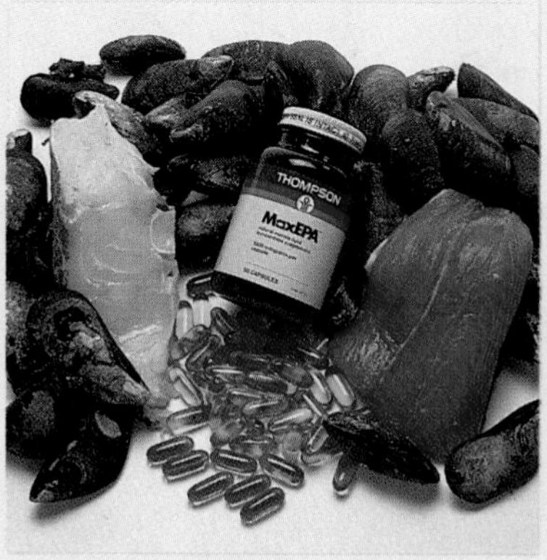

Seafoods are the major source of omega-3 fatty acids. Capsules containing these fatty acids are available, but they should be used with caution.

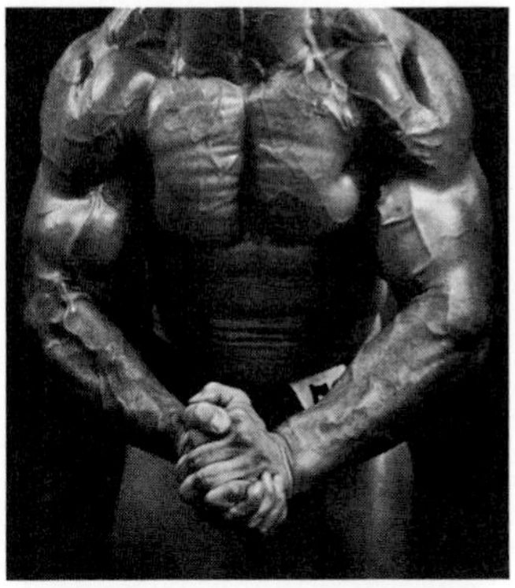

Some athletes, ignoring the health risks, use anabolic steroids to help them improve their performance.

include the sex hormones estrogen and testosterone and other hormones produced by the adrenal cortex—a tissue located in the adrenal gland that covers the top of the kidneys. There is hardly a body system that is not influenced by the steroid hormones. Their actions include increasing the formation of glucose, controlling sodium and potassium levels in blood, and promoting wound healing. There are "anabolic" steroids that act to build up muscle tissue and promote bone growth. (Unfortunately, steroid hormones have been abused by some athletes to increase body size and muscle mass. In healthy people, the use of certain types of steroid hormones increases the risk of cancer, sterility, and liver disease and causes anxiety and depression. Some ill effects of the hormones are not reversible and are life-threatening.[8]) Cholesterol is found in particularly high amounts in brain and nerve cell membranes. The presence of cholesterol in animal cell membranes means that it is found in both the fat and lean parts of animal products.

Food Sources of Cholesterol Cholesterol is present only in animals so it is exclusive to foods of animal origin (Table 7-5). It is a clear, oily liquid that cannot be seen in foods.

Foods don't have to be high in fat to be high in cholesterol. Liver and egg yolks are two of the richest sources of cholesterol, yet neither food is very high in fat. Beef is a moderate source of cholesterol, but it is often high in fat. Whole milk and bacon both contain a good deal of fat but not much

TABLE 7-5
Food sources of cholesterol

Food	Amount	Cholesterol, mg*
Animal Products		
brains	3 oz	>2,000
liver	3 oz	470
egg yolk	1	212
shrimp	3 oz	119
prime rib	3 oz	80
baked chicken (no skin)	3 oz	75
turkey (no skin)	3 oz	64
hamburger, regular	3 oz	60
pork chop, lean	3 oz	60
fish, baked (haddock, flounder)	3 oz	58
ice cream	1 c	56
sausage	3 oz	55
hamburger, lean	3 oz	50
whole milk	1 c	34
crab, boiled	3 oz	33
lobster	3 oz	29
cheese (cheddar)	1 oz	26
2%-fat milk	1 c	22
yogurt, low-fat	1 c	17
1%-fat milk	1 c	14
skim milk	1 c	7

*Recommended daily maximum intake for adults is 300 mg.

TABLE 7-6

Sources of cholesterol in the U.S. diet[24]

Food	% Of Total Cholesterol Intake
Eggs (egg yolk)	42
Beef, poultry, fish	38
Milk and milk products	15
Fats and oils	5

cholesterol. Most of the cholesterol consumed by people in the U.S. comes from egg yolks and meats with far less contributed by dairy products (Table 7-6). Beyond the fact that cholesterol is only found in animal products, it is hard to make generalizations about its food sources. You have to use a reference like Table 7-5 and check the nutrition labeling on food packages to learn the cholesterol content of foods.

Production of Cholesterol by the Liver A constant supply of cholesterol for hormone production and cell membranes is guaranteed by the liver; it's not necessary to depend on food sources of cholesterol for our supply. The liver produces cholesterol from fragments of saturated fatty acids. Under normal circumstances, the amount of cholesterol produced by the liver changes depending on the amount of cholesterol in the diet. In general, the amount of cholesterol produced by the liver decreases as intake of saturated fats and cholesterol increases. Adjustments made in the amount of cholesterol produced by the liver helps to keep blood cholesterol levels within a normal range. The liver's ability to regulate blood cholesterol content by cutting back on production is limited. Intakes of saturated fatty acids or cholesterol that are higher than the amount the liver can compensate for may result in high blood cholesterol levels.

Not everyone who has a high-fat or high-cholesterol diet develops high blood cholesterol levels, however. The reason for this is not known with certainty. It may be that some people's bodies break down cholesterol more effectively or that some people's livers produce less of it.

High blood cholesterol levels may exist for several reasons that are not related to diet. Cholesterol levels can be increased by genetic traits that cause the liver to produce an excessive amount of cholesterol and by certain drugs such as oral contraceptive pills and some drugs used for treating high blood pressure. People with a genetic tendency to form excessive cholesterol generally have higher blood cholesterol levels than do other people, even if they rigorously stick to diets designed to decrease their blood cholesterol.

A discussion of dietary fat and cholesterol, blood cholesterol, and heart disease follows our discussion of the lipoproteins. Certain types of lipoproteins are pivotal in the relationships between diet and heart disease.

Lipoproteins

Cholesterol is fat-soluble and must be made water-soluble so that it can be transported in blood. To meet this requirement, cholesterol and many other types of fat-soluble substances become attached to water-soluble "protein

lipoprotein: (*lipo* = "lipid" = fat) Water-soluble substance containing fat and protein molecules. The vast majority of lipids found in blood are lipoproteins.

phospholipids: (*phospho* = "phosphorus") Fatlike substances that contain fatty acids and phosphorus, and sometimes nitrogen. They are soluble in both water and fat. Lecithin is the most common phospholipid found in the body.

chylomicrons: (kī lō mī'krän) Tiny droplets containing triglycerides, phospholipids, cholesterol, and protein that are manufactured in the cells that line the small intestine. They serve to transport some of the end products of fat digestion to the heart and general circulation by way of the lymph system. They are just barely soluble in water.

carriers." When a fat or fatlike substance is combined with a protein carrier, the result is a **lipoprotein**. Lipoproteins contain mainly cholesterol, triglycerides, protein, and phospholipids (fats that are attached to phosphorus). If it weren't for the lipoproteins, fats circulating in the blood stream would rise to our heads and shoulders because they would float.

Four major types of lipoproteins transport fats and fatlike substances in the blood. They are classified by their density—their weight relative to the weight of other substances of equal volume. Lipoproteins containing a large proportion of fat and fatlike substances have low densities, whereas those containing relatively large amounts of protein have high densities. Figure 7-6 shows the proportion of cholesterol, triglycerides, protein, and **phospholipids** in each.[12]

- **Chylomicrons** are the least dense lipoprotein; they come close to floating in blood. They are packed with triglycerides and contain very little cholesterol or protein. Chylomicrons are responsible for transporting many of the end products of fat digestion through the blood.
- Very low density lipoproteins (VLDL) also consist primarily of triglycerides, but they contain less of them and are therefore slightly more dense than the chylomicrons. Very low density lipoproteins are produced

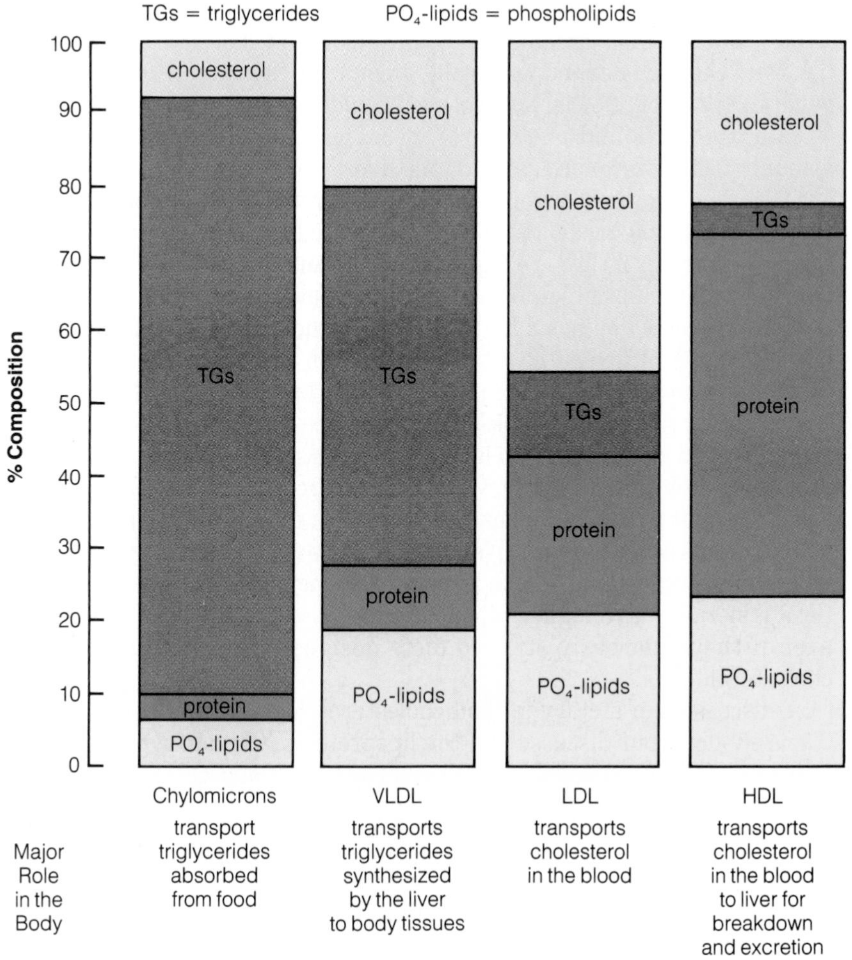

FIGURE 7-6

Composition and functions of the major classes of lipoproteins.

primarily by the liver and are used to transport triglycerides formed by the liver to fat and other cells. When very low density lipoproteins have transferred most of their content of triglycerides to cells, they become low-density lipoproteins.

- Low-density lipoproteins (LDL) contain the highest proportion of cholesterol of all the lipoproteins, and they are the major transporters of cholesterol in the blood. People who have high total blood cholesterol levels (a measure that includes the cholesterol content of all the lipoproteins) almost always have high levels of LDL.
- High-density lipoproteins (HDL) contain the largest amount of protein. They are considered the "good" lipoproteins. HDL removes cholesterol from the blood by transporting it to the liver, where it is broken down and eventually excreted.

Much of the concern about cholesterol and the lipoproteins that transport it in the blood is due to the strong association between blood levels of cholesterol and the risk of heart disease and stroke. Both disorders frequently result from **atherosclerosis**, a type of "hardening of the arteries" that is more likely to occur when blood cholesterol levels are high.

atherosclerosis: a type of "hardening of the arteries" in which plaque (cholesterol and other blood components) builds up in the walls of arteries. As the condition progresses, the arteries narrow, and the supply of blood to the heart, brain, muscles, and other organs and tissues is reduced.

Atherosclerosis

Atherosclerosis is the leading form of heart disease in the U.S. and the basic cause of some strokes. It results from the buildup of a solid material called *plaque* in the walls of arteries. The largest single component of plaque is cholesterol. The accumulation of cholesterol plaque within the walls of blood vessels causes the vessels to become narrower (Figure 7-7). If arteries become narrowed by 50% or more, symptoms of atherosclerosis appear. Two common symptoms are chest pains and shortness of breath. These symptoms are due to the reduced blood flow to the heart and lungs caused by the narrowed arteries. People who experience these symptoms are said to have *angina*. When one or more major arteries in the heart becomes plugged, a heart attack occurs. The stoppage in blood flow causes the affected part of the heart to stop functioning, and the heart may stop beating.

The reduced diameter of the arteries leading to the brain increases the chances that a blood clot will form and clog the vessel. If atherosclerosis

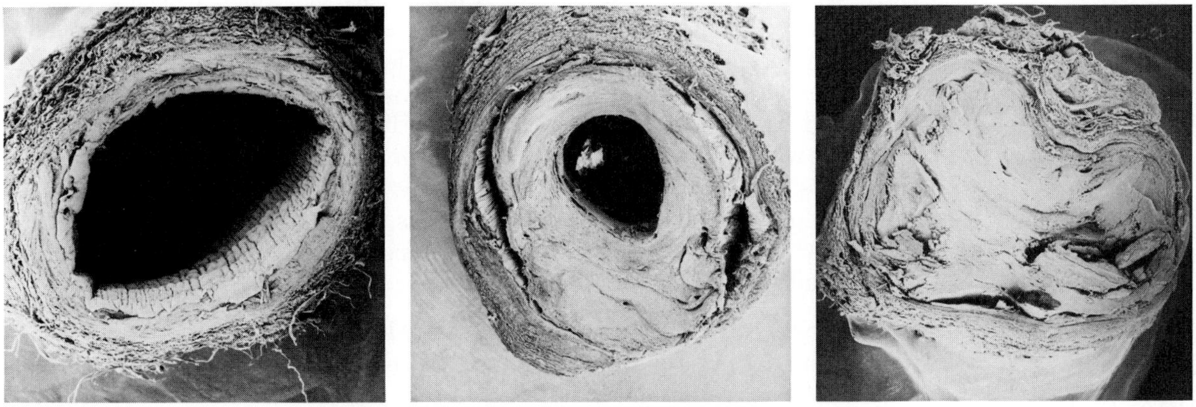

(a) (b) (c)

FIGURE 7-7
Scanning electron micrographs of cross sections of blood vessels varying in the degree of plaque formation. (a) A healthy vein. Note the various muscular layers. (b) Vessel whose capacity has been reduced by cholesterol deposits. (c) A totally blocked vessel.

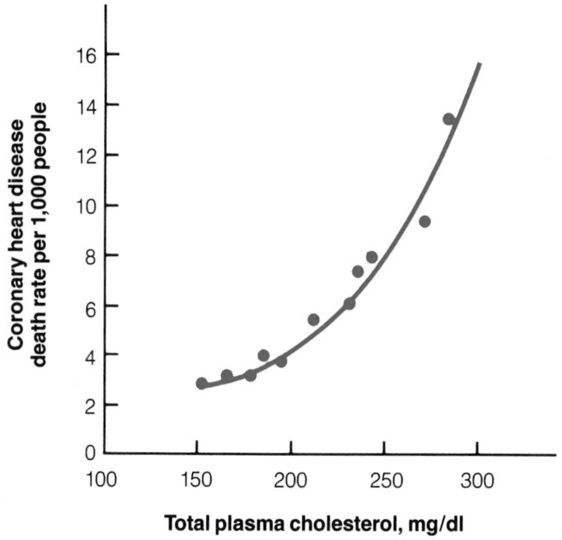

FIGURE 7-8
The relationship between blood cholesterol level and death from heart disease.

continues to progress, one or more of the arteries in the brain may become blocked. When this happens, a person experiences a *stroke*. The severity of a stroke depends on which part of the brain was denied blood and for how long.

Blood Cholesterol Levels and Atherosclerosis The likelihood of developing atherosclerosis and of dying from heart disease increases as blood cholesterol levels increase (Figure 7-8).[15] Approximately 40% of young adults in the U.S. have some degree of atherosclerosis,[10] and most adults have blood cholesterol levels that put them at risk for developing heart disease.[12] As illustrated in Figure 7-9, the average blood cholesterol levels of U.S. adults and youths are far above those associated with the lowest risk of developing heart disease. Total cholesterol levels of about 160 mg/dl in adults and 110 mg/dl in youths aged 5 to 18 correspond to lowest risks of developing heart disease. If you have had your blood cholesterol tested and want to know if the results may put you at risk, see Table 7-7. Blood cholesterol levels associated with low, moderate, and high risks of developing heart disease are presented there.

It should be stressed that an elevated cholesterol level does not guarantee that a person will develop heart disease or stroke. It means that the person's chances of developing them are greater than if his or her cholesterol level was lower. A small proportion of people who have severe atherosclerosis have never had a high cholesterol level, and some people with high cholesterol levels do not develop atherosclerosis or heart disease. People with high levels of HDL—the lipoprotein that lowers blood cholesterol level and protects against heart disease—may not develop atherosclerosis in spite of high blood cholesterol levels. A person's chances of developing heart disease are also increased by smoking, high blood pressure, and a family history of heart disease.

Lowering Blood Cholesterol Levels In general, people can lessen their risks of atherosclerosis, heart disease, and stroke by reducing their blood cholesterol levels.[11,13] Blood cholesterol reductions can be achieved by dietary changes and by drugs. Except for people with very high blood

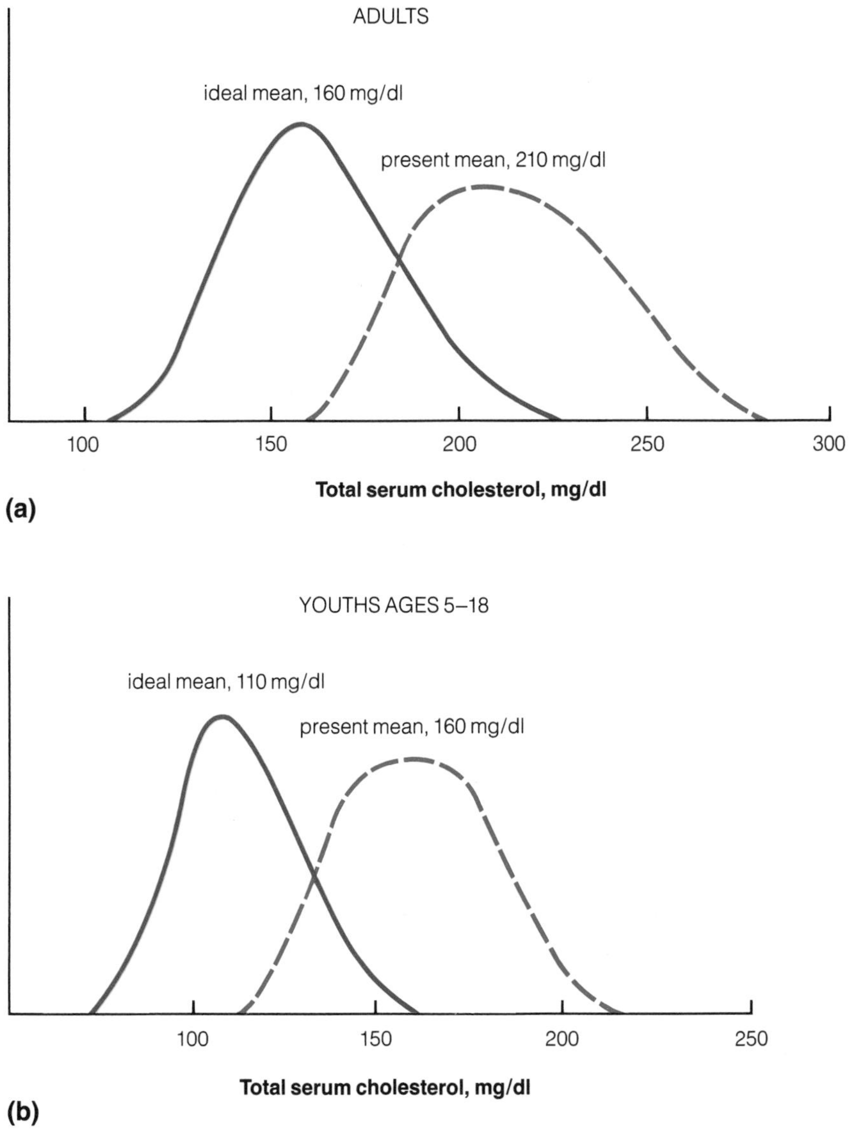

FIGURE 7-9
The difference between where serum cholesterol levels are and where they would be for low risk of heart disease among (a) adults and (b) youths.

TABLE 7-7
Blood cholesterol levels associated with the risk of developing heart disease by age group[30]

	Blood Cholesterol Level, mg/dl		
Age, years	Low Risk	Moderate Risk	High Risk
2–19	less than 170	170–185	185+
20+	less than 200	200–240	240+

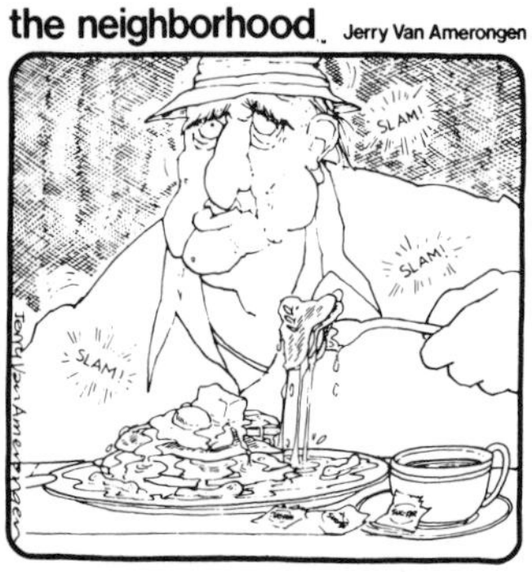

Half way through his "Hearty Man" breakfast, Dwayne thought he heard some of his smaller arteries slamming shut.

cholesterol levels, dietary changes are the recommended means of reducing cholesterol levels. Many of the drugs used to reduce cholesterol levels have side effects that make them worth the risks they present only for people who can't reduce their cholesterol levels by diet. In addition, the drugs are very expensive.

The type of diet that reduces blood levels of cholesterol in most people provides 30 percent or less of total calories as fat, 300 mg or less of cholesterol, and more polyunsaturated fats than saturated fats. Specifically, it is recommended that there be at least an even split between the amounts of saturated and polyunsaturated fats consumed; that is, that the ratio of the grams of polyunsaturated fats to the grams of saturated fats is one or greater.[14] Monounsaturated fats act to lower blood cholesterol levels, but to a lesser extent than do polyunsaturated fats.[15]

Two other approaches to reducing blood cholesterol are being recommended. One calls for eating fish at least twice a week. The other encourages the consumption of oat bran or products made from whole oats. Oat bran binds with cholesterol in the intestines and partially blocks its absorption. Consuming 2 tablespoons of oat bran a day has been found to lower blood cholesterol levels about as much as the cholesterol-lowering drugs.[16,17]

Of all the recommendations cited for a diet that reduces blood cholesterol levels (Table 7-8), the most common is to reduce saturated fat intake and limit total fat intake to less than 30 percent of total calories consumed. This makes a much larger dent in the blood cholesterol levels of most people than does reducing cholesterol intake or switching from saturated to polyunsaturated fats.[12,13] In light of all the publicity that cholesterol has gotten, this statement may seem strange, but it's true. Total dietary fat intake has a stronger influence on blood cholesterol levels in most people than does the intake of cholesterol. Table 7-9 will give you an idea of how a high-fat diet compares with a low-fat diet.

Major factors related to increasing HDL levels:
weight loss if overweight
physical fitness

Increasing HDL Levels Nutrition researchers have worked a long time trying to find a diet that helps increase HDL levels, which are not as easily modified by diet as is LDL, the lipoprotein that carries the most cholesterol. Low-fat diets do not increase HDL, and some research has shown that they actually decrease it.[12] Weight loss among people who are overweight and physical fitness are the major routes to increasing HDL levels.[19]

Phospholipids

emulsifying agent: A substance that will cause two liquids that are not soluble in each other to mix. An emulsifying agent allows a fat to mix with water, such as happens when bile causes the mixing of fat with digestive juices.

As we've said, phospholipids are fatlike substances that contain fatty acids attached to phosphorus and sometimes nitrogen. They are soluble in both water and fat, and they primarily function as **emulsifying agents** and as a component of cell membranes. The benefit of emulsifying agents is that they allow fat- and water-soluble substances to mix. This characteristic of phospholipids makes them well suited for helping dietary fats become soluble in water and acted upon by enzymes during digestion. The phospholipids in the lipoproteins just discussed work with protein carriers to make the transported triglycerides and cholesterol soluble in blood.

If it weren't for emulsifying agents, mayonnaise, for example, would "separate." The oil and water that are its basic components are held together in a smooth mixture (are *emulsified*) by the phospholipids contained in the egg yolk that is added. See Figure 7-10.

TABLE 7-8
Summary of dietary recommendations for reducing blood cholesterol levels

30% or less of total calories from fats
300 mg or less of cholesterol per day
P/S of 1 or greater
two or more fish meals per week
regular consumption of oat bran or products made from whole oats

TABLE 7-9
Comparison of the fat content of two menus

Meal	High-fat Menu	Lower-fat Menu
Breakfast	orange juice, 6 oz cornflakes, 1 c whole-wheat toast, 2 slices margarine, 2 t milk, 1 c	orange juice, 6 oz cornflakes, 1 c whole-wheat toast, 2 slices margarine, 2 t skim milk, 1 c
Lunch	cream of tomato soup, 1 c grilled cheese sandwich potato chips, 1 oz milk, 1 c	vegetable soup, 1 c cheese sandwich tomatoes, ½ c skim milk, 1 c
Snack	peanut butter, 2 T Ritz® crackers, 4	orange, 1 whole-wheat crackers, 4
Dinner	tossed salad, 1½ c salad dressing, 2 T fried chicken, 4 oz french fries, 1 c green beans, ½ c margarine, ½ t ice cream, 1 c milk, 1 c	tossed salad, 1½ c salad dressing, 2 T baked chicken, 4 oz boiled potatoes, 1 c green beans, ½ c margarine, ½ t ice milk, 1 c skim milk, 1 c

Food Constituent Analysis

	High-Fat Menu	Lower-Fat Menu
Calories	2,800	1,800
Carbohydrate, % of calories	38	53
Protein, % of calories	14	21
Fat, % of calories	48	29
P/S*	0.7	0.9
Cholesterol, mg	390	210

*P/S = ratio of the grams of polyunsaturated fats to the grams of saturated fats. A ratio of 1 or greater is recommended.

■
FIGURE 7-10
The beaker on the left contains water and oil. Note the layers. The beaker on the right contains an emulsion—mayonnaise—made by combining an egg with lemon juice, salad oil, and flavoring. The phosphate in the egg yolk served as the emulsifying agent.

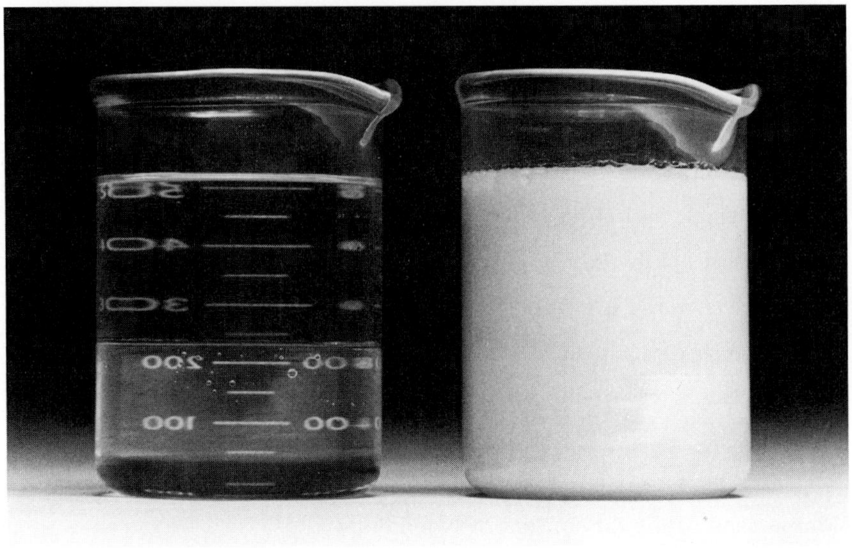

Waxes

waxes: Fat-soluble substances made from long-chain fatty acids and alcohol.

Waxes, too, are a type of fat. Like other fats, they contain a good deal of stored energy. (Think of the heat produced by wax candles.) Humans cannot digest wax, and the only way the body uses this type of fat is as a protective coating for the internal ear canal. Certain marine animals—sperm whales, for example—produce wax as a storage form of energy.

Artificial Fats

What do sucrose, long-chain fatty acids, and the proteins of egg whites and milk have in common? They are the basic ingredients of artificial fats.

The first artificial fat was discovered in the 1960s by accident. Researchers at a large company were attempting to develop a synthetic fat that could be absorbed easily by premature infants. Instead, the product developed wasn't absorbed well at all. It had the taste and texture of fat, but since it was not broken down by digestive enzymes or absorbed, it provided no calories. Although the researchers failed to develop the product they sought, they opened the doors to what has become a multimillion dollar industry.

Two artificial fats have now been developed, Olestra™ and Simplesse™. Both look and taste like fat and contain no cholesterol, but they have little else in common. Olestra is made by chemical reactions that tightly bind sucrose to long-chain fatty acids. The resulting chemical is a *sucrose polyester*. Olestra provides no calories, is heat-stable (so it can be used in cooked products), and may help reduce blood cholesterol levels.[9,20]

Simplesse can be produced from either egg white protein or cow's milk protein. It is partially digested by the body and provides 1⅓ calories per gram, one-seventh the calories provided by a gram of fat. Because it forms a gel when heated, Simplesse is not suitable for use in cooked products. Table 7-10 provides a comparison of Olestra and Simplesse.

Several side effects of artificial fats have been noted in human studies. It appears their use can decrease the absorption of the fat-soluble vitamins

■
TABLE 7-10
Comparison of two artificial fats

	Olestra	Simplesse
Basic ingredient(s)	Sucrose and long-chain fatty acids (sucrose polyester)	egg white protein or cow's milk protein
Caloric content	0	1⅓ calories per gram
Cholesterol content	0	0
Heat-stable?	yes	no
Food uses	Same as Simplesse plus cooking oils, shortenings, bakery products, snack foods	ice cream, yogurt, margarine, salad dressings, mayonnaise, cheese

(vitamins A and E, for example), and cause flatulence (gas), diarrhea, and other gastrointestinal upsets.[9,20]

Much remains to be learned about these products, because they have not yet been tested extensively in human studies. Questions yet to be answered include:

- Are they safe for all people?
- Do they help overweight individuals lose weight safely?
- Do they have positive or negative effects on overall diet quality?
- Do they increase the risk that people will develop deficiencies of fat-soluble vitamins?

Because artificial fats are classified as foods, rather than drugs, laboratory tests of their safety and effectiveness are not required. Nonetheless, it is likely that they will be tested so that questions posed by scientists and consumers about their safety can be answered.

■ ■ ■

DIGESTION AND ABSORPTION OF FATS

Digestion (Figure 7-11)

Lipases are the main enzymes involved in fat digestion. There are four major ones: lingual (tongue) lipase, gastric (stomach) lipase, pancreatic lipase, and intestinal lipase. Produced by glands located underneath the tongue, lingual lipase initiates the breakdown of fats in the mouth by splitting apart certain fatty acids. Since it is rendered inactive by the acid in the stomach, lingual lipase's role in fat digestion is short-lived and therefore limited.

Gastric lipase is produced by glands located in the wall of the stomach. It too has only a limited effect on fats. Gastric lipase breaks some of the triglycerides present into diglycerides, monoglycerides, glycerol, and fatty acids. A small proportion of the fatty acids that are split off from triglycerides are phospholipids, and some phospholipids are also consumed in

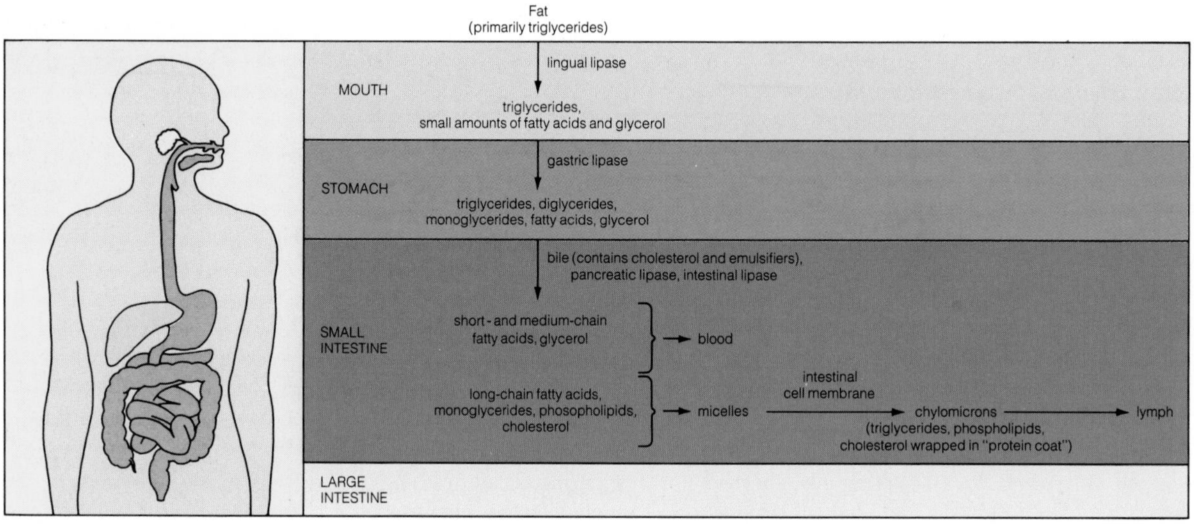

FIGURE 7-11
Overview of the digestion and absorption of fat.

foods. When churned together with fats in the stomach, the phospholipids partially emulsify the fats, which allows the fats to mix with water. This also allows the fats to come into contact with gastric lipase (which, like all digestive enzymes, is water-soluble) and facilitates the breakdown of fats.

Almost all of the breakdown of fats occurs in the small intestine. There the emulsification continues with the help of bile, a substance that is produced in the liver and stored in the gallbladder. Once made soluble in water, fats are easily broken down by pancreatic lipase, intestinal lipase, and other fat-splitting enzymes. The end products of fat digestion in the small intestine are fatty acids of various lengths, glycerol, phospholipids, cholesterol, and monoglycerides.

Normal fat digestion can be disrupted by several conditions. Diseases that affect the pancreas, such as pancreatitis (inflammation of the pancreas) and cystic fibrosis, reduce lipase production and lead to the incomplete digestion of fat. Intestinal infections that produce diarrhea may lead to the incomplete absorption of fats, because diarrhea causes foods to pass through the intestines quickly. Under normal circumstances, however, humans absorb about 95 percent of the fats that are consumed.

Absorption

The absorption of the end products of fat digestion is quite involved. Fatty acids of short and medium chain lengths and glycerol are absorbed into the cells lining the small intestines. Once inside these cells, the fatty acids are converted to water-soluble substances by becoming attached to protein carriers. After they become water-soluble, the short- and medium-chain fatty acids can be absorbed into blood vessels and transported to the liver. Since glycerol is water-soluble, it does not need a protein carrier to be absorbed into the blood.

The fate of long-chain fatty acids, most monoglycerides, phospholipids, and cholesterol is substantially different from that of the shorter-chain fatty acids and glycerol. On the surface of the lining of the small intestine, these substances are loosely combined into **micelles**, which pass into the cells of the lining. Once inside the cells, the micelles are repackaged into chylomi-

micelles: (mī sel′) Loosely bound molecules containing long-chain fatty acids, monoglycerides, phospholipids, and cholesterol. They are soluble in water.

crons (the least dense lipoproteins), which are barely soluble in water. The chylomicrons are absorbed into the lymph system, rather than into the blood. Lymph vessels that pick up nutrients from the small intestines "dump" them into the heart, and from there they enter the blood and general circulation.

Chylomicron levels in the blood increase dramatically after a person has eaten a high-fat meal. (See Figure 7-12.) Normally, enzymes in the liver break down the chylomicrons within a few hours. Because blood levels of chylomicrons remain elevated for several hours after a meal, the blood sample for a test to determine triglyceride levels should be drawn after a person has fasted for twelve hours.

The liver handles the triglycerides, fatty acids, and glycerol it receives in a number of ways:

- Triglycerides can be broken down into fatty acids and glycerol, or they can be sent to fat cells for storage.
- Fatty acids and glycerol can be reassembled into triglycerides, used to meet the energy needs of the liver, or sent back into the bloodstream for use by cells throughout the body.
- Fatty acids can also be used by the liver to make cholesterol and other fatlike substances.

Figure 7-13 summarizes the ways the body uses fats consumed in foods. The figure incorporates many of the functions of dietary fat and fatlike substances that have been discussed in this chapter.

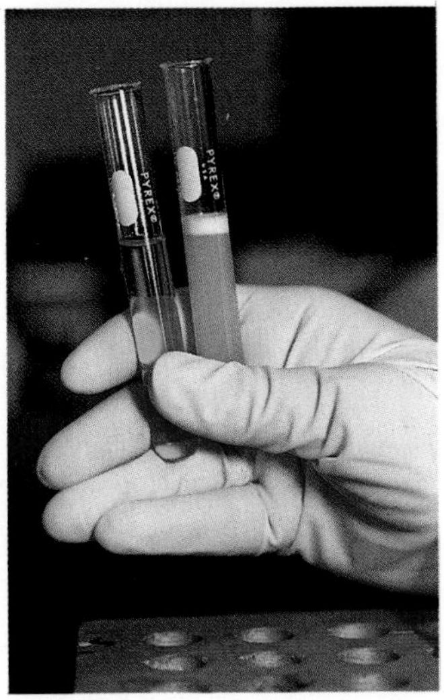

FIGURE 7-12

Blood plasma samples taken from a person while fasting *(left)* and after a high-fat meal *(right)*. Note the differing chylomicron layers at the top of the samples.

Energy Formation from Fatty Acids and Glycerol

As discussed in the section on nutrition and physical performance in chapter 3, fatty acids serve as our bodies' main source of energy when we are at rest or engaged in low levels of activity. Fatty acids are converted to energy in the **citric acid cycle**. Because glycerol can be converted to glucose, it enters the glycolysis pathway of energy formation.

citric acid cycle: A series of reactions in which specific forms of the energy nutrients are converted to carbon dioxide and water with a concomitant release of energy.

Optimal utilization of fatty acids for energy requires that the body have sufficient glucose to meet part of the energy need. If we consume far more fats than carbohydrates, or if our fuel supply is drawn from fat stores, our body must rely too heavily on fatty acids for energy. When that happens, some of the fatty acids that enter the citric acid cycle are not completely

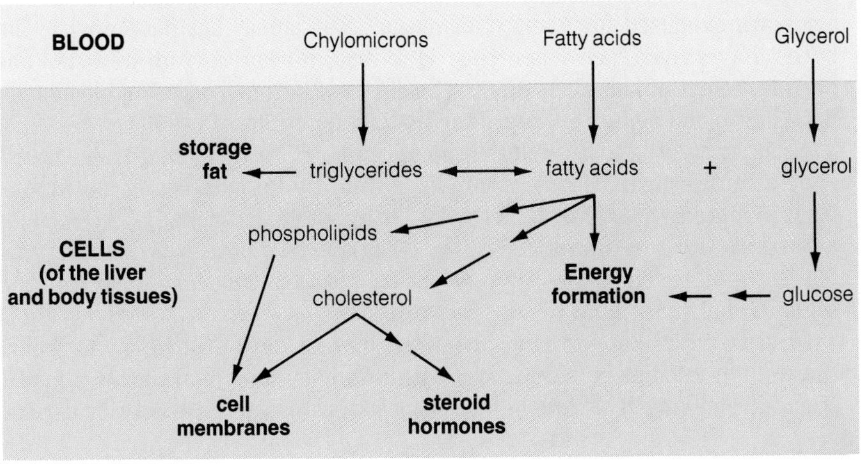

FIGURE 7-13

Major ways the body uses fats and fatlike substances received from foods.

BOX 7-2

WHY WHALES HAVE BAD BREATH

The "bad breath" symptom of ketosis holds for whales as well as humans. For most of the winter months whales live off the fat they stored during the summer. This exclusive use of body fat for fuel can make them unattractive diving partners for humans. One diver says that it's a good idea to be underwater if a whale surfaces nearby. This is because the air they exhale has a very offensive odor and it will coat your mask with a layer of grease. From a distance, however, the whales' ketosis does not tarnish their beauty.

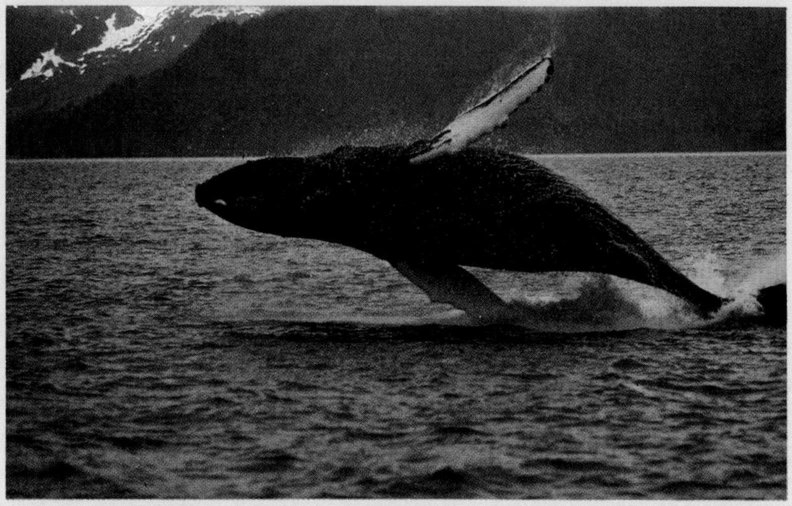

ketone bodies: A group of chemical by-products formed by incomplete utilization of fat for energy.

ketosis: A condition in which *ketone bodies*—breakdown products from fats used in energy formation—accumulate in the blood and urine; it results when people depend primarily on dietary fat or body fat stores for energy.

used up. By-products of the incomplete "burning" of fatty acids accumulate in the cells and eventually spill over into the blood. These by-products of the incomplete utilization of fatty acids are called **ketone bodies**. Low levels of ketone bodies in cells and the blood do not threaten health, but high levels do; they cause a condition known as **ketosis**.

Ketosis People with insulin-dependent diabetes who fail to take insulin, people on low-calorie–high-fat diets, and people who fast all develop ketosis. This is because their cells do not receive enough glucose, and fatty acids are overused for energy formation. The coma that people with diabetes may experience when they lack insulin results from ketosis. The harmful effect of ketosis is due to the effect of ketone bodies on blood acidity. High blood acidity disrupts the normal functions of cells.

Symptoms of ketosis include loss of appetite, fatigue, confusion, shortened attention span, thirst, and mild nausea. Bad breath is also a common, early symptom. (See Box 7-2.) The loss of appetite that usually accompanies ketosis has not gone unnoticed by the designers of weight-loss diets. A number of popular weight-loss approaches are based on low-carbohydrate, "ketogenic" diets that tend to suppress appetite.

Mild forms of ketosis can appear within two days after a low-carbohydrate–high-fat diet is begun, and within twenty-four hours after a fast is started. The length of time before ketosis develops and its severity depend on the person's glycogen stores and the amount of carbohydrate being consumed. Ketosis can generally be prevented by consuming 100 grams or more of carbohydrate a day.[21]

■ ■ ■

FOOD SOURCES OF FAT

Three types of food provide about 90 percent of the fat consumed in the U.S.: fats and oils (43%); beef, poultry, and fish (36%); and dairy products (12%).[24] The most concentrated sources of fats in the diet are fats such as butter, margarine, and oils. Many fast foods such as hamburgers, fried chicken, French fries, potato and taco chips, ice cream, and milk shakes also are high in fat. Nearly all vegetables are naturally low in fat—before butter and sauces are added to them. Other than avocados, fruits contain little fat. Table 7-11 lists food sources of fat and the percent of total calories supplied by fat.

Not all foods that are high in fat *look* it. Bacon and sausage appear fatty and they are, but what about nuts, milk chocolate, and cheese? They are also high in fat, but it is not so apparent. Dry-roasted nuts lack the oily shine that other roasted peanuts have, but if you crush a dry-roasted nut between two sheets of paper towel, you'll see quite a grease spot. You can't always tell the fat content of food by looking at it. Most of the fat we consume in food is invisible to the eye.

TABLE 7-11
Food sources of fat

		Fat Content	
Food	**Amount**	Grams	% Of Total Calories*
Fats and Oils			
butter	1 t	4	100
margarine	1 t	4	100
oil	1 t	4.7	100
mayonnaise	1 T	11	99
heavy cream	1 T	5.5	93
salad dressing	1 T	6	83
gravy	¼ c	14	77
salad dressing, low-cal	1 T	1	45
Meats and Eggs			
frankfurter	1 (2 oz)	17	83
bologna	1 oz	8	80
sausage	4 links	18	77
bacon	3 pieces	9	74
salami	2 oz	11	68

continued

TABLE 7-11, *continued*

Food	Amount	Fat Content: Grams	Fat Content: % Of Total Calories*
Meats and Eggs, *cont.*			
egg	1	6	68
pork, beef, or veal with fat	3 oz	18	62
hamburger, regular (20% fat)	3 oz	16.5	62
chicken, fried with skin	3 oz	14	53
Big Mac®	6.6 oz	31.4	52
Quarter Pounder with Cheese®	6.8 oz	28.6	50
Whopper®	8.9 oz	32	48
hamburger, lean (10% fat)	3 oz	9.5	45
TV dinner, pork	11 oz	21.9	43
pork, beef, or veal (lean)	3 oz	8	39
tuna in oil, drained	3 oz	7	38
chicken, baked, without skin	3 oz	4	25
flounder, baked	3 oz	1	13
shrimp, boiled	3 oz	1	9
tuna in water	3 oz	1	7
Dairy Products			
cheddar cheese	1 oz	9.5	74
whole milk	1 c	8.5	49
2% milk	1 c	5.0	32
1% milk	1 c	2.7	24
yogurt with fruit	1 c	2.6	10
skim milk	1 c	0.4	4
Other			
avocado	½	15	84
sunflower seeds	¼ c	17	77
peanut butter	1 T	8	76
peanuts	¼ c	17.5	75
potato chips	1 oz (13 chips)	11	61
chocolate chip cookies	4	11	54
french fries	20 fries	20	49
taco chips	1 oz (10 chips)	6.2	41
potatoes, mashed	½ c	4.5	41
potato, baked	1	0.2	1

*Recommended intake for adults is 30% or less of total calories. Diets that contain less than 30% of their total calories as fat include less than 34 grams of fat per 1,000 calories—for most adults, less than 78 grams of fat per day.

RECOMMENDED INTAKE OF FAT

With the exception of linoleic acid, the body can manufacture the fats it needs from carbohydrates and proteins. Consequently, there is no dietary requirement for fat, but there is one for linoleic acid. One to two percent of the total supply of calories should come from linoleic acid. Getting this amount is not a problem for most people; it is the most abundant polyunsaturated fatty acid in the U.S. diet. Americans consume an average of 5% of their total calories as linoleic acid.[22]

Although there is no RDA for fat, it is generally recommended that no more than 30% of the total calories consumed should come from fat, and that there should be at least an even split (a P/S ratio of at least 1) between the amount of polyunsaturated and saturated fats consumed.[23] (The P/S ratios for a variety of food sources of fat are given in Table 7-4.) Monounsaturated fats should make up about 10% of the total calories in a diet—or a third of a 30%-fat diet. On average, people in the U.S. consume 38% of their total calories as fat and consume more saturated fat than is recommended (Figure 7-14).[24]

The good news is that the fat intake of Americans is improving. The proportion of fat intake provided by vegetable oils is increasing, while that from animal fat is declining (Figure 7-15). Declines in the intake of animal fat have been accompanied by a 40% decline in heart disease the last 40 years.[25] The best news, however, would be evidence that *total* fat intake is decreasing. This goal is important because, in addition to concerns about heart

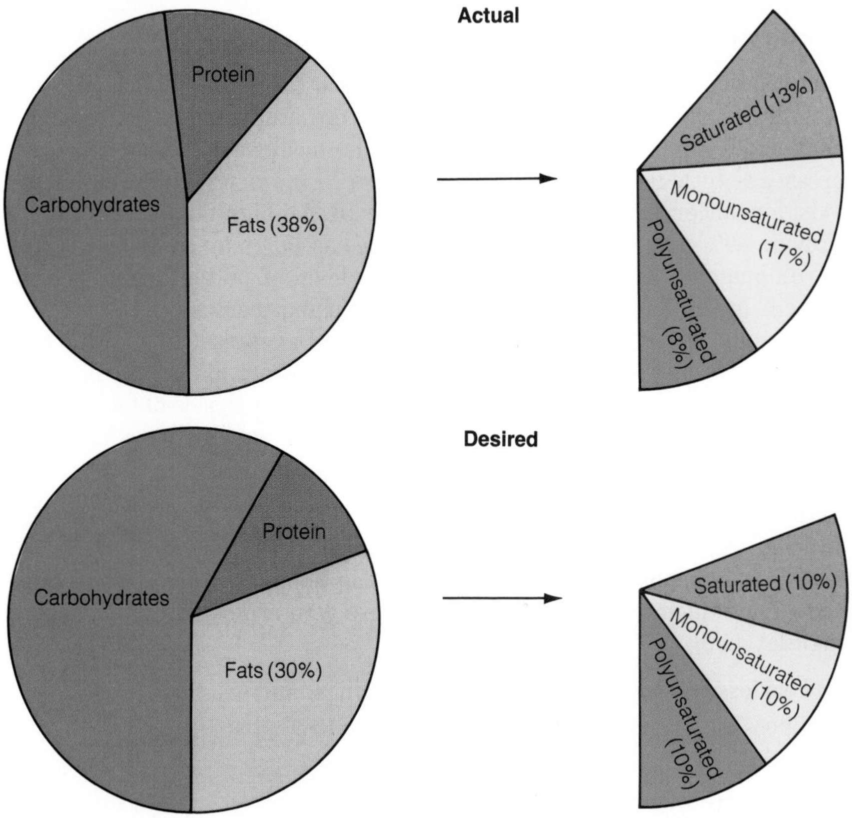

FIGURE 7-14
Actual and desired distribution of calories from fat.

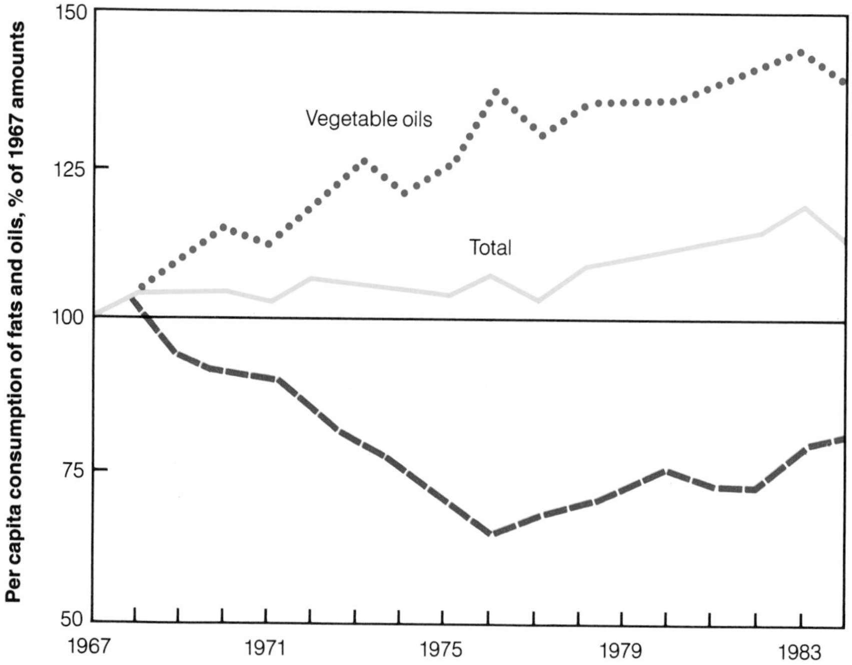

■
FIGURE 7-15
Overall changes in fat consumption in the U.S. since 1967.

disease and the high calorie content of fats, high fat intakes are also associated with the development of certain types of cancer. Unfortunately, the total fat content of the typical U.S. diet continues to be too high.

Dietary Fats and Cancer

The relationship between total fat intake and the development of cancer was first suspected in the 1940s,[26] and recent studies have confirmed it. Studies of populations have shown that the incidence of colon cancer increases as total fat intake increases (Figure 7-16). Very similar correlations exist for cancer of the breast.[27] It is suspected that high-fat diets (those that provide 40% or more of their total calories as fat) may contribute to the development of cancer by increasing the level of potentially toxic substances in the colon and, in females, by causing increased production of estrogens that may enhance tumor growth.[28] In contrast to the 30% total fat diet recommended for reducing the risk of heart disease, it has been suggested that diets containing 20% to 25% of total calories of fat would be best for reducing cancer risk.[29] In any event, the bottom line is that most Americans would probably be healthier if they consumed less fat.

Trimming Fat Intake How does one go about reducing total fat intake? It doesn't have to be very painful; rather small changes in food choices can lead to significant reductions in fat consumption. Here are some suggestions for reducing total fat intake for those who are currently consuming high-fat diets:

1. Use less butter, margarine, salad dressings, and oil.
2. Choose lean cuts of beef, such as flank and round steak.
3. Use low-fat dairy products.
4. Bake, broil, or microwave instead of frying foods.

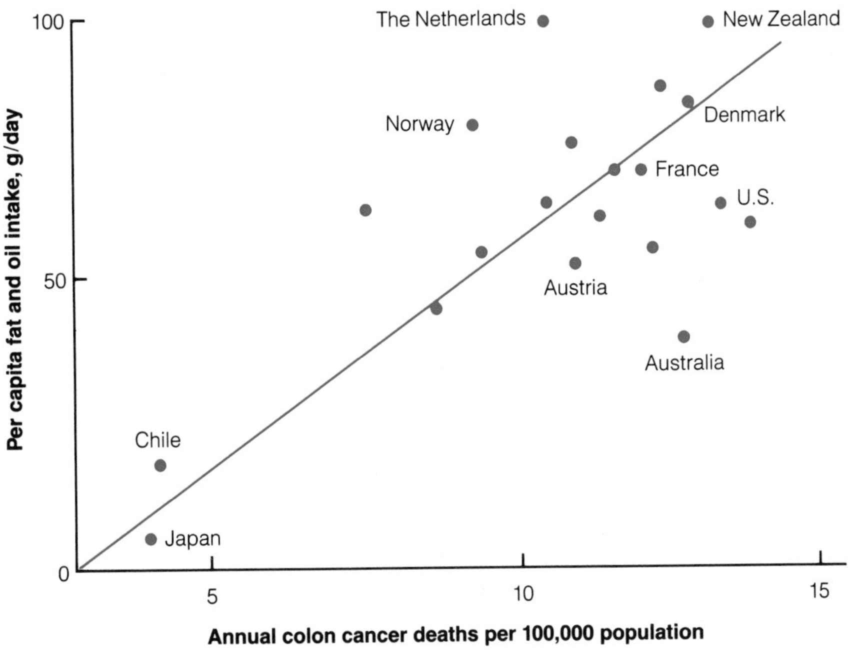

FIGURE 7-16
The relationship between a population's average fat and oil intake and death rates from colon cancer.

The exercises in Putting Nutrition Knowledge to Work will help you to assess the fat level of your diet and to identify some simple changes that will lower your fat intake.

COMING UP IN CHAPTER 8

In the next chapter, we begin our "tour" of the substances in food that make carbohydrates, proteins, and fats work for us—the vitamins and minerals. Although vitamins and minerals occur in foods in very small amounts, their roles in the body are large indeed.

REVIEW QUESTIONS

1. Like carbohydrates, fats consist of the elements ________, ________, and ________, but fats contain a higher proportion of the element ________.
2. Why do fats provide more than twice as much energy gram for gram than carbohydrates?
3. Cite three roles of dietary fat and three roles of body fat.
4. For healthy adults, the only known essential fatty acid is ________ ________.
5. What name change has been recommended for *triglycerides*?
6. Glycerol attached to two fatty acids forms a ________.
7. Glycerol attached to two polyunsaturated fatty acids forms a ________ ________.

8. A fatty acid that contains 12 or more carbons is considered a ________ ________-chain fatty acid.
9. Which is chemically weaker, a single bond or a double bond?
10. True or false: Saturated fats tend to be solid at room temperature, whereas unsaturated fats tend to be liquid at room temperature.
11. What types of food provide over 50% of their total fat content as saturated fats? What foods provide mainly polyunsaturated fats?
12. What two vegetable oils are high in saturated fats?
13. It has been recommended that Americans in general should consume fish more often and high-fat meats less often. What is the basis for this recommendation?
14. Name three adverse potential consequences of consuming high amounts of fish oils.
15. The harder the hydrogenated fat made from vegetable oils, the more ____________ fatty acids it contains.
16. What are the two major roles of cholesterol in the body?
17. Which food accounts for the largest proportion of cholesterol intake by Americans in general? What type of food is the second leading contributor to cholesterol intake?
18. Is cholesterol an essential nutrient?
19. Which type of diet is more likely to elevate blood cholesterol levels: a diet that is high in saturated fat or a high-cholesterol diet?
20. Name the four major types of cholesterol-containing lipoproteins. High levels of which one of these reduce the risk of developing heart disease, and high levels of which one increase the risk?
21. True or false: Most adults in the U.S. have blood cholesterol levels that put them "at risk" of developing heart disease.
22. True or false: Monounsaturated fats, like polyunsaturated fats, tend to lower blood cholesterol.
23. Give three examples of dietary advice that generally helps lower blood cholesterol if followed.
24. Low HDL levels can often be raised by ____________________________ and by ____________________________.
25. Where are most of the body's phospholipids located?
26. What digestive enzyme acts on fats in the stomach?
27. How does bile facilitate fat digestion?
28. Which end products of fat digestion are absorbed into blood vessels, and which are absorbed into the lymph system?
29. Diagram the major ways the body uses fats and fatlike substances received from food.
30. What are ketone bodies?
31. What is ketosis?
32. Why do people on very high fat diets or very low calorie diets or people with diabetes develop ketosis?
33. Three types of food account for about 90% of the fat consumed in the U.S. What are those types of food?

34. Two types of food account for the least fat consumed in the U.S. What are they?
35. What percentage of the total calories in a "lean" hamburger patty are fat calories?
36. What percentage of our total caloric intake should be provided by fat, according to recommendations?
37. High-fat diets have been associated with the development of ______ and ________ cancer.

Answers

1. Carbon, hydrogen, and oxygen; hydrogen.
2. Fats contain more carbon–hydrogen bonds, and carbohydrates contain more carbon–oxygen bonds. C–H bonds release more energy when broken than do C–O bonds.
3. Tables 7-1 and 7-2 provide the answers.
4. Linoleic acid.
5. Triacylglycerol.
6. Diglyceride.
7. Polyunsaturated fat.
8. Long.
9. Double bond.
10. It's true. As a matter of fact, the more double bonds contained in the fatty acids of a fat, the softer or more liquid it is at room temperature.
11. Refer to Table 7-4 for the answers.
12. Coconut oil and palm oil.
13. The answer is provided in Box 7-1.
14. Slowed blood clotting time (excessive bleeding), toxicities of vitamins A and D, intake of environmental contaminants.
15. Saturated.
16. Steroid hormone formation and as a component of cell membranes.
17. Eggs are number 1; meats are number 2.
18. No, it is produced by the liver.
19. A diet that is high in saturated fat.
20. Chylomicrons, VLDL (very low density lipoproteins), LDL (low-density lipoproteins), and HDL (high-density lipoproteins); high levels of HDL reduce the risk; high levels of LDL increase the risk.
21. True.
22. True.
23. See Table 7-8.
24. Losing weight if overweight, becoming physically fit.
25. In cell membranes.
26. Gastric lipase.
27. Bile emulsifies fats, thereby making fats partly soluble in water so they can be broken down by enzymes.

28. See Figure 7-11.
29. See Figure 7-13.
30. Fatty acid fragments that remain when fats are incompletely used to form energy.
31. A condition that results from abnormally high levels of ketone bodies in the blood.
32. In each case, ketosis develops because too little glucose is available to cells for energy formation, and the body must overrely on fats to meet energy needs.
33. Fats and oils; beef, poultry, and fish; and dairy products.
34. Fruits and vegetables.
35. 45%.
36. 30% or less.
37. Colon, breast.

■ ■ ■

PUTTING NUTRITION KNOWLEDGE TO WORK

1. Assume that your diet provided almost no carbohydrate, but plenty of protein and fat. (a) How would your body's need for glucose be met? (b) What would likely happen to your appetite on this type of diet? Why?

   (Answers: (a) They would be met in three ways: by converting stored glycogen to glucose, by converting certain amino acids to glucose, and by converting glycerol (generated by the breakdown of storage fat) to glucose. (b) Your appetite would probably decrease due to mild ketosis that results from the extensive use of fatty acids for energy formation.)

2. Here is the list of ingredients given on a package of wheat snack crackers: whole wheat, vegetable oil (coconut oil), salt. Are the crackers made from saturated or unsaturated fatty acids?

   (Answer: Refer to Table 7-4.)

3. After a full afternoon of studying for mid-term exams, you decide to go out for dinner at a fast-food restaurant. You order "the usual"—a quarter-pound cheeseburger (518 calories), an order of (20) French fries (220 calories), and a diet soda (0 calories). What percentage of the total calories consumed in this meal would come from fat? Use Table 7-13.

   (Answer: Total calories in the meal = 738; total grams fat = 48.6. Calories contributed by fat = 48.6 grams of fat × 9 calories per gram of fat = 437.4 calories. Percent of total calories as fat = 437.4 ÷ 738 = 0.593. Converting to a percent, 0.593 × 100 = 59.3%.)

4. Name a low-fat alternative for each of these high-fat foods.

   a. bacon
   b. bologna
   c. sausage
   d. ground beef
   e. salad dressing
   f. potato chips
   g. cream soup
   h. pastries and rich desserts

i. ice cream
j. milk
k. American cheese

(Answers: a. Canadian bacon, lean ham. b. chicken, turkey, turkey ham. c. lean ham or pork. d. ground turkey or extra-lean beef. e. low-calorie salad dressing, yogurt dressing. f. popcorn, pretzels (preferably low-salt), whole-grain cereals. g. broth-based soup. h. angel food cake, fruit. i. ice milk, frozen yogurt. j. skim milk, buttermilk. k. skim milk, low-fat mozzarella cheese.)

5. How do you score on fat? How often do you eat each of these types of food? less than once per week, 1 to 3 times a week, 4 to 6 times a week, or daily?

a. Fried or deep-fat-fried foods
b. Fatty meats such as bacon, sausage, luncheon meats, and heavily marbled steaks and roasts
c. Whole milk, high-fat cheeses, and ice cream
d. High-fat desserts such as pies, pastries, and rich cakes
e. Rich sauces and gravies
f. Salad dressings or mayonnaise
g. Whipped cream, table cream, sour cream, or cream cheese
h. Butter or margarine on vegetables

Is it time to cut back on foods that are high in fat? If you answered "4 to 6 times a week" or "daily" several times, you may have a high fat intake.

NOTES

1. W. E. M. Lands, Renewed questions about polyunsaturated fatty acids. *Nutrition Reviews* 44 (1986): 189–195.

2. D. Kromhout, E. B. Bosschiefer, and C. Lezenne-Coulander, The inverse relation between fish consumption and 20-year mortality from coronary heart disease, *New England Journal of Medicine* 312 (1985): 1205–1209.

3. F. N. Hepburn, J. Exler, and J. L. Weihrauch, Provisional tables on the content of omega-3-fatty acids and other fat components of selected foods, *Journal of the American Dietetic Association* 86 (1986): 788–793.

4. H. Carswell, Fish oil in anti-coronary heart disease swim, *Medical Tribune*, June 18, 1986.

5. M. Thorngren, E. Nilsson, and A. Gustafson, Plasma lipoproteins and fatty acid composition during a moderate eicosapentaenoic acid diet, *Acta Medica Scandinavica* 219 (1986): 23–28.

6. P. Singer, M. Wirth, et al., Blood pressure and lipid-lowering effect of mackerel and herring diet in patients with mild essential hypertension, *Atherosclerosis* 56 (1985): 223–235.

7. C. D. Turner and J. T. Bagnara, *General Endocrinology*, 5th ed. (Philadelphia: W. B. Saunders Co., 1971), 348–386.

8. *Physician's Desk Reference*, 41st ed. (Oradell, N.J.: Medical Economics Co., 1987).

9. R. W. Fallat, Short term study of sucrose polyester, a non-absorbable fat-like material as a dietary agent for lowering plasma cholesterol, *American Journal of Clinical Nutrition* 29 (1976): 1204–1205.

10. P. O. Kwitervoich, Jr., and K. M. Salz, Pediatric aspects of the diet-heart hypothesis, in *Infant and Child Feeding* (New York: Academic Press, 1981), 283–313.

11. D. F. Horrobin and M. S. Manku, How do polyunsaturated fatty acids lower plasma cholesterol levels? *Lipids* 18 (1983): 558–562.

12. E. J. Schaefer, D. G. Rees, and E. N. Siguel, Nutrition, lipoproteins, and atherosclerosis, *Clinical Nutrition* 5 (1986): 99–111.

13. A. C. Arntzenius and D. Kromhout, et al., Diet, lipoproteins, and the progression of coronary atherosclerosis, The Leiden Intervention Trial, *New England Journal of Medicine* 312 (1985): 805–811.

14. R. W. Mahley, Atherogenic hyperlipoproteinemia, *Medical Clinics of North America* 66 (1982): 375–402.

15. A. Keys, The diet and 15-year death rate in the Seven Country Study, *American Journal of Epidemiology* 124 (1986): 903–915.

16. B. P. Kinosian and J. M. Eisenberg, Cutting into cholesterol. Cost-effective alternatives for treating hypercholesterolemia, *Journal of the American Medical Association* 259 (1988): 2249–2254.

17. K. V. Gold and D. M. Davidson, Oat bran as a cholesterol-reducing dietary adjunct in a young, healthy population, *Western Journal of Medicine* 148 (1988): 299–302.

18. A. Nordoy, Dietary fatty acids, platelets, endothelial cells and coronary heart disease, *Acta Medica Scandinavica* (Supplement) 701 (1985): 15–22.

19. P. Hespel, Changes in plasma lipids and apoproteins associated with physical training in middle-aged sedentary men, *American Heart Journal* 115 (1988): 786–792.

20. S. M. Grundy and J. V. Anastasia, et al., Influence of sucrose polyester on plasma 1 lipoproteins and cholesterol metabolism in obese patients with and without diabetes mellitus, *American Journal of Clinical Nutrition* 44 (1986): 620–629.

21. R. A. Gelfand and R. S. Sherwin, Nitrogen conservation in starvation revisited: protein sparing with intravenous fructose, *Metabolism* 35 (1986): 37–44.

22. *Recommended Dietary Allowances*, 9th ed., Food and Nutrition Board, National Research Council (Washington, D.C.: National Academy of Sciences, 1980).

23. Dietary guidelines for Americans, 2nd ed., *Home and Garden* bulletin no. 232 (Washington, D.C.: U.S. Departments of Agriculture and Health and Human Services, 1985).

24. Nationwide Food Consumption Survey, report no. 85. Nutrition Monitoring Division, CSF 11 (Washington, D.C.: U.S. Department of Agriculture, 1985).

25. T. Thom, *Personal communication* (National Heart, Blood, and Lung Institute, Washington, D.C.), April 14, 1986.

26. A. Tannebaum, The genesis and growth of tumors. IV. Effects of a high-fat diet, *Cancer Research* 2 (1942): 468–475.

27. S. C. Newman, A. B. Miller, and G. R. Hove, A study of the effect of weight and dietary fat on breast cancer survival time, *American Journal of Epidemiology* 123 (1986): 767–774.

28. *Diet, Nutrition, and Cancer*, Committee on Diet, Nutrition, and Cancer. National Research Council (Washington, D.C.: National Academy of Sciences, 1982).

29. L. A. Cohen, Effect of varying proportions of dietary fat on the development of N-nitrosomethylurea-induced rat mammary tumors, *Anti-Cancer Research* 6 (1986): 215–218.

30. National Cholesterol Education Program, National Heart, Lung, and Blood Institute, Bethesda, Md., 1988.

CHAPTER

8

INTRODUCTION TO VITAMINS AND MINERALS

The decade was the 1920s. Horse-drawn carriages competed with cars for space on the roads, listening to the radio had become a major form of entertainment, and "My Blue Heaven" was a hit tune. World War I was over, and the Depression had not yet begun. It was a time of rapid growth for industries, cities, and the U.S. population—a "boom" period.

It was also a time when thousands of people were suffering serious health problems due to deficiency diseases; pellagra, the niacin-deficiency disease, and rickets, caused by a deficiency of vitamin D, were common. Thousands of people died from pellagra early in this century (Figure 8-1). Orthopedic wards in many city hospitals were largely occupied by children requiring treatment for bone deformities caused by rickets. Pellagra, rickets, and other serious deficiency diseases had captured the attention of the American people and had made them very aware of the importance of vitamins and minerals to health.

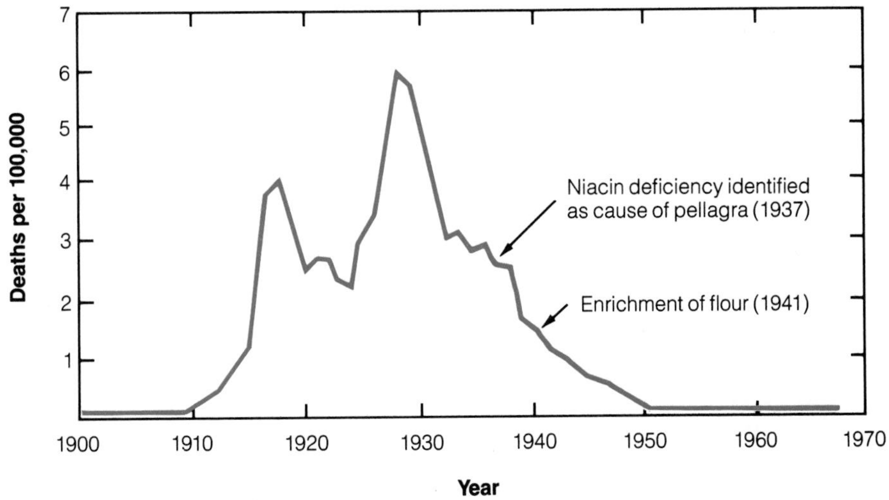

FIGURE 8-1
Pellagra death rates.

People's concerns about vitamins and minerals have changed substantially since the days of widespread deficiency diseases. Today, most Americans have access to a balanced variety of foods, and vitamin- and mineral-deficiency diseases are far less common. Vitamin- and mineral-deficiency diseases now occur so infrequently that when they do occur, they are apt to be diagnosed incorrectly or to be accurately diagnosed only after many other diseases have been ruled out.

Current concerns about vitamins and minerals center on the common occurrence of mild forms of deficiency, on toxicity diseases resulting from excessive use of vitamin and mineral supplements, and on the roles of vitamins and minerals in preventing chronic diseases and disorders. We are entering a new age in the study of vitamins and minerals—an age in which the emphasis is on the roles vitamins and minerals play in keeping people healthy, rather than just free from deficiency diseases.

VITAMIN AND MINERAL BASICS

Vitamins and minerals are sometimes referred to as *trace nutrients* and as *the micronutrients*. Humans need them in very small amounts, and they are present in foods in very small amounts. Nonetheless, very small amounts of these essential substances have profound effects on body functions.

How Vitamins and Minerals Are Similar

Vitamins and minerals share several characteristics:

- Both are found in small amounts in food.
- Both are needed in small amounts by the body.
- Neither is used as a source of energy.
- Both play important roles in the metabolism of carbohydrates, proteins, and fats.

The similarity that warrants the most discussion is the last one. A major function of many vitamins (the B-complex vitamins) and minerals is as activators of the enzymes involved in the metabolism of carbohydrates, proteins, and fats. Many of the problems that occur when too little or too much of a vitamin or mineral is available to the body are caused by faulty enzyme functioning.

Enzymes, Coenzymes, and Cofactors Vitamins and minerals serve as "switches" that turn on and off the hundreds of enzymes involved in carbohydrate, protein, and fat metabolism. An enzyme is "switched on" when its particular vitamin or mineral activator is present. When attached to its activator, an enzyme is able to transform specific raw ingredients into chemical substances needed by the body. When a sufficient supply of the substance produced by the activated enzyme is available, the activator detaches, thereby "turning off" the enzyme.

coenzyme: A form of a B-complex vitamin that activates an enzyme. Each B-complex vitamin has one or more coenzyme forms that activate specific enzymes.

Vitamins that activate enzymes are called **coenzymes** (Figure 8-2). All of the B-complex vitamins have coenzyme forms whose chemical structures are very similar to those of the respective vitamins. Like switches that turn

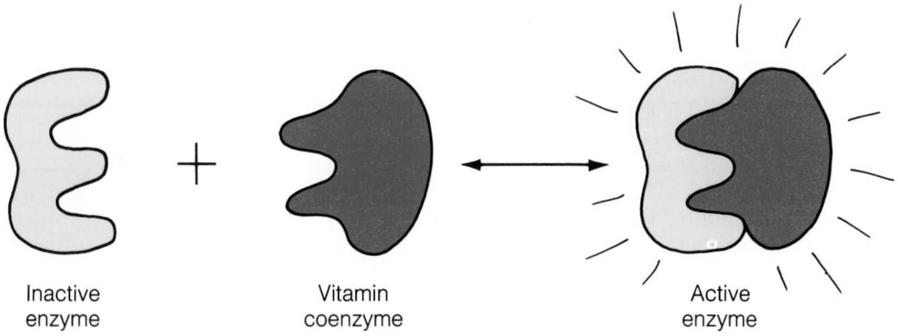

FIGURE 8-2
An enzyme is activated when a coenzyme attaches to it.

lights on and off, coenzymes are not destroyed when they are used, and they are used thousands of times.

Minerals that activate enzymes are called **cofactors**. Because they are minerals, cofactors have particular electrical charges and other properties. These charges and other metallic properties activate and deactivate particular enzymes in the body just as the coenzymes do. Some enzymes require both a coenzyme and a cofactor for activation. Enzymes are activated only by specific coenzymes and cofactors. An enzyme that requires a niacin coenzyme for activation, for example, is not activated by any other coenzyme.

cofactor: A chemical substance that activates a particular enzyme. Many minerals act as cofactors.

Is enzyme activity accelerated if a person consumes extra vitamins and minerals? No. High levels of vitamins and minerals do not improve or accelerate enzyme functions, because they do not cause an increase in enzyme levels. The mistaken notion that increased levels of vitamins and minerals in the diet can stimulate "lazy" enzymes has been advanced by people who sell vitamin and mineral supplements. Some of these people have gone so far as to add enzymes to products to make them more attractive to people who do not know that enzymes are broken down in the small intestine.

How Vitamins and Minerals Differ

Vitamins and minerals differ in many respects. Table 8-1 summarizes the differences. We discuss five key differences here.

Vitamins are organic substances, whereas minerals are inorganic substances. Organic substances can be assembled by living matter. Nearly all organic substances contain carbon, and most of them contain hydrogen and oxygen as well. Carbohydrates, proteins, fats, and vitamins are all organic. Vitamins are organic whether they are produced by a plant or in a test tube, because they are the same chemical substances. Vitamins, like other organic substances, are destroyed when their molecular structures are broken down.

organic substances: Chemical substances that arise from living matter. Almost all organic substances contain carbon.

inorganic substances: Chemical substances that may occur in nature but that cannot be produced by living matter.

Minerals, on the other hand, are inorganic substances; they cannot be produced by living matter. Minerals are elements, and the amount of each mineral on this planet is fixed. They cannot be created or destroyed by the human body; they can only be recycled.

Whereas a vitamin may have several molecular forms, the atomic structure of a mineral is specific to that mineral. Some vitamins occur in several molecular forms. For example, there is not just one vitamin B_6, but it has three chemically similar forms. Some vitamins have **provitamins**, compounds that chemically resemble the particular vitamin and

provitamin: A vitaminlike substance that is converted to a vitamin by metabolic reactions in the body.

TABLE 8-1

Differences between vitamins and minerals

Characteristic	Vitamins	Minerals
Chemical makeup	organic molecules (contain carbon)	inorganic atoms
	can be produced by living matter	not produced (can neither be created nor destroyed—only recycled)
	may have provitamins	no "prominerals"
	destructible	indestructible
	uncharged	carry a charge (are reactive)
Absorption	generally almost complete regardless of amount consumed	generally limited
	level of absorption unrelated to need	level of absorption may be related to need
Functions	as coenzymes (the B-complex vitamins)	as cofactors as structural components in nutrient transport in transmission of electrical impulses
Excretion	in urine	in feces and urine

which are converted to the vitamin by the body. Beta-carotene is a provitamin of vitamin A, for instance. On the other hand, minerals do not vary in composition; a mineral is always the same element.

A mineral carries an electrical charge and is thus more reactive than a vitamin. A single atom of a mineral typically does not have an equal number of protons and electrons; therefore, it carries a charge. Atoms that carry a charge are called **ions**. Minerals are attracted to ions that can supply the electrons or protons needed to neutralize their charge. Because of this property, minerals are reactive.

ion: An atom that carries an electric charge (positive or negative).

Most mineral elements carry a charge; for example, calcium (Ca^{++})*, fluorine* (F^{-})*, and iron* (Fe^{++} *or* Fe^{+++})*.*

Many of the functions of minerals are related to their reactivity. The charge carried by a mineral can result in relatively stable relationship, such as the bonding of calcium to phosphorous in bone, or to a temporary association, such as occurs among the minerals in body fluids. Minerals dissolved in body fluids continually combine with, and break away from other charged particles in the fluid. The processes of combining, uncombining, and moving results in the transmission of electrical impulses. Electrical impulses generated by minerals act to stimulate nerve and muscle cells and to transport nutrients across cell membranes. The beating of the heart, for example, is triggered by electrical impulses generated when certain minerals enter heart muscle cells. The change in charge between the outside and inside of the cells created by the movement of minerals stimulates cells to contract. Electrical currents generated by the movement of minerals across the membranes of muscle cells of the heart are recorded by electrocardiograms (EKGs). Abnormalities in the pattern of electrical activity signal pending or

Why is electrocardiogram *abbreviated* EKG? *The* K *is for* kardia, *Greek for "heart." An alternate, less frequently used abbreviation is* ECG.

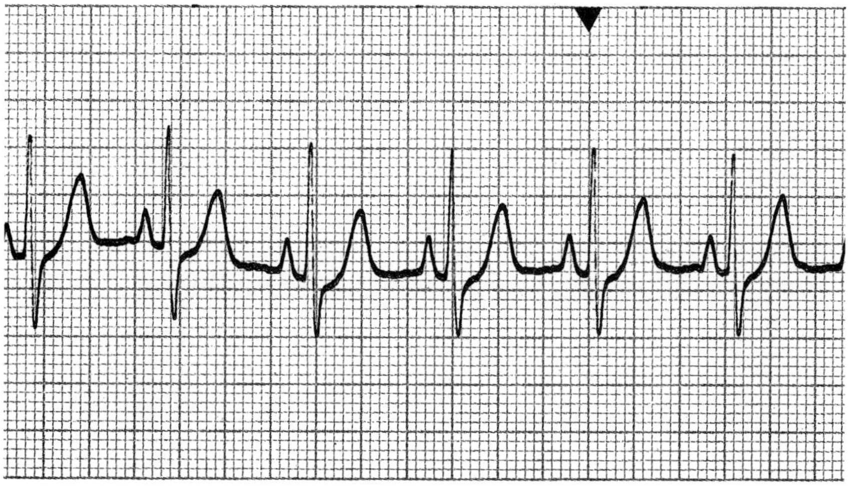

The electrical current measured by an EKG results from the movement of minerals across the membranes of the muscle cells in the heart.

past problems in the heart. Electroencephalograms (EEGs) similarly record electrical activity occurring in the brain.

Minerals become a component of body structures; vitamins do not. Minerals play a leading role as components of body structures. Bones, cartilage, toenails, and fingernails all contain minerals that substantially contribute to their hardness and strength. Vitamins participate in the manufacture of these structures through their function as coenzymes but do not become part of the structure.

Minerals tend to be absorbed less completely than vitamins. What you eat may not be what you get. Because minerals are reactive, they sometimes combine with other substances to form compounds that are not easily absorbed. Absorption of zinc, for example, can vary from 0 to 100 percent depending on what has reacted with it.[1] Populations that subsist primarily on whole grains (for example, people in certain countries in the Middle East) experience zinc deficiency more often than people who consume a more varied diet. Although adequate levels of zinc are present in the whole grains, only a small amount can be absorbed because the zinc is tightly bound to phytic acid, a natural component of whole grains.[2] Another example is the interaction between tea and iron. Drinking tea with a meal can decrease iron absorption by 50 percent or more. In the intestines, iron combines with the tannic acid contained in tea and forms a compound that cannot be absorbed.[3]

Not all interactions of minerals with other substances reduce the minerals' absorption. For example, vitamin C and alcohol increase iron absorption. The amount of vitamin C in 4 ounces of orange juice nearly quadruples the amount of iron that can be absorbed from plant foods consumed at the same time as the orange juice. (See Box 8-1.) Alcohol is a very strong "enhancer"; it can cause such excessive absorption of iron from iron-rich foods that iron overdose can result. (See Box 8-2.)

The differences in mineral absorption just described pertain to the **bioavailability** of minerals. *Bioavailability* refers to the difference in the amount of a mineral consumed and the amount absorbed. For example, if 100 mg of calcium are consumed and 20 mg are absorbed, the bioavailability of calcium in the food or diet tested is 20 percent.

bioavailability: The percentage of the total amount of a mineral consumed that is absorbed.

BOX 8-1

NAILING ORANGES

Before iron pills became available, one folk medicine method of preparing iron supplements called for inserting iron nails into oranges and letting an "iron brew" develop. After allowing time for the iron to interact with the vitamin C (ascorbic acid), the juice of the orange would be drunk as an iron tonic. Apples, although not high in vitamin C, also were used.

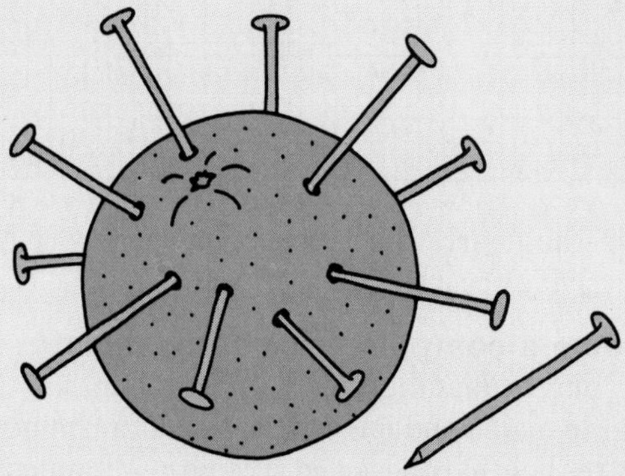

The old-fashioned way of making an iron supplement.

The bioavailability of minerals in food is important to people who are concerned about getting full value from the foods they eat. A parallel concern is for minimizing the losses of vitamins and minerals in food preparation.

Preserving the Vitamin and Mineral Content of Foods

Food storage and preparation techniques influence the vitamin and mineral content of food. Vitamins are much more vulnerable than minerals to losses during processing, storage, and cooking. The mineral content of foods is reduced somewhat by soaking or boiling them and by any cooking method that causes the food to lose fluids, since the fluids contain dissolved minerals. Minerals may also be lost during processing. The flour refining process, for example, removes grains' germs and outer coverings, both of which are good sources of various minerals.

BOX 8-2

ALCOHOL AND IRON OVERLOAD AMONG THE BANTUS

A traditional drink of the African Bantus is homemade beer brewed in large iron kettles. During the brewing process, the alcohol produced dissolves iron from the kettle and adds about 80 mg of highly absorbable iron to each quart of beer. Some of the tribesmen who regularly drink this beer develop hemosiderosis, a disease related to excessive levels of iron in the body.[4]

TABLE 8-2

Relative stability of vitamins during food storage and preparation

Stable	Unstable	Very Unstable
niacin	vitamin B_6	vitamin C
vitamin K	riboflavin	thiamin
vitamin B_{12}	pantothenic acid	folic acid
vitamin D	vitamin A	
	beta-carotene (a provitamin)	
	vitamin E	

Table 8-2 categorizes vitamins by their stability during food storage and preparation. As you can see, vitamin C, thiamin, and folic acid are the most fragile vitamins. The chemical structures of vitamins are broken down by exposure to:

- light
- acidity or basicity (**pH**)
- oxygen
- heat
- moisture

pH: A measure of how acidic or basic (alkaline) a solution is. The neutral point, where a solution is neither acidic nor basic, is pH 7. Acidity increases as pH drops from 7 to zero, and basicity increases as pH rises from 7 to 14. Reference points:
lemon juice 2.2
tomato juice 4.2
milk 6.6
water 7.0 (neutral)
seawater 8.0
ammonia 11.1

Until the 1960s, milk was generally sold in clear glass bottles. It was discovered, however, that the exposure of milk to light reduced its vitamin content. That finding led to the use of colored glass, fogged plastic, and cardboard milk containers.

The pH of the solution surrounding foods affects the stability of vitamins. Vitamin C, for example, is highly stable in acidic solutions such as orange juice and tomato juice, but slowly breaks down in a nearly neutral solution such as milk.

Major losses of vitamins often occur during cooking. Overcooking, keeping cooked foods hot for extended periods, cooking foods in too much water, and discarding cooking liquids all result in vitamin losses. (Overcooking vegetables is a nutritional misdemeanor; in addition to causing vitamin losses, it impairs their taste.) For example, when green beans and peas are kept hot for three hours, they lose more than half of their thiamin, riboflavin, and vitamin C.[5] Cooking vegetables in a large amount of water causes appreciable losses of water-soluble vitamins. Approximately one-third of the water-soluble vitamin content of boiled vegetables is thrown away when the water they were cooked in is poured down the drain.[6] Food

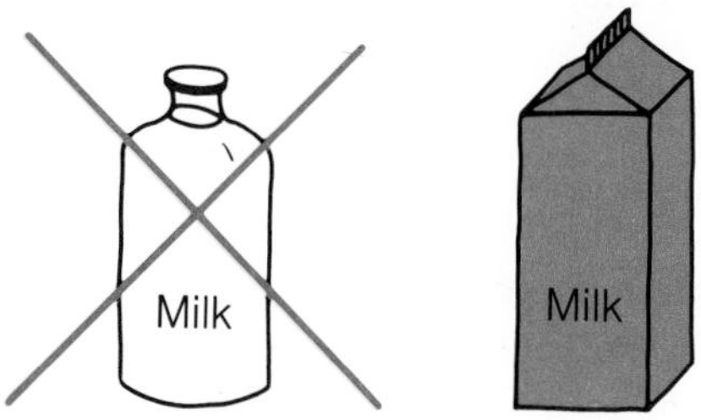

The discovery that vitamins in milk are destroyed by exposure to light led to the phasing out of clear-glass milk bottles.

TABLE 8-3

Food handling practices that preserve the vitamin and mineral content of food

Food Storage
Store foods for the shortest amount of time possible.
Select fresh and frozen products over heavily processed and canned products.
Store vegetables and fruits that do not need refrigeration in a cool, dry, clean place.
Wrap leftover perishable foods tightly and store in a refrigerator set just above 32°F.
Avoid the freeze–thaw–freeze cycle; this causes major losses of vitamin content.
Food Preparation
Don't overcook foods, especially vegetables. Cooked vegetables should still be a bit crunchy.
Microwave, stir-fry, steam, or broil foods, using just enough liquid to prevent scorching.
Serve foods as soon as they are prepared (or be the first one in the cafeteria line). Time meal preparation tasks so that all foods to be served are ready at the same time.

storage and preparation practices that preserve the vitamin and mineral content of foods are summarized in Table 8-3.

On the other hand, some foods gain vitamins and minerals during processing. How that happens is the subject of the next section.

enrichment: The replacement of thiamin, riboflavin, niacin, and iron lost during the refining of grains. The term applies only to grain products, and the levels of enrichment are regulated.

fortification: The addition of nutrients to foods. Nutrients used in fortification may or may not have been present in the food originally. There are no regulations governing the types of foods that may be fortified or the fortifying nutrients.

bran: The outermost covering of a whole grain. It is removed during refining.

germ: The nutrient- and fat-dense component of a whole grain. Because the unsaturated fats in the germ may break down during storage and cause the grain to become rancid, the germ is removed during refining.

ENRICHMENT AND FORTIFICATION OF FOODS

Vitamins and minerals are added to foods by enrichment and fortification. **Enrichment** replaces particular vitamins and minerals lost during the refining of grains. For example, bread that is made from refined flour is enriched. **Fortification** is simply the addition of nutrients to foods regardless of whether they were present in the food originally. Many foods—ranging from apple juice to cupcakes—are fortified with vitamins and minerals. Both processes were developed before World War II to help prevent the then-widespread deficiency diseases.[7] Today, many more products are fortified than enriched. Only refined-grain products are allowed to be labeled as "enriched," but any food may be fortified.

Enrichment

Enrichment would not be necessary if people consumed whole-grain foods. So, then, why are grains refined? Because many people prefer them that way. A wheat, oat, or rice grain contains a **bran** coating and a **germ** in

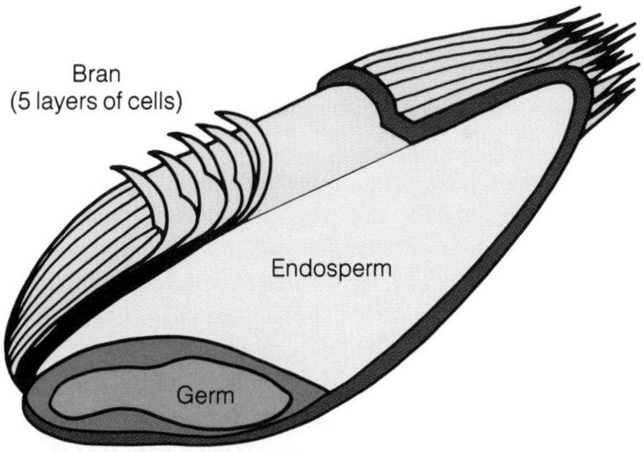

■
FIGURE 8-3
Gross composition of a grain of wheat. The *bran* provides dietary fiber. The *germ* contains protein, unsaturated fats, thiamin, niacin, riboflavin, iron, and other nutrients. The bran and germ are removed in the refining process. The *endosperm* contains starch grains embedded in a protein matrix.

addition to a starchy endosperm (Figure 8-3). Bran is tough and resists softening unless it is cooked for a long time. The germ, although rich in vitamins and minerals, contains unsaturated fatty acids, which become rancid with storage. The bran and germ portions of whole grains are removed during the refining process to improve the texture, cooking properties, and storage life of the grain.

The benefits of refining come with a high cost: lost nutrient content of the grains. Lost along with the bran and germ is much of the whole grain's content of dietary fiber, calcium, phosphorus, magnesium, zinc, vitamin B_6, pantothenic acid, and folic acid (Table 8-4). Thiamin, riboflavin, niacin, and iron content of grains is also lost in refining, and these four nutrients (only these four) are replaced by enrichment. The term *replaced* here is key. Enriched nutrients are added at levels that approximate the amount lost in refining.

enriched nutrients: thiamin, riboflavin, niacin, and iron.

enriched foods: wheat flour, cornmeal, grits, polished rice.

Enrichment does not replace all of the nutrients lost during refining, nor does it guarantee that the enriched nutrients won't be lost during food preparation. (See Box 8-3.) Nonetheless, it has reduced the incidence of thiamin, riboflavin, niacin, and iron deficiencies in the U.S.[8] As shown in Table 8-5, whole-grain and enriched breads contain greater amounts of the enriched nutrients than do refined, unenriched breads. (Box 8-4 clears up a sometimes confusing point about whole-grain products.)

■
TABLE 8-4
Comparison of the dietary fiber and nutrient content of 1 cup of whole-wheat flour and 1 cup of enriched white flour

Nutrient	Whole-Wheat Flour	Enriched White Flour
Dietary fiber	11.6 g	3.5 g
Calcium	50 mg	20 mg
Phosphorus	445 mg	100 mg
Magnesium	135 mg	30 mg
Zinc	2.9 mg	0.8 mg
Vitamin B_6	1.1 mg	0.07 mg
Pantothenic acid	1.3 mg	0.5 mg
Folic acid	46 mcg	20 mcg

SPRAY ON—RINSE OFF

A common method of enriching refined grains is "spraying" a mixture of thiamin, riboflavin, niacin, and iron on the starchy endosperm. Unfortunately, this coating of nutrients can be washed away by rinsing the grain or by cooking it in excess water. The traditional method of preparing rice in many countries consists of rinsing the rice thoroughly and then boiling it in more water than is absorbed. This method can result in the loss of over 50% of the "sprayed on" nutrients.[7] This is why the labels on many rice packages advise that the rice not be rinsed before cooking or drained after cooking.

TABLE 8-5
The difference enrichment makes in a slice of bread

	Enriched Nutrients, mg			
	Thiamin	Riboflavin	Niacin	Iron
Unenriched white bread	0.0	0.0	0.2	0.2
Enriched white bread	0.1	0.1	0.7	0.7
Whole-grain bread	0.1	0.3	0.8	0.8

THE *WHOLE* TRUTH

If the word *whole* does not appear on the label of a grain product, the product may be made from colored, refined flour or from a mixture of whole and processed grains. Breads and cereals labeled as whole-grain products must be made from grains whose bran coatings and germs have not been removed. If you want to be certain that you use whole-grain products, you must read labels.

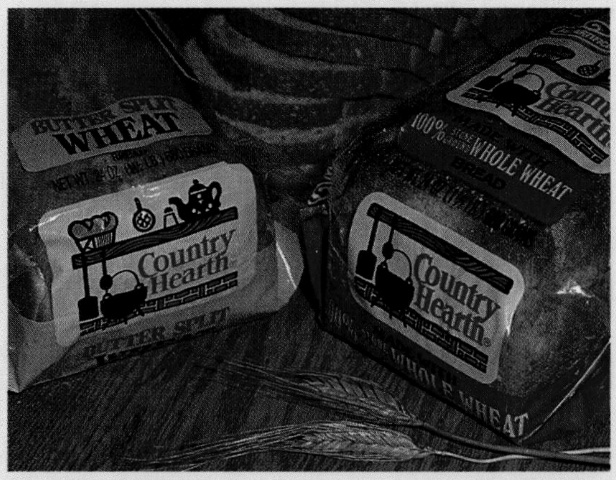

BOX 8-5

THE ORIGIN OF BREAKFAST CEREAL FORTIFICATION

In the 1940s, a General Mills employee noted that many families put a bottle of vitamin and mineral supplements on the breakfast table along with the milk, juice, and cereal. General Mills market research found that taking a supplement at breakfast time had become a routine for many families. It was reasoned that adding a vitamin and mineral supplement to breakfast cereals might improve sales. Apparently this reasoning was sound; the number of fortified breakfast cereals on the market today exceeds those that are not.

TABLE 8-6
Examples of fortified foods

Food Product	Fortification
Salt	iodine
Milk	vitamin D
Low-fat milk	vitamins A and D
Margarine	vitamin A
Water	fluoride
Infant cereals	iron
Breakfast cereals	vitamins, minerals, fiber
Yogurt, flour, and orange juice	calcium
Fruit drinks	vitamin C

Fortification

Early fortification efforts included adding iodine to salt, vitamin D to milk, vitamin A to low-fat milk and margarine, and iron to infant cereals. Fortification of each of these foods was implemented to protect people from specific deficiency diseases.[8] Fortification of foods with vitamins and minerals has spread far beyond the original intention of preventing deficiency diseases. See Table 8-6. Foods are now fortified for sales appeal rather than to correct specific dietary inadequacies. (Breakfast cereals are good examples; see Box 8-5.) Unlike enrichment, fortification is not limited to a few nutrients or to particular nutrient amounts, and no scientific justification is required for fortifying foods. It can be and has been overdone.

Fortification of foods has sometimes been overdone. In the 1950s, for example, oversupplementing foods with vitamin D was associated with an increased occurrence of hypercalcemia, the formation of hard calcium deposits in soft tissues such as the liver, kidneys, and lungs.[7]

Foods we consume are the major source of vitamins and minerals. But, as will be discussed in the next section, they are also available in bottles.

PILLS AS A SOURCE OF VITAMINS AND MINERALS

Overall, about 40 percent of Americans take vitamins or minerals in pill form, and sales of vitamin and mineral supplements are expected to increase by 15% annually during the 1990s.[9] For the most part, people use

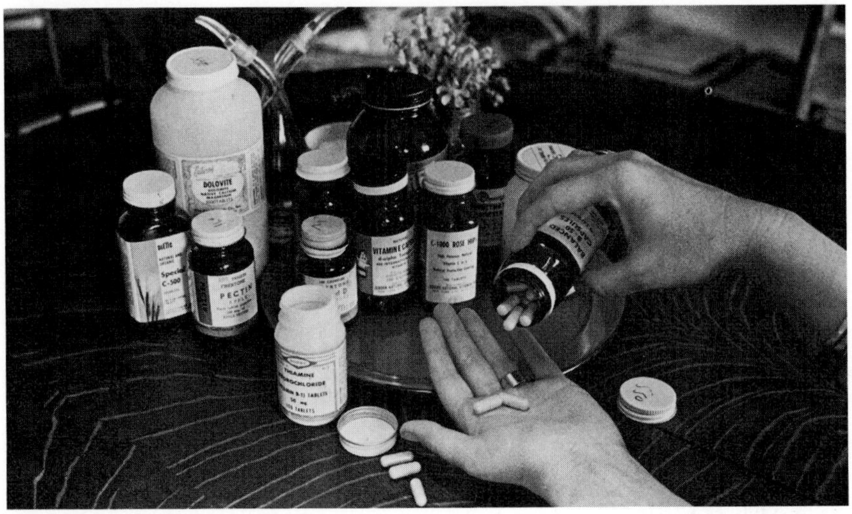

Supplements may or may not benefit the people who use them.

TABLE 8-7
Reasons people give for using supplements

"I'm sick and I hope it will help me get well."

"Why not?" (They may help me, and they won't hurt me.)

"I don't trust the quality of food supply."

"I hate vegetables."

"It's like insurance. I don't eat a balanced diet every day."

"I sell them."

"Someone said they prevent cancer [or heart disease or some other disease or health problem]."

"To help me cope with the stress in my life."

"Doctor's orders."

supplemental vitamins and minerals as a nutritional insurance policy—for protection against inadequate diets. Many people take them for specific reasons, such as for treating colds, improving their complexion, or giving them energy (Table 8-7). Most supplement users choose a single vitamin or mineral, and among those, vitamin C supplements are the most popular.[10] Pregnant women are the population group most likely to use supplements, and teenagers, the least likely (Table 8-8).[10,11]

Use of Supplements to Balance the Diet

A balanced diet is seldom achieved by taking a vitamin and mineral supplement. No supplement can provide 100 percent of all the nutrients a person needs daily, and most multivitamin and mineral supplements contain only 7 to 17 of the 40 essential nutrients. Even that level of nutrient variety is not available to many supplement users, because most people who take supplements choose supplements of specific, individual nutrients. Some supple-

■

TABLE 8-8

Vitamin and mineral supplement users in the United States[10,11]

Population Group	Percentage Who Use Regularly or Occasionally
Pregnant women	80–90
Breast-feeding women	80
World-class athletes	72
Elderly	27–98
Lacto-ovovegetarians	55–85
Infants	45
High-school athletes	44
College students	43
Women	41
Registered nurses	38
Registered dietitians	37
Men	33
Teenage females	21
Teenage males	12

ments include biotin, molybdenum, and pantothenic acid—micronutrients that are very rarely in short supply in diets. Some supplements contain substances that are not essential and that have never been shown to be related to deficiency diseases or improvement in health.[12] For example, bottles of "rutin" pills can be purchased in some grocery and health food stores. What is rutin? An unneeded substance that costs $4.95 per bottle.

Several studies have shown a mismatch between the vitamin and mineral supplements that are taken and those that are in short supply in diets.[13,14] Supplements are often taken by people whose dietary intakes of the vitamins and minerals contained in the supplements are already adequate. At the same time, people with deficient intake levels of particular nutrients may fail to select the supplements that could correct the deficiencies.

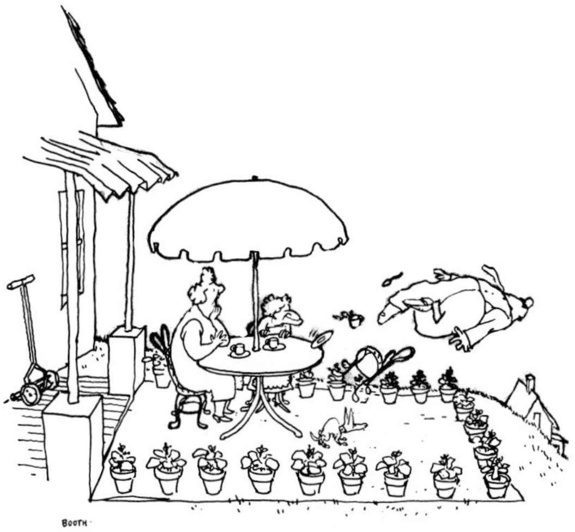

"Oh-oh! There go Papa's timed-release vitamins!"

Although it has not been shown that healthy people with well-balanced diets benefit from supplements,[15] vitamin or mineral supplementation is beneficial in some situations. Table 8-9 summarizes these situations. In cases where faulty diets have produced a need for supplements, dietary improvements should go hand-in-hand with supplement use.

Choice of Supplements

Hundreds of supplements and supplement combinations are available over-the-counter. Depending on the type and amount of vitamins and minerals included, a supplement can represent money ill-spent, a benefit, or an overdose risk. The primary health concerns related to supplement use are the dangers of overdosing and of using them for self-treatment of diseases for which they are ineffective.

High doses (those exceeding 2 times the U.S. RDA) of certain vitamins and minerals can precipitate toxic reactions if they are habitual. Vitamins D and A, selenium, iodine, and other trace elements are of particular concern, because their margins of safety above the U.S. RDAs are narrow.

megadose: Dosage level of a vitamin or mineral that exceeds 10 times the U.S. RDA.

Megadoses Vitamin and mineral supplements that exceed 10 times the U.S. RDA are considered **megadoses** and are the supplements most likely to lead to overdose. Megadoses of vitamins and minerals exceed the level the body can use for normal nutrient functions. Instead of promoting the normal functions of vitamins and minerals, megadose supplements may negate them and produce adverse effects totally unrelated to the vitamin or mineral's normal functions.[16]

TABLE 8-9
Situations in which vitamin and mineral supplements may be beneficial

Situation	Supplement Type
Oral contraceptive use	folic acid, vitamin B_6
Pregnancy	iron, folic acid
Diagnosed deficiency disease (e.g., anemias)	as indicated
Vegan diets	B_{12}, vitamin D, zinc, iron
Osteoporosis	calcium, vitamin D, fluoride
Chronic dieting	multivitamin and mineral
Use of drugs that interfere with the micronutrients (e.g., some antihypertensives and antibiotics)	as indicated by type of drug
Diseases that produce malabsorption (e.g., cystic fibrosis, celiac disease)	multivitamin and mineral, or as indicated
Inadequate diets due to food allergies, alcoholism, or a narrow selection of food types	multivitamin and mineral, or as indicated by type of deficiency signs

It has been suggested that because of the druglike effects of very high levels of intake, supplements that contain megadoses of vitamins and minerals should be sold only on a prescription basis. With a few exceptions, it is legal to formulate and sell vitamin and mineral supplements at any dosage level.[17]

Labeling of Supplements

The labels of vitamin and mineral supplement containers are generally very informative. Some of the information on labels is required by law, and some is listed at the manufacturers' discretion. Figure 8-4 shows a label of a popular multiple-vitamin and mineral supplement. All supplement labels must

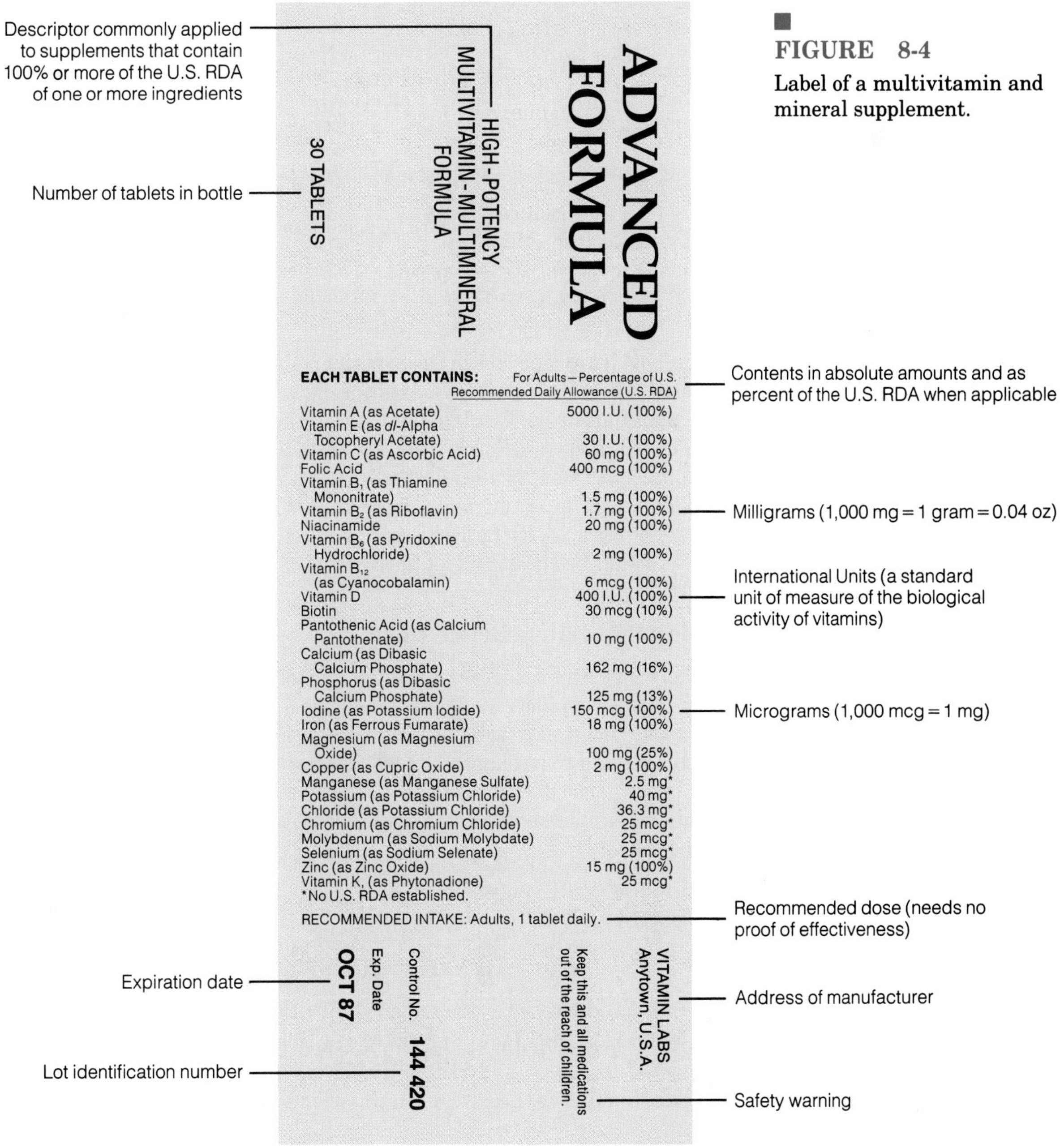
Descriptor commonly applied to supplements that contain 100% or more of the U.S. RDA of one or more ingredients
Number of tablets in bottle
ADVANCED FORMULA
HIGH-POTENCY MULTIVITAMIN-MULTIMINERAL FORMULA
30 TABLETS
EACH TABLET CONTAINS:
For Adults—Percentage of U.S. Recommended Daily Allowance (U.S. RDA)
Vitamin A (as Acetate) 5000 I.U. (100%)
Vitamin E (as dl-Alpha Tocopheryl Acetate) 30 I.U. (100%)
Vitamin C (as Ascorbic Acid) 60 mg (100%)
Folic Acid 400 mcg (100%)
Vitamin B1 (as Thiamine Mononitrate) 1.5 mg (100%)
Vitamin B2 (as Riboflavin) 1.7 mg (100%)
Niacinamide 20 mg (100%)
Vitamin B6 (as Pyridoxine Hydrochloride) 2 mg (100%)
Vitamin B12 (as Cyanocobalamin) 6 mcg (100%)
Vitamin D 400 I.U. (100%)
Biotin 30 mcg (10%)
Pantothenic Acid (as Calcium Pantothenate) 10 mg (100%)
Calcium (as Dibasic Calcium Phosphate) 162 mg (16%)
Phosphorus (as Dibasic Calcium Phosphate) 125 mg (13%)
Iodine (as Potassium Iodide) 150 mcg (100%)
Iron (as Ferrous Fumarate) 18 mg (100%)
Magnesium (as Magnesium Oxide) 100 mg (25%)
Copper (as Cupric Oxide) 2 mg (100%)
Manganese (as Manganese Sulfate) 2.5 mg*
Potassium (as Potassium Chloride) 40 mg*
Chloride (as Potassium Chloride) 36.3 mg*
Chromium (as Chromium Chloride) 25 mcg*
Molybdenum (as Sodium Molybdate) 25 mcg*
Selenium (as Sodium Selenate) 25 mcg*
Zinc (as Zinc Oxide) 15 mg (100%)
Vitamin K1 (as Phytonadione) 25 mcg*
*No U.S. RDA established.
RECOMMENDED INTAKE: Adults, 1 tablet daily.
Contents in absolute amounts and as percent of the U.S. RDA when applicable
Milligrams (1,000 mg = 1 gram = 0.04 oz)
International Units (a standard unit of measure of the biological activity of vitamins)
Micrograms (1,000 mcg = 1 mg)
Recommended dose (needs no proof of effectiveness)
VITAMIN LABS
Anytown, U.S.A.
Keep this and all medications out of the reach of children.
Control No. 144 420
Exp. Date
OCT 87
Expiration date
Lot identification number
Address of manufacturer
Safety warning

FIGURE 8-4

Label of a multivitamin and mineral supplement.

TABLE 8-10

Guidelines for selecting over-the-counter vitamin and mineral supplements

1. Supplements labeled *megadose, therapeutic,* or *high-potency* are likely to contain levels of vitamins and minerals that exceed the body's ability to use them, and may precipitate toxic overdosing. Pass them by for lower-dose levels.

2. Select supplements that contain vitamins and minerals recognized as essential. The listing of para-amino benzoic acid (PABA), inositol, and enzymes included on labels should serve as a strong clue that the product contains unneeded substances.

3. Examine the label for the percentage of the U.S. RDA of each micronutrient included. Select the one that has a balance of vitamins and minerals that does not exceed 100% of the U.S. RDA.

4. Buy the least expensive supplement that meets the criteria in number 3. *Natural* and *organic* are sales terms. The average markup on vitamins is 43%, but some health food stores mark up some supplements as much as 500%.

5. Note the expiration date on the label.

indicate how many pills are in the container, the vitamins and minerals that are included and their doses, an expiration date, and the name and address of the manufacturer. The labels or packaging must not state unproven health claims about the micronutrients contained, but manufacturers are free to present this type of information anyplace else.

Guidelines for selecting over-the-counter vitamin and mineral preparations are presented in Table 8-10. For most people, foods—not supplements—should be the source of nutrients.

Supplements versus Better Diets

It is likely that Americans would benefit far more from a healthier selection of foods than from increased supplement use. The major nutritional problems in the U.S. today are not vitamin and mineral deficiencies; they are problems related to a reliance on foods that are high in fat, cholesterol, and salt at the expense of high-fiber, low-calorie, nutrient-dense foods. Vitamin and mineral supplements cannot solve these dietary problems, but dietary changes can.

REVIEW QUESTIONS

1. Name three characteristics shared by vitamins and minerals.
2. A major role of many vitamins, particularly the B-complex vitamins, is to act as ____________ that activate enzymes. Minerals, on the other hand, function as ____________ in enzyme activation.

3. Vitamins and minerals differ in five key ways. What are they?
4. What is the major difference between organic and inorganic substances?
5. Name two "stable" and two "very unstable" vitamins.
6. The chemical structure of vitamins can be broken down by exposing them to acidic or basic pH, air, heat, __________, and __________.
7. List three storage guidelines and three preparation guidelines for minimizing vitamin and mineral losses.
8. __________ refers to the addition of nutrients to foods, whereas __________ refers to the replacement of (four) nutrients to refined grain products.
9. Name four types of foods that are fortified.
10. List five situations in which the use of vitamin and/or mineral supplements may be beneficial.

Answers

1. Both vitamins and minerals are found in small amounts in food; are needed in small amounts by the body; cannot be used as a source of energy; and they play important roles in carbohydrate, protein, and fat metabolism.
2. Coenzymes, cofactors
3. See Table 8-1.
4. "Organic" chemical substances arise from living matter, such as the energy nutrients and vitamins. "Inorganic" chemicals cannot be produced by living matter.
5. Refer to Table 8-2 for the answers.
6. Light, moisture.
7. Table 8-3 holds the answers.
8. Fortification, enrichment.
9. See Table 8-6 for a list of fortified foods.
10. Table 8-9 lists the situations.

■ ■ ■

PUTTING NUTRITION KNOWLEDGE TO WORK

1. Assume that you saw a sign in a drugstore announcing that "organic calcium" tablets were on sale. Is that possible?

   (Hint: Are minerals organic?)
2. Let's say you consumed 10 mg of zinc but that only 1 mg was absorbed. What's the bioavailability of the zinc?

   (Hint: What percent of 10 mg is 1 mg?)
3. Martha loves beef liver and ate 6 6-ounce portions of it over a three-day period. Is she likely to develop an iron overdose from eating that much liver?
4. The U.S. RDA for calcium is 1000 mg (1 gram). John took a supplement that contains 4000 mg of calcium. Would that constitute a megadose?

NOTES

1. W. Mertz, Trace elements, *Contemporary Nutrition* 3 (1978):1–2.
2. A. S. Prasad, Discovery and importance of zinc in human nutrition, *Federation Proceedings* 43 (1984):2829–2834.
3. E. R. Monsen and J. L. Balintfy, Calculating dietary iron bioavailability: refinement and computerization, *Journal of the American Dietetic Association* 80 (1982):307–311.
4. W. Mertz, Mineral elements: New perspectives, *Journal of the American Dietetic Association* 77 (1980):258–263.
5. M. K. Head, Nutrient losses in institutional food handling, *Journal of the American Dietetic Association* 65 (1974):423–427.
6. Conserving the nutrient value of foods, Home and garden bulletin no. 90 (Washington, D.C.: U.S. Department of Agriculture, 1980).
7. F. J. Levinson, Food fortification in low-income countries: A new approach to an old standby, *American Journal of Public Health* 62 (1972):715–718.
8. "The nutritive quality of processed foods: General policies for nutrient additions," *Nutrition Reviews* 40 (1982):93–96.
9. M. L. Stewart, Appendix of individual nutrient intake distributions for vitamin/mineral supplement use: A telephone survey of U.S. adults (Springfield, Va.: National Technical Information Service, 1985).
10. J. T. McDonald, Vitamin and mineral supplement use in the United States, *Clinical Nutrition* 5 (1986):27–33.
11. L. O. Schulz, Factors influencing the use of nutritional supplements by college students with varying levels of physical activity, *Nutrition Research* 8 (1988):459–466.
12. S. P. Gourdine, W. W. Traiger, and D. S. Cohen, Health food stores investigation, *Journal of the American Dietetic Association* 83 (1983):286–290.
13. J. P. Koplan, J. L. Annest, et al., Nutrient intake and supplementation in the United States (NHANES II), *American Journal of Public Health* 76 (1986): 287–289.
14. R. P. Farris, J. L. Cresanta, et al., Dietary studies of children from a biracial population, *Journal of the American College of Nutrition* 4 (1985):539–552.
15. M. A. Dubick and R. B. Rucker, Dietary supplements and health aids: Critical evaluation, *Journal of Nutrition Education* 15 (1983):47–53 and123–127.
16. Food and Nutrition Board, National Research Council, *Recommended Dietary Allowances*, 9th ed. (Washington, D.C.: National Academy of Sciences, 1980).
17. A. Forbes, *Proceedings* of Conference on Government Regulations and Nutrition Alternatives (Vitamin Nutrition Information Service, Port St. Lucie, Fla., 1981), 24–32.

CHAPTER

9

WATER-SOLUBLE VITAMINS

If people had known then what we know now, *vitamines* would not have been the name given to the newly discovered, essential components of food. Perhaps *vita* (Latin, "life") would have stuck, but *amine* would not have been used. The first vitamin discovered contained an amine, a nitrogen-containing compound. Subsequent investigations revealed that many "vitamines" did *not* contain nitrogen, which made *amine* inappropriate for them. To lessen the mistake, the *e* was dropped from *vitamin.* In order to keep the new discoveries straight, they were lettered in alphabetical order. (There were some mistakes, as Box 9-1 points out.) Later, as the vitamins' chemical characteristics became more clear, names were assigned to them to eliminate the confusion in the lettering and numbering system. In most cases, the letters have had more staying power than the chemical names, perhaps because they are easier to remember. For example, *vitamin* B_{12} is more memorable than *cyanocobalamin.*

BOX 9-1

WHAT HAPPENED TO VITAMIN F?

The lettering system for vitamins went awry after vitamin A was identified. Isolating vitamins from foods in the early 1900s was a crude process, and errors were made. For example, what was thought to be vitamin B turned out to be several different vitamins; hence the origin of the "B-complex" vitamins.

Many suspected vitamins were given letters or subscript numerals and then later found not to be essential. Today we have the lettered vitamins A, B_1, B_2, B_3, B_6, B_{12}, C, D, E, and K. What happened to vitamins B_4, B_5, and B_7 through B_{11}, and to vitamins F, G, H, I, and J? Eventually it was learned that they are not needed in the human diet. The vitamins initially labeled as H, M, S, W, and X were all found to be the same one (biotin), and the letters assigned to them had to be dropped from use. (Running out of alphabet letters was a primary reason for giving newly discovered vitamins chemical names.)

TABLE 9-1

Water- and fat-soluble vitamins and their chemical names

Water-Soluble Vitamins	Fat-Soluble Vitamins
the B-complex vitamins	vitamin A (retinol)
thiamin (vitamin B_1)	vitamin D (cholecalciferol)
riboflavin (vitamin B_2)	vitamin E (tocopherol)
niacin (vitamin B_3)	vitamin K (phylloquinone, menaquinone)
vitamin B_6 (pyridoxine)	
folacin (folic acid)	
vitamin B_{12} (cyanocobalamin)	
biotin	
pantothenic acid (pantothenate)	
vitamin C (ascorbic acid, ascorbate)	

To date, 13 essential vitamins have been identified, each of which is soluble in either water or fat (see Table 9-1). Provitamins—vitaminlike chemicals that are converted to the actual vitamin in the body—have been identified for 3 vitamins: niacin, vitamin A, and vitamin D. Vitamin B_{12} is the vitamin discovered most recently; it was identified in 1948.

CHARACTERISTICS OF VITAMINS

Water-soluble and fat-soluble vitamins differ in several respects. In addition to their solubility difference, they differ in their functions and in the extent to which they can be stored in the body (Table 9-2).

Water-Soluble Vitamins

The B-complex vitamins function as coenzymes in reactions that lead to the formation of energy, proteins, fats, and other substances in the body. The fat-soluble vitamins—vitamins A, D, E, and K—do *not* function as coenzymes. They perform a wide variety of other roles, including promoting bone formation and protecting cell membranes from damage.

With the exception of vitamin B_{12}, the water-soluble vitamins are stored in low amounts in the body. Any surpluses received in foods or supplements are excreted in the urine. These low levels of body stores mean that foods containing the water-soluble vitamins should be consumed daily. It also means that deficiencies of the water-soluble vitamins develop rather quickly, sometimes within weeks after the intake of the vitamins has stopped. For the same reason, overdose reactions to them develop relatively soon after the overdoses occur and disappear quickly.

Fat-Soluble Vitamins

Fat-soluble vitamins are stored by the body for varying lengths of time. High intakes on some days balance out the low intakes of other days. The

TABLE 9-2

Comparison of the general characteristics of water- and fat-soluble vitamins

	Water-Soluble Vitamins	Fat-Soluble Vitamins
Solubility	water	fats, oils
Function	coenzymes	not as coenzymes
Potential for building body stores	low*	medium to high
Deficiency	rapid onset (weeks to months)	slow onset (months to years)
Overdose reaction	rapid onset, short duration (hours to days)	slow onset, long duration (days to months)

*Vitamin B_{12} is an exception; it is a water-soluble vitamin that can be stored in high amounts in the body.

body's ability to store the fat-soluble vitamins makes it possible to prevent deficiency diseases by giving large doses of them periodically. Vitamin A, for example, has been given in large doses to children in some areas of the world where vitamin A deficiency is common. The injection builds up enough of a store to meet the children's need for vitamin A for six months. Deficiencies of the fat-soluble vitamins generally develop slowly because they can be stored.

Overdose reactions to the fat-soluble vitamins occur when the storage sites in the body are filled and the excess overflows into the blood, liver, bones, and other tissues. Since the overflow is not readily excreted, high levels of the fat-soluble vitamins can remain in the body and disrupt the normal functions of cells. Generally, overdose reactions to excessive levels of the fat-soluble vitamins develop more slowly, last longer, and are more serious than overdose reactions to the water-soluble vitamins.

Box 9-2 discusses some "vitamin imposters"—substances that are marketed as being essential or beneficial to human health but, in fact, are not.

THIAMIN (VITAMIN B_1)

For centuries, **beriberi** plagued populations of people whose diets were high in polished rice. This thiamin-deficiency disease was recognized in China as early as 2600 B.C., but it was not until the early 1900s that the cure was found.[1] The cure consisted of adding the rice polishings—the bran and germ portions of the grain—to the diet. Nearly all of the thiamin content of whole grains is in the outer covering and the germ. Today, polished and refined grains are generally enriched with thiamin and three other nutrients that are lost in substantial amounts in processing.

beriberi: The thiamin-deficiency disease.

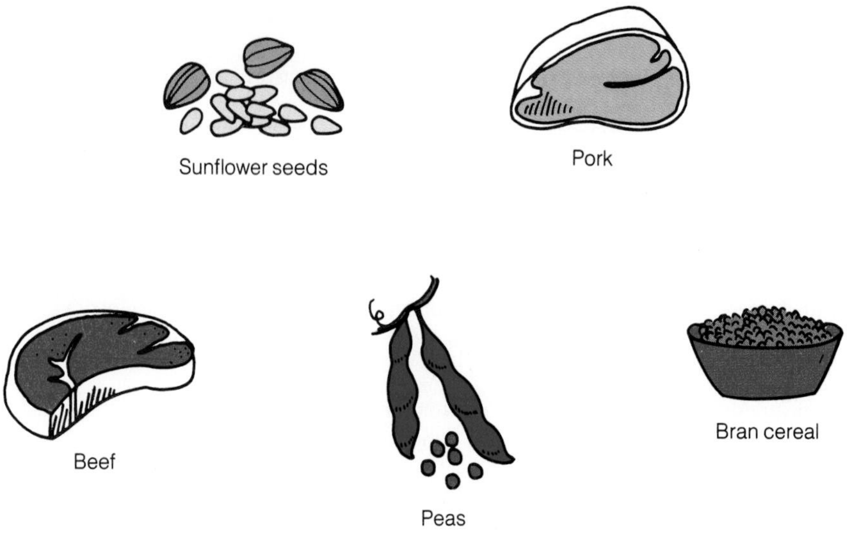

Thiamin occurs in grains and meats.

Functions

glucose, alcohol $\xrightarrow{\text{thiamin}}$ energy

Thiamin plays a role in energy metabolism, a subject frequently referred to in chapter 3. Thiamin's coenzymes and those of riboflavin and niacin (which we will discuss next) play key roles in reactions that lead to the formation of energy. Energy is needed for growth, physical movement, nerve functioning, and most other body processes. Consequently, these three vitamins have a broad influence on health. Thiamin specializes in activating enzymes involved in the formation of energy from glucose. It also is used in the formation of energy from alcohol.

Sources

Before grain products were enriched in the U.S., meat, poultry, and fish were the largest contributors of thiamin to American diets. Although these are still important sources, enriched grain and cereal products are now the leading food sources of thiamin.[2]

Many plants and animals require thiamin for energy metabolism, and thiamin is contained in a wide assortment of foods. See the list of good food sources of thiamin in Table 9-3. Notice that only milk and milk products are not represented in the list.

Recommended Intake

Most American diets provide at least the RDA for thiamin of 1.4 mg for males and 1.0 mg per day for females 23 to 50 years old.

Due to its central role in energy metabolism, the need for thiamin is greater with high-calorie diets. An athlete who consumes 4,000 calories a day requires about twice as much thiamin for energy metabolism as an office manager whose caloric intake is 1,800 a day. The increased need for thiamin that accompanies high-calorie diets is generally provided by the foods that are consumed. The thiamin requirement may be less than 1 mg per day for people on calorie-restricted diets.[3]

TABLE 9-3
Food sources of thiamin

Food	Amount	Thiamin, mg*
Meats		
pork roast	3 oz	0.8
beef	3 oz	0.4
ham	3 oz	0.4
liver	3 oz	0.2
Nuts and Seeds		
sunflower seeds	¼ c	0.7
peanuts	¼ c	0.1
almonds	¼ c	0.1
Grains		
bran flakes	1 c	0.6
macaroni	1 c	0.2
rice	1 c	0.2
bread	1 slice	0.1
Vegetables		
peas	½ c	0.3
lima beans	½ c	0.2
corn	½ c	0.1
broccoli	½ c	0.1
potato	1	0.1
Fruits		
orange juice	1 c	0.2
orange	1	0.1
avocado	½	0.1

*RDAs for adults aged 23–50 are 1.4 mg for males and 1.0 mg for females.

Deficiency Tissue stores of thiamin are limited and will become depleted within three to four weeks of a dietary deficiency. About 50 percent of the RDA is needed to prevent the development of beriberi, the thiamin-deficiency disease.[4]

People at risk of thiamin deficiency:
those whose diets consist primarily of refined, unenriched grain products
alcohol abusers

Beriberi occurs rarely in the U.S., since most grain products are enriched with thiamin.[3] Nonetheless, thiamin deficiency is still found among people who consume refined, unenriched grains as staple foods,[5] and among alcoholics. Alcoholics absorb thiamin poorly and yet have a great need for it due to thiamin's role in energy formation from alcohol.[6]

The first symptoms of thiamin deficiency are behavioral changes such as mental confusion, loss of appetite, irritability, and the expression of vague fears.[7] The behavioral disturbances are followed by a loss of sensation in the arms and legs, irregular heartbeat, muscular weakness, and eventually,

Beriberi *translates to "I cannot, I cannot"; people with the disease cannot walk.*

BOX 9-2

"VITAMINS" THAT AREN'T

Not every substance labeled a "vitamin" really is one. Each substance listed here is purported to be a vitamin or an essential organic substance by someone, and these substances are added to supplements and cosmetic products.

- bioflavonoids (vitamin P)
- choline
- gerovital H-3
- hesperidin
- inositol
- laetrile (vitamin B_{17})
- lecithin
- lipoic acid
- nucleic acids
- pangamic acid (vitamin B_{15})
- para-amino benzoic acid (PABA)
- provitamin B_5 complex
- rutin

None of these substances is a vitamin: none of them is required in our diets; deficiency diseases do not result from low intakes of *any* of them, and "extra" intakes of them have *not* been shown to be beneficial.

Nonetheless, the benefits of these "vitamin imposters" continue to be extolled. Inositol is promoted for preventing hair loss, gerovital H-3 for slowing down the aging process, and lecithin for "burning away" excess body fat.[1] Laetrile, a cyanide-containing component of apricot pits, has been used illegally *and ineffectively* to treat cancer. In an attempt to circumvent regulations controlling the sale of drugs, laetrile was labeled as a vitamin by some enterprising people.

Some of these nonvitamins, however, do have some value to humans. For example, although nutritionists have been unable to identify an essential function of PABA, it makes a fine sunscreen.

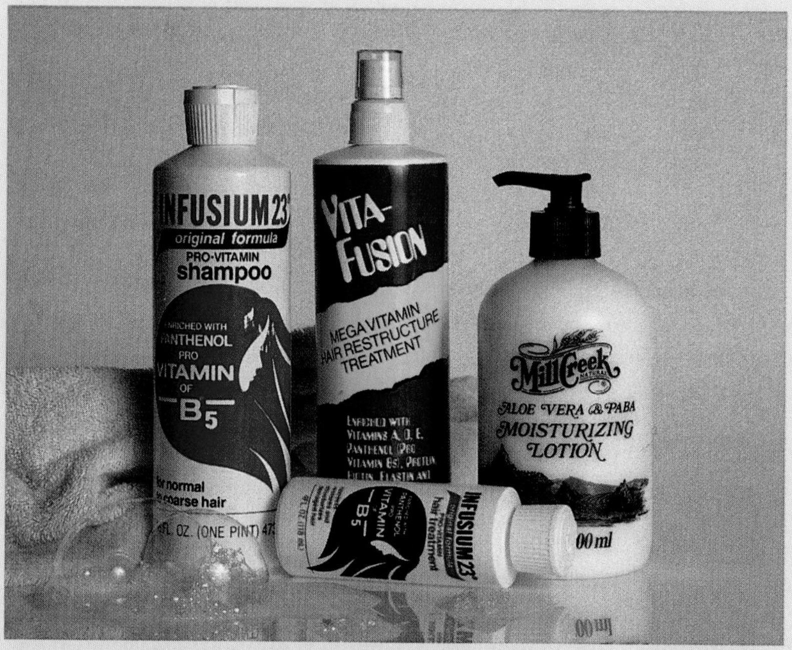

Bogus vitamins help to sell cosmetic products.

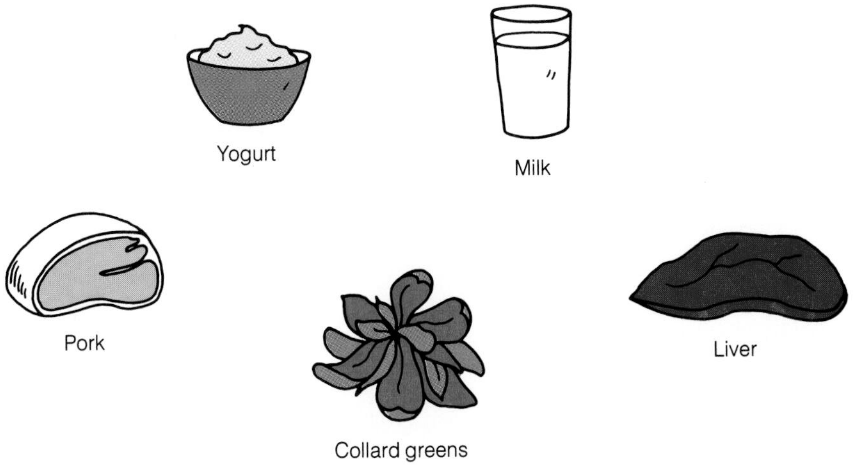

Good sources of riboflavin.

paralysis and heart failure. It is easy to understand why beriberi has been a dreaded disease throughout history.

Toxicity Toxic reactions from overdoses of thiamin are rare, but they can be caused by injections of the vitamin. The symptoms of thiamin toxicity are severe. They include convulsions, headache, weakness, paralysis, and irregular heartbeat. Thiamin supplements have not been associated with the development of toxicity symptoms.

RIBOFLAVIN (VITAMIN B_2)

In the late 1800s, the search began for the compound that gave certain enzymes a fluorescent yellow color. The search finally ended in 1933. The bright yellow substance contained in what was frustratingly referred to as the "old yellow enzymes" was identified as riboflavin. Because it formed coenzymes, it was added to the growing list of B-complex vitamins.

Functions

Riboflavin naturally occurs in foods in two coenzyme forms. Both serve to activate enzymes involved in the formation of energy from the breakdown of carbohydrates, proteins, and fats.

carbohydrates, proteins, fats $\xrightarrow{\text{riboflavin}}$ energy

Sources

Dairy products are the leading source of riboflavin in the U.S. diet, followed by meats and whole- and enriched-grain products. Only a few vegetables are good sources of riboflavin, most of them of the "dark green and leafy" type. Table 9-4 lists food sources of riboflavin.

Recommended Intake

The RDA for adult females and males 23–50 years of age is 1.2 mg and 1.6 mg, respectively. The meager amount of riboflavin stored in the body is

■
TABLE 9-4
Food sources of riboflavin

Food	Amount	Riboflavin, mg*
Milk and Milk Products		
milk	1 c	0.5
2% milk	1 c	0.5
low-fat yogurt	1 c	0.5
skim milk	1 c	0.4
yogurt	1 c	0.1
American cheese	1 oz	0.1
cheddar cheese	1 oz	0.1
Meats and Eggs		
liver	3 oz	3.6
pork chop	3 oz	0.3
beef	3 oz	0.2
egg	1	0.2
tuna	½ c	0.1
Vegetables		
collard greens	½ c	0.3
broccoli	½ c	0.2
spinach, cooked	½ c	0.1
Grains		
macaroni	1 c	0.1
bread	1 slice	0.1

*RDAs for adults aged 23–50 are 1.2 mg for females and 1.6 mg for males.

depleted within a month if intakes fall below 1.2 mg per day.[3] Health problems caused by a deficiency of riboflavin become noticeable with habitual intakes of less than 50% of the RDA.[7]

Deficiency Riboflavin deficiency occurs throughout many parts of the world.[5] People in the U.S. are generally spared because they consume enough dairy products, meats, and grain products to meet the need for riboflavin.

ariboflavinosis: (*a*, "without"; *osis*, "abnormal condition") The riboflavin-deficiency disease.

People at risk of developing ariboflavinosis:
- *vegans and others who consume small amounts of milk, cheese, and meats*
- *alcohol abusers*
- *users of tranquilizers and antidepressants*
- *individuals with thyroid disease*
- *newborns receiving phototherapy for jaundice*

The riboflavin deficiency disease is **ariboflavinosis.** Due to riboflavin's broad role in energy metablism, ariboflavinosis disrupts a wide array of normal body functions. Common signs of riboflavin deficiency include decreased growth, cracks around the nose, reddening of the eyes, inflammation and soreness of the lips and tongue, and greasy, scaly skin eruptions. Scars at the corners of the mouth are a classic sign of previous ariboflavinosis (Figure 9-1).

Riboflavin deficiency may result from a low intake of milk, cheese, and meats, from strict vegetarian diets (the *vegan* diet), alcoholism, from the abuse of certain tranquilizers and antidepressants, and from thyroid disease. Some newborns who have undergone phototherapy for the treatment of jaundice have developed ariboflavinosis due to the destruction of riboflavin in the blood by the fluorescent lights.[9]

Riboflavin deficiency due to poor diets rarely occurs by itself. Most diets that are deficient in riboflavin are also low in protein, a number of other vitamins, and some minerals.

Toxicity Riboflavin appears to be nontoxic, even when taken in high amounts. High intakes of riboflavin are rapidly excreted by the body.

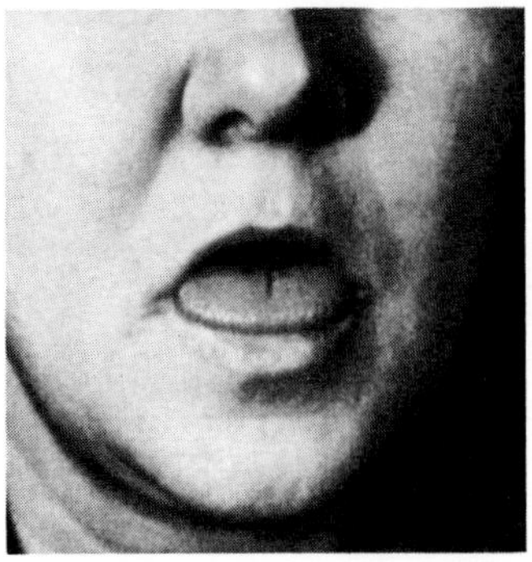

FIGURE 9-1

These scars at the corners of the mouth indicate a history of riboflavin deficiency.

NIACIN (VITAMIN B_3)

In 1914, U.S. Public Health Service bacteriologist Joseph Goldberger was dispatched to the southern United States. His mission was to discover the cause of pellagra, a common and horrible disease that can result in insanity and death. Twenty years later it would be shown to be due to niacin deficiency, but Goldberger expected to find a bacterial cause of what was then thought to be an infectious disease.[10]

Goldberger noted that pellagra was most prevalent among poor people and children in orphanages, and that it was not spread by contact. He also noted dramatic differences in the diets of the poor and the well-off; poor people's diets tended to consist of cornmeal, grits, fat back, and molasses and little meat or milk. People with higher incomes consumed more milk, meat, and vegetables. The observation that the orphanage children who did

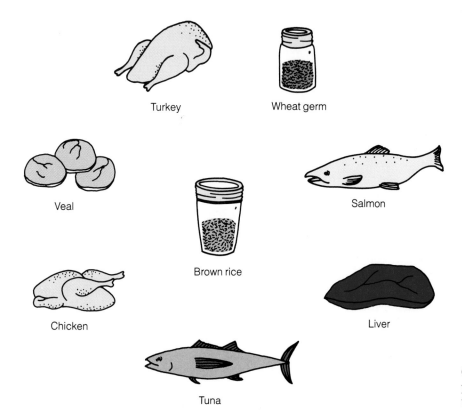

Turkey
Wheat germ
Veal
Salmon
Brown rice
Chicken
Liver
Tuna

Good sources of niacin and its provitamin, the amino acid tryptophan.

not get the disease were the ones who were known to have raided the milk and meat supplies at night provided a strong clue that the disease was related to diet.

In dramatic fashion, Goldberger disproved the notion that pellagra was an infectious disease. He, his wife, and fourteen volunteers received injections of the blood of people with pellagra. Not one of them developed pellagra, and the search for the dietary cause of the disease intensified.[11] It took until 1937 to identify niacin deficiency as the culprit. The prevalence of pellagra declined rapidly in the U.S. as dietary intakes improved.[10]

Functions

glucose $\xrightarrow{\text{niacin}}$ energy
fatty acid units $\xrightarrow{\text{niacin}}$ fatty acids
$H_2 + O \xrightarrow{\text{niacin}}$ water

Like thiamin and riboflavin, niacin plays a critical role in energy metabolism. Its two coenzymes accept energy released during the breakdown of glucose and transfer it to ADP. These coenzymes are also used in fatty acid synthesis and in processes that lead to the formation of a major end product of energy metabolism, water.

Sources

60 mg tryptophan = 1 mg niacin

The food sources of niacin include those that contain either the vitamin or its provitamin, the essential amino acid tryptophan. Niacin is the only known vitamin whose provitamin is an amino acid. It takes 60 mg of tryptophan to yield 1 mg of niacin. Tryptophan is the least abundant essential amino acid, and it makes an important contribution to niacin status only in people whose diets provide ample amounts of high-quality protein. In the U.S. in general, more than half of people's niacin requirement is met by consuming high-quality animal protein.[13] When the content of high-quality proteins in diets is inadequate, tryptophan is used to form body proteins, rather than niacin.

Meats are the leading sources of niacin and tryptophan (Table 9-5). The tryptophan content in a serving of fish, turkey, chicken, beef, or pork can contribute 2 to 7 milligrams of niacin in addition to the niacin already present. Notice in the table that liver contains a very high amount of tryptophan. If all of the tryptophan in liver could be converted to niacin, a 3-ounce serving would provide 43 mg of niacin!

Milk and milk products contain only a trace of niacin (less than half a milligram per serving), but they are included in the table because of their tryptophan content. Although three glasses of milk contain only a fraction of a milligram of niacin, the 336 mg of tryptophan present in the milk can be converted to 5.6 mg of niacin.

Whole- and enriched-grain products are poor sources of tryptophan, but they contain niacin. The amount of niacin present in a single serving of whole-grain or enriched rice, bread, pasta, or other grain product is small, but the amount is significant because these foods tend to be eaten often.

The bulk of the niacin requirement in this country is met by tryptophan consumption. Approximately 75% of our intake of niacin comes from tryptophan supplied by the high-quality protein in our diets.[12] As seen in Table 9-5, the best sources of niacin are meats, including fish, chicken, beef, and pork. Meats are generally good sources of tryptophan as well as niacin, and even small amounts of these foods contribute substantially to niacin intake.

TABLE 9-5
Food sources of niacin and its provitamin, tryptophan

Food	Amount	Niacin, mg*	Tryptophan, mg
Meats			
liver	3 oz	14.0	1,766
tuna	½ c	10.3	238
turkey	3 oz	9.5	291
chicken	3 oz	7.9	311
salmon	3 oz	6.9	229
veal	3 oz	5.2	399
beef (round steak)	3 oz	5.1	297
pork	3 oz	4.5	313
haddock	3 oz	2.7	155
scallops	3 oz	1.1	252
Milk and Milk Products			
cottage cheese	½ c	trace	156
Swiss cheese	1 oz	trace	114
whole milk	1 c	trace	112
cheddar cheese	1 oz	trace	91
colby cheese	1 oz	trace	87
Grains			
wheat germ	1 oz (¼ c)	1.5	76
brown rice	½ c	1.2	25
noodles, enriched	½ c	1.0	37
rice, white, enriched	½ c	1.0	23
bread, enriched	1 slice	0.7	26

*RDAs for adults aged 23–50 are 18 mg for males and 13 mg for females.

Recommended Intake

To account for the potential contribution of tryptophan in meeting niacin requirement, the RDAs for niacin are given as "niacin equivalents" (NEs). One NE equals 1 milligram of niacin or 60 milligrams of tryptophan. Thus, the RDAs include the contribution of tryptophan in meeting the dietary allowances for niacin.

The niacin RDAs are 18 mg NE for adult males and 13 mg NE for adult females. An average intake of 13 mg or more is needed to maintain the body's limited stores of this vitamin.[3]

Deficiency

Signs of **pellagra**, the niacin-deficiency disease, develop within about two months when niacin intakes are less than 50% of the RDA.[13] The average U.S. diet supplies 16–34 mg NE, and pellagra is now rare in this country.

pellagra (*pelle*, "skin"; *agra*, "rash") The niacin-deficiency disease, which is accompanied by characteristic changes in the skin.

Pellagra remains a public health problem in some countries, particularly those that rely on corn as the staple food.[5] Corn contains niacin, but in a

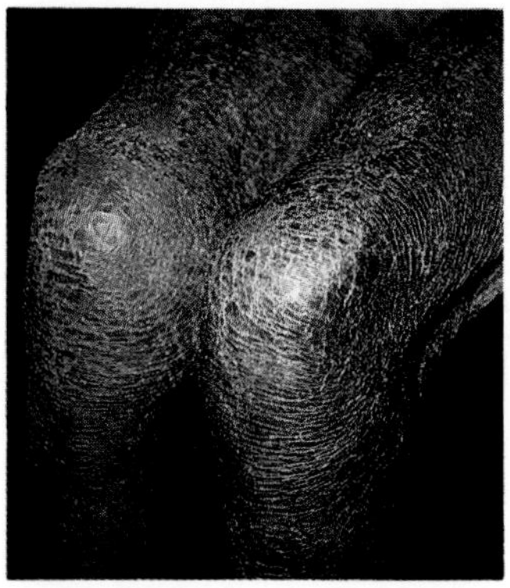

FIGURE 9-2
Dry, scaly skin accompanies pellagra.

dermatitis: (*dermis*, "skin"; *itis*, "inflammation") Inflammation of the skin.

dementia: (from Latin *dementare*, "to make insane") A deteriorative mental state.

bound form that cannot be absorbed. The treatment of cornmeal with lye that is customary in many Latin American cultures effectively liberates the niacin from its bound form.

Victims of pellagra suffer what has been called "the four D's": **dermatitis**, diarrhea, **dementia**, and death. Dermatitis is the most characteristic sign of niacin deficiency. Although all skin surfaces are dry and scaly, skin exposed to light develops a reddish rash (Figure 9-2). This distinctive rash led to the early designation of pellagra as "the illness of the sun."[11] The dementia caused by pellagra can be severe. During the early 1900s, when pellagra was common in this country, a number of hospitals were devoted to the care of pellagra victims who had become insane. Weight loss and weakness (which could be called "the two W's") also are classic signs of pellagra.

Toxicity

Niacin toxicity has been caused by long-term intakes as low as 2½ times the RDA.[8] The most obvious sign of mild niacin overload is a temporary flushing of the skin. Nausea, low blood pressure, rapid heartbeat, fainting, hypoglycemia, and liver damage have been reported with niacin intakes exceeding 3 grams per day over a period of time.[3]

Awareness of the signs of niacin toxicity has increased over recent years due to the number of cases seen in hospital emergency rooms. Although the symptoms of niacin toxicity quickly subside when people stop using high-dose niacin supplements, people experiencing the toxic reactions are likely to feel that their life is on the line and they seek care immediately. (See Box 9-3).

BOX 9-3

REPORT OF AN OUTBREAK OF NIACIN TOXICITY

On December 17, 1980, 18 (42%) of 43 persons in a nursing home in northern Illinois developed facial flushing and/or a rash, most commonly on the face or upper arms, within 15–30 minutes of eating breakfast. Symptoms lasted an average of approximately 50 minutes. Eggs, toast, coffee, orange juice, milk, and cornmeal mush had been served at the meal. The cornmeal mush was the only food known to have been eaten by all ill individuals. Nursing home personnel had noted that the mush appeared to be a slightly different color than usual.

Samples of cornmeal used to make the mush were tested by the Food and Drug Administration (FDA) and were found to contain >1,000 mg of niacin per pound. (The recommended level for this product is 16–24 mg per pound.) When the cornmeal was received from the distributor it was poured out of packages and stored in an unlabeled, large plastic container in the nursing-home kitchen. It has not been possible to identify the source of contamination of the cornmeal involved in the outbreak.

Niacin is a common additive in commercially available cornmeal. In this outbreak, if the source of the excess niacin was at the manufacturing plant, it may have resulted from inadequate mixing or measurement of the additive during processing.

Source: The Morbidity and Mortality Weekly Report, January 16, 1981, published by the Centers for Disease Control, Atlanta, Georgia.

Much of what is known about niacin toxicity stems from the use of high doses for the experimental treatment of conditions such as schizophrenia and high blood-lipid levels. The dementia produced by pellagra resembles that found in schizophrenia, but niacin has not been demonstrated to be effective in treating schizophrenia.[14] High levels of niacin—in the range of 3 to 6 grams per day—are known to lower blood cholesterol and triglyceride levels. The simultaneous occurrence of niacin toxicity symptoms, however, has eliminated such high doses of niacin from consideration as an agent for lowering blood lipid levels in the future.[15,16]

■ ■ ■

VITAMIN B_6 (PYRIDOXINE)

Vitamin B_6 was isolated in the 1930s from the group of vitamins originally thought of as "vitamin B." Investigations conducted over the next thirty years showed that there was not one vitamin B_6, but three naturally occurring forms of the vitamin. The most commonly referred to active form of vitamin B_6 is pyridoxine.

Functions

The coenzymes of vitamin B_6 activate a large number of enzymes (more than sixty of them), the vast majority of which are involved in protein metabolism. Enzymes involved in the conversion of the amino acid tryptophan to niacin and to the neurotransmitter serotonin require a vitamin-B_6 coenzyme. Many other examples of reactions involving amino acids could be given to demonstrate the broad influence of vitamin B_6 on protein metabolism.

amino acids $\xrightarrow{\text{vitamin } B_6}$ proteins, neurotransmitters

The active forms of vitamin B_6 are found in meats, legumes, and green and yellow vegetables.

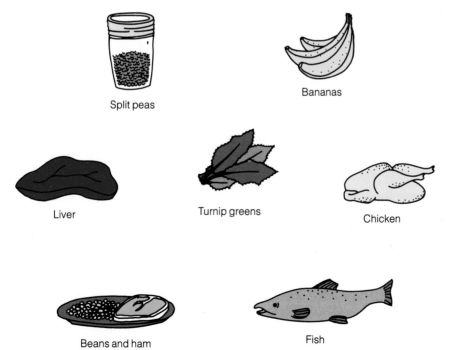

Sources

Meats are the leading source of vitamin B_6 in the U.S. diet (Table 9-6). Dried beans and peas, eggs, and a few types of fruits and vegetables also contribute to vitamin B_6 intake. Foods that contain only low amounts of vitamin B_6 are milk, cheese, and grains, and they are not listed in Table 9-6. Nonetheless, if they are consumed regularly, these foods contribute significantly to meeting vitamin B_6 needs.[2]

Recommended Intake

The adult RDAs for vitamin B_6 of 2.0 mg and 2.2 mg per day for females and males, respectively, is at the upper limit of the amount typically consumed in the U.S. These levels closely approximate the level needed to maintain normal vitamin functions; they include only a small "margin of safety."[3]

TABLE 9-6

Food sources of vitamin B_6

Food	Amount	Vitamin B_6, mg*
Meats and Eggs		
liver	3 oz	0.8
salmon	3 oz	0.7
other fish	3 oz	0.6
chicken	3 oz	0.4
ham	3 oz	0.4
hamburger	3 oz	0.4
veal	3 oz	0.4
egg	1	0.3
pork	3 oz	0.3
beef	3 oz	0.2
Legumes		
split peas	½ c	0.6
dried beans (cooked)	½ c	0.4
Fruits		
banana	1	0.6
avocado	½	0.4
watermelon	1 c	0.3
Vegetables		
turnip greens	½ c	0.7
brussels sprouts	½ c	0.4
potato	1	0.2
sweet potato	½ c	0.2
carrots	½ c	0.2
peas	½ c	0.1

*RDAs for adults aged 23–50 are 2.0 mg for females and 2.2 mg for males.

Deficiency The name given to vitamin-B_6 deficiency is quite straightforward: *vitamin-B_6 deficiency*. Mental changes, including depression and confusion, are the earliest symptoms of the deficiency in adults. As the deficiency becomes more severe, disturbances in protein metabolism eventually lead to convulsions and other serious disturbances of the nervous system.

A vivid picture of deficiency symptoms in infants was obtained in 1951 when vitamin B_6 was inadvertently omitted from a commercial infant formula. The symptoms shown by the infants who had been fed the formula were strikingly similar to those that had been seen in vitamin-B_6-deficient laboratory animals: vomiting, weight loss, hyperirritability, and convulsions.[3] The formula was withdrawn from the market as soon as the mistake was noted.

Certain groups within the U.S. population are at risk for vitamin-B_6 deficiency. Women using oral contraceptive pills for more than two or three years are more likely to become vitamin-B_6 deficient than women who do not use the pill.[17] Decreased levels of vitamin B_6 may cause depression among oral contraceptive users.[18] Adolescent girls and pregnant women share the risk of vitamin B_6 deficiency.[19,20] One study of 583 adolescent girls in Southern states identified vitamin B_6 deficiency among 13% of the sample.[19]

People at risk of developing vitamin-B_6 deficiency:
- *oral contraceptive users*
- *adolescent girls*
- *pregnant women*

Vitamin B_6 has been used to treat premenstrual syndrome (PMS), even though there is no evidence that vitamin B_6 deficiency is responsible for any aspect of the syndrome. Very high levels of vitamin B_6 (50 times the RDA) have been reported to alleviate such symptoms as the swelling, anxiety, and headaches that precede menstruation in some women.[21] The levels of vitamin B_6 that have been used to treat premenstrual syndrome fall into the potentially toxic category.

Toxicity Vitamin B_6 was once considered a highly nontoxic vitamin. As vitamin B_6 supplementation grew in popularity, however, so did knowledge about toxic dose levels and symptoms. Daily intakes exceeding 25 times the RDA are associated with the development of burning, shooting, and tingling pains in the arms and legs; clumsiness; and numbness.[22] Severe nervous-system problems have been reported with vitamin B_6 intakes that exceed 2 grams per day.[23] Vitamin B_6 is no longer regarded as nontoxic.

FOLACIN (FOLIC ACID)

Folacin is one of the most difficult vitamins to isolate from foods. It is very fragile—because it is easily destroyed by heat—and it is present in only trace amounts in food. Problems with finding it, and then not destroying it in isolating it from the other chemical substances in food, delayed its discovery. It was not until the early 1940s that folacin was isolated from dark green vegetables.

Functions

Folacin's coenzymes play a central role as activators of enzymes involved in DNA replication and the synthesis of proteins from amino acids. Without sufficient folacin, DNA cannot replicate normally, and cells do not receive

$$1 \text{ DNA} \xrightarrow{\text{folacin}} 2 \text{ DNA}$$

$$\text{amino acids} \xrightarrow{\text{folacin}} \text{proteins}$$

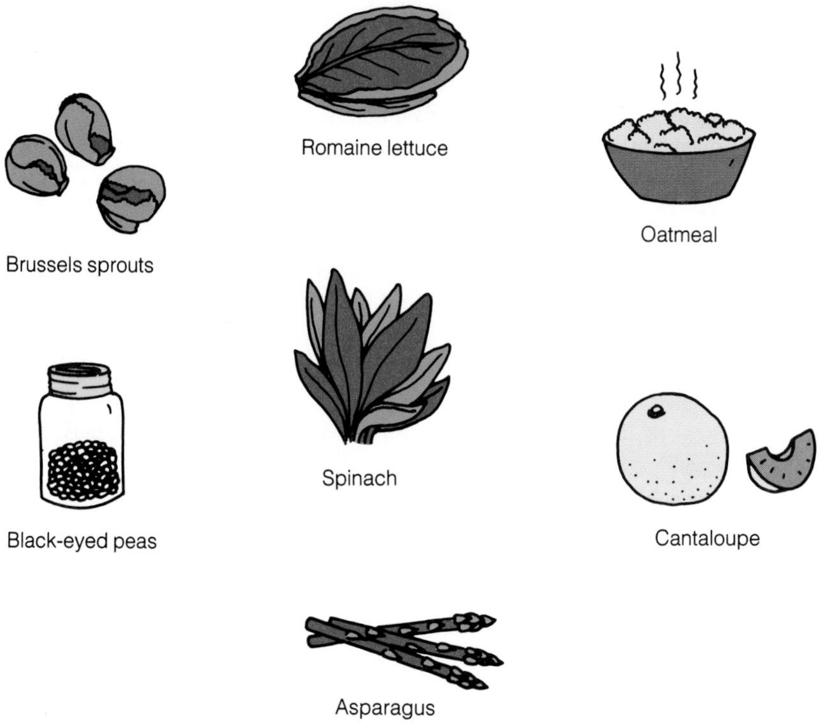

Good sources of folacin.

the protein they need to maintain normal functions. The influence of folacin on cell division and the manufacture of proteins makes it a particularly important vitamin for growth.

Sources

The name *folacin* was derived from the Latin word *folia* for "leaves." Many of the best sources of folacin are darkly colored, leafy plants. Asparagus, brussels sprouts, spinach, romaine lettuce, collard greens, and broccoli are all key sources of folacin. These, and other good sources of folacin are listed in Table 9-7. Note that cantaloupe, citrus fruits, and whole grains also provide notable levels of the vitamin.

Folacin that can be absorbed occurs in foods in both a free form and in combination with other substances. The chemical procedure used to assess folacin content generally measures only the free form. Consequently, nutrient composition tables tend to underestimate the total folacin content of food by approximately 60%.

Recommended Intake

The adult RDA for folacin is set at 400 mcg (0.4 mg) for both males and females. (See Box 9-4.) A minimum of 100 mcg of folacin per day is needed to maintain normal blood levels.[3] The average folacin content of U.S. diets is about 600 mcg, but diets that include lots of vegetables and fruits can provide as much as 1 to 2 mg.[24]

Deficiency The most characteristic sign of folacin deficiency is large, irregularly shaped red blood cells (Figure 9-3). Normally, red blood cells increase in size in preparation for DNA replication and cell division. Without

TABLE 9-7
Food sources of folacin

Food	Amount	Folacin, mcg*
Vegetables		
asparagus	½ c	120
brussels sprouts	½ c	116
black-eyed peas	½ c	102
spinach, cooked	½ c	99
romaine lettuce	1 c	86
lima beans	½ c	71
peas	½ c	70
collard greens (cooked)	½ c	56
sweet potato	½ c	43
broccoli	½ c	43
Fruits		
cantaloupe	¼	100
orange juice	1 c	87
orange	1	59
Grains		
oatmeal	½ c	97
wheat germ	¼ c	80
wild rice	½ c	37

*RDAs for adults aged 23–50 are 400 mcg (0.4 mg) for both males and females.

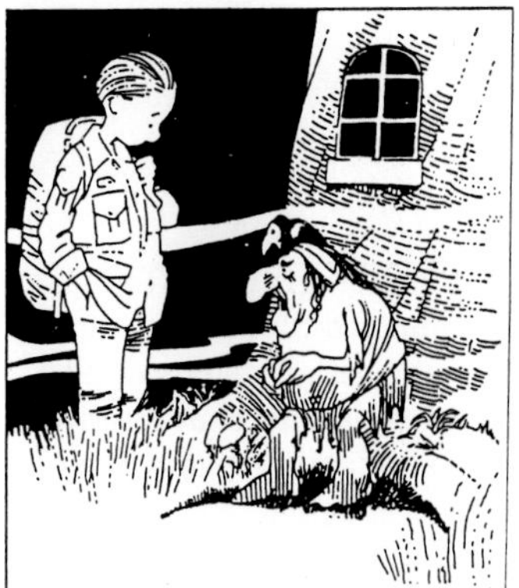
"You've seen those cute little Keebler elves who make cookies? Well, I can broccoli!"

© Richard Guindon

adequate folacin, however, DNA does not replicate, and cells fail to divide. The large, abnormally shaped red blood cells that result when cells fail to divide are called **megaloblasts**, and the folacin-deficiency disease is referred to as *megaloblastic anemia.* The sequence and timing of events in the development of folic-acid deficiency is shown in Figure 9-4.[25] It takes about two months for a dietary deficiency of folacin to cause cells to become large and abnormally shaped, and five months for a full-blown case of megaloblastic anemia to develop.

megaloblasts: Large, irregularly shaped red blood cells. They are found in cases of folacin deficiency and vitamin-B_{12} deficiency.

Other cells, such as those that line the cheeks and gastrointestinal tract, are also affected by folacin deficiency. Since these cells "turn over," or replace themselves more frequently than do red blood cells, a deficiency of

BOX 9-4

HOW MUCH IS 400 mcg?

The amount of folacin required each day by humans—400 mcg—is so small that it is hard to visualize. Think about the amount of sugar in a single packet; sugar packets typically contain about a teaspoonful. That amount of folacin would meet your RDA for thirty years! You would need to eat 18,500 cups of asparagus, one of the best sources, to get a teaspoonful of folacin.

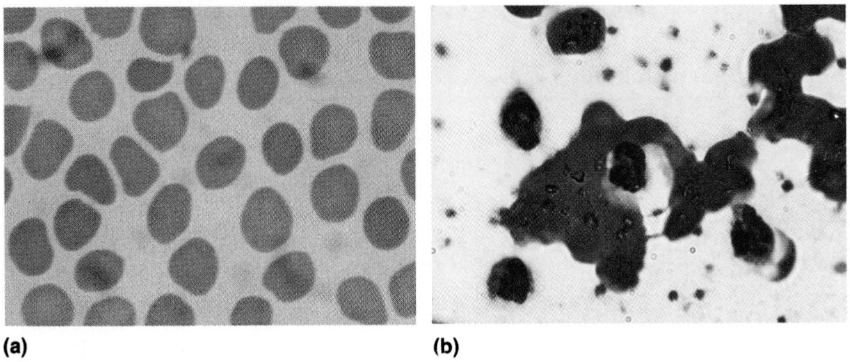

FIGURE 9-3
Photomicrographs of *(a)* normal red blood cells and *(b)* the abnormally shaped red blood cells that characterize megaloblastic anemia due to a folacin deficiency. Magnification × 1,000.

folacin can be observed earlier in samples of cells from these tissues. Folacin deficiency also can produce such psychological effects as irritability and "paranoid" behavior. Children with folic acid deficiency fail to grow.

People at risk of developing folacin deficiency:
infants, children
pregnant women
oral contraceptive users
alcoholics
anticonvulsant users

Certain groups within the U.S. population are at risk of developing folacin deficiency, most notably, poorly nourished children and pregnant women. These groups are vulnerable because they have high requirements for the vitamin for growth and protein synthesis. It has been estimated that perhaps one-third of all pregnant women in the world develop folic-acid deficiency.[26] Women taking oral contraceptive pills, alcohol abusers, and long-term users of anticonvulsants (such as Dilantin) are also at risk of folacin deficiency.

Toxicity Dose levels of folacin for over-the-counter sale are limited to 400 mcg, which makes it relatively inconvenient to consume a massive amount. Dose levels are limited because supplemental folacin may mask the signs of vitamin-B_{12} deficiency. We will return to this topic in the next section.

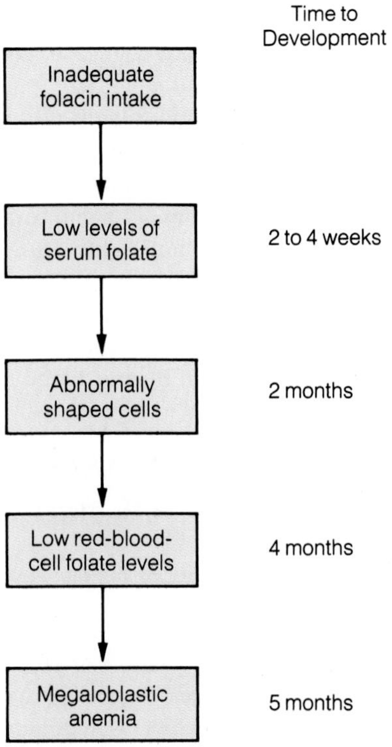

FIGURE 9-4
Sequence and timing of events in the development of dietary folacin deficiency.

Experimentally induced folacin toxicity has been produced with doses of 15 mg per day (about 38 times the RDA). Symptoms of overdose do not represent serious problems, but they include such aggravations as diarrhea, sleep disturbances, and irritability. Very high doses—3 grams per day or more—can produce fever, body pain, and other ill effects.[25]

■ ■ ■

VITAMIN B_{12} (CYANOCOBALAMIN)

Vitamin B_{12}, required in the smallest amounts of the essential nutrients, is the most recently discovered vitamin (1948). Vitamin B_{12} represents a family of similar chemical substances, of which cyanocobalamin (*cyano*, "dark blue"; *cobalamin*, "cobalt-containing") is the most common naturally occurring form. Its crystals are a beautiful dark blue color.

Vitamin B_{12} is not a typical vitamin. Unlike other vitamins, it:

- is produced only by microorganisms
- occurs nearly exclusively in foods of animal origin
- contains the mineral cobalt
- requires a carrier for absorption
- is not freely absorbed (Absorption depends on body B_{12} storage levels.)

Animals obtain B_{12} by ingesting either microorganisms or foods previously supplied with B_{12} by microorganisms. Some animals obtain vitamin B_{12} from bacterial production of the vitamin in their intestinal tracts. (Human intestines do not appear to be occupied by B_{12}-producing microorganisms.) Plants do not require vitamin B_{12}, nor do they produce it.

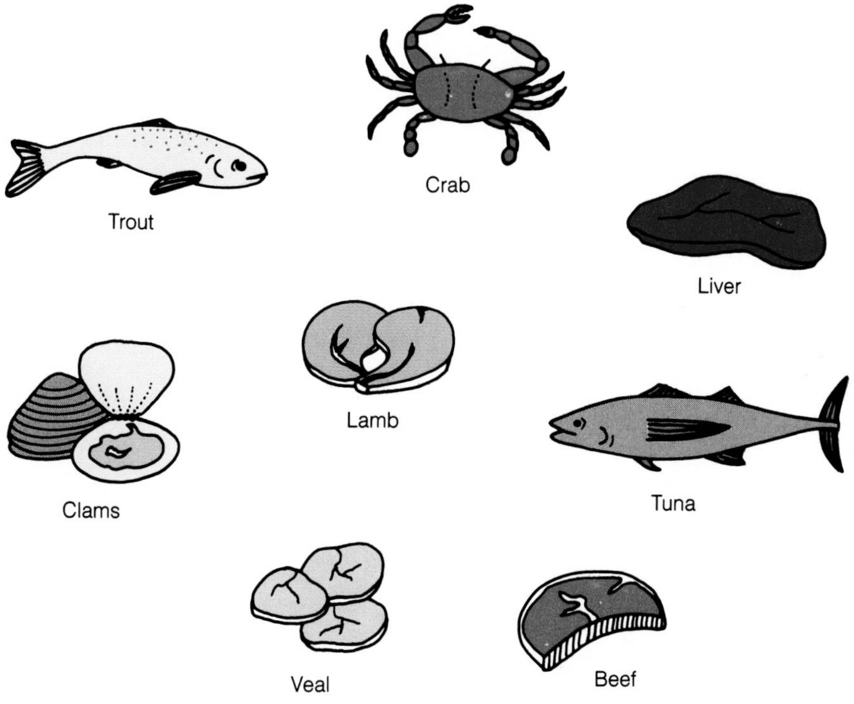

Good sources of vitamin B_{12}.

intrinsic factor: A protein produced by the stomach that facilitates the absorption of vitamin B_{12} in the small intestine.

A small amount of B_{12} is absorbed in the lower part of the small intestine by simple diffusion. Absorption of the remaining 99% is facilitated with the help of a carrier. **Intrinsic factor**, a protein produced by the stomach, combines with the vitamin and "escorts" it to special intrinsic factor–vitamin B_{12} (IF-B_{12}) receptors on the surface of the small intestine. The IF-B_{12} receptors also serve to regulate the amount of B_{12} that enters the bloodstream. When vitamin B_{12} storage levels are high, the number of IF-B_{12} receptors is low, thus limiting the amount of B_{12} that is absorbed.[27]

Functions

fatty acid units $\xrightarrow{\text{vitamin } B_{12}}$ fatty acids

amino acids $\xrightarrow{\text{vitamin } B_{12}}$ proteins

The coenzymes of vitamin B_{12} are involved in the metabolism of fatty acids and amino acids that leads to the formation and maintenance of components of nerve, blood, and other cells. The coenzymes of vitamin B_{12} and folacin function together to activate the enzymes involved in cell division. Vitamin B_{12} is required in the series of reactions that precede the use of folacin in DNA replication. Without vitamin B_{12}, folacin cannot perform its role in protein synthesis, even if folacin is available. Thus, a vitamin-B_{12} deficiency may appear to be a folacin deficiency.

Sources

Nearly all of the vitamin B_{12} in U.S. diets is supplied by the B_{12} coenzymes found in meats, milk and milk products, and eggs.[2] (See Table 9-8.) Plants do not naturally contain B_{12}, but trace amounts are sometimes present in them due to contamination by microorganisms. Fermented foods, such as

TABLE 9-8
Food sources of vitamin B_{12}

Food	Amount	Vitamin B_{12}, mcg*
Meats and Eggs		
liver	3 oz	6.8
trout	3 oz	3.6
beef	3 oz	2.2
clams	½ c	2.0
crab	3 oz	1.8
lamb	3 oz	1.8
tuna	½ c	1.8
veal	3 oz	1.7
hamburger, regular	3 oz	1.5
egg	1	0.6
Milk and Milk Products		
skim milk	1 c	1.0
milk	1 c	0.9
yogurt	1 c	0.8
cottage cheese	½ c	0.7
American cheese	1 oz	0.2
cheddar cheese	1 oz	0.2

*The RDA for adults aged 23–50 is 3.0 mcg for both females and males.

tofu and soy sauce, and products that contain yeast provide very small amounts of vitamin B_{12}—far too little to include them in Table 9-8.

Recommended Intake

A little vitamin B_{12} goes a long way; the adult RDA of 3 mcg per day is so small that you would need a microscope to see it. An average daily intake of 2 mcg is needed to prevent or cure vitamin B_{12} deficiency.[26]

Deficiency Before vitamin B_{12} was identified, it was known that a substance contained in liver cures **pernicious anemia**, a progressive and potentially fatal disease. The substance eventually isolated from liver that is responsible for the cure is vitamin B_{12}. The scientific importance of this discovery was recognized with the award of Nobel Prizes to several scientists involved in the research.

pernicious anemia: (pernicious means destructive, fatal) A severe form of anemia characterized by an increase in the size, and a decrease in the number of red blood cells. Symptoms include degenerative changes in nerve cells and impaired functioning of the nervous system.

Vitamin-B_{12} deficiency can result from a number of causes:

- inadequate vitamin B_{12} intake due to the avoidance of meats, dairy products, and eggs
- inadequate production of intrinsic factor by the stomach
- chronic malabsorption problems

Vitamin-B_{12} deficiency is most often due to either a low intake of animal products or to a lack of intrinsic factor.[25] Thus, vegans, people who genetically lack the ability to produce intrinsic factor, and people who have had part of their stomach removed are most vulnerable to vitamin-B_{12} deficiency.

Because the body can store three to five years' worth of vitamin B_{12}, there is a large time lag between the onset of poor diet or absorption and the development of deficiency symptoms. The first signs of vitamin-B_{12} deficiency are numbness and tingling in the hands and feet. As the deficiency progresses, red blood cells become enlarged, just as they do in folacin deficiency. Moodiness, confusion, depression, delusions and even overt psychoses may develop. If left untreated, vitamin-B_{12} deficiency can result in irreparable nerve damage and death.

People at risk of developing vitamin-B_{12} deficiency:
vegans
people who lack the ability to produce intrinsic factor
people who have undergone stomach surgery

Both vitamin-B_{12} deficiency and folacin deficiency are characterized by megaloblasts, which can lead to misdiagnosis—a vitamin-B_{12} deficiency may be erroneously diagnosed as a folacin deficiency based on the shape of red blood cells—and thus to the wrong treatment. Folacin, when mistakenly given for a vitamin B_{12} deficiency, brings about an improvement in red blood cells, but it has no effect on the nerve damage produced by the B_{12} deficiency. Because of the improvement in red blood cells, the damage that is

BOX 9-5

THE B_{12} BOOST

Vitamin B_{12} has sometimes been referred to as the "pick me up" vitamin. In the 1960s and 1970s, B_{12} injections were commonly used to give elderly people an "energy lift." Although many of the recipients swore by the value of the treatment, it was not scientifically shown to be beneficial to health. The practice of giving B_{12} injections ended abruptly when health insurers decided that their policies did not cover the treatment.[14]

occurring to nerves may be overlooked and may thus proceed to an irreversible stage. To reduce the possibility of masking vitamin-B_{12} deficiency with folacin, federal law limits over-the-counter folacin supplements to 400 mcg (0.4 mg).

Treatment for vitamin-B_{12} deficiency depends on its cause. If inadequate dietary intake is the cause, adding meats, milk, and eggs to the diet or using B_{12} supplements will cure and prevent the deficiency. Vitamin-B_{12} deficiency caused by inadequate production of intrinsic factor must be treated with periodic B_{12} injections. (B_{12} injections have been used as "body energizers," as Box 9-5 points out.) Injections of vitamin B_{12}, rather than pills, are used when a lack of intrinsic factor is the primary cause of the deficiency, since the vitamin B_{12} in pills is not absorbed if intrinsic factor is not produced by the stomach.

Toxicity Vitamin B_{12} appears to be nontoxic, even when taken in doses as large as 100 mg.[27] Absorption of B_{12} rapidly declines with high intakes of supplemental vitamin B_{12}.

BIOTIN

Before it was isolated from foods, biotin was commonly called the "egg-white injury factor." It was well-known that laboratory animals given raw egg whites as their sole source of protein develop dermatitis and muscle problems, and that if the egg whites are cooked, these problems do not appear. It was reasoned that raw egg whites contain an essential nutrient that is bound to a substance that is destroyed by heat. Avidin, a protein in egg white that is broken down by heat, was found to be the "binder" of the

Biotin is found in nuts, eggs, milk, and some vegetables and fruits.

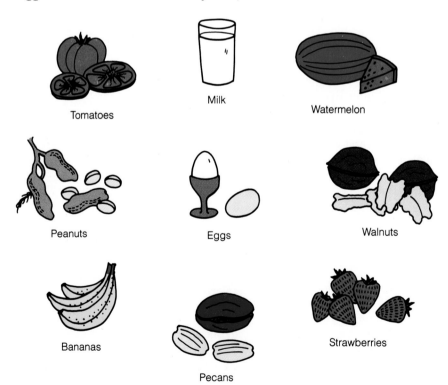

essential nutrient, biotin. "Egg-white injury factor" was relabeled *biotin* and was classified as a B-complex vitamin.

Functions

By activating enzymes involved in splitting and rearranging glucose, amino acids, and fatty acid molecules, the coenzyme biotin plays major roles in energy production and in the synthesis of nonessential amino acids and fatty acids.

glucose $\xrightarrow{\text{biotin}}$ energy

amino acid$_1$ $\xrightarrow{\text{biotin}}$ amino acid$_2$

fatty acid units $\xrightarrow{\text{biotin}}$ fatty acids

Sources

There are few "rich" food sources of biotin, but it is found in small amounts in most foods. As shown in Table 9-9, nuts, eggs, milk, and certain fruits and vegetables are good sources of biotin.

TABLE 9-9
Food sources of biotin

Food	Amount	Biotin, mcg*
Nuts		
peanuts	¼ c	120
walnuts	¼ c	90
pecans	¼ c	80
peanut butter	1 T	60
Eggs		
egg yolk	1	70
egg white	1	20
Milk	1 c	50
Fruits		
strawberries	1 c	60
watermelon	1 c	60
banana	1	50
cantaloupe	¼	40
grapefruit	½	30
raisins	¼ c	20
peach	1	20
Vegetables		
tomato	1	50
potato	1	40
zucchini	½ c	30
corn	½ c	20
spinach, cooked	½ c	20

*The provisional RDA for adults is 100–200 mcg. Provisional RDAs are listed in Table II of the RDAs inside the cover of this book. They are the "estimated safe and adequate daily dietary intakes."

Biotin is also produced by bacteria in the large intestine. Although the extent of absorption of the biotin produced by bacteria is not known, part of the human requirement for the vitamin may be met by these bacteria.

Recommended Intake

The provisional RDA for adults is 100–200 mcg a day, a level of intake at least six times the amount needed to prevent deficiency.[28] (The "provisional" RDA is the "estimated safe and adequate daily intake level" reported in Table II of the RDAs.) Low intakes of biotin have not been reported in the U.S.[3]

Deficiency Biotin deficiency rarely occurs outside of experimental studies that intentionally produce it. Humans given 6 raw egg whites per day develop dermatitis due to biotin deficiency within 3 to 4 weeks, and experience mental changes, muscle pain, nausea, and loss of appetite after 5 weeks. The symptoms disappear within 5 days after biotin is given.[29]

Toxicity Even in doses exceeding 100 times the RDA, biotin is remarkably safe.[30]

■ ■ ■

PANTOTHENIC ACID (PANTOTHENATE)

Pantothenic *is derived from the Greek* panto, *meaning "all."*

Soon after pantothenic acid was isolated from yeast, it was discovered in at least trace amounts in a wide variety of foods. It is indeed fortunate that pantothenic acid is widely available in foods, because it is needed for metabolic reactions that occur everywhere in the body.

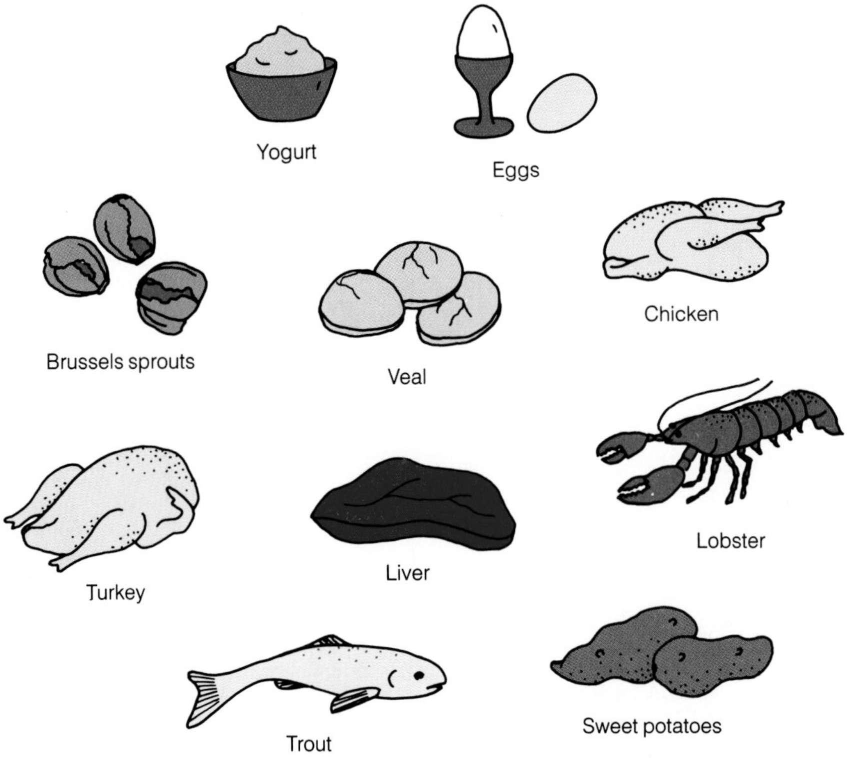

Good sources of pantothenic acid.

Functions

Pantothenic acid is the main component of "coenzyme A," a critically important coenzyme in the release of energy from glucose, the formation of glucose from amino acid (gluconeogenesis), and the synthesis of fatty acids. Its importance in nutrient metabolism is pervasive.

glucose $\xrightarrow{\text{pantothenic acid}}$ energy

amino acids $\xrightarrow{\text{pantothenic acid}}$ glucose

fatty acid units $\xrightarrow{\text{pantothenic acid}}$ fatty acids

Sources

Pantothenic acid is hard to avoid in foods. Table 9-10 lists some of the best food sources, but many other foods also contain pantothenic acid. A varied diet that includes sufficient amounts of the other B-complex vitamins is almost guaranteed to provide enough pantothenic acid.[3]

Recommended Intake

The provisional RDA is 4–7 mg of pantothenic acid for adults. On average, U.S. diets supply 7 mg per day.[31]

TABLE 9-10
Food sources of pantothenic acid

Food	Amount	Pantothenic Acid, mg*
Meats and Eggs		
liver	3 oz	6.0
trout	3 oz	1.7
egg	1	1.6
lobster	3 oz	1.3
turkey	3 oz	1.0
chicken	3 oz	0.9
veal	3 oz	0.9
beef (round steak)	3 oz	0.4
Milk and Milk Products		
yogurt	1 c	1.3
milk	1 c	0.7
Legumes		
dried beans, cooked	½ c	0.7
Vegetables		
brussels sprouts	½ c	1.1
sweet potato	½ c	1.0
broccoli	½ c	0.3
corn	½ c	0.2
Fruits		
Banana	1	0.5

*The provisional RDA for adults is 4–7 mg.

Deficiency Pantothenic-acid deficiency almost never occurs among people who eat enough food to avoid starvation. Deficiency in humans has been experimentally induced, and the symptoms include headache, fatigue, reduced growth, "burning feet," and a wide range of other symptoms related to its broad functions.

Toxicity Adverse symptoms of diarrhea and edema (water retention) can be induced with massive doses of pantothenic acid—10 to 20 grams per day.[32] Like biotin, it is a highly nontoxic vitamin.

VITAMIN C (ASCORBIC ACID)

Why humans, unlike most animals, developed a requirement for a dietary source of vitamin C is one of the great unsolved mysteries of science; most animals manufacture vitamin C from glucose. Humans, guinea pigs, monkeys, fruit-eating bats, and a few other animals require vitamin C because they lack the enzyme needed to convert glucose to vitamin C.

The chemical name for vitamin C is derived from Latin a scorbutus, *meaning "without scurvy."*

Vitamin C was not discovered until 1928, but its deficiency disease, scurvy, has been known for hundreds of years. Most cases of scurvy stem from a dietary lack of fruits and vegetables. In earlier times, ocean voyagers, explorers, and soldiers were among those most likely to develop scurvy. Outbreaks of scurvy had such devastating effects on populations that the lack of vitamin C is thought to have influenced the course of history. Many military campaigns were abruptly ended by outbreaks of scurvy among soldiers when they had depleted their supply of fruits and vegetables.[33] The lack of fruits and vegetables during winter months and periods of famine also precipitated epidemics of scurvy.

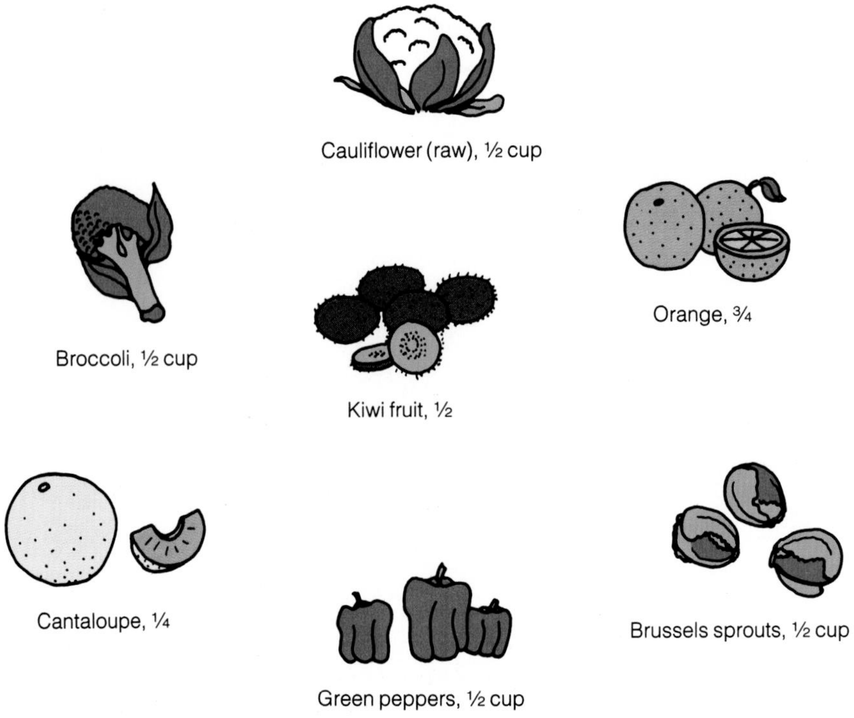

A day's supply of vitamin C is contained in each of these foods.

BOX 9-6

▪▪▪▪▪▪▪▪▪▪▪▪
DISCOVERING THE CURE FOR SCURVY

In 1740, Admiral George Anson of the British navy set sail on a voyage around the world with six ships and 1,955 men. He returned four years later with only the lead ship and 904 men. Outbreaks of scurvy had claimed the lives of nearly half of the sailors. These losses are said to have inspired James Lind to find a cure for scurvy.

Among the various treatments that Lind administered to sailors who developed scurvy, oranges and lemons were found to be most effective in curing it. It is said that the sailors who received the oranges and lemons felt such relief that ships' supplies of the fruits were often stolen, gorged upon, and hoarded.

Lind waited seven years to publish the results of his experiment, and it was not until almost fifty years later that lime juice or lemon juice was prescribed for all British sailors.[33] The use of lime juice by British sailors led to their being nicknamed "Limeys."

It was known as early as the 1500s that extracts of pine needles would cure scurvy, and 200 years later, that oranges, limes, and lemons would provide prompt recovery from the disease. (A quick history of the discovery of the cure for scurvy is presented in Box 9-6). In spite of this knowledge, epidemics of scurvy continued to occur. Scurvy was rampant among soldiers in the Civil War and it threatened the lives of sailors until the early twentieth century.

Functions

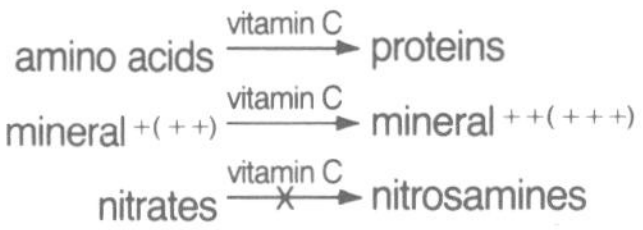

Vitamin C functions in protein synthesis in two ways. It changes the charge of iron so that it can be readily absorbed, and it serves as an antioxidant. These roles are discussed individually.

$$\text{amino acids} \xrightarrow{\text{vitamin C}} \text{proteins}$$
$$\text{mineral}^{+(++)} \xrightarrow{\text{vitamin C}} \text{mineral}^{++(+++)}$$
$$\text{nitrates} \xrightarrow[\times]{\text{vitamin C}} \text{nitrosamines}$$

Vitamin C participates in the construction of protein from amino acids by accepting hydrogen atoms that are released when amino acids combine. Many of the reactions involved in *collagen* formation, for example, require vitamin C. This structural component of bones, muscles, blood vessels, and cartilage develops abnormally in the absence of vitamin C.

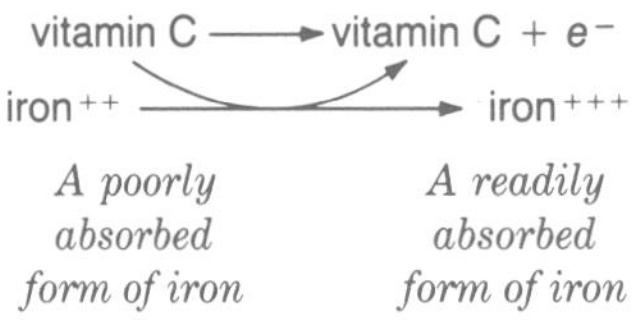

Changing the Charge of Iron Vitamin C promotes iron absorption by "pulling" electrons away from iron present in the gastrointestinal tract. The change takes iron from a "plus 2" state (iron^{++})to a "plus 3" state (iron^{+++}). By means of this action, vitamin C converts a poorly absorbed form of iron into one that is readily absorbed. (The ability of vitamin C to improve the bioavailability of dietary iron was discussed in chapter 8.)

$$\text{vitamin C} \longrightarrow \text{vitamin C} + e^-$$
$$\text{iron}^{++} \longrightarrow \text{iron}^{+++}$$

A poorly absorbed form of iron *A readily absorbed form of iron*

Role as an Antioxidant Vitamin C is one of a number of **antioxidants** present in cells that protect molecules from **oxidation**. Molecules that undergo oxidation either gain oxygen or lose electrons. Most oxidation reactions that occur in the body—such as the formation of water by the combination of oxygen and hydrogen—are a normal part of metabolism. Other

antioxidant: A substance that delays or prevents oxidation.

oxidation: The addition of oxygen to (or the removal of electrons from) a molecule.

Cured with Water, Salt, Sugar, Sodium phosphate, Sodium ascorbate (Vitamin C), Sodium nitrite.

Vitamin C is added to some smoked and cured meat products that contain nitrates to help protect against nitrosamine formation.

types of oxidation reactions, however, can have harmful consequences. Some molecules become highly unstable when oxidized and cause damage to nearby molecules.

Oddly enough, vitamin C protects molecules from oxidation by being highly susceptible to oxidation itself. Oxidizing agents are more likely to react with oxidation-prone vitamin C than they are with other, more stable molecules. Although the process destroys vitamin C, it serves the purpose of protecting other molecules from damage due to oxidation.

Vitamin C is much more susceptible to oxidation than are beta-carotene and vitamin E, two other vitamin antioxidants. It has been called the "antioxidants' antioxidant," because of the way it functions to protect both beta-carotene and vitamin E from oxidation.

In its role as an antioxidant, vitamin C blocks the formation of nitrosamines from nitrates. Nitrates are commonly added to smoked and cured meats to protect them against spoilage and enhance their flavor. In the absence of vitamin C, nitrates tend to combine with amino acids present in the small intestine and form nitrosamines. Exposure of the gastrointestinal tract to nitrosamines has been associated with the development of certain types of cancer, but nitrates themselves appear to be harmless.[36] Meat packers have recently begun fortifying bacon, sausages, and other nitrate-containing meat products with vitamin C to protect against nitrosamine formation.

Vitamin C as Therapy Several therapeutic applications have been proposed for supplemental vitamin C. It has been used to:

- prevent colds and to aid in their treatment,
- increase iron absorption among people with iron-deficiency anemia, and
- "acidify" urine for the prevention of certain types of kidney and bladder infections among people susceptible to them.

The most effective applications are the use of vitamin C to increase iron absorption and acidify urine for the prevention of urinary-tract infections.[8]

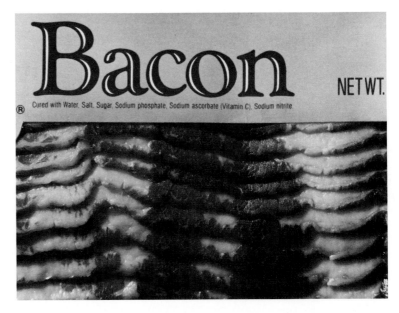

TABLE 9-11
Food sources of vitamin C

Food	Amount	Vitamin C, mg*
Fruits		
kiwi fruit	1, or ½ c	108
orange juice	6 oz	87
orange	1	85
cantaloupe	¼	63
grapefruit juice	6 oz	57
cranberry juice	½ c	54
grapefruit	½	51
strawberries	½ c	48
watermelon	1 c	31
grape juice	½ c	29
raspberries	½ c	18
Vegetables		
green peppers (raw)	½ c	95
cauliflower (raw)	½ c	75
broccoli (cooked)	½ c	70
brussels sprouts	½ c	65
collard greens	½ c	48
cauliflower (cooked)	½ c	30
potato	1	29
tomato (raw)	½	23

*The RDA for adults aged 23–50 is 60 mg.

High intakes of vitamin C may produce mild antihistamine effects that help to reduce the severity of colds.[34,35]

Vitamin C and Cancer At the present, there is no strong evidence that vitamin C prevents cancer. A few studies have indicated that vitamin C protects against the development of some types of cancer, whereas other studies have shown no relationship or even harmful effects.[36,37,38] Vitamin C appears to have no benefit in the treatment of advanced cancer.[39] Nonetheless, because of its antioxidant functions and its ability to block nitrosamine formation, few scientists rule out the possibility that vitamin C may be beneficial in protecting against the development of certain types of cancer.

Sources

Vitamin C is found in abundant quantities in certain fruits and vegetables (Table 9-11), but it occurs in very small amounts in meats, dairy products, and grain products. One fruit, the Australian green plum (perhaps the most sour tasting fruit in existence), contains 882 mg of vitamin C per ounce.[40] That's enough vitamin C to fulfill your dietary need for it for two weeks.

Single servings of oranges, orange juice, cantaloupe, grapefruit, green peppers, cauliflower, broccoli, and brussels sprouts contain a day's supply of vitamin C for adults. Although citrus fruits are the best known sources of vitamin C, they are by no means the only rich source of vitamin C.

Other sources of vitamin C such as potatoes and cabbage can make substantial contributions to the vitamin C requirement if eaten often. Early in this century, potatoes supplied more than a third of the vitamin C consumed by Americans. Potatoes now supply less than one-sixth of the total U.S. vitamin C intake.[2] Potato consumption by the Irish and the preference for cabbage among the British have been credited for preventing massive outbreaks of scurvy during times of food shortage in Ireland and England.

Recommended Intake

Although the adult RDA for vitamin C is 60 mg for both males and females, scientific opinion about how much vitamin C we should consume is far from settled. The RDA for vitamin C has fluctuated widely in the various editions of the RDAs—from a low of 30 mg to a high of 150 mg. Although it is known that 10 mg of vitamin C daily is enough to prevent scurvy, the optimal amount of vitamin C for protection against infection, and possibly cancer, is unknown.[33] The variations in the vitamin C RDA reflect the continuing controversies surrounding the issue of how much is needed for optimal health.

It is known that certain conditions increase the need for vitamin C. These include:

- cigarette smoking
- oral contraceptive use
- emotional and physical stress[3]

Of these conditions, emotional and physical stress (such as injuries, high environmental temperature, and others) increase vitamin C utilization the most, by as much as three to four times normal.[41]

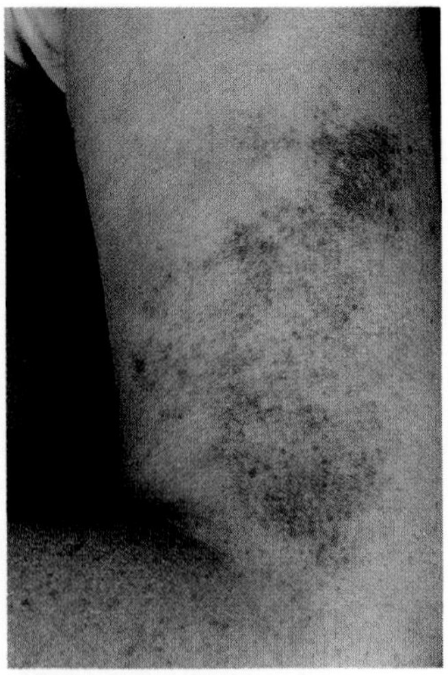

FIGURE 9-5
Vitamin-C deficiency causes blood vessels to become weak. Small hemorrhages result when weakened blood vessels break.

Deficiency Vitamin-C deficiency occurs within one to two months after the onset of a sustained dietary deficiency, and it will eventually lead to death if not corrected. The most obvious signs of vitamin-C deficiency result from the failure of collagen to form normally. The abnormal collagen formed during the time of vitamin-C deficiency causes poor bone and teeth development, a weakening of the blood vessels, and delayed wound healing. Small hemorrhages—areas of bleeding—develop spontaneously during vitamin-C deficiency, producing blood clots and irregularly shaped black and blue marks under the skin (Figure 9-5). Hemorrhages also occur in blood vessels located around organs and in the muscles. As the deficiency advances, classic symptoms of scurvy become apparent: tender, sore gums that bleed easily and loss of hair and teeth. With severe vitamin-C deficiency, there is increased hemorrhaging around the joints and the stomach, heart, and other organs; movement becomes very painful; and the person may experience bouts of hysteria and depression. The sudden death observed in severe cases of scurvy is likely due to internal bleeding.

The year-round availability of fruits and vegetables in the U.S. has made vitamin C deficiency rare, but it occasionally does occur. (Box 9-7 gives an example.) Infants given cow's milk as the sole source of nutrition, elderly people on limited diets, and people who stop using high doses of vitamin C supplements abruptly are at risk of developing scurvy.

BOX 9-7

A PERPLEXING CASE OF INFANT IRRITABILITY

A very concerned mother took her nine-month-old baby to a public health clinic because he had no appetite, was irritable, and cried whenever he was held or touched. Scurvy was suspected, but that possible explanation was dismissed when the mother said that she gave the baby a bottle of orange juice each morning. Further questioning eventually uncovered the cause of the baby's problems. The mother had been conscientiously boiling the baby's orange juice to sterilize it, thereby destroying most of the vitamin C in the juice.

"Rebound scurvy" is the vitamin C–deficiency disease that develops when high-dosage vitamin C supplements are stopped suddenly. The body becomes conditioned to excreting high levels of excess vitamin C and it appears to continue to excrete it at a high rate even after intake levels are decreased.[33] Infants born to women taking high doses of vitamin C (more than 1 gram per day) are at high risk of developing rebound scurvy within the first few weeks after birth if they are not supplemented with vitamin C.[42] Such infants can be successfully treated for rebound scurvy by being given decreasing dose levels of supplemental vitamin C.

People at risk of developing vitamin-C deficiency:
- *infants born to women taking high doses of vitamin C during pregnancy*
- *infants fed only cow's milk*
- *heavy cigarette smokers*
- *long-term oral contraceptive users*
- *users of high-dosage vitamin-C supplements who stop taking them abruptly*

Toxicity The body is partially protected from overdoses of vitamin C by limits on how much can be absorbed. As shown in Figure 9-6, absorption of vitamin C decreases markedly with increasing intake. Unabsorbed excess

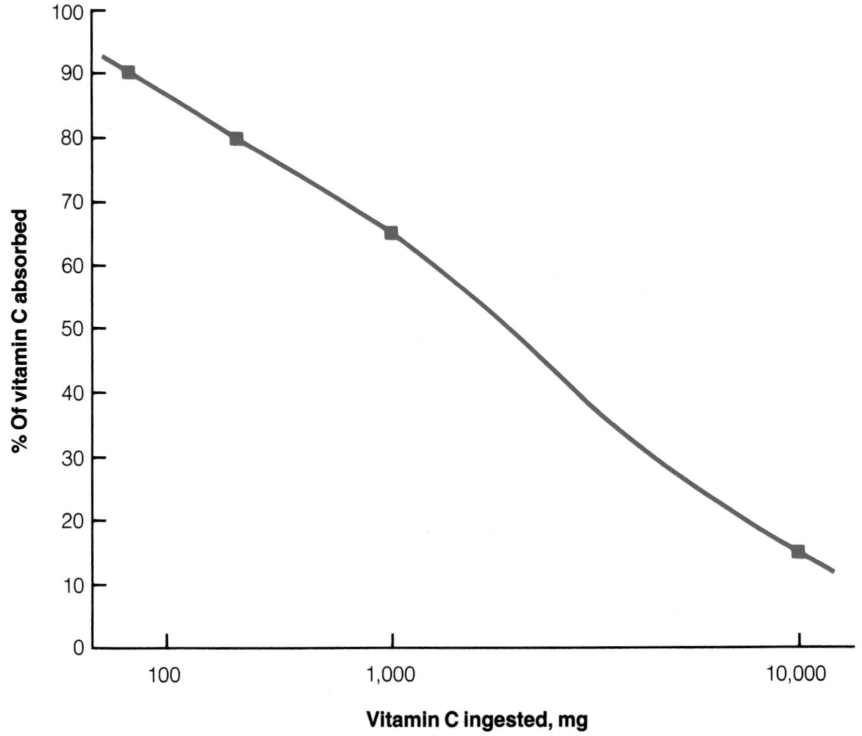

FIGURE 9-6
Vitamin C absorption at increasing levels of intake.

vitamin C causes some problems in the intestines. Diarrhea, nausea, and abdominal cramping result when intake is more than 2 grams per day. (Many ardent vitamin C users regard these as mere nuisances.)

Absorbed vitamin C that cannot be used or stored is excreted in the urine. However, high blood levels of vitamin C can have adverse effects. They may contribute to the formation of kidney stones and they may precipitate abortion in pregnant women.[33] The results of blood and urine tests for glucose may be "muddled" by supplemental vitamin C: because glucose and vitamin C are very similar in chemical structure, they can be difficult to distinguish in tests for glucose.

■ ■ ■

COMING UP IN CHAPTER 10

The four fat-soluble vitamins are presented next. To help remember which of the vitamins are fat-soluble, mentally visualize the term *DEKA* for vitamins D, E, K, and A. In chapter 10, however, the fat-soluble vitamins are discussed in the order of their listing in the RDA tables, so we start with vitamin A and its provitamin, beta-carotene.

■ ■ ■

REVIEW QUESTIONS

1. Match each vitamin with its alternate name.

	Vitamin	Alternate Name
_____	vitamin D	a. vitamin B_3
_____	pantothenic acid	b. folic acid
_____	vitamin B_6	c. vitamin B_1
_____	thiamin	d. retinol
_____	niacin	e. cyanocobalamin
_____	folacin	f. cholecalciferol
_____	riboflavin	g. vitamin B_2
_____	vitamin C	h. pyridoxine
_____	vitamin B_{12}	i. tocopherol
_____	vitamin E	j. phylloquinone
_____	vitamin K	k. pantothenate
_____	vitamin A	l. ascorbic acid

2. Which vitamins in the left-hand column in question 1 are B-complex vitamins?
3. Which vitamins in the left-hand column in question 1 are fat-soluble?
4. List four major differences between water-soluble and fat-soluble vitamins.
5. To which vitamin can tryptophan, an amino acid, be converted?
6. Explain why the effects of excessive intakes of thiamin, riboflavin, and niacin are short-term.
7. Milk used to be sold in clear-glass bottles, but now it's packaged in opaque plastic containers or cardboard cartons. The change was made to protect one nutrient from destruction due to exposure to ultraviolet light. Which nutrient?

Answers

1. From top to bottom: f, k, h, c, a, b, g, l, e, i, j, d.
2. B-complex vitamins: pantothenic acid, vitamin B_6, thiamin, niacin, folacin, riboflavin, vitamin B_{12}. (Biotin is the eighth B-complex vitamin.)
3. Vitamins D, E, K, and A (Remember the *DEKA* memory aid.)
4. See Table 9-2.
5. Niacin (60 milligrams of tryptophan yield 1 milligram of niacin).
6. Excess amounts of water-soluble vitamins are excreted in the urine and do not remain in the body very long.
7. Riboflavin.

■ ■ ■

PUTTING NUTRITION KNOWLEDGE TO WORK

1. While you are home for the holidays you spend an evening with Uncle Max and Aunt Hilda. Although they are pleased to learn that you're doing well in college, they think you look tired and worn out. Before you return to college, they give you a gift: a bottle of nutrient supplements to "pick you up." The bottle label states that the supplement contains:

PABA	niacin	chlorine
thiamin	pantothenic acid	biotin
riboflavin	pangamic acid	inositol

   a. How many "nonvitamins" does the supplement contain?

   (Table 9-1 will help you answer this question).

   b. All of the vitamins contained in the supplement are involved in energy formation. Assuming that you're in good nutritional health, why would the supplement *not* give you an energy burst?

   (Your answer should include information about the effect of "extra" vitamins on enzyme function.)

2. Assume that you have only enough money to buy one kind of vegetable at the grocery store and that you want a vegetable that is a good source of both vitamin B_6 and folacin. Consult Tables 9-6 and 9-7 to make your choice. If the store doesn't have that vegetable, what else could you buy that would be a good source of both of these vitamins?
3. Suppose you have been a "strict" vegetarian for five years and are concerned about your vitamin B_{12} intake. While in a health food store, you notice a bottle of vitamin B_{12} supplements. You purchase them and take one of the 10-microgram tablets each day for a year. At the end of the year, you are diagnosed as having pernicious anemia. Propose one likely reason why the supplement did not prevent this vitamin-B_{12} deficiency disease.

   (Hint: Consider the other causes of vitamin-B_{12} deficiency.)

4. Compared to biotin and pantothenic acid, vitamin C has relatively few good food sources. How often do you consume a standard serving of the sources of vitamin C listed in Table 9-11?

5. Cow's milk contains about 2 mg of vitamin C per cup. Suggest why the vitamin C content of cow's milk is so low.

   (Hint: Do calves require vitamin C?)

6. Cases of vitamin-C deficiency are frequently noticed first by dentists. Why is this?

   (Hint: What happens to gums with a vitamin-C deficiency?)

NOTES

1. Some facts and myths of vitamins, *FDA Consumer*. DHHS publication no. (FDA) 79–2117, (Rockville, Md.: Food and Drug Administration, 1981).
2. S. O. Welsh and R. M. Marston, Review of trends in food use in the United States, 1909 to 1980, *Journal of the American Dietetic Association* 81 (1982):120–125.
3. *Recommended Dietary Allowances*, 9th ed., Food and Nutrition Board, National Research Council (Washington, D.C.: National Academy of Sciences, 1980).
4. M. S. Bamji, Transketolase activity and urinary excretion of thiamin in the assessment of thiamin: Nutrition status of Indians, *American Journal of Clinical Nutrition* 23 (1970):52–58.
5. N. S. Scrimshaw, Nutrition and preventive medicine, in *Public Health and Preventive Medicine*, 12th ed., ed. J. M. Last (Norwalk, Conn.: Appleton-Century-Croft, 1986), 1515–1542.
6. C. M. Leevy and H. Baker, Vitamins and alcoholism, *American Journal of Clinical Nutrition* 21 (1968):1325–1328.
7. C. S. Lo, Riboflavin status of adolescent southern Chinese, *Human Nutrition Clinical Nutrition* 39 (1985):297–301.
8. D. R. Miller and K. C. Hayes, Vitamin excess and toxicity, in *Nutritional Toxicology*, ed. J. N. Hathcock (New York: Academic Press, 1982), 81–133.
9. M. C. Linder, Nutrition and metabolism of vitamins, in *Nutritional Biochemistry and Metabolism*, ed. M. C. Linder (New York: Elsevier, 1985), 75.
10. G. A. Goldsmith, Niacin: Antipellagra factor, hypocholesterolemic agent, *Journal of the American Medical Association* 194 (1965):147–154.
11. W. J. Darby, K. W. McNutt, and E. N. Todhunter, Niacin, *Nutrition Reviews* 33 (1975):289–297.
12. M. K. Horwitt, Niacin, in *Modern Nutrition in Health and Disease*, eds. R. S. Goodhardt and M. E. Shils (Philadelphia: Lea and Febiger, 1973), 198–202.
13. J. R. Moran and H. L. Green, The B vitamins and vitamin C in human nutrition, *American Journal of Diseases of Children* 133 (1979):308–314.
14. M. A. Dubick and R. B. Rucker, Dietary supplements and health aids: A critical evaluation—Part 1: Vitamins and minerals, *Journal of Nutrition Education* 15 (1983):47–53.
15. Coronary Drug Project Research Group, Clofibrate and niacin in coronary heart disease, *Journal of the American Medical Association* 231 (1975):360–381.
16. R. H. Knopp, J. Ginsberg, et al., Contrasting effects of unmodified and time-release forms of niacin on lipoproteins in hyperlipidemic subjects, *Metabolism* 34 (1985):642–650.
17. S. L. Ink and L. M. Henderson, Vitamin B_6 metabolism, *Annual Review of Nutrition* 4 (1984):455–470.
18. V. Wynn, P. W. Adams, et al., Tryptophan, depression, and steroidal contraception, *Journal of Steroid Biochemistry* 6 (1975):965–970.
19. J. A. Driskell, A. J. Clark, et al., Vitamin B_6 status of Southern adolescent girls, *Journal of the American Dietetic Association* 85 (1985):46.
20. J. A. Driskell, A. J. Clark, and S. W. Moak, Longitudinal assessment of vitamin B_6 status in Southern adolescent girls, *Journal of the American Dietetic Association* 87 (1987):307–310.

21. M. J. Williams, R. I. Harris, and B. C. Dean, Pyridoxine treatment for premenstrual syndrome, *Journal of International Medical Research* 13 (1985): 174–179.

22. K. Dalton, Pyridoxine for premenstrual syndrome (letter to the editor), *Lancet* ii (1985):1168–1169.

23. H. Schaumburg, Sensory neuropathy from pyridoxine abuse: A new megavitamin syndrome, *New England Journal of Medicine* 309 (1983):8–9.

24. C. E. Butterworth, Jr., R. Santini, Jr., and W. B. Frommeyer, Jr., The pteroylglutamate composition of American diets as determined by chromatographic fractionation, *Journal of Clinical Investigation* 42 (1963):1929–1939.

25. V. Herbert, Folic acid and vitamin B_{12}, in *Modern Nutrition in Health and Disease*, eds. R. S. Goodhardt and M. E. Shils (Philadelphia: Lea and Febiger, 1973), 221–244.

26. V. Herbert, The five possible causes of all nutrient deficiency: Illustrated by deficiencies of vitamin B_{12} and folic acid, *American Journal of Clinical Nutrition* 26 (1973):77–88.

27. T. C. Campbell, R. G. Allison, and C. J. Carr, *Feasibility of identifying adverse health effects of vitamins and essential minerals in man*, (Bethesda, Md.: Federation of American Societies for Experimental Biology, 1980).

28. D. M. Mock, D. L. Baswell, et al., Biotin deficiency complicating parenteral alimentation: diagnosis, metabolic repercussions, and treatment, *Journal of Pediatrics* 106 (1985):762–769.

29. K. S. Roth, Biotin in clinical medicine: A review, *American Journal of Clinical Nutrition* 34 (1981):1967–1974.

30. M. Lipton, R. B. Mailman, and C. B. Nemeroff, Vitamins, megavitamin therapy, and the nervous system, in *Nutrition and the Brain*, eds. R. J. Wurtman and J. J. Wurtman (New York: Raven Press, 1979).

31. P. C. Fry, H. M. Fox, and H. G. Tao, Metabolic response to a pantothenic acid deficient diet in humans, *Journal of Nutrition Science and Vitaminology* 22 (1976):339–346.

32. R. S. Harris and S. Lepkovsky, Pantothenic acid in *The Vitamins: Chemistry, Physiology, Pathology*, Vol. 2., eds. W. H. Sebrell, Jr., and R. S. Harris (New York: Academic Press, 1954), 591.

33. R. E. Hodges and E. M. Baker, Ascorbic acid in *Modern Nutrition in Health and Disease*, eds. R. S. Goodhart and M. E. Shils (Philadelphia: Lea and Febiger, 1973), 245–255.

34. J. L. Coulehan, K. S. Reisinger, et al., Vitamin C prophylaxis in a boarding school, *New England Journal of Medicine* 290 (1974):6–10.

35. T. R. Karlowski, T. C. Chalmers, et al., Ascorbic acid for the common cold: A prophylactic and therapeutic trial, *Journal of the American Medical Association* 231 (1975):1038–1042.

36. P. M. Newberne and V. Suphakarin, Nutrition and cancer: A review with emphasis on the role of vitamins C and E and selenium, *Nutrition and Cancer* 5 (1983):107–119.

37. S. L. Ramney, Plasma vitamin C and uterine cervical dysplasia, *American Journal of Obstetrics and Gynecology* 151 (1985):976–980.

38. S. Fukushima, Promoting effects of sodium L-ascorbate on two-stage urinary bladder carcinogenesis in rats, *Cancer Research* 43 (1983):4454–4457.

39. C. G. Moertel, High-dose vitamin C versus placebo in the treatment of patients with advanced cancer who have had no prior chemotherapy, *New England Journal of Medicine* 312 (1985):137–141.

40. J. C. Brand, U. Cherikoff, et al., Nutrients in important bush foods, *Proceedings of the Nutrition Society of Australia* 7 (1982):50–54.

41. M. E. Visagie, J. P. Duplessis, and N. F. Laubscher, Effect of vitamin C supplementation on black mine-workers, *South African Medical Journal* 49 (1975):889–892.

42. W. A. Cochrane, Over-nutrition in prenatal life: A problem? *Canadian Medical Association Journal* 931 (1965):893–899.

CHAPTER 10

FAT-SOLUBLE VITAMINS

Four of the 13 vitamins known to be essential for human health are soluble in fat. The fat-soluble vitamins (the "DEKA" vitamins) were all discovered between 1913 and 1929. Vitamin A was discovered in the midst of World War I. The discovery of vitamin E occurred in 1929, the year of the Wall Street crash that ushered in the worldwide Great Depression. The fat-soluble vitamins became recognized during the same era as talking movies, plastics, and Henry Ford's assembly line.

The discoveries and laboratory syntheses of the fat-soluble vitamins were followed by intense investigations into the effects of these vitamins on health and disease. Although many health problems have been solved as a result, research continues, and it is certain that the investigations will produce additional benefits to human health and to the science of human nutrition. There is much more work yet to be done.

The fat-soluble vitamins are located in the parts of plants and animals that contain fat, such as the germ portions of whole grains, the fat component of cell membranes, and fat storage cells. No single food or single food type is a good source of all of the fat-soluble vitamins; each tends to be found in a particular assortment of foods. Thus, a varied diet is needed to assure sufficient levels of the fat-soluble vitamins.

Our presentation of the fat-soluble vitamins begins with the first vitamin discovered, vitamin A, and its provitamin, beta-carotene.

VITAMIN A (RETINOL) AND BETA-CAROTENE

Vitamin A holds the distinctions of being the first vitamin discovered (in 1913) and of having more chemical versions than any other vitamin. More than 1,500 derivatives of retinol, the primary naturally occurring form of vitamin A, have been manufactured. The pharmaceutical industry produces tons of retinol and its related chemical forms for use in supplements, animal feeds, fortified foods, and products for treating acne and wrinkles.

Most of the vitamin A in American diets is in the form of its provitamin, beta-carotene. Colorful vegetables, particularly the dark green, yellow, and orange ones, are generally excellent sources of vitamin A.

The names of the primary form of vitamin A and its major provitamin reflect a major function and a food source of the vitamin, respectively. *Retinol* was designated as the chemical name for vitamin A when its effect on the retina of the eye was discovered. *Carotene* is derived from the German word for carrots, a major source of the provitamin.

At least ten types of carotenes can be converted to vitamin A by the body, of which beta-carotene is the most important. It is the most common type of carotene found in foods, and it yields far more vitamin A per unit weight than any of the other carotenes do. Although it was long thought that only retinol is used by the body, new knowledge reveals a potentially important role of beta-carotene in the prevention of cancer.[1]

Functions

Eat your carrots! They're good for your eyes.
—Mom, 1968, 1969, 1970, . . .

Three major functions have been identified for vitamin A, and one for beta-carotene. Vitamin A plays a major role in vision, in the maintenance of **epithelial tissue**, and in bone growth. Beta-carotene functions as an antioxidant.

epithelial tissue: The outermost layer of cells that form the surface of the skin and eyes, and the lining of the respiratory, reproductive, and gastrointestinal tracts.

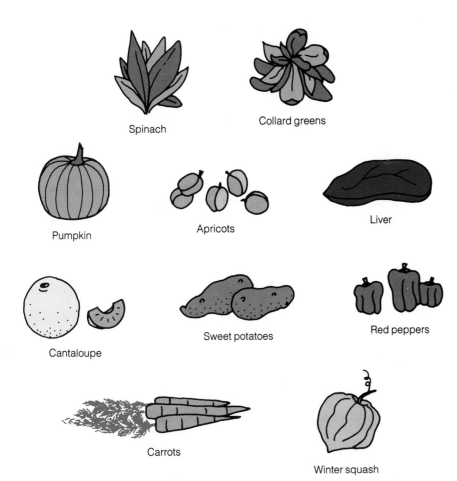

Vision Vitamin A affects vision through two separate mechanisms: it makes vision in dim light possible, and it protects the outer eye.

Vitamin A is found in large amounts in the retina of the eye—the layer of cells that line the inside of the eye (Figure 10-1). The retina is a light-sensitive structure that receives the images formed by the lens and transfers the images to the brain via the optic nerve. The cells of the retina contain "rods" and "cones." Rods function to adjust vision for sight in dim light, and cones detect the color of light. The rods contain **rhodopsin**—a light-sensitive substance formed from retinal (a form of vitamin A)—and opsin—a protein. Vision in dim light requires the production of rhodopsin, whereas vision in normal light does not (Figure 10-2). Without sufficient vitamin A, the retina cannot produce enough rhodopsin, and vision in dim light is impaired (Box 10-1).

rhodopsin: The light-sensitive component of the rods in the retina. It is produced when retinal, a form of vitamin A, combines with the protein opsin. It is also called *visual purple.*

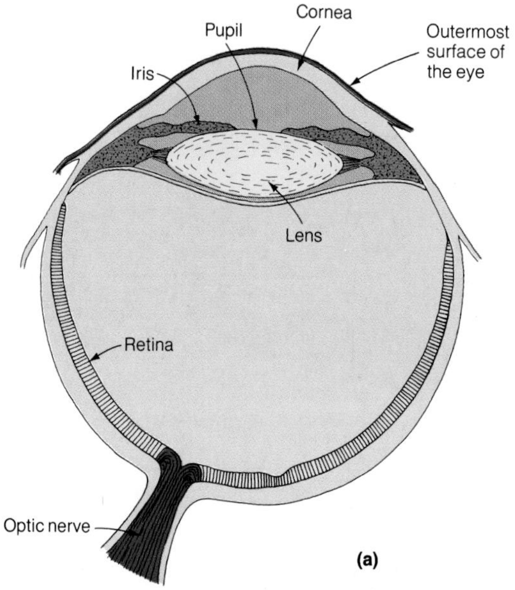

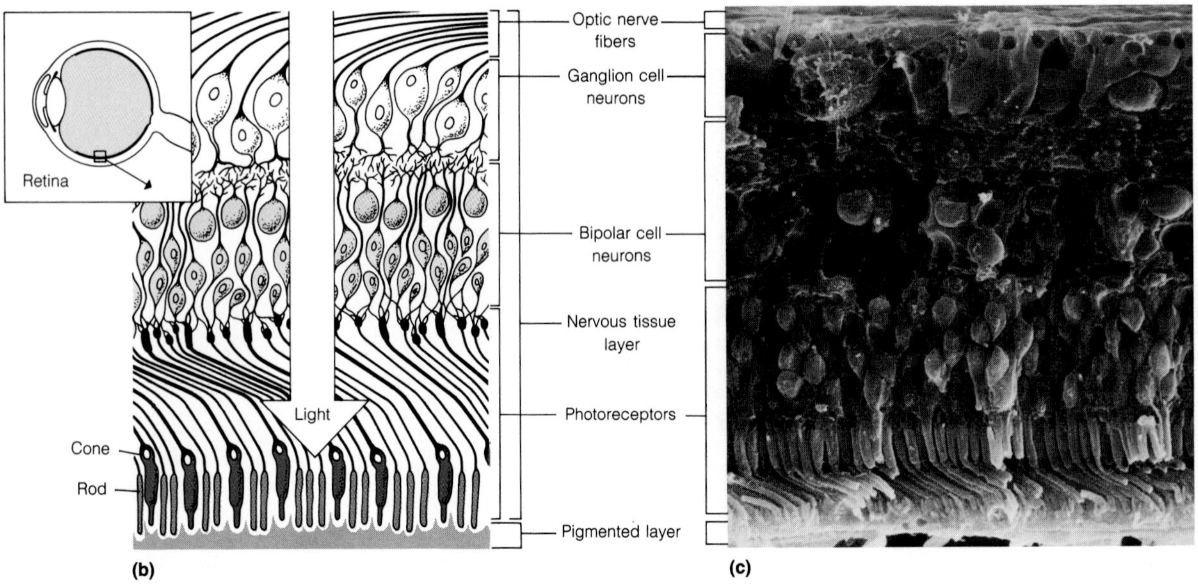

FIGURE 10-1

(a) Diagram of the structure of the eye. Note the location of the retina. (b) Diagram and (c) electron micrograph of the components of the retina.

BOX 10-1

LIGHTS OUT!

How often do you walk from a brightly lit room to one that is dimly lit and notice that it takes your eyes a few seconds to adjust to the lower level of light? During those few seconds, the rods in your retina cells are adjusting to the decrease in light by producing rhodopsin.

The retinas of people with vitamin-A deficiency fail to make the adjustment, and those persons are "blinded" in dim light.

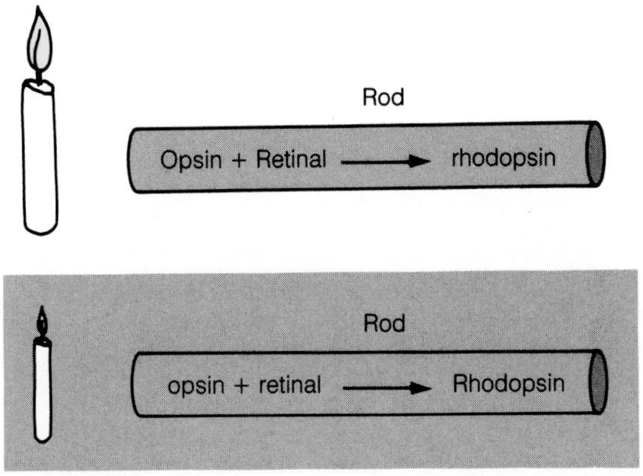

FIGURE 10-2
Rhodopsin formation in the rods of the retina makes vision in dim light possible.

Epithelial Tissue Maintenance Vitamin A is also needed for the maintenance and **differentiation** of epithelial tissue—the cells that form the outermost layer of the skin and eyes and the linings of the respiratory, reproductive, and gastrointestinal tracts. Epithelial-tissue cells secrete mucus and other protective substances and transmit sensory stimuli to the nervous system.

differentiation: The development of cells that function differently than the parent cells.

Epithelial cells are subjected to a good deal of wear and tear and must be replaced frequently. Replacement of epithelial cells requires the generation of new cells that can perform the particular specialized functions. The process of growing cells that have specialized functions from cells that do not perform the functions is known as *cellular differentiation.*

The role of vitamin A in maintaining and differentiating epithelial cells accounts for many of the problems that occur with vitamin-A deficiency. Lack of vitamin A interferes with epithelial cell growth. Old cells are not replaced and they become dry and crusty. Mucus production is also decreased by vitamin-A deficiency. This causes the linings that mucus is supposed to cover to dry out and become susceptible to infections.

The failure of epithelial cells to differentiate normally in vitamin-A deficiency may be a factor in cancer development.[2] The finding that approximately 50 percent of all fatal cancers start with abnormal differentiation of epithelial cells has made vitamin A a prime target of study in cancer research. Although vitamin A does not appear to be effective in halting the spread of established cancer, it is believed that it may prevent the initiation of cancer.[3]

Functions of vitamin A:

dim light $\xrightarrow{\text{vitamin A}}$ vision

$\text{cell}_1 \xrightarrow{\text{vitamin A}} \text{cell}_2$

bone $\xrightarrow{\text{vitamin A}}$ bone growth

oxidizing agent $\xrightarrow[\times]{\text{beta-carotene}}$ cell membrane damage

BOX 10-2

VITAMIN-A TREATMENT OF ACNE

The similarity between the pimplelike protrusions produced by both vitamin-A deficiency and acne led to the testing of vitamin A in its retinol form for the treatment of acne. Large amounts of the vitamin proved to be effective for treating cystic acne, a severe form of the disorder,[5] but many side effects made retinol treatment risky.

Very high doses of vitamin A—60 to 100 times the adult-male RDA—are necessary for treating severe acne, and these dosage levels were found to produce vitamin-A toxicity. To avoid this, less toxic forms of vitamin A were tested. Retinoic acid emerged as the form that cured most cases of acne without producing toxicity symptoms.

Even though retinoic acid is much less toxic than retinol in high amounts, it may cause problems if used by pregnant women. Vitamin-A toxicity and birth defects have been observed among newborns of women who used retinoic acid for acne treatment during pregnancy.

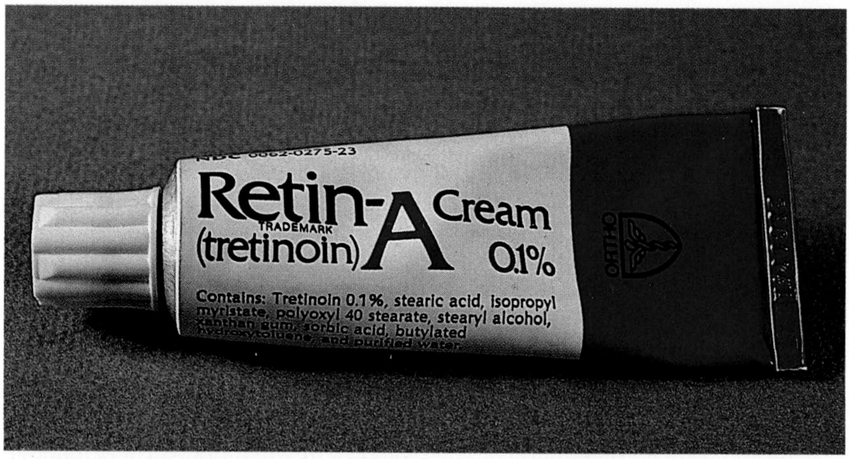

There really is a drug that can diminish skin wrinkling. It's Retin-A™, a substance derived from vitamin A, and it is sold only by prescription.

Vitamin A and the Skin Vitamin A and its derivatives are used for treating acne and other skin disorders involving epithelial tissue.[4] Large doses of vitamin A appear to reduce local infections that occur with certain types of acne. A potential side effect of using vitamin A for treating acne is vitamin-A toxicity. (See Box 10-2.)

A derivative of vitamin A that diminishes wrinkles in many people has been discovered. The product is Retin A™. It appears to work by improving the process by which cells are replaced. Retin A is available on a prescription basis only and should only be taken under the supervision of a physician. It should not be taken by women who are or may become pregnant.

Vitamin A and Bone Growth How vitamin A influences bone growth is unclear, but the abnormal bone growth of children with vitamin-A deficiency is well-known. Some bones, such as the skull, stop growing, whereas other bones grow excessively. The growth of boney structures in unusual places, such as the ears, also has been observed in vitamin-A deficiency.[3] These results point to an important role of vitamin A in regulating bone growth.

BOX 10-3

BETA-CAROTENE AND CANCER

Beta-carotene may inhibit the spread of cancer by stabilizing **singlet oxygen**. Singlet oxygen (O) consists of one atom of oxygen—rather than the usual two (O_2). Singlet oxygen is highly reactive with molecules, particularly unsaturated fatty acids, in their vicinity. Disruptions in the double bonds of unsaturated fatty acids by singlet oxygen yield **free radicals**, atoms that have become reactive because they have given up electrons to singlet oxygen. Free radicals remain reactive until they are deactivated by an antioxidant such as vitamin E. If allowed to "propagate," free radicals damage many unsaturated fatty acids in cell membranes, and that may decrease cells' resistance to cancer.

Beta-carotene is a very effective deactivator of singlet oxygen. Deactivation of singlet oxygen helps to retard the formation of free radicals. Thus, beta-carotene may provide protection against the development of cancer by protecting cells from disruption by singlet oxygen and free radicals.[7]

The effectiveness of beta-carotene in cancer prevention is currently being tested by 20,000 physicians. Half of the doctors are taking 30 mg of beta-carotene every other day, and the other half are taking a placebo. Since cancer generally takes more than a decade to develop, it will be years before it is known whether beta-carotene supplements protect against cancer.

singlet oxygen: A high-energy, highly reactive form of oxygen. Singlet oxygen participates in reactions that yield free radicals.

free radicals: Atoms within molecules that have become highly reactive because they have lost electrons due to oxidation by singlet oxygen or another oxidizing agent. The double bonds in unsaturated fatty acids are particularly susceptible to oxidation and, therefore, to free radical formation.

Beta-Carotene as an Antioxidant Beta-carotene plays a role in the maintenance of normal cell functions through its role as an antioxidant. By neutralizing substances that are highly reactive and harmful to cell membranes, beta-carotene prevents damage to cells and cellular functions. The protective effects of beta-carotene may even extend to cancer prevention (Box 10-3).

Sources

Vitamin A and its provitamins are found in relatively few foods. Eighty to ninety percent of the vitamin A consumed in the U.S. comes from only 50 foods, most of them vegetables that are rich in beta-carotene.[6] Of the animal sources of vitamin A, only liver can be considered to be a rich source, and that's because the liver is the main storage site for vitamin A in animals. A three-ounce serving of liver provides a nine-day supply of vitamin A. One-half cup of carrots, sweet potatoes, or spinach supplies more than enough beta-carotene to meet one day's need. The major sources of beta-carotene and vitamin A are listed in Table 10-1.

Plants containing carotenes can be recognized easily by their deep yellow color. Some dark green vegetables are also good sources of carotene, but their dark color hides the lighter shades of the carotenes. The carotenes in spinach can be seen in a faded part of a leaf, and the carotene colors in sweet peppers increase as the vegetable matures and goes from green to dark orange. The darkness of the yellow of egg yolks and butter is determined by the amount of carotene in the respective animals' diets. Nonetheless, since not all carotenes are converted to vitamin A, the vitamin-A value of egg yolks, butter, and other foods cannot be estimated by color alone.

TABLE 10-1
Food sources of beta-carotene and vitamin A

Food Source of Beta-Carotene	Amount	Vitamin A, IU*
Vegetables		
carrot, raw	1 med.	7,900
sweet potato	½ c	7,850
pumpkin	½ c	7,840
spinach, cooked	½ c	7,300
collards, cooked	½ c	6,030
winter squash	½ c	4,200
red peppers	½ c	2,225
broccoli	½ c	1,900
Fruits		
cantaloupe	¼	5,400
apricots, canned	½ c	2,260
papaya	½ c	1,595
watermelon	2 c	1,265
peaches, canned	½ c	1,115
nectarine	1	1,001
Food Source of Vitamin A (Retinol)	**Amount**	**Vitamin A, IU**
Meats and Eggs		
liver	3 oz	45,400
crab	½ c	1,680
egg yolk	1 med.	590
Milk and Cheese		
whole milk	1 c	330
fortified skim milk	1 c	330
American cheese	1 oz	330
Swiss cheese	1 oz	320
2% milk	1 c	210
unfortified skim milk	1 c	10
Fats		
butter	1 t	160
margarine (fortified)	1 t	160

*The RDAs for adults 23–50 years of age are 4,000 IU (800 mcg RE) for females and 5,000 IU (1,000 mcg RE) for males.

Recommended Intake

1 Retinol Equivalent (RE) = 5 IU vitamin A

The unit of measurement for vitamin A was formerly International Units (IU). Although the use of IU is still common, the use of *Retinol Equivalents (RE)* is preferred because it includes retinol and its provitamin, beta-carotene. One RE equals 5 IUs of vitamin A.

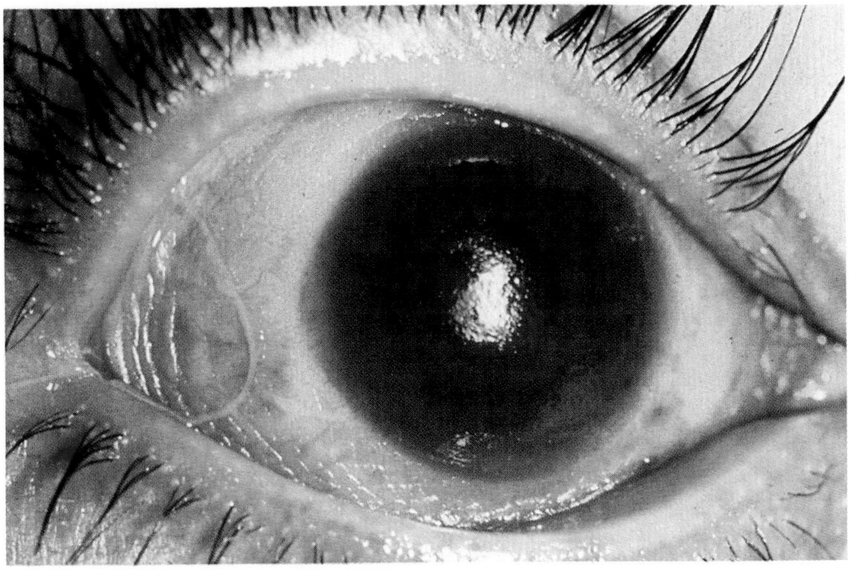

FIGURE 10-3
Xerophthalmia resulting from vitamin-A deficiency is a major cause of blindness in some developing countries. The covering of the eye dries out, hardens, and becomes susceptible to infection.

The RDA for females 23–50 years of age is 4000 IU (800 mcg RE), and for males it's 5000 IU (1000 mcg RE). Well-nourished people have a three- to five-month store of vitamin A, and severe vitamin-A deficiency is rare in the U.S.

Deficiency The symptoms of vitamin-A deficiency are closely related to its roles in vision, the maintenance of epithelial tissues, and bone growth.

Night blindness, an early symptom of vitamin-A deficiency, was described in AD 325 to exist "when vision is good in the day time, declines after sunset, and disappears at night."[8] Today, key indicators of vitamin-A deficiency among children in developing countries are stumbling at twilight and the inability to find objects in dimly lit homes.

It was known in ancient times that liver would cure night blindness. Although the juice of liver and fish oils were applied directly to the eye as treatment, it was eventually recognized that ingestion of food sources of vitamin A provided the most effective cure.[8]

Vitamin-A deficiency also causes the epithelial tissue covering the eye to become dry and thick, and to provide little resistance to infections. A condition called **xerophthalmia** (or "dry eye") develops if the deficiency is not corrected (Figure 10-3). Vision is partially or totally lost in cases of xerophthalmia. The steps in the development of xerophthalmia are summarized in Figure 10-4.

Vitamin-A deficiency is the leading cause of blindness in some developing countries. An estimated 500,000 children are blinded each year due to xerophthalmia. Many more children experience infectious diseases and stunted growth because of vitamin-A deficiency.[9] A supplement of the amount of vitamin A a child needs yearly costs less than a quarter. Unfortunately, the complexities of distributing the vitamin to high-risk children in developing countries have prevented the worldwide elimination of vitamin-A deficiency.

People at greatest risk of developing vitamin-A deficiency are malnourished children whose diets consist almost exclusively of starchy foods and people who have long-lasting infectious diseases, fat absorption problems, and liver disease.

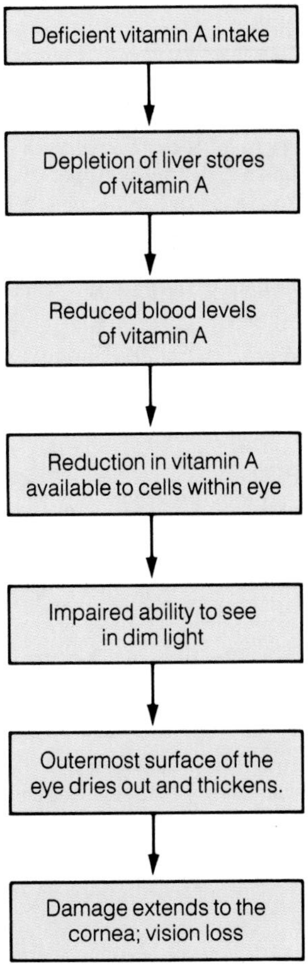
Deficient vitamin A intake
Depletion of liver stores of vitamin A
Reduced blood levels of vitamin A
Reduction in vitamin A available to cells within eye
Impaired ability to see in dim light
Outermost surface of the eye dries out and thickens.
Damage extends to the cornea; vision loss

FIGURE 10-4
The progression of vitamin-A deficiency.

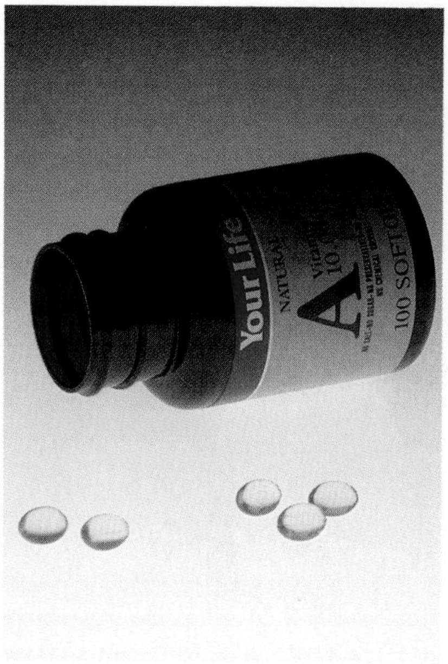

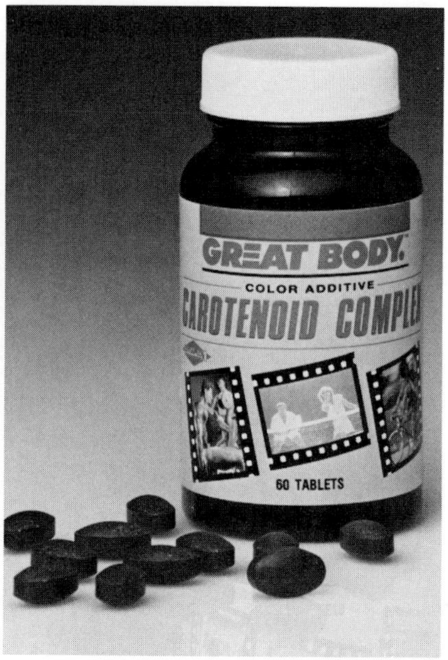

(Left) Each of these tablets contains about 10,000 IU of vitamin A. Regular consumption of 2 tablets per day by children, or 3 tablets per day by adults, may lead to the development of hypervitaminosis A.

(Right) Carotene "tanning pills."

xerophthalmia: (zir′ äf thal′ mē ə) "Dry eyes"; a condition caused by vitamin-A deficiency. If not corrected in its early stages, it can lead to permanent blindness; generally accompanied by chronic infections of the eyes.

People at risk of developing vitamin-A deficiency:
- *malnourished infants and young children*
- *people with prolonged cases of infectious disease*
- *people who are unable to absorb fat*
- *people with cirrhosis and other liver diseases*

hypervitaminosis A: The vitamin-A toxicity disease.

carotenemia: Yellowish discoloration of the skin caused by excessive intake of carotene; also called hypercarotenemia.

Vitamin A Toxicity Vitamin A, but not beta carotene, is highly toxic if it is taken in large amounts. The vitamin-A toxicity disease is known as **hypervitaminosis A.** It can be produced by ingesting large amounts of polar bear or seal liver as previously discussed, or more commonly, by the excessive use of vitamin-A supplements. In children, 3,600 REs (18,000 IUs) taken daily for a period of months can cause hypervitaminosis A. Adults are more resistant to vitamin-A toxicity than are children; daily intakes of 4,000 to 5,000 RE (20,000 to 25,000 IU) for 8 to 12 months can produce vitamin-A toxicity symptoms. Doses of vitamin A in excess of 200,000 RE (1,000,000 IU) produce hypervitaminosis A in a matter of days.[10] Vitamin-A toxicity has been identified among people treating themselves for acne with retinol.

People with vitamin-A toxicity have blurred vision, pain in the bones and joints, headaches, dry skin, and a poor appetite. The symptoms of advanced vitamin-A toxicity are so similar to those of a brain tumor that some patients have been sent to surgery before the misdiagnosis has been recognized.[11]

Carotene Overdose Excessively high intake of carrots, sweet potatoes, and beta-carotene supplements does not cause hypervitaminosis A; it causes a condition known as **carotenemia**. The major effect of carotenemia is a yellowing of the skin. This feature of carotene overdose has led to the use of carotene in "tanning pills."[12]

The yellow coloration of the skin produced by carotenemia is very similar to that occurring with jaundice. In cases of carotenemia, however, the whites of the eyes do not become yellow. Skin coloration returns to normal within two to six weeks after the intake of carotene-rich foods returns to normal.

Carotenemia is generally not regarded as hazardous to health. Recently, however, carotenemia has been found to produce temporary infertility in women.[13]

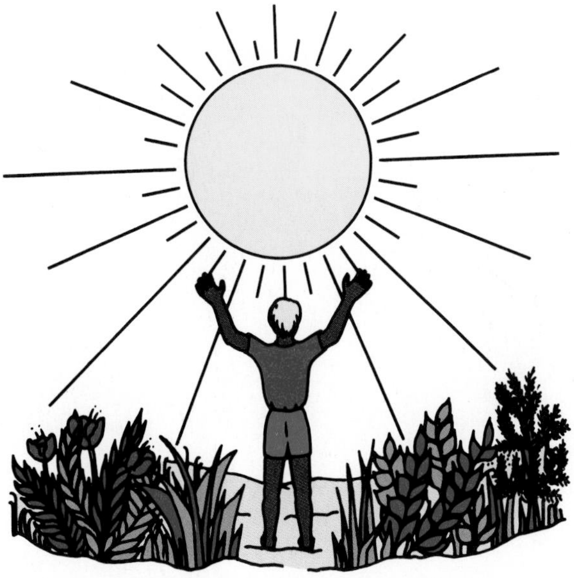

Vitamin D has been called the "sunshine vitamin."

VITAMIN D (CHOLECALCIFEROL)

What do you get when you combine a cholesterol-like compound with ultraviolet light from the sun? You get "the sunshine vitamin." Vitamin D is formed in human skin when its provitamin, 7-dehydrocholesterol, absorbs energy from ultraviolet light emitted by the sun (Figure 10-5). The vitamin D formed in other animals is similarly produced when a provitamin of vitamin D is exposed to ultraviolet light.

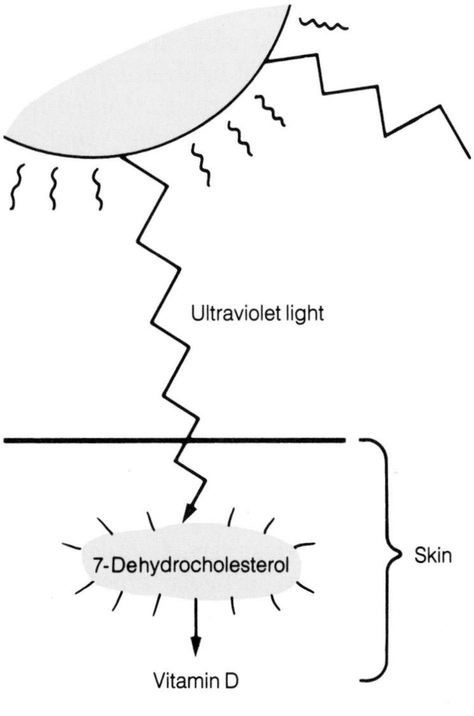

FIGURE 10-5
When the vitamin D provitamin, 7-dehydrocholesterol, in the skin is exposed to ultraviolet light, vitamin D is formed.

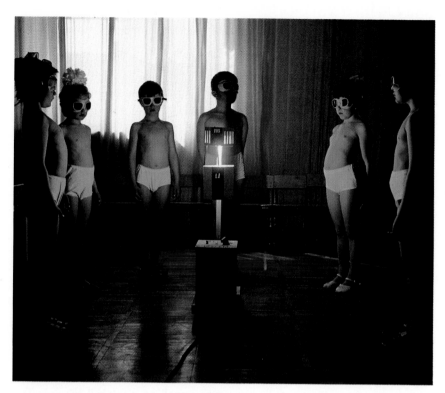

Children in the USSR receive periodic doses of ultraviolet light as a vitamin-D supplement.

Very few foods contain measurable amounts of vitamin D, and many people don't get enough exposure to sunlight to produce the level needed. To prevent vitamin-D deficiency, especially among populations who get little direct exposure to sunlight, certain foods have been fortified with vitamin D. Milk has been selected as the food to be fortified with vitamin D in the U.S. In Great Britain and Scandinavia, margarine has been chosen. In the Soviet Union, no foods are fortified with vitamin D. Rather, children receive periodic exposures to ultraviolet light. Another source of vitamin D is emerging in the United States marketplace. Cereal manufacturers have begun to add vitamin D, along with the many other nutrients, to some breakfast cereals.

Functions

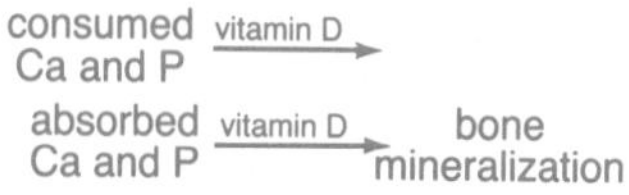
consumed Ca and P
vitamin D
absorbed Ca and P
vitamin D
bone mineralization

Vitamin D's importance in human nutrition lies in its role of making calcium and phosphorus available for use by the body. It does this in two ways: by increasing the absorption of calcium and phosphorus, and by promoting the incorporation of calcium and phosphorus into bones.

Vitamin D influences calcium and phosphorus absorption by stimulating DNA to produce "transport proteins." These proteins bind to calcium and phosphorus and greatly increase their absorption by the small intestine. If transport proteins are not available, only very small amounts of calcium and phosphorus can be absorbed. In this respect, vitamin D is an unusual vitamin. Stimulating DNA to produce particular types of proteins is a function generally performed by hormones. (Vitamin D has been called the vitamin that "acts like a hormone.") Vitamin D affects the mineralization of bone by stimulating the uptake of calcium and phosphorus by bone cells.

TABLE 10-2
Food sources of vitamin D

Food	Amount	Vitamin D, IU*
Milk		
milk (fortified whole, lowfat, or skim)	1 c	100
Fish and Seafoods		
salmon	3 oz	340
tuna	3 oz	150
shrimp	3 oz	127
Organ Meats		
beef liver	3 oz	42
chicken liver	3 oz	40
Eggs		
egg yolk	1	27

*The RDAs for adults aged 23–50 are 200 IU (5 mcg of cholecalciferol) for both males and females.

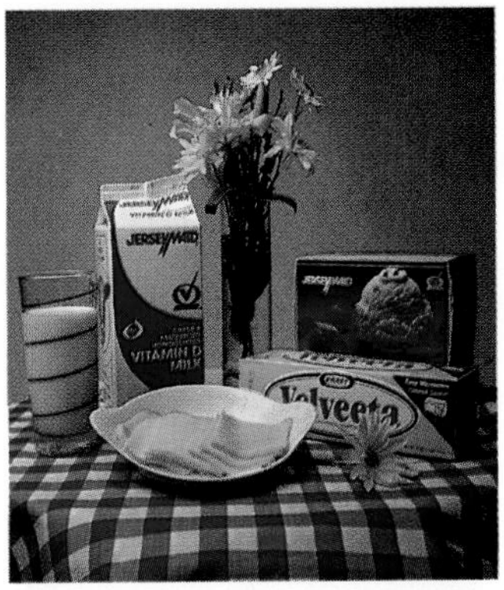

Milk is fortified with vitamin D in the U.S.; products made from milk usually are not.

Sources

Except for a few types of fish and fish oils, few foods are good sources of vitamin D. In fact, most foods do not contain any vitamin D. As shown in Table 10-2, liver, eggs, and butter contain some vitamin D, but not nearly as much as vitamin-D-fortified milk. (Milk contains very little vitamin D if it is not fortified.)

By law, milk processed in the U.S. must be fortified with 400 IU of vitamin D per quart. Milk from which cheese, yogurt, ice cream, and other dairy products are made is not required to be fortified with vitamin D, and it seldom is. Consequently, people who do not drink milk and who depend on other dairy products for the nutrients that milk provides may not get enough vitamin D. Without adequate exposure to the sun, or the consumption of foods that provide vitamin D, calcium and phosphorus in the diet will be less well absorbed and poorly utilized by the body.

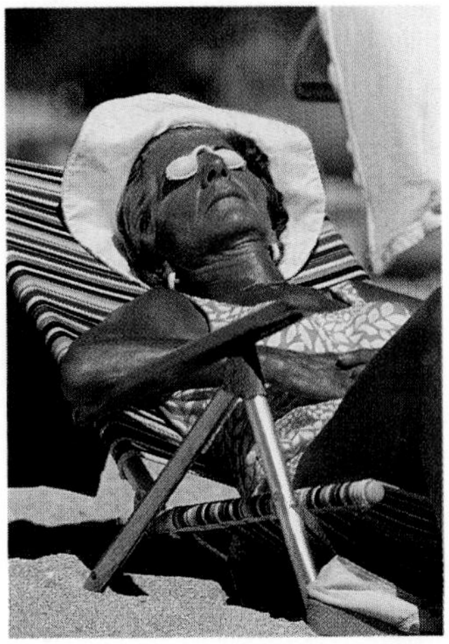

The Sun as a Source of Vitamin D The RDA for vitamin D can be obtained simply by exposing the skin to sunlight. How much exposure does it take? It depends upon how darkly colored the person's skin is and how much skin is exposed. Adults with light skin can get the RDA for vitamin D by exposing their hands, arms, and face to sunlight for about 15 minutes twice a week. About 10,000 IU of vitamin D are produced when most of the body is exposed to the sun until a mild sunburn results. People with dark skin require longer periods of exposure to the sun, because less ultraviolet light penetrates dark skin.[14] (Box 10-4 gives more information about ultraviolet light.)

There is a limit to how much vitamin D can be produced in the skin. The production of vitamin D stops when 15 to 20 percent of the original provi-

BOX 10-4

ULTRAVIOLET LIGHT BLOCKERS

Materials such as glass and clear plastic may allow sunlight to pass through, but they block ultraviolet wavelengths. Thus, skin cells cannot produce vitamin D if the sunlight they receive comes through a window.

What about the light from light bulbs? Can it be used to stimulate vitamin-D production in the skin? No. Ordinary light bulbs do not emit ultraviolet wavelengths. Actually, that's a good thing for humans, because the ultraviolet range of the spectrum causes sunburn.

tamin stores in the skin have been converted. Consequently, you cannot receive an overdose of vitamin D by too much being produced in your skin.[14] (But you *can* overdose on sunshine. Excessive exposure of the skin to ultraviolet rays has been related to the development of a particular type of skin cancer.)

Recommended Intake

1 mcg cholecalciferol
= 1 mcg vitamin D
= 40 IU vitamin D

Dietary sources of vitamin D are needed only by people who fail to get enough direct exposure to sunlight. Food sources are important for people who stay indoors during the winter months, or who for other reasons are seldom exposed to the sun.

The unit for measuring vitamin D has recently been switched from IU of vitamin D to micrograms of cholecalciferol. Five mcg of cholecalciferol is equivalent to 200 IU of vitamin D, the RDA level for adult males and females.

rickets: The vitamin-D deficiency disease in children.

osteomalacia: The vitamin-D deficiency disease in adults.

Deficiency Vitamin-D deficiency results from a lack of skin exposure to sunlight, a low dietary intake of vitamin D, or a combination of these. It can also be caused by rare genetic disorders that reduce the body's ability to use calcium, phosphorus, or vitamin D.

Before the fortification of milk and other foods with vitamin D, the deficiency in children was widely prevented by "sunning" them regularly during the winter and by giving them periodic doses of cod liver oil. (Many people who grew up in the first half of this century recall the routine of taking a spoonful or dropperful of the strange-tasting substance.)

The vitamin-D-deficiency disease has two names. When it occurs in children, it is called **rickets**; when it develops in adults, it is called **osteomalacia**. Whether it occurs in children or adults, the basic problem produced by the deficiency is the same—soft, fragile bones. Without vitamin D, calcium and phosphorus are poorly absorbed, and bones fail to mineralize normally. The bones in the legs of children with rickets become bowed by the weight of the body (Figure 10-6). In adults, the loss of calcium and phosphorus from bones causes them to become porous and to break easily. Figure 10-7 summarizes the consequences of vitamin-D deficiency.

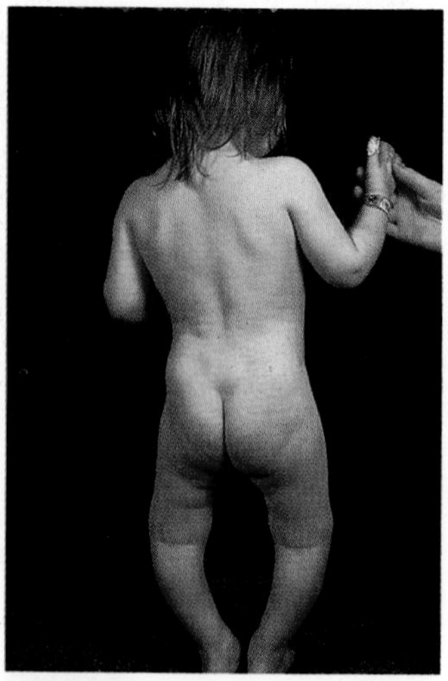

FIGURE 10-6
An outward sign of rickets is bone malformation.

Vitamin-D deficiency may also contribute to the development of osteoporosis. Both osteomalacia and osteoporosis lead to the demineralization of bones. Osteoporosis, however, is generally more closely associated with a long-term deficiency of calcium than of vitamin D.

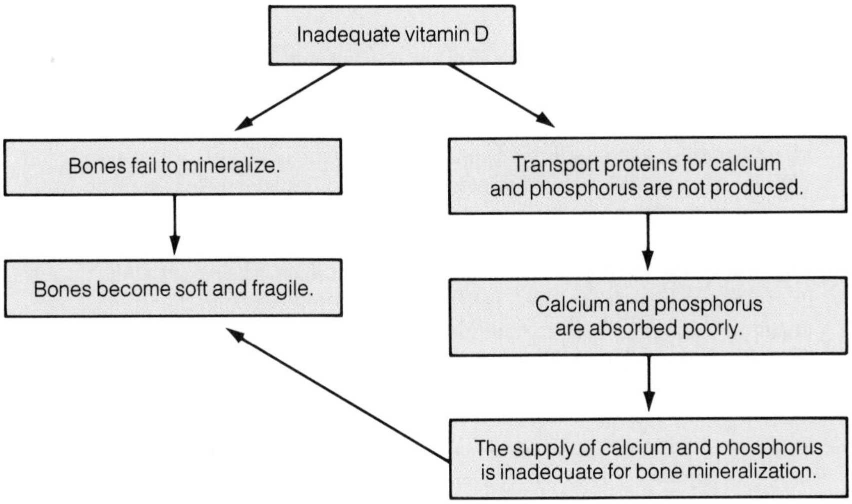

FIGURE 10-7
The major consequences of vitamin-D deficiency.

Rickets still emerges occasionally in the U.S. Between 1974 and 1978, 24 cases of rickets were diagnosed in Philadelphia. The affected children had been eating a vegetarian diet and wearing the long, hooded garments required by the practices of their religion. Low dietary intake of vitamin D combined with little exposure to the sun led to the development of rickets in these children. All of the children improved after they were given vitamin D, but their growth remained unusually slow.[15]

Rickets is also occasionally observed among breast-fed infants. Breast milk contains low amounts of vitamin D, and breast-fed infants can develop rickets if they are not exposed to sunlight.[16]

People at risk of developing vitamin-D deficiency:
- *those who get little exposure to direct sunlight or who consume inadequate amounts of vitamin-D-fortified milk*
- *breast-fed infants whose mothers are deficient in vitamin D*

Toxicity Vitamin D is the most toxic of all vitamins. Supplement doses as low as 2 times the RDA for children and 10 times the RDA for adults can produce vitamin-D toxicity. Excess vitamin D in the blood causes calcium to be deposited in soft tissues of the heart, kidney, and brain. Seizures, disorientation, joint pain, and many other problems are caused by overdoses of vitamin D.[17] Early scientific experiments with vitamin-D supplements in children were quickly stopped when it was observed that high doses of vitamin D led to permanent mental retardation.

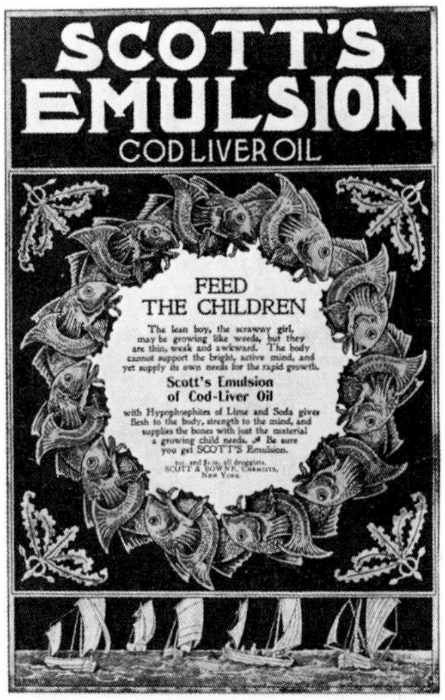

Before milk was fortified with vitamin D, many parents gave their children cod liver oil during the winter as a precaution against rickets.

VITAMIN E (TOCOPHEROL)

After vitamin E was discovered in 1929, animal studies showed it to have a profound influence on reproduction, muscle development, and the longevity of certain types of cells. These findings led many people to believe that vitamin E held strong promise for curing a number of human diseases. Unfortunately, few of the spectacular effects of vitamin E in laboratory animals have been shown to occur in humans (Box 10-5). Nonetheless, vitamin E is still an intriguing vitamin. A nagging suspicion exists among scientists that the vitamin has important applications in human nutrition and health, but that we just have not yet been able to discover them. Scientists working with vitamin E have called it "the elusive vitamin" and "the vitamin in search of a disease."

BOX 10-5

VITAMIN E AND REPRODUCTION

Controversy surrounding vitamin E began shortly after it was discovered. One of the first observed effects of vitamin-E deficiency in laboratory rats was the failure to reproduce successfully. The problems associated with reproduction quickly vanished when the rats were given vitamin E.

Consequently, vitamin E came to be promoted as "the sex vitamin." Even its chemical name, *tocopherol*, reflects this; it is derived from the Greek words meaning "bringing forth in childbirth." Nonetheless, research has yet to establish a direct relationship between vitamin E and human reproduction.

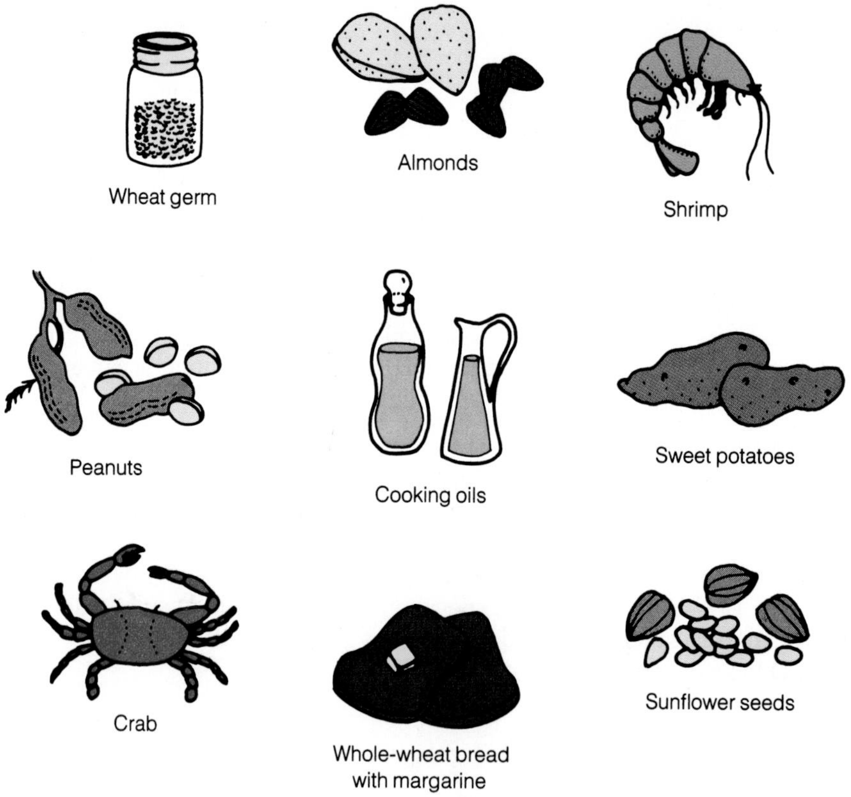

Sources of vitamin E.

Although at least ten forms of vitamin E occur in foods, just one of them, "alpha tocopherol," accounts for practically all of our dietary intake. Beta, gamma, delta, and other tocopherols (each assigned a letter of the Greek alphabet) are less common, and their vitamin-E value is less than alpha tocopherol's.

Functions

The fat-soluble vitamin E is found wherever unsaturated fatty acids are present—in vegetable oils, nuts and other oily foods, in the body's fat stores, and in the fat contained in cell membranes. It functions to protect

BOX 10-6

TASTE-TESTING FOR OXIDIZED FATTY ACIDS

You probably have some personal experience with oxidized fatty acids. Have you ever tasted margarine or butter that has been left out of the refrigerator too long on warm summer days, or eaten french fries that tasted like they were cooked in old oil? If so, you know the rancid flavor of fats that have been oxidized. Prolonged exposure of vitamin E to heat and oxygen destroys it. Without vitamin E available to act as an antioxidant, the unsaturated fatty acids in oils and solid fats become oxidized, and "turn rancid."

the fragile unsaturated fatty acids from attack by oxygen and the destructive effects of oxidation. (Box 10-6 explains one of these destructive effects.) Whether it be the oil contained in soybeans or that in cell membranes, vitamin E serves the same purpose: it acts as an antioxidant.

unsaturated fatty acids —(vitamin E, ✕)→ oxidized, broken-down fatty acids

Unsaturated fatty acids need protection against oxidation because they contain double bonds, which are weaker—more likely to give up electrons—than single bonds. Exposure of oxygen or singlet oxygen to an unsaturated fatty acid causes the loss of electrons from the double bonds in the unsaturated fatty acid, and the formation of free radicals. As described earlier, free radicals are highly reactive and proceed to cause damage to nearby unsaturated fatty acids. The chain reaction of free-radical damage causes terrific havoc in cells: broken down by free radicals, the unsaturated fatty acids in cell membranes lose their ability to regulate chemical traffic into and out of cells. Total disruption in cell functions results.

Vitamin E, present in the fat layer of cell membranes, prevents the spread of free radicals. It donates electrons to the free radicals and thereby prevents damage to unsaturated fatty acids (Figure 10-8). Unlike vitamin

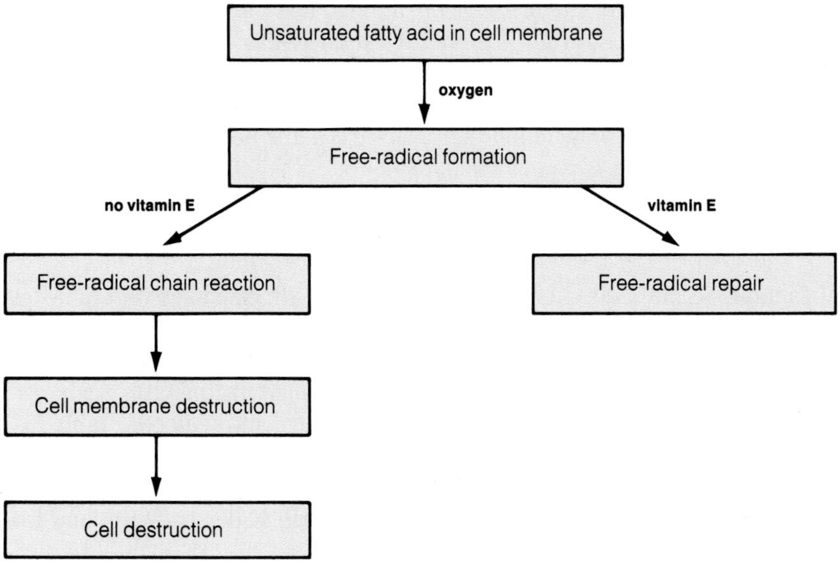

FIGURE 10-8
Sequence of events in the oxidation of unsaturated fatty acids.

C, vitamin E is not destroyed by its antioxidation activities. Vitamin E stays intact and can function repeatedly in antioxidation reactions.

Vitamin E and Air Pollution Vitamin E contained in lung cell membranes provides an important barrier against the harmful effects of air pollutants such as ozone and nitrogen dioxide. These pollutants can cause damage by oxidizing the unsaturated fatty acids in the cells that line the lungs. Vitamin E provides the body's first line of defense against cell damage due to oxidizers in the air.

Inadequate intake of vitamin E promotes the development of pollution-caused respiratory diseases. It has been suggested that people living in cities where air pollution is high may benefit from increasing their intake of vitamin-E-rich foods.[4]

Vitamin E and Diseases Extensive but unproven claims have been made for vitamin E as a treatment for hardening of the arteries. Investigations into this and into the role of vitamin E in heart diseases continue. These investigations have been spurred on by the finding that supplemental vitamin E may be useful for treating intermittent claudication, a condition caused by hardening of the arteries in the legs.[4] Poor circulation in the legs results, which produces pain in the calf muscles when walking.

Vitamin E has also been used for treating fibrocystic breast disease, a disease that is relatively common among women in the U.S.[19] The condition is characterized by the development of painful, fibrous knots in the breast. Fibrocystic breast disease appears to occur among women who drink a lot of (undecaffeinated) coffee and women who are long-term users of asthma medications containing caffeine. A sharp reduction in caffeine intake is the treatment of choice for many cases of fibrocystic breast disease, but vitamin E supplementation has also been used. The use of supplements containing 200 to 400 IU of vitamin E for three to four months may relieve the condition in some women.[4]

Fibrocystic breast disease was once thought to increase a woman's chances of developing cancer of the breast. Recent evidence suggests that this is probably not the case.[19] It is important, however, that any knots or lumps that develop in the breast be examined and identified.

Due to its role as an antioxidant, vitamin E has been singled out for cancer studies. Many studies examining vitamin E and cancer development have been completed, and none has shown a strong relationship between them. It is generally concluded that if there is a link between vitamin E and cancer in humans, it is a very weak one.[21]

Sources

Vitamin E accompanies unsaturated fatty acids, which makes vegetable oils and products made from them particularly rich food sources. Vegetable oils, margarine, and salad dressings contribute over 70 percent of the vitamin E consumed in the U.S.[21] Other foods containing unsaturated fatty acids, and therefore vitamin E, are nuts, seeds, whole grains, and seafoods. Table 10-3 shows examples of food sources of this vitamin. One food you will not see on the list is oysters. Although considered by some people to be a potent source of vitamin E, oysters contain only 0.1 mg vitamin E per half-cup, and few people consume a half-cup of oysters in a meal.

TABLE 10-3
Food sources of vitamin E

Food	Amount	Vitamin E mg α-TE*	Vitamin E IU
Oils			
oil	1 T	4.5	6.7
mayonnaise	1 T	2.3	3.4
margarine	1 T	1.8	2.7
salad dressing	1 T	1.5	2.2
Nuts and Seeds			
sunflower seeds	¼ c	18.2	27.1
almonds	¼ c	8.5	12.7
peanuts	¼ c	3.3	4.9
cashews	¼ c	0.5	0.7
Vegetables			
sweet potato	½ c	4.6	6.9
collard greens	½ c	2.1	3.1
asparagus	½ c	1.4	2.1
spinach, raw	1 c	1.0	1.5
Grains			
wheat germ	2 T	2.8	4.2
whole-wheat bread	1 slice	1.7	2.5
white bread	1 slice	0.8	1.2
Seafood			
crab	3 oz	3.0	4.5
shrimp	3 oz	2.4	3.7
fish	3 oz	1.6	2.4

*RDAs for adults 23–50 years of age are 8 mg α-TE (12 IU) for females and 10 mg α-TE (15 IU) for males.

Recommended Intake

Starting in 1980, the RDAs for vitamin E have been given in milligrams of alpha-tocopherol equivalents, abbreviated *mg α-TE*. One mg α-TE roughly equals 1.5 IU of vitamin E. The adult RDAs are 8 mg α-TE for females and 10 mg α-TE for males, or 12 IU and 15 IU, respectively. The average U.S. diet supplies 8 to 11 mg α-TE (12 to 16 IU of vitamin E) per day.[21]

1 mg α-tocopherol equivalent (TE) ≈ 1.5 IU vitamin E

Deficiency Two groups within the U.S. population are at risk of vitamin-E deficiency: premature infants and people who are not able to absorb fat. In many cases, premature infants are born before their bodies have built up a store of vitamin E. For this reason, premature infants are generally given

People at risk of developing vitamin-E deficiency:
premature infants
persons who absorb fat poorly

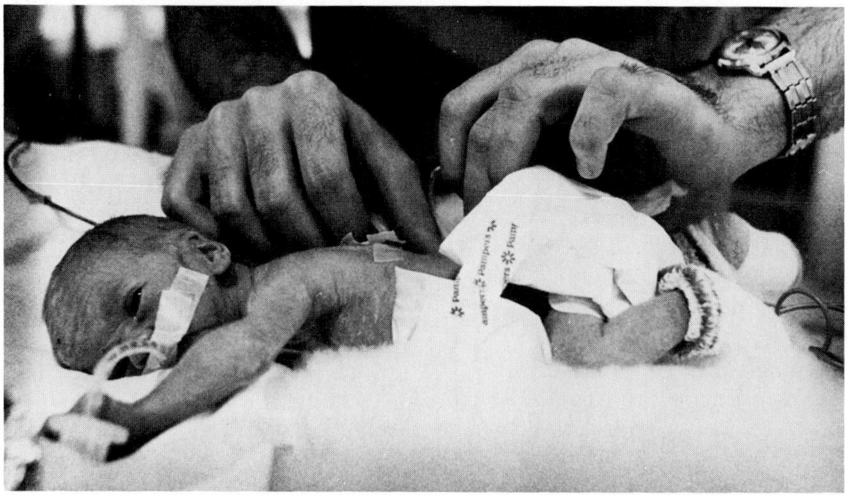

Many premature infants are born with vitamin-E deficiency because their bodies have not built up a store of vitamin E.

supplements of vitamin E to prevent a deficiency. Diseases such as cystic fibrosis that cause fats to be poorly absorbed also reduce the absorption of fat-soluble vitamins, including vitamin E. Those vitamins contained in foods are excreted along with the fat that is not absorbed.

Vitamin-E deficiency is diagnosed by a blood test. If a vitamin-E deficiency exists, red blood cell membranes break down easily when exposed to oxygen or another oxidizing agent. All of the adverse consequences of vitamin-E deficiency appear to be due to changes that occur in the cell membranes.

Toxicity Only very large amounts of vitamin E produce overdose symptoms. If taken for a year or more, a daily dose of 1,000 IU of vitamin E will produce excessive bleeding, impair wound healing, and cause depression in some people.[22] Few people taking between 100 and 800 IU per day develop any signs of overdose.[23]

VITAMIN K (PHYLLOQUINONE, MENAQUINONE)

The discovery of vitamin K stemmed from the observation that chicks fed a fat-free diet would bleed excessively if they were injured. When deficiencies of the then-known fat-soluble vitamins were shown not to cause the bleed-

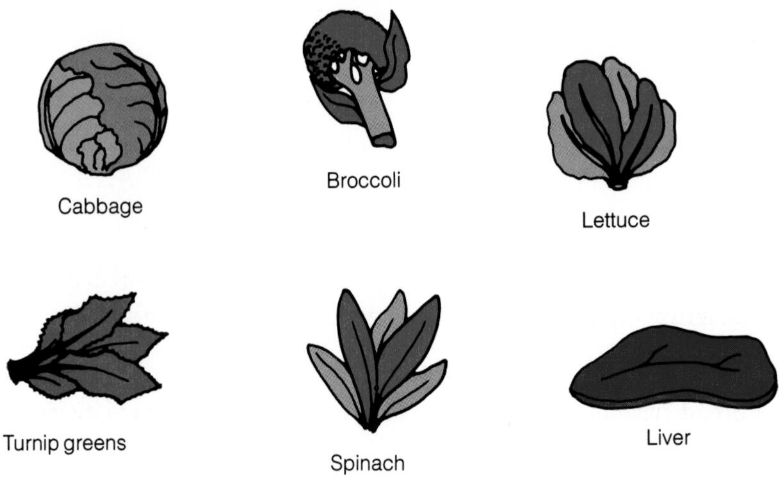

Green leafy vegetables and liver are excellent dietary sources of vitamin K.

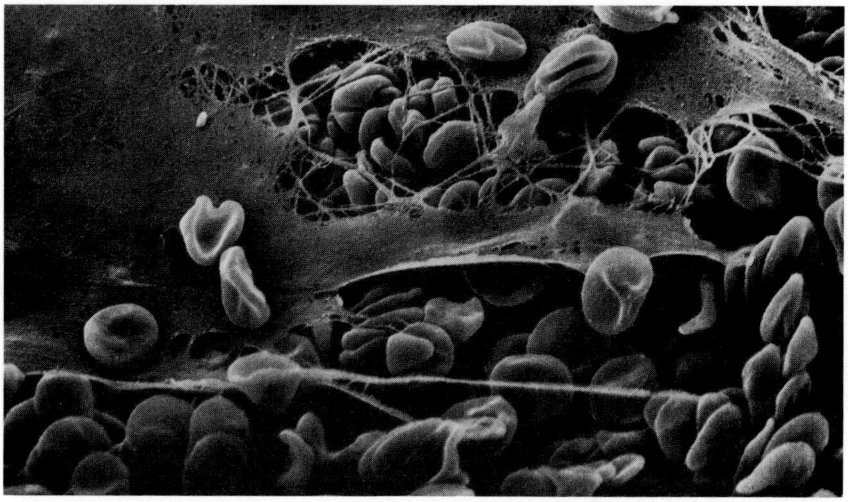

FIGURE 10-9
Scanning electron micrograph of a blood clot. Note the fibrin "net" or "web." Vitamin K stimulates the production of fibrin.

ing, it became apparent that yet another fat-soluble substance might be essential for humans. The German scientist who identified the new vitamin called it *Koagulierung* ("coagulation") vitamin, which is why it came to be called *vitamin K*. It was found to be required by humans as well as by a variety of animals. Vitamin K acts to stimulate the synthesis of prothrombin and three other blood-clotting factors needed to produce fibrin, the chemical substance that actually stops the bleeding (Figure 10-9).

Two naturally occurring forms of vitamin K exist. Phylloquinone (fil′ ō kwin′ ōn), vitamin K_1, occurs in foods, and menaquinone (men′ a kwin′ ōn), vitamin K_2, is produced by bacteria in the large intestine. Vitamin K has so far escaped popular use. It is rarely included in multivitamin supplements or fortified foods.

Sources

Humans obtain vitamin K from two sources: foods and bacteria. About half of the needed vitamin K is produced by bacteria normally present in the upper part of the large intestine. (See Figure 10-10.)

Green leafy vegetables are by far the best food sources of vitamin K (Table 10-4). Some meats are moderate sources of the vitamin. Other than these, few foods can be considered good sources of vitamin K.

Recommended Intake

The provisional adult RDA for vitamin K is 70 to 140 mcg. Typical U.S. diets provide 300 to 500 mcg per day—much more than is required.[21]

People at risk of developing vitamin-K deficiency:
newborns that have not received vitamin K injections
long-term antibiotics users

Deficiency Only two groups of people are at risk of developing vitamin-K deficiency: newborns who are not given vitamin K after birth, and people who take antibiotics for extended periods. Infants are born with a low supply of vitamin K and have not yet acquired the intestinal bacteria that will produce it. As a precaution against uncontrolled bleeding, newborns are routinely given an injection of vitamin K.

Long-term antibiotic therapy kills most of the bacteria that inhabit the gut, and with them goes the bacterial source of vitamin K. One study

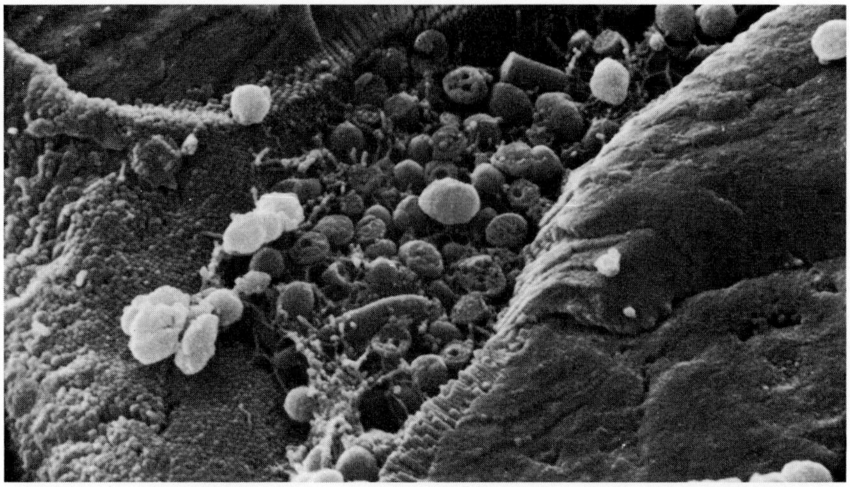

■
FIGURE 10-10
Electron micrograph (magnification × 7,112) of a colony of bacteria in a fold of the large intestine. Note the brushlike microvilli of the surrounding epithelial cells.

showed that 31 percent of patients with gastrointestinal disorders that required the long-term use of antibiotics developed vitamin-K deficiency.[23]

People with vitamin-K deficiency bruise easily; their bodies may be literally covered with black and blue marks. Bruises develop when small areas of hemorrhage that are normally clotted off quickly after a "bump" continue to bleed. Uncontrolled bleeding also occurs among people with hemophilia, a genetic disease that is not related to vitamin-K deficiency.

Toxicity Phylloquinone and menaquinone, the two naturally occurring forms of vitamin K, do not appear to cause toxic reactions if taken in large amounts. On the other hand, a synthetic form of vitamin K called *menadione* does cause toxic reactions. Menadione is water-soluble and thus useful for people who cannot absorb fat. If taken in high amounts, menadione can cause liver damage and excessive bleeding. Thus, it is used only when the fat-soluble forms of vitamin K cannot be absorbed and is available only with a doctor's prescription.

■
TABLE 10-4
Food sources of vitamin K

Food	Amount	Vitamin K, mcg*
Vegetables		
turnip greens	½ c	546
broccoli	½ c	168
lettuce	½ c	108
cabbage	½ c	105
spinach	½ c	75
asparagus	½ c	48
Meats		
liver	3 oz	77
ham	3 oz	13

*The provisional RDA for adults is 70–140 mcg.

COMING UP IN CHAPTER 11

The topic switches to minerals in chapter 11. You will be introduced to their functions, food sources, recommended levels of intake, and problems related to consuming too little and too much of them. You will also become acquainted with some of the health issues that surround calcium, iron, sodium, fluoride, and other minerals.

REVIEW QUESTIONS

1. Which fat-soluble vitamins have provitamins?
2. Why was vitamin A named *retinol*?
3. Which fat-soluble vitamin is *least* widely distributed in foods?
4. Reconsider the steps in the development of vitamin-A deficiencies presented in Figure 10-4. What events (that is, steps) precede the development of blindness?
5. Cite two reasons for fortifying milk with vitamin D.
6. Why do people who take antibiotics for long periods of time (a month or more) risk developing vitamin-K deficiency?
7. Overdoses of which two fat-soluble vitamins are associated with the greatest threats to health?
8. Which two fat-soluble vitamins function as antioxidants?

Answers

1. Vitamins A and D.
2. Because it is found in high amounts in the retina of the eye and it functions in vision.
3. Vitamin D.
4. See Figure 10-4.
5. Milk is commonly consumed by growing children, who have a high need for vitamin D. Also, milk is a good source of calcium, and vitamin D facilitates the absorption of calcium.
6. Antibiotics kill bacteria in the large intestine that produce part of our supply of vitamin K.
7. Vitamins A and D.
8. Vitamin A (beta-carotene) and vitamin E.

PUTTING NUTRITION KNOWLEDGE TO WORK

1. Do you consume enough vitamin A? Refer to Table 10-1 and note how often you consume one or more servings of a good source of vitamin A or beta-carotene.

2. Although cheese is made from milk, it contains only a very small amount of vitamin D. State why cheese does not contain the level of vitamin D you might expect of a milk product.
(Hint: Do both milk and *cheese have to be fortified with vitamin D?)*
3. If you received all of the vitamin D you needed each day from vitamin D fortified milk, how many cups of milk would you need to meet your RDA for vitamin D?
4. Whole grain breads contain more vitamin E per one ounce slice than does white bread. State why there's a difference in the vitamin E content of these two types of bread.
(What happens to the germ component of wheat when it's processed?)
5. Since the diets of Americans in general include less animal fat and more vegetable sources of fat than in the past, what would you expect has happened to the level of vitamin E intake, and the need for vitamin E? *(Clue: Both intake and need have changed in the same direction.)*

NOTES

1. M. S. Menkes and G. W. Comstock, et al., Serum beta-carotene, vitamins A and E, selenium, and the risk of lung cancer, *New England Journal of Medicine* 315 (1986):120–124.

2. D. S. Goodman, Vitamin A and retinoids in health and disease, *New England Journal of Medicine* 310 (1984):1023–1031.

3. L. Schoeff, Vitamin A, *American Journal of Medical Technology* 49 (1983):447–452.

4. L. Oversen, Vitamin therapy in the absence of obvious deficiency: What is the evidence? *Drugs* 27 (1984):148–170.

5. Effects of isotrentinoin on plasma lipids and lipoproteins, *Nutrition Reviews* 44 (1986):196–198.

6. A. U. Pickle and A. M. Hartman, Indicator foods for Vitamin A assessment, *Nutrition and Cancer* 7 (1985):3–23.

7. G. W. Burton and K. U. Ingold, Beta-carotene: An unusual type of lipid antioxidant, *Science* 224 (1984):569–573.

8. G. Wolf, Vitamin A in *Nutrition and the Adult*, eds. R. B. Alfin-Slater and D. Kritchevsky (New York: Plenum Press, 1980), 97–203.

9. J. Perisse and W. Placchi, Geographical distribution and recent changes in world supply of vitamin A, *Food and Nutrition* (Roma) 6 (1980):21–27.

10. D. R. Miller and K. C. Hayes, Vitamin excess and toxicity in *Nutrition Toxicology*, ed. J. N. Hathcock (New York: Academic Press, 1982), 81–133.

11. Some facts and myths of vitamins, *FDA Consumer*, DHHS publication no. (FDA)79–2117 (Rockville, Md.: Food and Drug Administration, 1981).

12. L. Fenner, The tanning pill, a questionable inside dye job, *FDA Consumer* 16 (1982):23–24.

13. E. Kemmann, S. A. Pasquale, and R. Skaf, Amenorrhea associated with carotenemia, *Journal of the American Medical Association* 249 (1983):926–929.

14. M. D. Holick, Vitamin D synthesis by the aging skin, in *Nutrition and Aging,* Vol. 5, eds. M. Hutchinson and H. N. Munro (Orlando, Fla., Academic Press, 1986),45–58.

15. S. Bachrachy, J. Fisher, and J. S. Parks, An outbreak of vitamin D deficiency rickets in a susceptible population, *Pediatrics* 64 (1979):871–877.

16. D. V. Edidin, and L. L. Levitsky, et al., Resurgence of nutritional rickets associated with breast feeding and special dietary practices, *Pediatrics* 65 (1980): 232–235.

17. M. A. Dubick and R. B. Rucker, Dietary supplements and health aids: A critical evaluation—Part 1: Vitamins and minerals, *Journal of Nutrition Education* 15 (1983):47–53.
18. C. K. Chow, Nutritional influences on cellular antioxidant defense systems, *American Journal of Clinical Nutrition* 32 (1979):1066–1081.
19. S. M. Love, R. S. Gelman, and W. Silen, Fibrocystic "disease" of the breast: A nondisease? *New England Journal of Medicine* 307 (1982):1010–1014.
20. P. M. Newberne and V. Suphakarn, Nutrition and cancer: A review, with emphasis on the role of vitamins C and E and selenium, *Nutrition and Cancer* 5 (1983):107–119. (See also *The Surgeon General's Report on Nutrition and Health*, 1988, pp.218–219.)
21. *Recommended Dietary Allowances*, 9th ed., Food and Nutrition Board, National Research Council (Washington, D.C.: National Academy of Sciences, 1980).
22. M. A. Dubick, Dietary supplements and health aids: A critical evaluation, *Journal of Nutrition Education* 15 (1983):123–127.
23. S. D. Krasinski and R. M. Russell, et al., The prevalence of vitamin K deficiency in chronic gastrointestinal disorders, *American Journal of Clinical Nutrition* 41 (1985):639–643.

CHAPTER 11

MINERALS I

The periodic table (Figure 11-1) lists the known elements that make up everything that exists above, below, and on earth. Of the 109 elements in the table, at least 20 are known to be required for building the human body and keeping it healthy, and 15 of the 20 must be obtained in the diet (Table 11-1). The other 5—oxygen, carbon, hydrogen, nitrogen, and sulfur—are abundant in the carbohydrates, proteins, and fats we eat, in the air we breathe, or in the water we drink. Oxygen, carbon, hydrogen, and nitro-

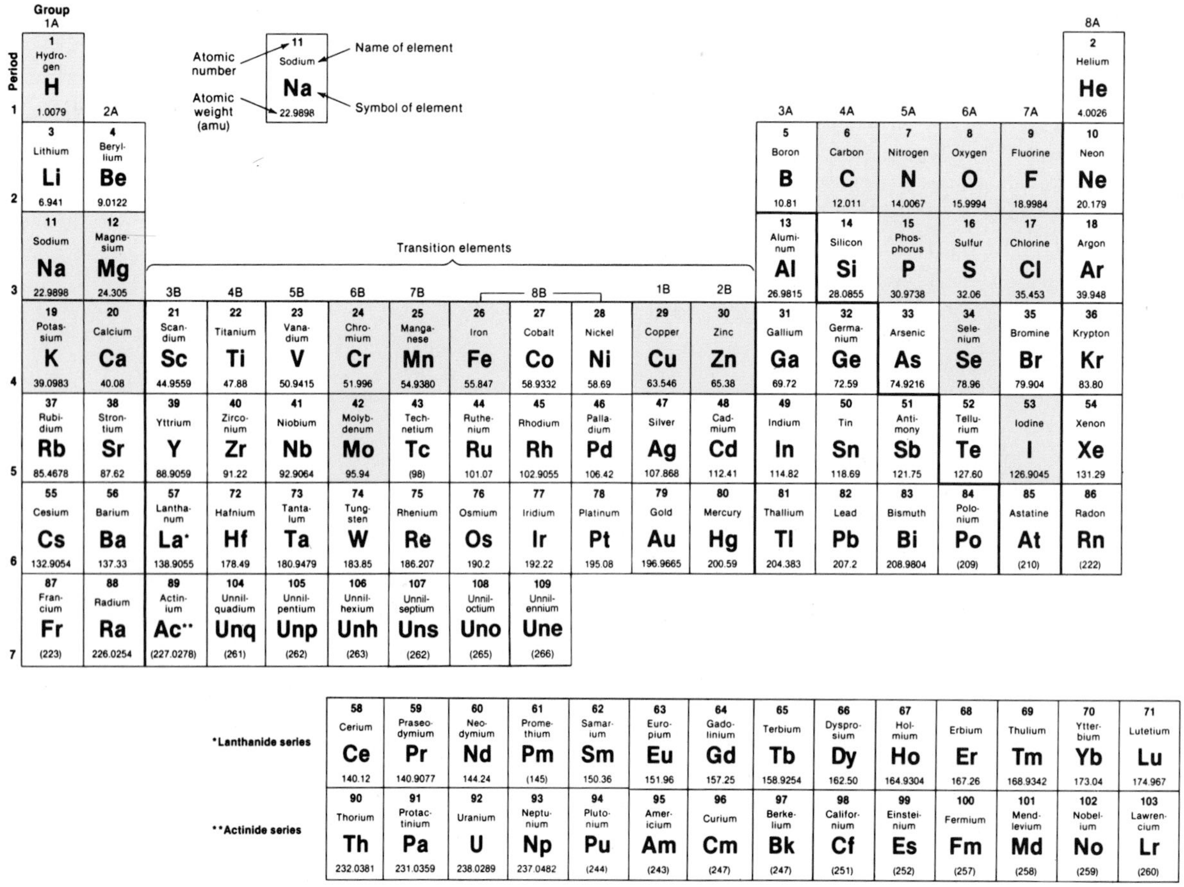

FIGURE 11-1
The periodic table of elements. The 20 elements required by humans are shown in green.

■
TABLE 11-1

Essential mineral elements for which RDAs have been assigned (The abbreviation for each mineral is in parentheses.)

RDAs	Provisional RDAs*
calcium (Ca)	copper (Cu)
phosphorus (P)	manganese (Mn)
magnesium (Mg)	fluoride (F)
iron (Fe)	chromium (Cr)
zinc (Zn)	selenium (Se)
iodine (I)	molybdenum (Mo)
	sodium (Na)
	potassium (K)
	chloride (Cl)

*"Estimated safe and adequate daily dietary intakes," commonly referred to as *provisional RDAs*.

gen are considered the "bulk" minerals, because they are found in large amounts in the body (see Figure 11-2).

Humans require substantially greater amounts of minerals than of vitamins, and foods generally contain much larger amounts of minerals. If you added up the adult RDAs for the 15 essential minerals, the total amount would approximately fill a tablespoon. The amount of vitamins calculated from the adult RDAs would total only one one-hundredth of that amount. Minerals are needed in greater amounts because, unlike vitamins, they serve as components of body structures such as bones and teeth, and they are found in relatively large amounts in blood and other body fluids.

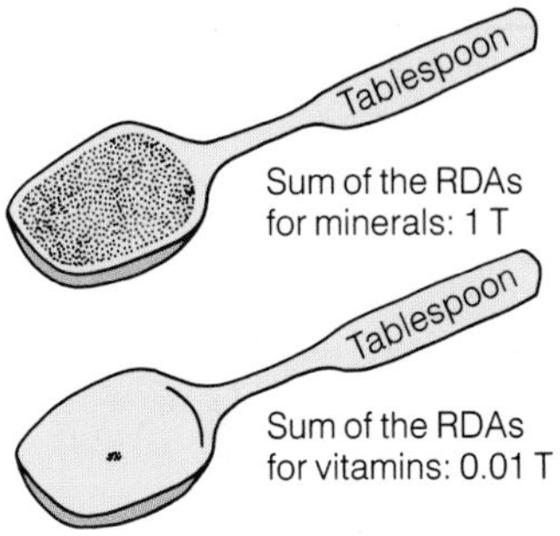

The list of essential minerals will probably be expanded in the future. It is expected that microscopic amounts of nickel, vanadium, and even arsenic will be shown to be required by humans in the not-too-distant future.

This book devotes two chapters to the essential minerals and presents them in the order they are listed in the RDA tables—and in Table 11-1. This

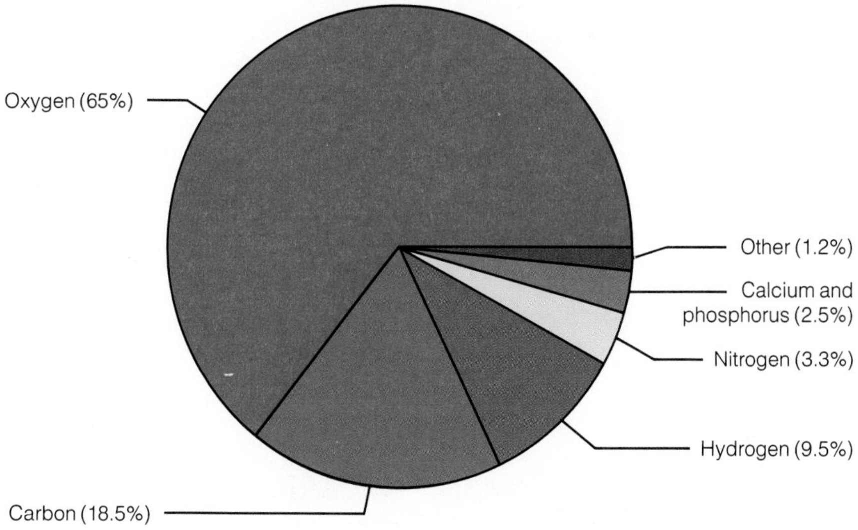

■
FIGURE 11-2

Mineral composition of the human body. The "other" category includes potassium, sodium, sulfur, chlorine, iron, zinc, magnesium, iodine, and other minerals.

chapter discusses the 6 minerals included in Table 1 of the RDAs. Chapter 12 discusses the 9 minerals for which "estimated safe and adequate daily dietary intakes"—provisional RDAs—have been established. Nutrients with provisional RDAs are listed in Table 2 of the RDA tables. There is nothing provisional about our requirement for these 9 minerals. It's simply that less is known about how much of them humans require for health.

CALCIUM (Ca)

Calcium has become very popular in the United States. It is widely regarded as the "anti-osteoporosis" mineral. The "calcium craze" began in the early 1980s, when the consensus of scientific opinion changed from regarding osteoporosis as an inevitable problem of aging to seeing it as related to the long-term adequacy of calcium intake. Lifelong adequate intakes of calcium are now viewed as the key to preventing osteoporosis.[1]

Concern about osteoporosis is reflected in people's calcium supplement use and food-buying practices in the U.S. In the mid 1980s, sales of calcium supplements were increasing by 33 percent a year and were expected to exceed 270 million dollars in yearly sales by 1990.[2] Average consumption of low-fat milk and dairy products is increasing, and more and more food products are being fortified with calcium. Food manufacturers have responded to consumer demand for high-calcium foods by adding the mineral to an array of products, including diet soft drinks, milk products, orange juice, breakfast cereals, and flour.

Functions

The role of calcium in preventing osteoporosis is now widely appreciated, and we will return to this important topic later in the chapter. But calcium also performs other functions that help to keep the body alive and functioning well. Calcium is needed to stimulate nerve impulses and muscle contrac-

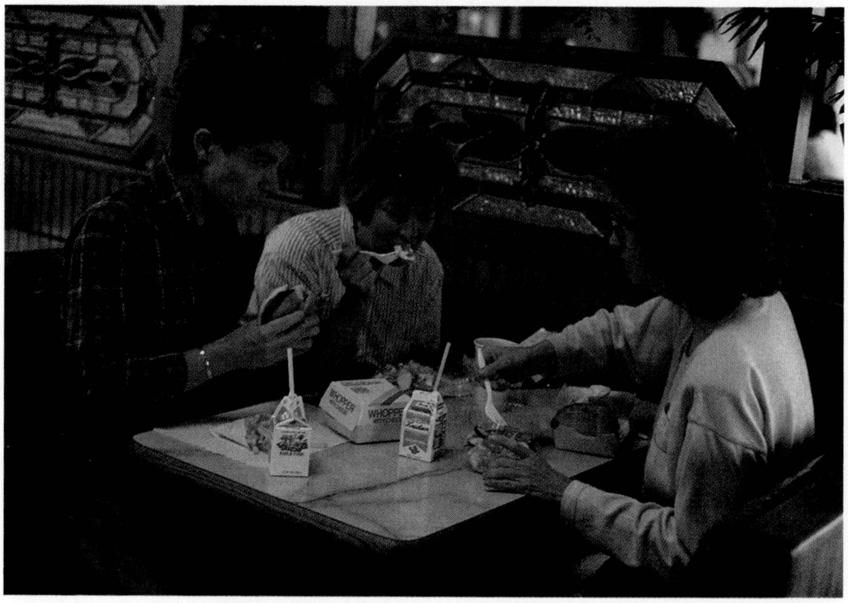

News about calcium and osteoporosis is changing the way Americans eat.

tions, and it is an essential cofactor in blood coagulation. About 99 percent of the three pounds of calcium contained in the adult body is located in the bones, and the remaining one percent is in the blood and the fluids that surround cells.

As with the other minerals, calcium's property of carrying a charge is basic to its functions. As an ion, calcium interacts with ions of opposite charge in its environment. The interactions of calcium with other ions result in the formation of crystals, and in the initiation of electrical currents and specific chemical reactions. The ability of calcium to form crystals with other minerals is essential to its role in bone formation. Its ability to transmit an electrical charge across cell membranes accounts for its effectiveness in stimulating nerve impulses and muscle contractions. Calcium's role as an enzyme cofactor in the chain of reactions that lead to blood coagulation is also related to its property of being charged.

Functions of calcium:
bone mineralization
nerve impulse transmission
muscle contraction
blood coagulation

Of all the functions of calcium, its role in bone formation and maintenance is of greatest concern to public health. This function is singled out for further discussion here in order to explain calcium's role in promoting bone health and preventing osteoporosis.

Calcium and Bone Formation Bone is not as solid and metabolically inactive as it may look. Bone is living tissue that is infiltrated by blood vessels, nerves, and specialized cells. About half of the content of bone is water, and half is made up of solids. The "solid" part of bones is a network of strong protein fibers (the "protein matrix") embedded with mineral crystals (Figure 11-3). Calcium is by far the most abundant mineral in bones. It forms crystals with phosphorus and, to a lesser extent, with carbon, magnesium, and other minerals during bone formation. The combination of the tough protein matrix with the mineral crystals makes bone very strong yet shock-absorbant and slightly flexible.

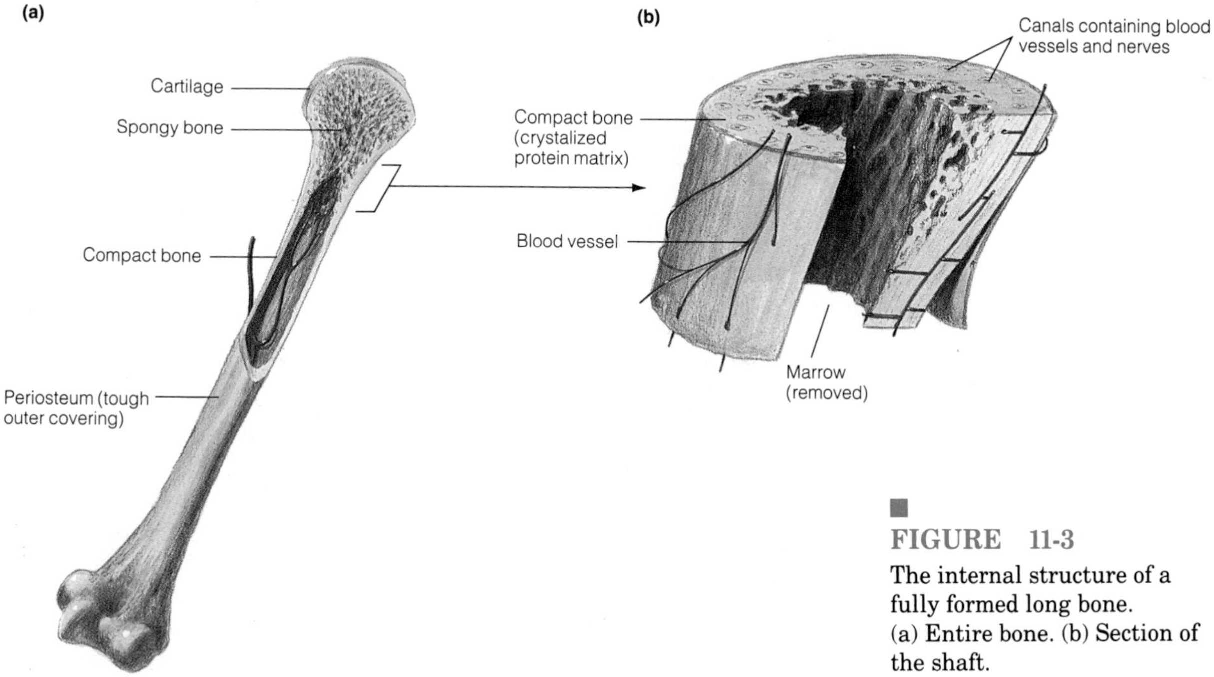

FIGURE 11-3
The internal structure of a fully formed long bone.
(a) Entire bone. (b) Section of the shaft.

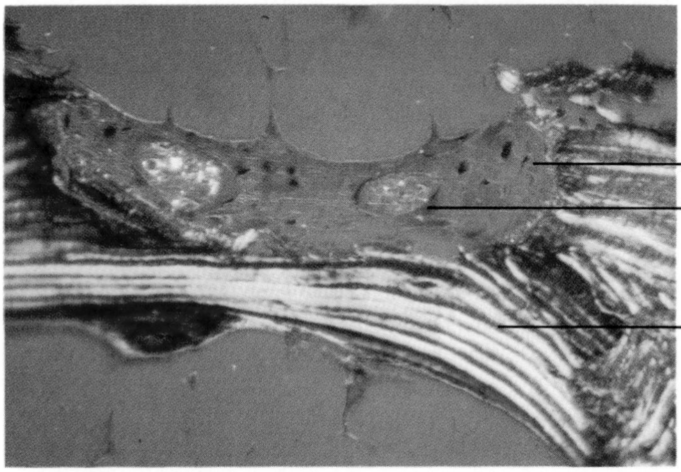

FIGURE 11-4
Photomicrograph of an osteoclast. This large, sausage-shaped cell is actively dissolving the bone tissue beside it. Osteoblasts (*not shown*) are cells that form bone tissue.

The teeth, which constitute a particular type of bone tissue, have the same properties as other bone plus an additional feature: they have a hard outer coating of enamel that does not contain blood vessels or nerve cells. It serves to protect the teeth from destruction by bacteria and the rigorous chewing and grinding that they must withstand. In this chapter, the term *bone* refers to both skeletal bones and teeth.

remodeling: The breakdown and build up of bone tissue.

Bones slowly but continually go through a repair and replacement process known as **remodeling**. During remodeling, the old protein matrix is replaced with newly synthesized protein, and the minerals are recycled. A continual supply of nutrients is needed to support the activities of bone cells in forming and maintaining bone tissue.

osteoblasts: (*osteo* = "bones"; *blast* = "germinating, growing") Bone cells that cause bone to form.

osteoclasts: (*clast* = "breaking, destroying") Bone cells that cause the breakdown of bone.

The processes of bone formation and breakdown are directed by two types of bone cells: **osteoblasts** cause bone to form, and **osteoclasts** cause breakdown (Figure 11-4). Osteoblasts produce the protein that makes up the matrix around which minerals are deposited. The protein of the matrix chemically attracts calcium and other minerals contained in the mixture of nutrients supplied to bone tissue. Once inside the protein matrix, the minerals form crystals that embed in the matrix. The protein matrix continues to mineralize until it becomes filled with mineral crystals.

Certain hormones and physical activity are known to affect the activity of osteoblasts. For example, estrogen and growth hormone increase bone formation, and physical inactivity decreases it. (The relationship between physical activity and osteoporosis is explored in Box 11-1.) Osteoblast activity is also triggered by bone fractures; these bone-forming cells become very active when a bone breaks. Osteoblasts at the site of a break respond to a fracture by secreting large quantities of the protein needed to build new protein matrix. This new protein matrix attracts minerals, which deposit as crystals. As a result, broken bones are usually repaired within a few weeks to a month.

Osteoclasts play a role in bone health by, oddly enough, destroying the protein matrix. Osteoclasts secrete enzymes that break down the protein in the matrix for the purpose of renewing it. Lost with the matrix are the minerals embedded in it. Once released from the matrix, calcium and phosphorus return to the nutrient mixture from which they came and are circulated throughout the body in the blood. Most of the calcium and phosphorus

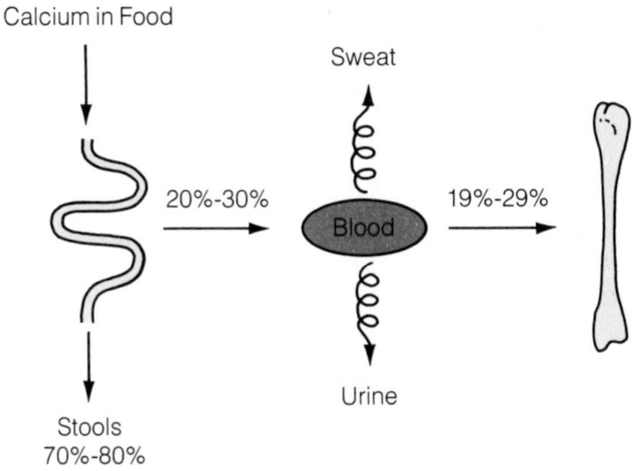

FIGURE 11-5
The body absorbs 20% to 30% of the calcium consumed in most foods. Of the amount absorbed, some (1%) is transported by the blood to nerves and muscles, and a tiny amount is lost in sweat and urine. Most of it (19% to 29% of that absorbed) is used to build and maintain bones.

that is lost from bone will be used again to form new bone. But, some of it will be diverted to carry out the other functions of these minerals, and small amounts will be lost in the feces, urine, and sweat (Figure 11-5). Failure to replace calcium, whether due to dietary causes or other reasons, can eventually lead to the demineralization of bones and to **osteoporosis**.

osteoporosis: (*osteo* = "bones"; *poro* = "porous"; *osis* = "abnormal condition") A condition characterized by porous bones; due to the loss of minerals from the bones.

Osteoporosis Approximately twenty million adults in the U.S. have osteoporosis, and one million of them have suffered a fracture of the wrist, hip, or other bone because of the disease.[1] One out of 4 women and 1 in every 8 men in the U.S. will develop osteoporosis. The risk of developing osteoporosis greatly increases among women after **menopause**, the period in life when a woman's estrogen level falls and her ability to reproduce ends (Figure 11-6). Many women over 90 years of age have experienced a fracture due to osteoporosis.[1] The consequences of osteoporosis are much more serious than bone fractures, however. Nearly 20 percent of elderly people who experience a hip fracture die from complications within six months.[3] Osteoporosis is the twelfth-leading cause of death in the U.S.[3,4]

menopause: The period of a woman's life when her physiological ability to reproduce ends; generally occurs between the ages of 45 and 52 and is accompanied by decreased levels of estrogen.

Osteoporosis becomes a painful disease over time, reducing the quality of life and causing a dramatic increase in the need for medical care. The nation's total health care bill for treating the disease and its complications amounts to over four billion dollars a year.[5] Because it is associated with

BOX 11-1

PHYSICAL ACTIVITY, BODY WEIGHT, AND BONE FORMATION

The amount of bone produced in the human body is determined by a number of factors, including the person's physical activity level and body weight. For reasons yet unknown, bone formation is stimulated when pressure is applied to the bone. When the physical strain on bones is increased, the osteoblasts become more active, thus accelerating the formation of bone. As a result, bones of physically active persons and heavy persons tend to be thicker and stronger than the bones of inactive and light people. Bones that are not used at all—such as the bones of a leg in a plaster cast or those of people who are bedridden—lose calcium and phosphorus, and they slowly decrease in size and strength.

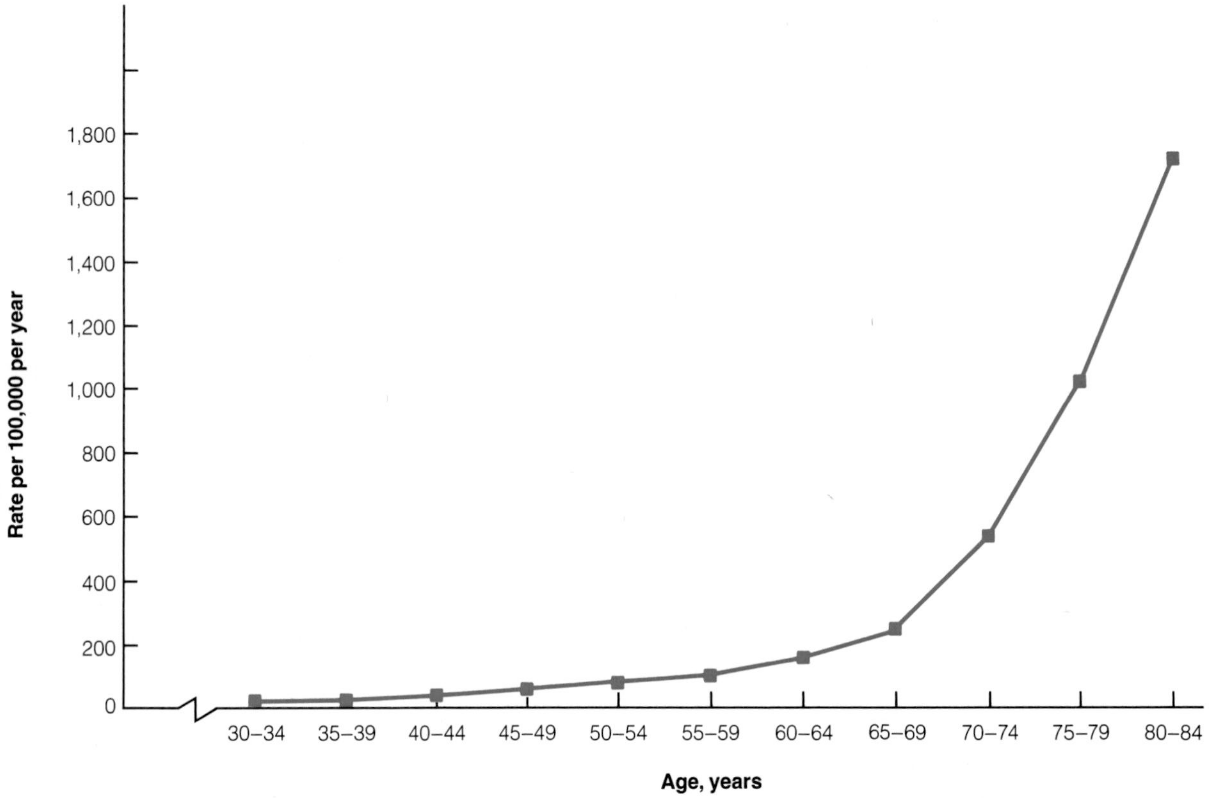

FIGURE 11-6
Estimated annual age-specific incidence of hip fracture among white females in the United States.

Risk factors for osteoporosis:
menopause (loss of estrogen)
low calcium intake
poor calcium absorption
high levels of calcium excretion
physical inactivity
inadequate vitamin D
thinness

aging, the importance of osteoporosis as a personal and public health problem will intensify as the U.S. population ages—unless we become more successful at preventing and treating the disease.

Cross-cultural comparisons of the incidence of osteoporosis strongly suggest that osteoporosis is not an inevitable consequence of aging. Women in the U.S. are 10–20 times more likely to develop osteoporosis than women of similar age in several other countries.[4] Women living in countries where osteoporosis is not a major public health problem appear to have more highly mineralized or denser bones than U.S. women. How dense bones become and stay depends on a number of factors, including the adequacy of calcium and vitamin D intakes, estrogen availability, and habitual physical activity level.

Building Dense Bones Bone formation begins early in life—during the fourth to sixth week of gestation—and does not stop until well into adulthood (Figure 11-7). Bones grow in length and width up to about age 20, and then, although they stabilize in size, they continue to mineralize until about age 30. The peak bone density achieved at around age 30 has been found to be an important predictor of osteoporosis. In general, the denser the bones become, the less likely it is that osteoporosis will develop later in life. Bone size and density normally remain fairly stable from age 30 to the mid 40s. After that, bones tend to demineralize and weaken with increasing age. An inch or two of height is generally lost during old age due to the compacting of weakened bones in the spine, and a "dowager's hump" may form. By the age of 90, the typical U.S. female's bones are half as dense as they once were.[1]

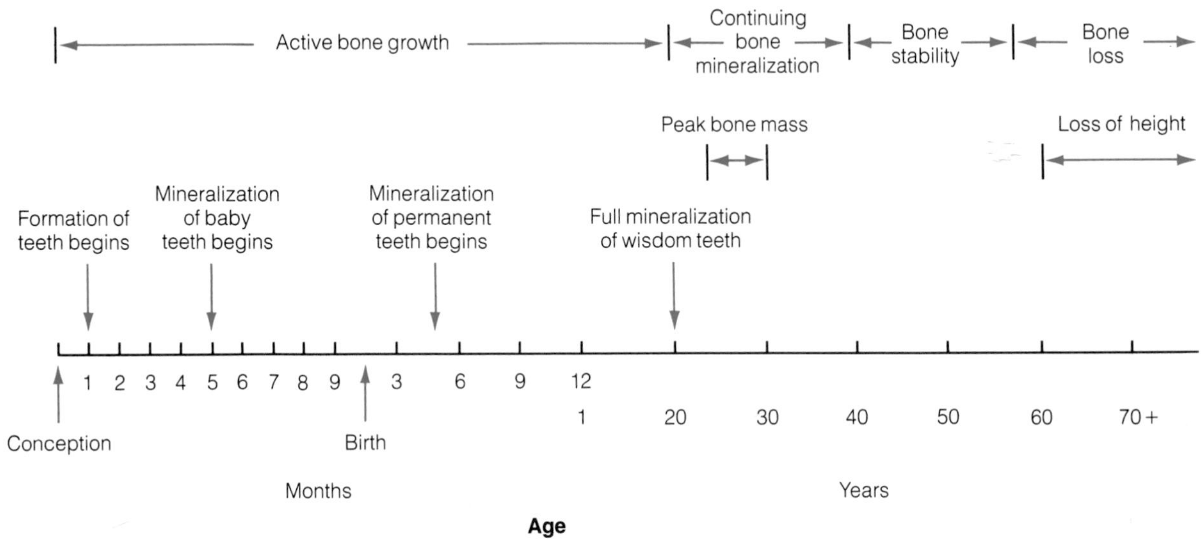

■ **FIGURE 11-7**
The life cycle of teeth and bone formation and loss in humans.

Some thinning of bone with aging occurs in most people. The extent of the loss, however, can be lessened in both women and men by lifelong dietary adequacy of calcium.[6] Adequate calcium intakes appear to be especially important during the first 30 years of life, when bones are increasing in mineral content and peak bone density is being established.[7] It is much easier for the body to mineralize bone that is forming and developing than it is to remineralize bones that have undergone extensive demineralization.

Scientists have yet to find a treatment that will totally reverse bone demineralization once it is established. Current recommendations call for treating osteoporosis that occurs after menopause with 1,000–1,500 mg of calcium daily. Small doses of estrogen and progesterone, as well as calcium

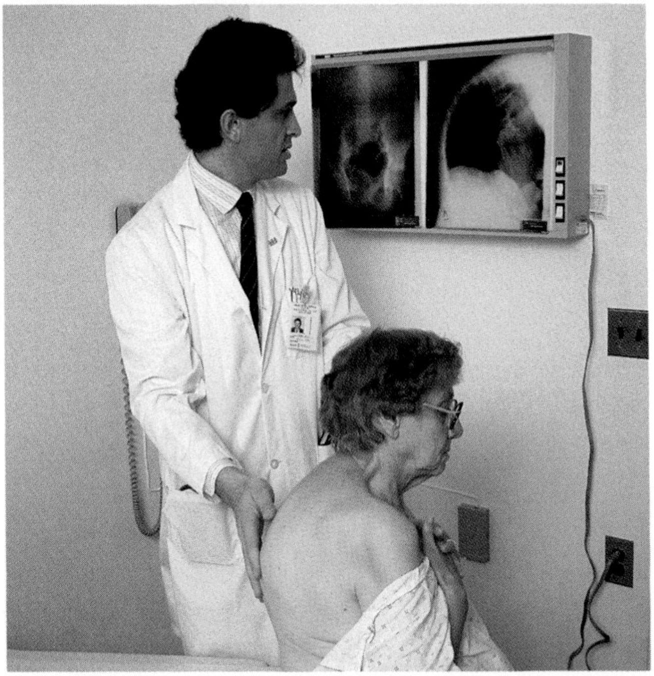

Our society has come to regard the stooped appearance of elderly women as a normal phenomenon of aging. Actually, "dowager's hump" can generally be prevented.

TABLE 11-2
Prevention and treatment of osteoporosis

Prevention
daily intake of 800 to 1,000 mg of calcium
adequate vitamin D
regular exercise
Treatment
estrogen/progesterone treatment in postmenopausal women who experience appreciable bone loss
intake of 1,000 to 1,500 mg of calcium per day
regular exercise
adequate vitamin D

supplements, are recommended for advanced cases of osteoporosis.[3] The effectiveness of calcium in reducing bone loss is enhanced by the concurrent consumption of the adult RDA of vitamin D,[8] and by regular, weight-bearing exercise.[5] Approaches to preventing and treating osteoporosis are summarized in Table 11-2.

Sources

Actually, the richest source of calcium is alligator meat. About 3½ ounces of it contain 2,130 mg of calcium.[15]

Most of the calcium supplied by the diets of Americans comes from milk and milk products (Table 11-3). (Growing calves have a high need for calcium, so cows' milk contains a high amount of it.) Milk, cheese, yogurt, ice cream, puddings, and other foods made from milk are all good sources of calcium. Chocolate milk, too, is a good source of calcium. Although it was once thought that the oxalic acid content of chocolate binds with the calcium in milk and reduces its availability, it is now known that as much calcium is absorbed from chocolate milk as whole milk.[11]

Only a few nonmilk foods—for example, spinach, collard greens, and tofu—contain much calcium, and substantially less calcium is absorbed

TABLE 11-3
Sources of calcium in the U.S. diet[10]

Food Category	Percentage of Total Calcium Consumed
Milk and milk products	73
Fruits and vegetables	9
Meat, poultry, and fish	4
Grain products	4
Potatoes	1
"Other"	9

TABLE 11-4
Food sources of calcium

Food	Amount	Calcium, mg*
Milk and Milk Products		
low-fat yogurt	1 c	415
low-fat yogurt with fruit	1 c	315
skim milk	1 c	300
1% milk	1 c	300
2% milk	1 c	298
3.25% milk (whole)	1 c	288
Swiss cheese	1 oz	270
cheddar cheese	1 oz	205
frozen yogurt	1 c	200
cream soup	1 c	186
pudding	½ c	185
ice cream	1 c	180
ice milk	1 c	180
American cheese	1 oz	175
custard	½ c	150
cottage cheese	½ c	70
low-fat cottage cheese	½ c	69
Vegetables		
collard greens, cooked	½ c	110
spinach, cooked	½ c	90
broccoli	½ c	70
Legumes		
tofu	½ c	155
dried beans, cooked	½ c	50
lima beans	½ c	40

*The RDA for adults 23–50 years of age is 800 mg.

from these foods than from milk. For example, the average amount of calcium absorbed from spinach is 5%, compared to an average of 28% from milk.[12] Table 11-4 lists food sources of calcium.

Recommended Intake

The RDA for calcium for adults 23–50 years of age is 800 mg (0.8 g). Most U.S. adults consume about half that amount.[13] The gap between the RDA and actual intake is wider still for postmenopausal women. It is estimated that the typical postmenopausal woman needs 1,200–1,500 mg of calcium per day but consumes only 475 mg.[14] The bottom line is that most women and many men in the U.S. do not consume enough calcium to prevent gradual losses in bone calcium content.[4]

Why are calcium intakes among adult women so far below the RDA? A major reason is that many women stop drinking milk after their teen years

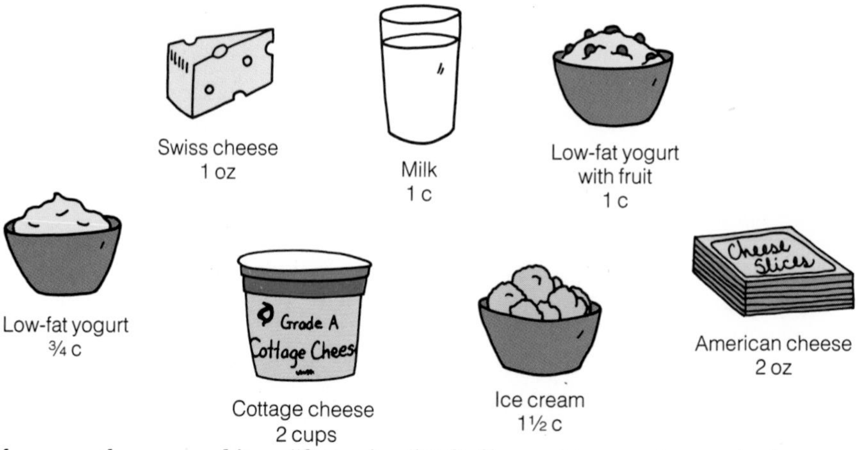
Swiss cheese
1 oz
Milk
1 c
Low-fat yogurt
with fruit
1 c
Low-fat yogurt
¾ c
Grade A
Cottage Chees
Cottage cheese
2 cups
Ice cream
1½ c
Cheese
Slices
American cheese
2 oz

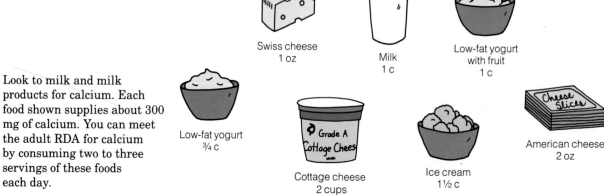

Look to milk and milk products for calcium. Each food shown supplies about 300 mg of calcium. You can meet the adult RDA for calcium by consuming two to three servings of these foods each day.

because they regard it as "fattening."[16] Coffee and tea are increasingly preferred after the teen years, and come to take over milk's place as the mealtime beverage. Men also tend to consume less milk with age, but they do not experience the bone loss that comes with menopause in women, and their higher bone masses are protective against osteoporosis.[1]

To avoid the calories in milk and other dairy products, many women turn to zero-calorie calcium supplements (Box 11-2). With the recent public notice given to the importance of adequate calcium intakes, these nonfood sources of calcium are increasingly being used as substitutes for milk and milk products. Although the supplements may bring calcium intakes up, they may shortchange people on the other nutrients they would get from milk and milk products. Figure 11-8 compares the nutrient content of milk and a calcium supplement.

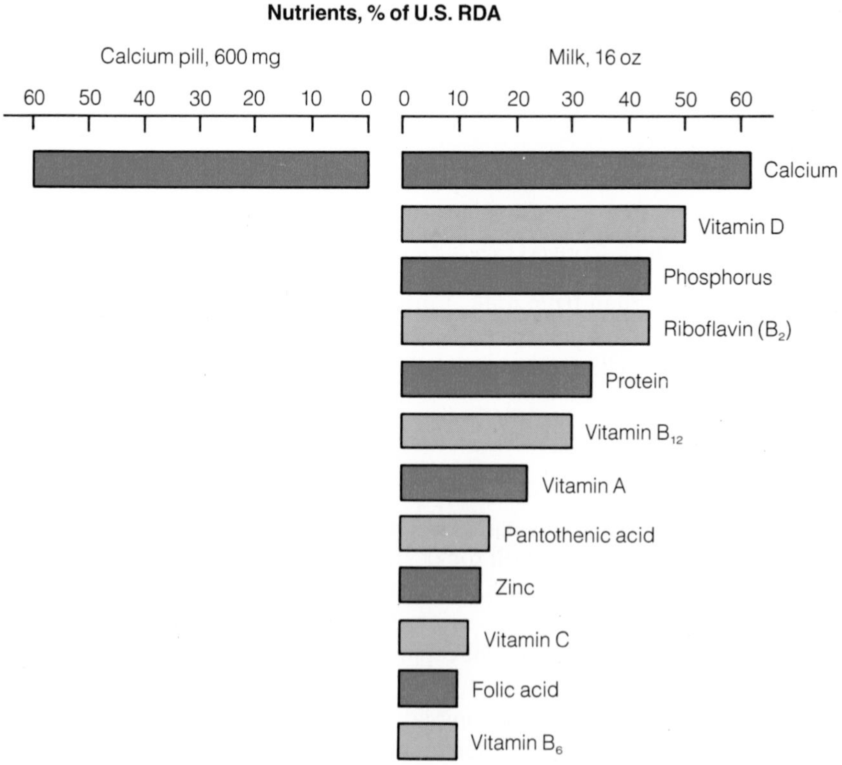
Nutrients, % of U.S. RDA
Calcium pill, 600 mg
Milk, 16 oz
60 50 40 30 20 10 0
0 10 20 30 40 50 60
Calcium
Vitamin D
Phosphorus
Riboflavin (B_2)
Protein
Vitamin B_{12}
Vitamin A
Pantothenic acid
Zinc
Vitamin C
Folic acid
Vitamin B_6

FIGURE 11-8
Comparison of some of the nutrients provided by a calcium pill and by two cups of milk.

BOX 11-2

SUPPLE-MENTAL CALCIUM

Calcium is needed in rather large amounts each day—amounts that are difficult to incorporate into a tablet that can be swallowed by humans. The challenge is complicated by the fact that calcium supplements cannot be 100% calcium. Calcium must be combined with other substances in order to increase its chemical stability. The most common calcium supplement is calcium carbonate, which is only 40% carbon by weight.

Processed oyster shells and animal bones are also used as calcium supplements. Because these "natural" sources of calcium contain many minerals in addition to calcium, a tablet of the size that can be more or less easily swallowed contains only about 250 mg of calcium. Some of the other mineral ingredients in these "natural" supplements are causes for concern. Some calcium supplements made from shells and bones contain excessive amounts of mercury and lead.[17] Furthermore, much of the calcium in shells and bones is in the form of calcium phosphate, the main type of mineral crystals in bone tissue and one of the least easily absorbed forms of calcium. This bioavailability problem is another disadvantage of this type of calcium supplement.

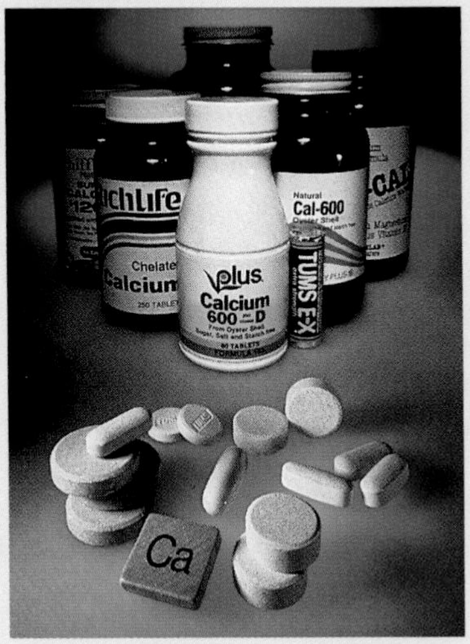

Some sources of supplemental calcium.

Antacids have become a very popular, although expensive route to calcium supplementation. Pharmacists and others have expressed concern about the habitual use of antacids among people who have no need for them. Antacids lower the acidity of fluids in the stomach, and habitual use may lower the acidity to levels that interfere with normal digestion and nutrient absorption. Calcium is one of the nutrients whose absorption is decreased by lower-than-normal levels of acidity in the stomach. Routine use of antacids as calcium supplements may pose a particular risk for the elderly, since stomach acidity generally declines during old age, and antacids may aggravate existing digestive problems.

Vitamin D, which is needed for the absorption of calcium, is only occasionally included in calcium supplements. When it is included, it is sometimes done so in irrational amounts. One calcium supplement on the market contains 112 mg of calcium and 400 IU of vitamin D in each tablet. To get the U.S. RDA of *calcium* from this supplement, a person would have to take 9 tablets, which would provide 3,600 IU of vitamin D—a huge overdose.

If calcium supplements are required, it is generally recommended that calcium carbonate be used, rather than supplements made from shells or bones.[17] The shift from food sources of calcium to supplements should not be made without considerable thought. Food sources of calcium are generally rich in a variety of other nutrients that can contribute substantially to a well-balanced diet.

Milk and milk products can be relatively high calorie sources of calcium, depending on the type of product selected. The more fat in the dairy product, the higher the caloric cost of the calcium that is obtained. The key to obtaining calcium at reasonable caloric costs is to choose low-fat milk and dairy products. Skim milk and low-fat yogurt are calorie bargains (see Table 11-5). You can get around 900 mg of calcium from 3 cups of skim milk for 270 calories. That's a 56% savings in calories over a similar amount of whole milk. A 6-ounce serving of low-fat yogurt has the same number of calories as a cup of cornflakes, and it provides one-half the adult RDA for calcium. Pudding, ice cream, and cottage cheese also are good sources of calcium, but they are calorically more expensive than low-fat milk and milk products.

TABLE 11-5

Caloric cost of 300 mg calcium from milk and milk products

Food	Amount that Provides Approximately 300 mg of Calcium	Calories
skim milk	1 c	90
1% milk	1 c	102
low-fat yogurt	¾ c	110
Swiss cheese	1¼ oz	138
2% milk	1 c	140
3.25% milk (whole)	1 c	160
cheddar cheese	1½ oz	175
American cheese	2 oz	220
low-fat yogurt with fruit	1 c	225
pudding	1½ c	240
cream soup	1 c	248
cottage cheese, low-fat	2 c	324
frozen yogurt	1½ c	324
milk shake	1¼ c	336
ice cream	1½ c	403
cottage cheese, regular	2 c	480

Deficiency The effects of dietary calcium deficiency on calcium functions vary. Bone formation and maintenance are affected the most, and the critical roles of calcium in maintaining normal nerve impulses, muscle contractions, and blood coagulation are affected least by calcium deficiency. A deficiency of calcium for these latter three functions would immediately threaten life, but it takes years for a loss of calcium from bones to jeopardize health. The body ensures the availability of calcium for nerve impulses, muscle contractions, and blood coagulation by tightly controlling blood calcium levels. Neither a low nor a high intake of calcium makes much difference in the blood calcium level. When dietary calcium is inadequate, the body draws upon the calcium in bones to maintain normal blood levels. The body protects itself from high intakes of calcium by limiting the amount that is absorbed.

Although the blood calcium level is remarkably stable, a few conditions will cause it to decrease or increase. Overdoses of vitamin D and a few rare genetic disorders and diseases cause abnormalities in blood calcium level. Both low and high blood calcium levels produce repetitive and uncontrolled nerve impulses and muscle spasms called **tetany**. Tetany is a condition in which contracted muscles fail to relax.

tetany: A condition in which muscles contract but fail to relax.

As explained in chapter 10, calcium deficiency tends to go hand-in-hand with vitamin-D deficiency. Vitamin-D deficiency decreases calcium absorption as well as the incorporation of calcium into bones.

Another effect of low calcium intake has been suggested by some recent research findings. Although the findings are controversial, it is reported that people who consume adequate amounts of calcium are less likely to develop hypertension than those who do not (Box 11-3).

Toxicity Calcium intakes as high as 2 grams per day do not appear to affect blood calcium levels, but the high levels of unabsorbed calcium that

BOX 11-3

IS CALCIUM INTAKE RELATED TO HYPERTENSION?

Maybe.

Research results suggesting that habitually low intakes of dietary calcium may be related to the development of hypertension[19,20] came as quite a shock to many scientists. After all, research up to the time these studies were published firmly pointed an accusing finger at sodium. Why would low calcium intakes and not high-sodium diets be related to hypertension in these studies?

Additional research has helped to answer this question, but the final word is not in yet. Analysis of data from several studies undertaken since the initial reports failed to show any effect of dietary calcium on blood pressure. It is generally concluded that it is vastly premature to recommend using calcium supplements to prevent or treat hypertension. It is not premature, however, to recommend that people with hypertension limit their salt intake if it is high.

result from such intakes tend to increase the bacterial production of gas and cause other gastrointestinal disturbances.[18] Although the amount of calcium absorbed decreases as calcium intake increases, a higher-than-normal level of calcium absorption can be forced by an overly generous dietary supply of vitamin D. Cases of **hypercalcemia**—a high level of blood calcium—have been identified in people taking two or more grams of calcium along with 1,000 IUs of vitamin D per day on a regular basis. Some people's bodies respond to high doses of calcium and vitamin D by forming calcium stones in the kidneys.

hypercalcemia: Above-normal levels of calcium in the blood.

A new concern about the potential for calcium overdose stems from the increasing availability of calcium-fortified foods and the popular use of calcium supplements and antacids. For the first time, many people in the U.S. are consuming high amounts of calcium. The results of this "uncontrolled experiment" will not be known for some time, but it is possible that long-term excessive intakes of calcium might decrease the absorption of other minerals, promote kidney stone formation, and perhaps cause other problems. Although the trend toward greater calcium intakes is a healthy one, the dietary goal should be to consume *adequate*, rather than excessive, amounts of calcium.

PHOSPHORUS (P)

Although phosphorus is perhaps best known as a component of friction matches (and the odor it produces when a match is lit), it is a very common constituent of food. Nearly 85% of the two pounds of phosphorus in the adult body is combined with calcium in bones. The rest of the body's phosphorus is found in the blood, the fluid that surrounds cells, and inside cells.

Functions

Most of the body's phosphorus, as we've said, is located in bones. Just as with calcium, however, the small amount that is outside the bones is involved in some critical functions. Phosphorus is a component of the genetic

Dietary sources of phosphorus. What type of food is missing from this picture? Only fruits tend to be poor sources of phosphorus.

Functions of phosphorus:
component of bone
component of DNA, RNA, ADP, and ATP
activates glucose for use in energy formation
component of certain lipids in the body

materials DNA and RNA and of the high-energy molecules ADP and ATP. Phosphorus serves in the preparation of glucose for the glycolysis phase of energy formation; both ADP and ATP must be combined with phosphorus before they can be used by cells to form energy. Many lipids in the body are combined with phosphorus and are called phospholipids. (Chapter 7 contains a discussion of this type of lipid.) The acid form of phosphorus, phosphoric acid, is soluble in both water and fat. Phosphoric acid alters the solubility of lipids, which allows them to stay in solution in body fluids. Lecithin and various types of lipoproteins—including chylomicrons, very low density lipoproteins (VLDL), low-density lipoproteins (LDL), and high-density lipoproteins (HDL)—all contain phosphoric acid. The presence of phosphoric acid contributes to the water-solubility of these substances. Phospholipids are found in high amounts in cell membranes and in cells of the brain and nervous system.

Sources

Phosphorus is widely distributed in nearly all foods; only fruits tend to contain low amounts (Table 11-6). About a third of the total U.S. intake of phosphorus comes from milk and milk products. Meats, grains, and vegetables are the other major sources (Table 11-7).

Flavored, carbonated beverages are a small but growing source of dietary phosphorus. Phosphoric acid is added to them as a preservative. Average consumption of soft drinks in the U.S. is increasing, and they now are consumed in higher amounts than any other beverage.[21]

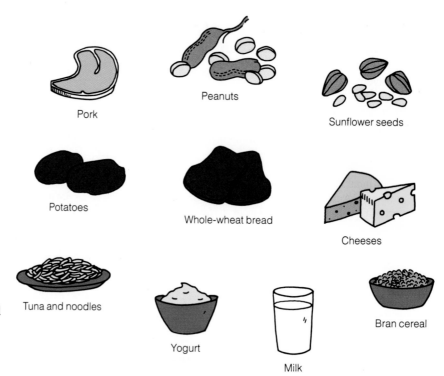

TABLE 11-6
Food sources of phosphorus

Food	Amount	Phosphorus, mg*
Milk and Milk Products		
yogurt	1 c	327
skim milk	1 c	250
whole milk	1 c	250
cottage cheese	½ c	150
American cheese	1 oz	130
Meats		
pork	3 oz	275
hamburger	3 oz	165
tuna	3 oz	162
lobster	3 oz	125
chicken	3 oz	120
Nuts and Seeds		
sunflower seeds	¼ c	319
peanuts	¼ c	141
pine nuts	¼ c	106
peanut butter	1 T	61
Grains		
bran flakes	1 c	180
shredded wheat	2 lg. biscuits	81
whole-wheat bread	1 slice	52
noodles	½ c	47
rice	½ c	29
white bread	1 slice	24
Vegetables		
potatoes	1 med.	101
corn	½ c	73
peas	½ c	70
french fries	½ c	61
broccoli	½ c	54
Other		
milk chocolate	1 oz	66
cola	12 oz	51
diet cola	12 oz	45

*The RDA for both male and female adults aged 23 to 50 is 800 mg.

TABLE 11-7
Sources of phosphorus in the U.S. diet

Food Category	Percentage of Total Phosphorus Intake
Milk and milk products	30
Meats	27
Grains and cereals	20
Vegetables and fruits	9
Other (eggs, beans, nuts, beverages)	14

Recommended Intake

The RDAs for phosphorus for adult males and females aged 23–50 years is 800 mg, the same level assigned to calcium. In contrast with calcium, however, phosphorus is widely available in foods, and a dietary lack of it almost never occurs. The average daily intake of phosphorus in the U.S. is 1,500 to 1,600 mg,[22] and the average appears to be increasing.[23]

The Calcium-to-Phosphorus Ratio Before the mid 1970s, the nutrition literature warned against diets containing more phosphorus than calcium. The ideal ratio of dietary calcium to phosphorus was thought to be 2:1; that is, twice as much calcium as phosphorus.[24] It was reasoned that since bones contain twice as much calcium as phosphorus and because high phosphorus levels reduce calcium absorption, people should consume more calcium than phosphorus to achieve the proper balance for bone health.

Phosphoric acid is added to soft drinks as a preservative.

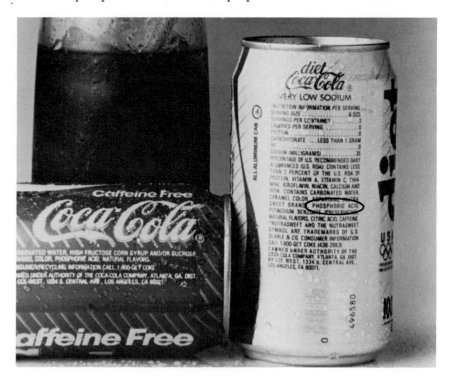

Research findings now indicate that maintaining a 2:1 calcium-to-phosphorus ratio may not be necessary. Bone formation and maintenance appear to proceed normally when the ratios are 2:1 to 1:2.[25] Current U.S. intake ratios average between 1:1.4 and 1:1.8, both within the acceptable range.[26]

Deficiency Phosphorus deficiency is very rare and is only known to occur among alcohol abusers, people with kidney disease, and habitual users of antacids—particularly those made from aluminum hydroxide. Some antacids reduce stomach acidity by binding phosphorus. In the process, however, the antacids render phosphorus unavailable for absorption. People with low blood levels of phosphorus feel weak and confused and experience pain in their bones and joints.[27]

Toxicity High intakes of phosphorus produce muscle tetany, a condition that has been observed among infants who are given only cow's milk during the first few weeks of life. Cow's milk contains twice the phosphorus of human milk and many infant formulas, and it can produce what is referred to as "cow's milk tetany" among very young infants. Adults appear to be able to tolerate up to 2 grams of phosphorus per day without consequence.[23]

MAGNESIUM (Mg)

Magnesium is a brilliant white metal that occurs in abundance in nature. An adult human body contains around an ounce of magnesium (about 5 teaspoons' worth), most of it located in the bones and muscles.

Plants are dietary sources of magnesium.

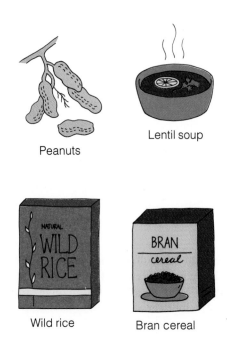

Functions

Functions of magnesium:
component of bone
transmission of nerve and muscle impulses
enzyme cofactor in energy formation
enzyme cofactor in protein synthesis
enzyme cofactor in calcium utilization

Magnesium has several functions in the human body. Like calcium, it is a component of bone (although a very minor one compared to calcium) and is involved in the transmission of impulses among nerve cells and muscle cells. Magnesium is also required as a cofactor by certain enzymes involved in the formation of energy and proteins and in the utilization of calcium. Magnesium's role as a cofactor in calcium utilization is particularly important. Without magnesium, the enzyme that facilitates the passage of calcium across cell membranes fails to act. This reduces the cells' uptake of calcium and results in symptoms of both calcium deficiency and magnesium deficiency.

Sources

Magnesium is widely distributed in both plant and animal products, but plants are by far the richer sources (Table 11-8). Breads and cereals, dried beans, nuts, and vegetables such as bean sprouts and black-eyed peas are among the best sources of magnesium. Although meats, milk, and cheese contain relatively little magnesium compared to plant sources, they can make an important contribution to magnesium intake if consumed regularly. As Table 11-9 shows, people in the U.S. get magnesium from a wide assortment of foods.

Recommended Intake

The RDA has been set at 300 mg magnesium per day for adult females and at 350 mg for males. Intakes of magnesium in the U.S. tend to be marginally sufficient.[28] Intakes below 220 mg per day eventually produce magnesium deficiency in adults.[27]

People at risk of developing magnesium deficiency:
alcohol abusers
people with diseases that cause malabsorption
people who are critically ill

Deficiency Most cases of magnesium deficiency in the U.S. result from diseases that reduce magnesium absorption or increase its excretion.[29] Alcohol abusers and people with gastrointestinal disorders that cause malabsorption are at high risk of developing a deficiency.[30] The diagnosis of magnesium deficiency among critically ill people in general is quite common. One study found that magnesium deficiency was a problem for 20% of the people admitted to a medical intensive care unit.[31]

The signs of magnesium deficiency are as diverse as its functions. They include muscle spasms, irregular heartbeat, convulsions, confusion, and personality changes. Since a deficiency of magnesium reduces calcium utilization, people with a magnesium deficiency also show signs of calcium deficiency.[29]

Toxicity Supplemental doses of magnesium are not very toxic in healthy people. The human body has two control mechanisms that protect it against magnesium overdose. First, the amount of magnesium that is absorbed in the intestine automatically decreases as magnesium intake increases (Figure 11-9); and second, the kidneys are able to excrete excess amounts of magnesium rapidly. Although high intakes of magnesium do not build up in the blood and cause problems, the presence of 3 to 5 grams of it in the intestine causes diarrhea.[32]

TABLE 11-8
Food sources of magnesium

Food	Amount	Magnesium, mg*
Legumes		
lentils, cooked	½ c	134
split peas, cooked	½ c	134
tofu	½ c	130
black-eyed peas	½ c	58
lima beans	½ c	32
Nuts		
peanuts	¼ c	247
cashews	¼ c	93
almonds	¼ c	80
Grains		
Bran Buds®	1 c	240
wild rice, cooked	½ c	119
fortified breakfast cereal	1 c	85
wheat germ	2 T	45
Vegetables		
bean sprouts	½ c	98
spinach, cooked	½ c	48
Milk and Milk Products		
milk	1 c	30
cheddar cheese	1 oz	8
American cheese	1 oz	6
Meats		
chicken	3 oz	25
beef	3 oz	20
pork	3 oz	20

*The RDAs for adults 23–50 years of age are 300 mg for females and 350 mg for males.

TABLE 11-9
Sources of magnesium in the U.S. diet

Food Category	Percentage of Total Magnesium Intake
Grains, breads, and cereals	21
Vegetables	17
Milk and milk products	16
Meats	15
Other (eggs, beans, nuts, fruits)	31

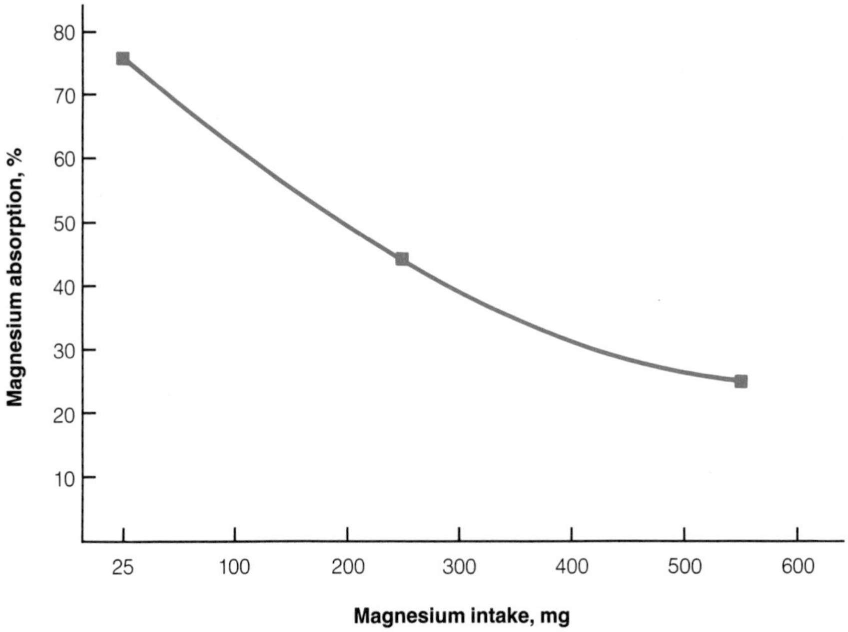

FIGURE 11-9
Magnesium absorption decreases as magnesium intake increases.

IRON (Fe)

Iron's chemical abbreviation is Fe; *it abbreviates the Latin word for the mineral,* ferrum.

What is the first thought that crosses your mind when you read the word *iron*? Students majoring in architecture are likely to think of a strong building material. A geologist might think of the many different types of rocks that contain iron. But to many nutritionists, the word automatically elicits thoughts about iron deficiency.

Iron deficiency continues to be a major public health problem. It is the most common nutrient deficiency in the U.S. and affects 10% to 20% of the world's population.[33] Although it causes few deaths worldwide, iron deficiency contributes to ill health and impaired performance for millions of people.

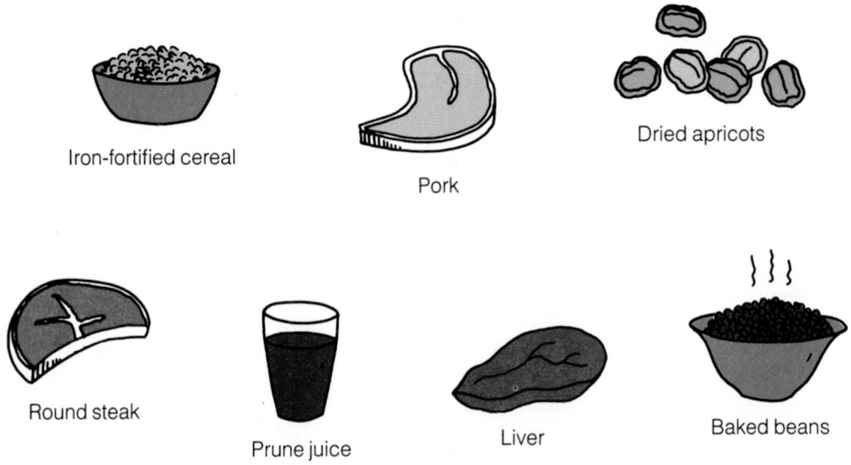

Dietary sources of iron. Iron is abundantly distributed in nature in rocks, but good food sources of iron are rare.

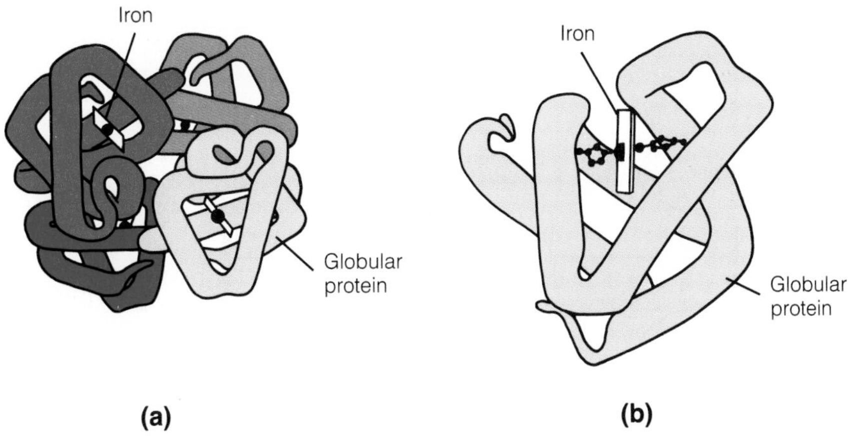

FIGURE 11-10
Molecular structure of *(a)* hemoglobin and *(b)* myoglobin, the two major iron-containing proteins in the body.

Functions

Most of the iron in the human body is incorporated in the proteins **hemoglobin** and **myoglobin**. Hemoglobin is the primary component of red blood cells, and myoglobin is a major protein of muscle cells (Figure 11-10). A small amount of the body's iron serves as a cofactor for enzymes involved in energy metabolism. Some iron is generally present in the liver and in bone marrow as **ferritin**, the storage form of iron. Altogether, the body's content of iron totals about 4 grams—approximately the weight of a penny.

hemoglobin: The iron-containing protein of red blood cells.

myoglobin: The iron-containing protein in muscle cells.

ferritin: The storage form of iron; most of the body's iron is stored in the liver and bone marrow.

Iron's Role in Hemoglobin and Myoglobin The iron in hemoglobin and myoglobin functions to provide oxygen to cells and to remove carbon dioxide from them. Oxygen is needed in large amounts by cells for the aerobic (oxygen-requiring) pathway of energy formation, the citric acid cycle (chapter 3). The end products of the citric acid cycle are ATP, water, and carbon dioxide. The carbon dioxide that is formed becomes toxic if it accumulates in the cells, and it does not accumulate if the iron contained in hemoglobin removes it from them.

Functions of iron:
- *transport of oxygen and carbon dioxide in hemoglobin and myoglobin*
- *enzyme cofactor in energy metabolism*

Iron contained in the hemoglobin component of red blood cells loosely attaches to oxygen when blood circulates through the lungs. The oxygen remains attached to the iron as it moves throughout the circulatory system until it passes near cells that need oxygen for energy formation. Those cells chemically pull oxygen away from the iron in the hemoglobin. The unbound reactive iron that remains immediately combines with carbon dioxide, a waste product of the citric acid cycle, and transports it to the lungs, where it is released (Figure 11-11). By repeating this oxygen pick-up and drop-off process, iron delivers about a quart of oxygen to cells each minute. (The combination of iron with oxygen or carbon dioxide also serves a "colorful" role; see Box 11-4.)

Muscle cells require more oxygen than most other types of cells because they produce large amounts of energy for physical movement. Myoglobin, which can trap the oxygen delivered by hemoglobin to muscle cells, store it, and release it for energy formation when needed, acts to increase the supply of oxygen that is available to muscles.

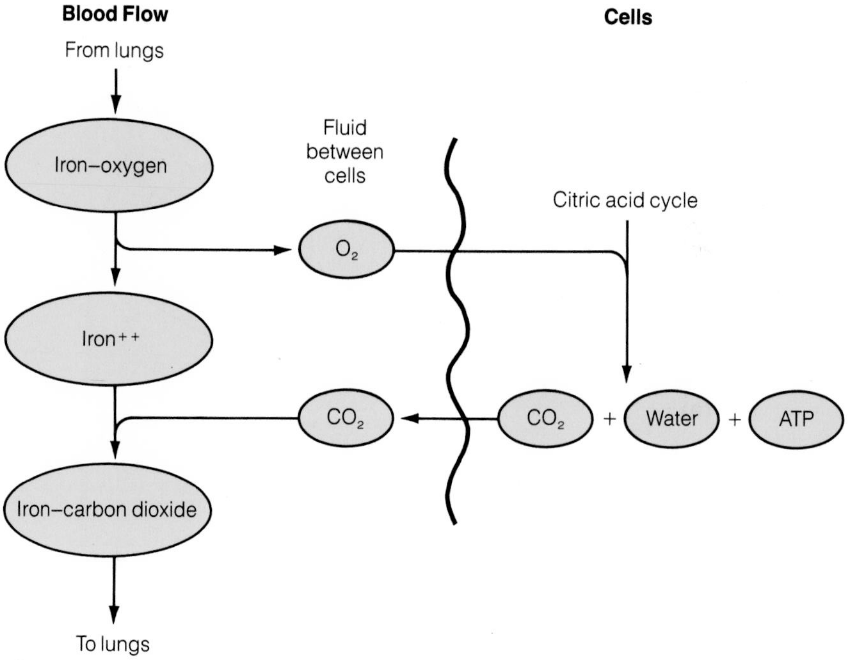

FIGURE 11-11
The role of iron in transporting oxygen to cells and carbon dioxide away from cells.

Food Sources

While nearly all foods contain iron, few foods contain very much of it. With the exception of a limited number of foods such as liver and prune juice, the "good" food sources of iron provide only 10% to 20% of the adult female RDA per serving (Table 11-10). Because iron is found in small amounts in most foods, diets containing a few good iron sources still provide only about 6 mg of iron per 1,000 calories consumed.[34] This situation means that most men can get the 10 mg of iron recommended for them each day, but it leaves many women with deficient intakes. The 18 mg of iron recommended for women is difficult to obtain from the low level of calories most women consume. Women in particular need good food sources of iron. (A food preparation method that can help you increase your iron intake is explained in Box 11-5.)

BOX 11-4

BLOOD RED

Why is blood red? Because oxygen is attached to the iron in the hemoglobin in it.

Hemoglobin is a reddish substance that varies from bright red to dark red depending on how much oxygen is attached to its iron. Blood leaving the lungs is saturated with oxygen and thus bright red. On its route back to the lungs, blood becomes darker in color, reflecting the substitution of carbon dioxide for oxygen on the iron atoms in hemoglobin. The blood vessels that carry oxygenated blood away from the lungs are called *arteries*. The darker-colored blood vessels (like the ones that are visible on the back of your hand), which carry carbon-dioxide-ladened blood back to the lungs, are called *veins*.

TABLE 11-10
Food sources of iron

Food	Amount	Iron, mg*
Meat and Meat Alternates		
liver	3 oz	7.5
round steak	3 oz	3.0
hamburger, lean	3 oz	3.0
baked beans	½ c	3.0
pork	3 oz	2.7
white beans	½ c	2.7
soy beans	½ c	2.5
pork and beans	½ c	2.3
lima beans	½ c	2.2
black-eyed peas	½ c	1.7
fish	3 oz	1.0
chicken	3 oz	1.0
Grains		
iron-fortified breakfast cereals	1 c	8.0 (4–18)
oatmeal (fortified)	1 c	8.0
bagel	1	1.7
English muffin	1	1.6
rye bread	1 slice	1.0
whole-wheat bread	1 slice	0.8
white bread	1 slice	0.6
Fruit		
prune juice	6 oz	7.0
dried apricots	½ c	2.5
prunes	5 med.	2.0
raisins	¼ c	1.3
plums	3 med.	1.1
Vegetables		
spinach, cooked	½ c	2.3
peas	½ c	1.6
asparagus	½ c	1.5

*RDAs for adults aged 23 to 50 are 10 mg for males and 18 mg for females.

The low amount of iron contained in most foods, and the common problem of iron deficiency has led to the addition of iron to cereals through enrichment and fortification. As a result, grain products have become a leading source of iron in the U.S. diet. About one-third of our total dietary iron comes from grain products, another third from meats, and the remaining third from a broad variety of foods (Table 11-11).[10]

Absorption of Iron Iron is not readily absorbed by the human intestinal tract. Factors such as the bioavailability of iron in foods, the types of foods eaten together, and the body's level of iron stores all influence iron absorption.

■
TABLE 11-11
Sources of iron in the U.S. diet

Food Category	Percentage of Total Iron Intake
Grains, breads, and cereals	35
Meats	32
Other (vegetables, beans, nuts, eggs)	33

heme iron: Iron attached to the hemoglobin and myoglobin in animal tissues. About 40% of the total amount of iron in meats is in this form.

nonheme iron: Iron that is not bound to hemoglobin or myoglobin. In plants, iron is usually bound to phytates.

Iron exists in foods in two forms: heme iron and nonheme iron. **Heme iron** is supplied by the hemoglobin and myoglobin that occur in meats. It is more readily absorbed than nonheme iron, because enzymes in the small intestine are able to digest these two proteins and free the iron they contain. On the other hand, **nonheme iron** is generally attached to substances in foods that resist digestion. Thus, it is less available to the body. In general, 10% to 20% of heme iron is absorbed, and only 1% to 8% of nonheme iron is absorbed (Figure 11-12).[38]

The low bioavailability of nonheme sources of iron can be illustrated with these examples:

- Both a 3-ounce hamburger and a cup of asparagus contain around 3 mg of iron. Because of the difference in the bioavailability of iron, however, 20 times as much iron can be absorbed from the hamburger as from the asparagus.

■
FIGURE 11-12
Average percentage of iron absorbed from selected foods by normal adults.

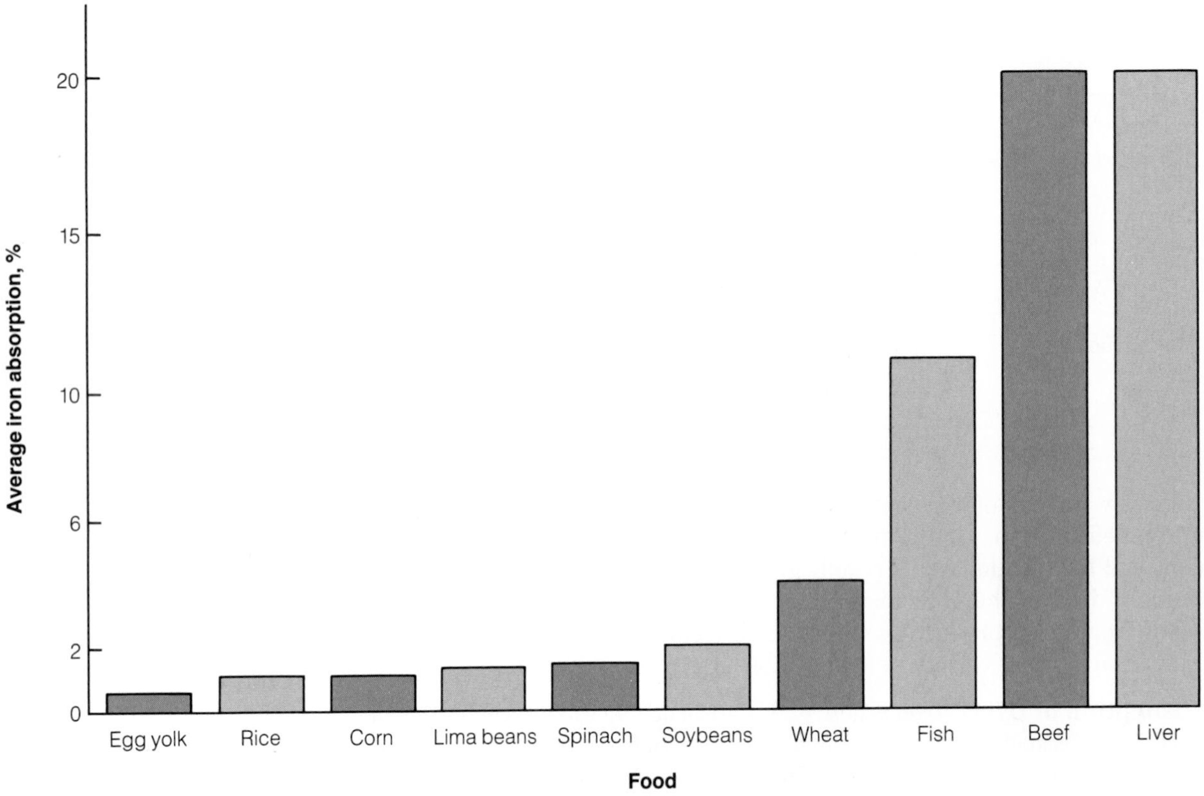

- Drinking tea with meals containing plant sources of iron further reduces the amount of iron that is absorbed.
- Eggs contain a fair amount of iron—about 1 mg per egg—but the iron in eggs is tenaciously bound to substances that resist digestion and block iron absorption.[36] Although food composition tables would indicate that eggs are a fairly good source of iron, they actually are not because so little of their iron is absorbed.
- The iron contained in iron-fortified cereals is in the form of poorly absorbed nonheme iron. The bioavailability of iron added to fortified cereals is about the same as it is for iron that occurs naturally in the cereal.[37] So, for example, only about 1% of the iron that is added to rice or corn and about 4% of the iron that is added to wheat products is available for absorption.

The absorption of nonheme iron is increased when vitamin C–rich foods are consumed along with plant sources of iron. Vitamin C converts the nonheme iron to a more absorbable form during digestion. Vitamin C is such a potent enhancer of iron absorption that it is thought that inadequate intakes of it may contribute substantially to the development of iron deficiency.[39,40] In general, good levels of iron absorption can be expected if daily diets contain meats, or contain about 75 mg of vitamin C if meats are not consumed.[40]

The body is not able to excrete high levels of absorbed iron, and iron can become toxic if it is allowed to accumulate in blood and tissues. The body partially protects itself from the harmful effects of high iron levels by limiting the amount that is absorbed. It also protects itself (to an extent) from iron deficiency by increasing the amount that is absorbed when the body's stores of iron are low. The amount of iron absorbed from foods can range from 2% when iron stores are high to over 30% when iron stores are depleted (Figure 11-13). The body's ability to regulate iron absorption provides a good deal of protection against iron deficiency and overdose in most situations.

Recommended Intake

The RDA for iron for females aged 23 to 50 is 18 mg; for males it is 10 mg. The RDAs for iron assume that people eat both meats and plants, and that an average of 10% of the iron consumed will be absorbed. People who get

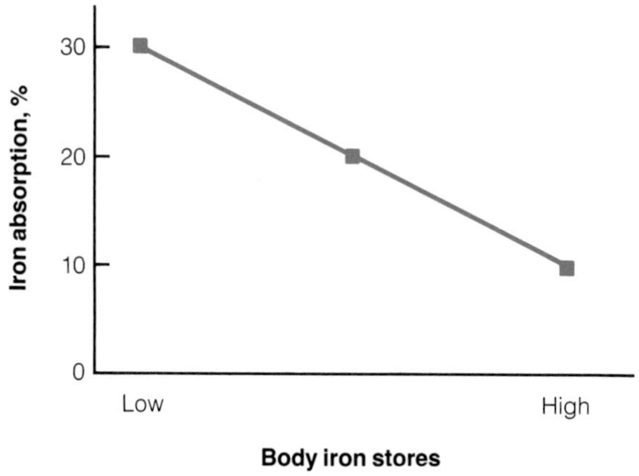

FIGURE 11-13
Iron absorption decreases as body stores of iron increase.

BOX 11-5

A DEPARTMENT OF DEFENSE RECIPE FOR IRON FORTIFICATION

About thirty years ago, a group of nutrition experts was brought together by the Department of Defense to study the adequacy of diets of military personnel. One component of the dietary assessment specifically addressed the adequacy of iron intake. Samples of foods prepared at various military bases were sent to a central laboratory for analysis of their iron content.

The experts were surprised to find that the amount of iron in foods from some of the bases was substantially higher than the foods prepared at other military bases. The reason for this unexpected result became clear when it was discovered that foods prepared in cast-iron pans, rather than glass cookware, contained unusually high levels of iron.[35] It was further noted that acidic foods extracted a good deal more iron from cast-iron pans during the cooking than nonacidic foods.

Cast-iron pans are not used as much as they once were in American kitchens, so their contribution to iron intake has declined. Cast-iron pans are heavy and they rust if they are not "seasoned." You can season cast iron by lightly coating the inside of the pan with vegetable oil and then heating the pan for a few minutes on the range or in the oven. This process may need to be repeated several times to season a pan to the point where foods do not stick to it. The pans must be reseasoned each time they are washed with dish detergent.

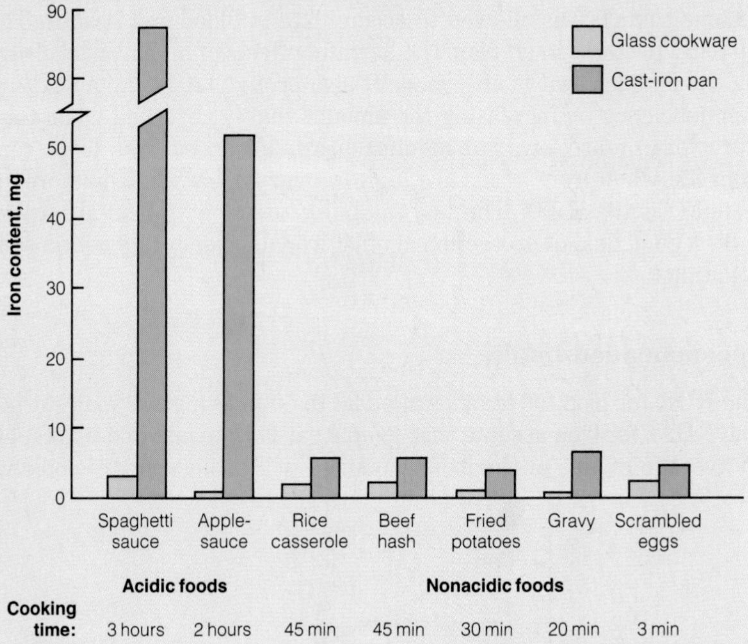

Iron content of 3½ ounces of food cooked in glass cookware and cast-iron pans.

most of their iron from meats need less than the RDA, and those who rely primarily on plant sources of iron may need more than the RDA.

Women need more iron than men, and they are much more likely to become iron deficient.[42] Throughout their reproductive years (roughly between the ages of 12 and 50) women lose an average of 1.5 mg of iron per day due to blood losses occurring with menstruation.[40] A good deal of iron is also

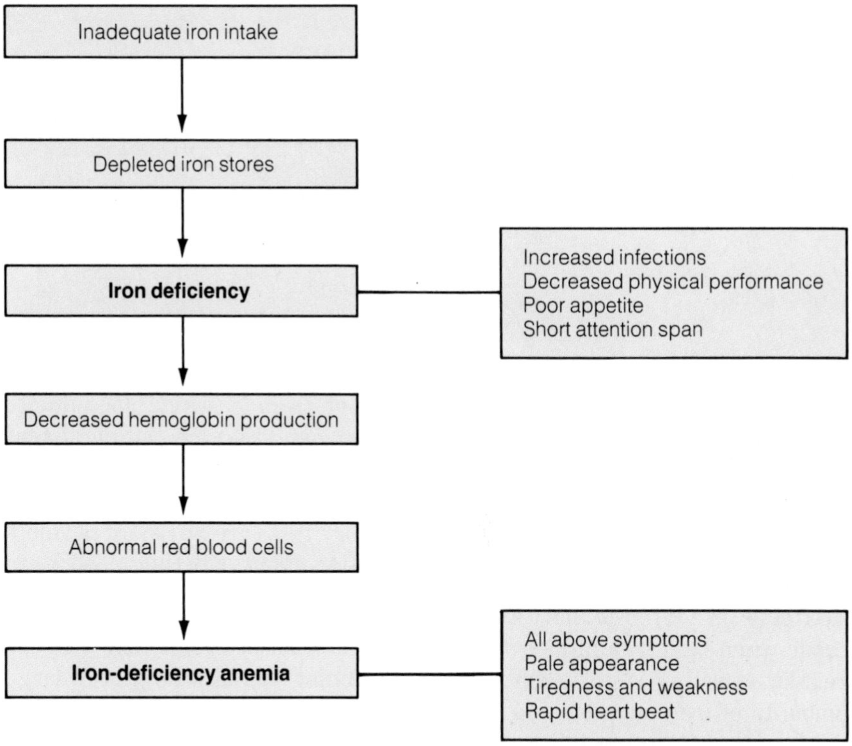

FIGURE 11-14
Progression of the development of iron-deficiency anemia due to inadequate iron intake.

needed during pregnancy, increasing further the iron need of many women. Except for pregnancy, when iron supplements are recommended, women can generally meet their iron requirements by consuming a diet that regularly includes meat and plant sources of iron along with adequate amounts of vitamin C.

Deficiency Iron deficiency continues to be a public health problem in the U.S., especially among pregnant women, young children, and teenagers; up to 20% of pregnant women, 14% of teenagers, and 9% of children aged 1 to 2 years are iron-deficient.[44] Studies show that people in low-income families are more likely to develop iron deficiency than others.

People at risk of developing iron deficiency:
pregnant women
young children
teenagers

Problems stemming from a lack of iron occur in two stages; the first stage is referred to as "iron deficiency," and the second, iron-deficiency **anemia**. Iron deficiency is diagnosed when iron stores are absent and the body does not have quite as much iron as it needs to function normally (Figure 11-14). Effects of iron deficiency include reduced resistance to infection, physical sluggishness, poor appetite, and shortened attention span.[45,46] Iron-deficiency anemia occurs when the available iron is insufficient for normal hemoglobin production. Without sufficient iron, red blood cells become pale and small and contain little hemoglobin (Figure 11-15). The body cells of people with iron-deficiency anemia do not receive enough oxygen. These people's skin is pale, they feel tired and weak, and their hearts beat rapidly in attempting to supply more oxygen to cells.

anemia: A condition in which the body's content of red blood cells, or the amount of hemoglobin within the cells, is lower than normal. There are many types of anemia, including the genetic sickle-cell anemia and those caused by deficiencies in vitamin B_{12} and folic acid. Iron-deficiency anemia, however, is the most common.

The diagnosis of iron deficiency is often based on measurements of the amount of hemoglobin in red blood cells. Hemoglobin values below 13 grams per 100 ml of blood in men and below 12 mg in women generally lead to diagnoses of iron deficiency.[47]

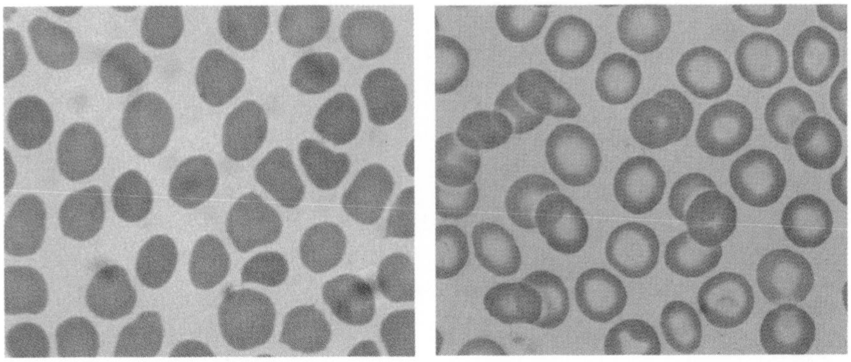

FIGURE 11-15

(a) Normal red blood cells.
(b) Red blood cells of a person with iron-deficiency anemia. The cells in (b) contain less hemoglobin and therefore less oxygen.

Major causes of iron deficiency:
inadequate iron intake
inadequate iron absorption
blood loss

Iron deficiency and its anemia also develop from losses in blood due to injury or disease. Injury-caused hemorrhaging and the slow but persistent losses of blood that occur with bleeding ulcers often produce anemia. People who donate blood too often and those who have conditions that require frequent drawing of blood samples for laboratory tests are at risk of developing anemia.[36] (Box 11-6 gives some information about donating blood.)

Toxicity The iron-toxicity disease is referred to as *iron poisoning*. It can occur when high iron intakes (over 75 mg per day) are combined with the regular consumption of alcohol.[36] Iron poisoning can also develop if large amounts of iron supplements are taken in a short period of time. Single doses of over 12 grams of iron in women and over 17 grams in men produce iron poisoning.[48] The excess iron that enters the blood cannot be excreted and it deposits in tissues. Because the iron that deposits in tissues is reactive, it causes damage to cells and impairs the functions of tissues and organs. Recently, iron overload has been associated with an increased risk of certain types of cancer in men.[49] Acute iron overload can lead to death, and it does so at least 2,000 times each year in the U.S.[50]

Iron overdose is a leading cause of hospitalization of young children in the U.S. (Table 11-12). It most often results from the ingestion of iron supplements found in the home. (Iron supplements containing 120 mg of iron are commonly prescribed during pregnancy, and they sometimes end up stored on the shelves of medicine cabinets where toddlers may find them.) The lethal dose of iron for a two-year-old is about 3 grams, the amount present in 25 pills that contain 120 mg of iron each.[48]

TABLE 11-12

Accidental overdoses of chemical substances by children up to age four in the U.S.[50]

Substance	Cases per 100,000 Children
Aspirin and substitutes	12.7
Solvents/petroleum products	11.2
Tranquilizers	9.9
Iron supplements	8.7
Corrosives and caustics	7.4

BOX 11-6

DONATING BLOOD

The adult human body contains about 21 cups of blood. Blood donations are generally a pint (2 cups). Thus, a blood donor gives about a tenth of his or her total supply. Healthy people generally can donate blood four times a year without harmful consequences. As a precaution, blood banks screen all potential donors' blood. If the iron content is found to be low, blood is not drawn from that person that day.

■ ■ ■

ZINC (Zn)

Zinc was not recognized as an essential nutrient until 1958. Before that, zinc had been thought of as toxic to humans. The primary experience scientists had previously had with zinc and health was zinc toxicity, which occurred in workers who processed zinc ores. Studies of zinc toxicity ultimately led to the identification of a dietary requirement for zinc and to the consequences of zinc deficiency. Zinc deficiency is now recognized as a cause of poor growth among children in many parts of the world, including some locations in the U.S.[51]

Functions

Zinc is a component of more than 200 enzymes, most of which are involved in protein and DNA synthesis. It is not an enzyme cofactor. Rather, zinc is incorporated into the structure of the enzymes, and enzyme levels decrease if zinc is not available when the enzymes are produced. Reduced levels of

Functions of zinc:

$$\text{amino acids} \xrightarrow{\text{zinc}} \text{proteins}$$

$$\text{DNA}_1 \xrightarrow{\text{zinc}} \text{DNA}_2$$

Dietary sources of zinc.

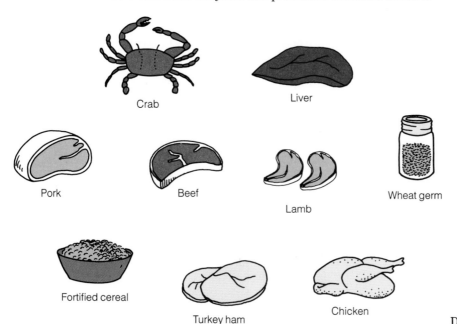

the zinc-containing enzymes cause a slowdown in protein synthesis and cell division. Consequently, normal growth and the repair and maintenance of tissues depend on an adequate supply of zinc.

Food Sources

The richest food sources of zinc—as well as iron—are meats. (See Table 11-13 and Box 11-7.) Many other foods contain small amounts of zinc, and their contribution to our total zinc intake largely depends on how frequently we consume them. Milk and milk products are the second-leading source of dietary zinc (Table 11-14), not so much because they are rich sources but because we tend to consume them often.[10]

In contrast, grains are a leading source of zinc in countries where little meat is eaten. Grains such as rice, corn, wheat, bulgar, and millet are major dietary sources of zinc in many countries. Whether zinc is primarily supplied by plants or by meats is an important issue, because the zinc in foods is not equally well absorbed.

Bioavailability of Zinc If the quality of food sources of zinc were graded, meats would be grade-A sources, and plants would be grade-B sources. Much of the zinc in meats is present in zinc-containing enzymes. This zinc is detached during digestion, which makes it available for absorption. On the other hand, the zinc contained in grains, beans, and other plants is less readily separated from the substances to which it is attached during digestion. Consequently, only a small amount of the zinc in plant foods becomes available for absorption. (See Figure 11-16.)

If the thought has crossed your mind that this discussion of zinc bioavailability sounds a lot like what you read about iron, go to the head of the class. The factors that affect zinc absorption are very similar to those that affect iron absorption.

Zinc Absorption and Iron Supplements Iron supplements in doses of 30 mg or more have recently been found to cause a decrease in zinc absorption.[52] The common use of iron supplements by pregnant women and infants (people with a high need for zinc because of the amount of protein synthesis

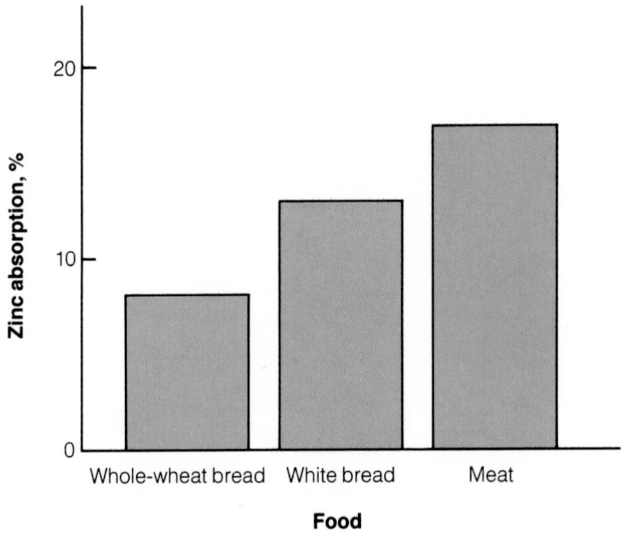

FIGURE 11-16
Absorption of zinc from three food sources.

TABLE 11-13
Food sources of zinc

Food	Amount	Zinc, mg*
Meats		
liver	3 oz	4.6
beef	3 oz	4.0
crab	½ c	3.5
lamb	3 oz	3.5
turkey ham	3 oz	2.5
pork	3 oz	2.4
chicken	3 oz	2.0
Legumes		
dried beans (cooked)	½ c	1.0
split peas (cooked)	½ c	0.9
Grains		
fortified breakfast cereals	1 c	1.5–4.0
wheat germ	2 T	2.4
brown rice	1 c	1.2
oatmeal	1 c	1.2
bran flakes	1 c	1.0
white rice	1 c	0.8
Nuts and Seeds		
pecans	¼ c	2.0
cashews	¼ c	1.8
sunflower seeds	¼ c	1.7
peanut butter	2 T	0.9
Milk and Milk Products		
cheddar cheese	1 oz	1.1
milk (whole)	1 c	0.9
American cheese	1 oz	0.8

*The RDA for adults aged 23–50 is 15 mg.

TABLE 11-14
Sources of zinc in the U.S. diet[10]

Food Group	Percentage of Total Dietary Supply of Zinc
Meats	46
Milk and milk products	21
Grains and cereals	13*
Fruits and vegetables	6
Other foods	14

*Grains and cereal products contributed 26% of the total supply of zinc in 1909–13.

BOX 11-7

OCTOPUS ANYONE?

Some seafoods that are excellent sources of zinc are not included in Table 11-13 because they are rarely eaten in the U.S. Some of them are listed here, along with their zinc content.

Seafood	Zinc, mg
octopus, 3 oz	37.7
squid, 3 oz	37.7
oysters (raw), 2	33.1
anchovies, 3 oz	15.6

occurring in their bodies) has led to concern about the effects of iron supplements on zinc status. Zinc and iron compete for the same absorption sites on the surface of the small intestine. If iron is present in higher amounts than zinc (which can occur when iron supplements are taken), iron will occupy most of the absorption sites and thereby crowd zinc out. The influence of iron supplements on decreasing zinc absorption can be lessened by taking iron supplements between meals or by lowering the dosage of iron.[52]

Recommended Intake

It has been estimated that only 8% of U.S. diets provide the adult RDA for zinc of 15 mg per day.[53] On average, people in the U.S. consume about 10 mg of zinc each day[55]—enough to meet their day-to-day needs, but not enough to maintain zinc stores.[53] Vegetarians need to consume considerably more than the 15 mg of zinc per day recommended because of the poor bioavailability of zinc in plant food sources.[56]

Deficiency Zinc deficiency is fairly prevalent throughout the world. In the U.S., mild forms of zinc deficiency have been identified in 2% to 3% of infants and children.[57] These mild deficiencies cause slow growth and poor appetite.[51] Zinc deficiency associated with the use of iron supplements during pregnancy has also been observed in the U.S.[52]

Severe zinc deficiencies have profound effects on growth, susceptibility to infection, and sexual maturation. The striking effects of severe zinc deficiency were first identified in studies of Iranian and Egyptian dwarfs. Although the men studied were in their early twenties, they had the physical appearance and sexual maturation level of ten-year-old boys. All of the men's diets were high in cereals and beans and very low in meats. (Zinc deficiency was suspected because laboratory studies a few years earlier had demonstrated that zinc deficiency produces similar results in animals.) Supplementation with zinc produced a rapid recovery in growth and sexual maturation in all of the men.[51]

Toxicity

> *Zinc may be only a poor relation of gold in the mineral world, but in the health food market it has financial clout.*
>
> *Consumer Reports*, January 1980

Zinc has been widely—and inappropriately—promoted as an antistress, cold-curing, virility-promoting mineral. Although these claims are false, they have made the use of zinc supplements very attractive to many people. Unfortunately, the negative effects of zinc supplements have received little publicity. Self-medication with zinc at levels greater than 15 mg per day is unwise because of the potentially adverse effects of high levels of zinc on blood lipids.[59] Supplemental zinc at doses of about the adult RDA level appear to block the effect of exercise on increasing body levels of HDL-cholesterol[60] (the lipoprotein you want to have in high amounts in your blood). Doses of zinc of 150 mg per day or more raise LDL-cholesterol[61] (the one you do not want to go up) and produce a drop in HDL-cholesterol.[59] (LDL- and HDL-cholesterol were discussed in chapter 7.)

IODINE (I)

The story behind iodine is rich and intriguing. Shortly after it was discovered in 1811, it became a very popular remedy. It was used in vapors and pills to "cure" a wide assortment of illnesses. In French hospitals, strips of gauze saturated with iodine were hung from the ceilings (like flypaper) to rid the air of germs. Iodine was thought to be so protective against disease

Iodine *is derived from the Greek* ioeidēs, *"violet in color."*

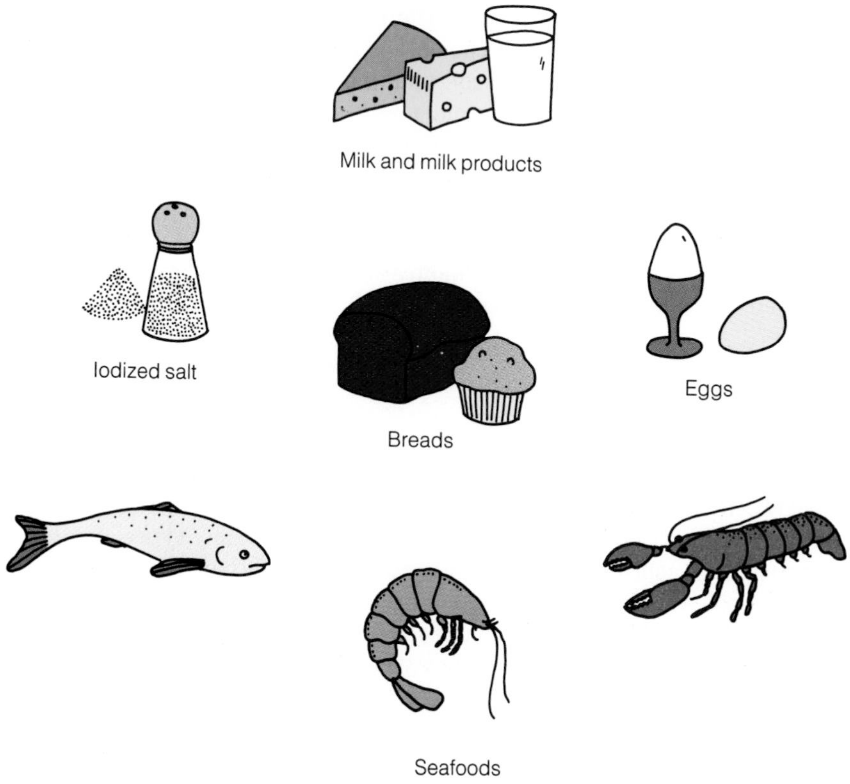

Seafoods are good sources of iodine, but most of the iodine in our diets comes from the intentional and unintentional addition of iodine to foods.

BOX 11-8

THE ACCIDENTAL DISCOVERY OF THE IODINE-CONTAINING THYROID HORMONES

Our knowledge of the role of iodine in the body has grown out of a laboratory mistake made in 1895. Eugene Baumann, a German scientist, was attempting to analyze the protein content of thyroid tissue. His usual procedure was to extract the protein with sulfuric acid. One day, however, he picked up nitric acid by mistake and added it to the thyroid mixture. To his astonishment, the characteristic violet fumes of iodine gas swirled up from the mixture. Thus began the discovery of the role of iodine in the thyroid.

that some people hung a bottle of it around their necks.[62] Iodine is still widely used as a disinfectant in medicinal lotions and cleansing solutions.

In addition to its property of destroying germs, iodine is known for its deficiency disease, **goiter**. Iodine-deficiency goiter has been a public health problem since at least as early as 3000 B.C.[63] The treatment for the deficiency, iodine-rich foods or extracts, has been known for hundreds of years, and yet the disease still affects millions of people in developing countries.[64]

goiter: Enlargement of the thyroid gland. When it is caused by a dietary lack of iodine, the disease is called *iodine-deficiency goiter*.

Functions

Although iodine is distributed throughout the body, it is concentrated in the thyroid gland, a pink "pad" of tissue wrapped around the front of the esophagus and windpipe at the base of the neck. The thyroid is the only tissue known to require iodine, and the only known role of iodine is in the formation of two important, iodine-containing hormones. (Box 11-8 tells how iodine was discovered in the thyroid.)

Iodine-containing thyroid hormones regulate the rate of energy metabolism and protein synthesis in cells. During growth, these hormones increase the pace at which energy and protein are formed by cells; when growth is not occurring, they decrease the rates. Without sufficient iodine, insufficient amounts of the thyroid hormones are produced, and growth and development are slow and abnormal.

Sources

The sea is the source of most of the iodine that enters the food chain and eventually the diet. Plants from the sea that are rarely eaten in the U.S. (seaweed, for example) are the only naturally rich sources of dietary iodine. Table 11-15 lists our most important food sources. Many types of ocean fish and shellfish contain moderate amounts of iodine. Other than these sources, most foods are naturally low in iodine. The iodine content of foods such as eggs, meats, and milk and milk products depends on the amount of iodine contained in the animal feed and on whether iodine was added to the foods during processing. Iodine is added to foods in several ways. It is purposefully added to salt, and it incidentally ends up in milk, bread, and some colored foods.

TABLE 11-15
Food sources of iodine

Food	Amount	Average Iodine Content, mcg*
Iodized salt	1 t	570
Seafoods	3 oz	56
Egg	1 large	37
Milk and milk products	8 oz	29
Vegetables	½ c	27
Meats	3 oz	22

*The RDA for adults aged 23–50 is 150 mcg.

Iodized salt has been available in the U.S. since 1924. It was introduced to halt **endemic** goiter in sections of the country referred to as the "goiter belt." Figure 11-17 shows areas of North America where goiter was unusually prevalent during the 1920s. The widespread use of iodized salt by people in the goiter belt led to a decline in goiter, and today it is rare in the U.S. About 50% of the salt sold in the U.S. is iodized, and on average, people receive about 150 mcg of iodine from iodized salt each day.[65] The addition of iodine to salt is voluntary, and the word *iodized* is clearly printed on the packaging of salts that are iodized.

endemic: A disease or condition that recurs continuously among a significant number of people within a population. Protein–calorie malnutrition and goiter are examples of endemic problems in some countries. Iron deficiency and obesity are endemic problems in the U.S.

Iodine incidentally ends up in foods by three major routes. It is widely employed by the dairy industry to disinfect the vats in which milk is pasteurized. Some of the iodine in the disinfectant adheres to the vats and enters the milk. Iodine is also used to improve the texture of bread dough by many commercial bakeries, and it is a component of food dyes such as Red number 3. Iodized salt and incidental sources of iodine are the major contributors to the iodine intake of people in the U.S.[66]

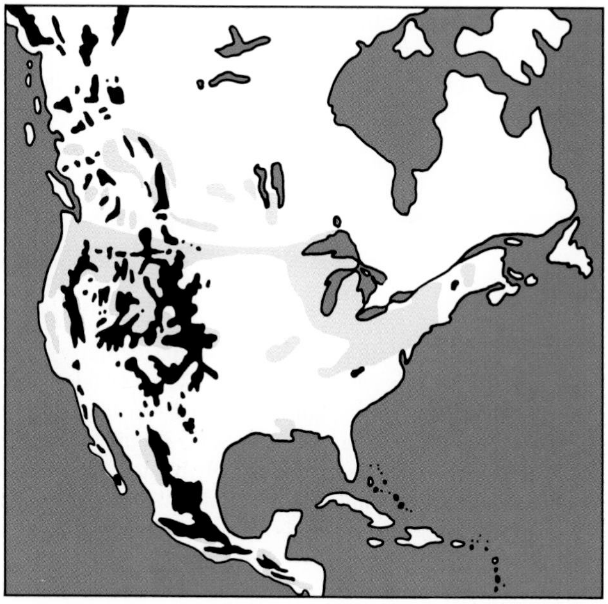

FIGURE 11-17
Regions of endemic goiter in North America in the early twentieth century (*violet areas*). Dark areas represent mountainous regions.

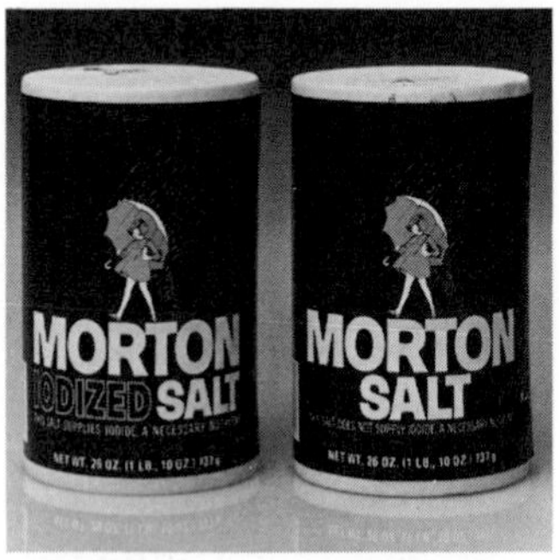

Iodized salt and incidental sources of iodine are the major contributors to the iodine intake of people in the United States.

Recommended Intake

Average daily intakes of iodine in the U.S. range from 4 to 13 times the adult RDA of 150 mcg.[62,68] Intakes of 2,000 mcg or less are probably safe, but ideally, diets should not contain more than 300 mcg.[62,67]

More iodine is available in the U.S. food supply today than there was just twenty years ago. The current issue is whether we might be getting too much iodine.[66,68] Although no solid evidence exists to show that the current levels of iodine intake are hazardous to health, some experts are expressing warnings with regard to further increases in iodine intake in the U.S.[67]

Deficiency Cases of goiter tend to "cluster" in areas where the soil content of iodine is very low and where iodine-fortified products are not used.[64] For example, over 40 million people living in areas of India with a poor soil content of iodine and no access to iodized salt have iodine-deficiency goiter.[64] India has instituted a program for iodizing all salt produced in the country by 1992.

An extreme example of the clustering of goiter cases has been noted among two nearby villages on the Congo River. The upstream village had a very high rate of goiter; over 80% of the population was affected. In contrast, few of the residents of the other village—on the other side of the river—developed goiter. What accounted for the difference? Iodine was being leached from the soil of the upstream village during heavy rains and floods. In effect, iodine was being removed from one bank of the river and being deposited on the bank downstream.[69]

cretinism: A condition in which the thyroid fails to function normally in the fetus and infant. Cretinism is characterized by small stature and mental retardation. When related to iodine deficiency, it is called *endemic cretinism.*

Goiter can also be caused by genetic disorders and thyroid diseases. Consumption of foods containing goitrogens (substances that induce goiter formation) may contribute to the development of goiter, as well. It is doubtful that humans consume sufficient cabbage, turnips, rutabagas, and other sources of goitrogens to cause goiter, but consumption of these foods may accentuate the effects of low iodine intakes.

Iodine deficiency can have serious consequences. Women who are iodine-deficient during pregnancy may deliver infants with a condition known as **cretinism**. This condition causes permanent reductions in physical growth and mental development. Older children and adults who experience iodine deficiency are constantly tired, have puffy hands and face, are not mentally alert, and show the classic sign of goiter—an enlarged thyroid gland (Fig-

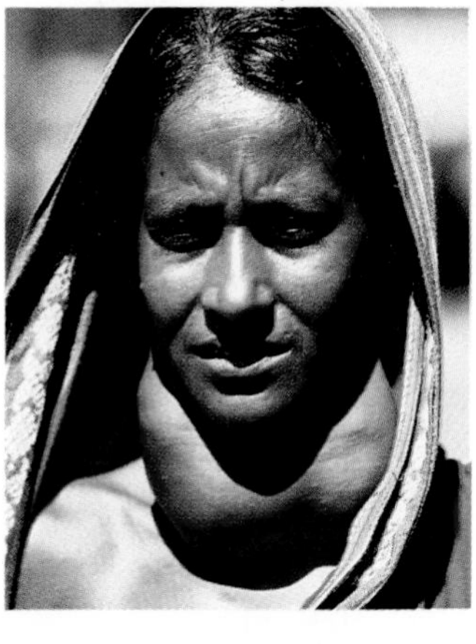

FIGURE 11-18
This Bangladesh woman suffers from goiter, the iodine-deficiency disease.

BOX 11-9

HISTORICAL NOTES ABOUT GOITER

Over the centuries, goiter has been one of the most persistent, widespread human diseases. It is a particularly obvious disease because of the visibly enlarged thyroid gland. Being visible, goiter has attracted attention. In some cultures, goiter was once considered a mark of beauty; in others it was thought to be a punishment for robbing the graves of saints. Napoleon appears to have found it particularly bothersome. He is reported to have been highly disturbed when a large number of recruits from the mountainous areas of France could not enter his army because their necks were too large to fit the uniform.[69]

ure 11-18). The enlarged thyroid does not decrease in size after the iodine deficiency has been corrected. (Some historical notes about goiter are given in Box 11-9.)

Toxicity Long-term intakes of more than 2,000 mcg of iodine per day are toxic and cause goiter. Yes, that's right; an enlarged thyroid results from excessive intakes of iodine just as from low intakes. Furthermore, the eyes of people with iodine toxicity appear to be bulging from their sockets, and the people may be very thin and "high-strung" or anxious.

Epidemics of iodine overdose have occurred in countries where iodine fortification of foods has been overdone and in Japan among people who have consumed high amounts of seaweed.[66,70]

epidemic: The appearance of a disease or condition that attacks many people within a population at the same time. Outbreaks of polio earlier in this century and the recent spread of acquired immune deficiency syndrome (AIDS) are examples of epidemics in the U.S.

■ ■ ■

REVIEW QUESTIONS

1. Define *remodeling*.
2. The cells that cause bones to form are the ____________, whereas those that cause the breakdown of bone are the ____________.
3. Name a hormone that increases bone formation.
4. List three environmental factors associated with the development of osteoporosis.
5. Phosphorus is widely distributed in foods, with one exception. What type of food tends to be a poor source of phosphorus?
6. What types of food are the leading sources of magnesium?
7. People with a deficiency of magnesium also show signs of ____________ deficiency.
8. Why do meats tend to be good sources of iron?
9. On average, approximately how many milligrams of iron are contained in 1,000 calories of a varied diet?
10. List two factors that affect iron absorption.

Answers

1. The breakdown and build up of bone tissues. The process maintains bone health.
2. Osteoblasts; osteoclasts.
3. Estrogen, growth hormone.
4. Dietary intake of calcium and vitamin D, physical activity.
5. Fruits.
6. Plants such as legumes, nuts, and grains.
7. Calcium.
8. Because they contain hemoglobin and myoglobin, iron-containing proteins found in muscle tissue.
9. 6 mg.
10. The form of the iron in food (either heme or nonheme); the body's need for iron; the presence of substances in food that bind iron and render it unavailable for absorption; the presence of vitamin C or alcohol in a meal.

PUTTING NUTRITION KNOWLEDGE TO WORK

1. How many cups of cooked beans would a 23-year-old woman need to eat each day if beans were her only dietary source of calcium?

   (See the RDA table inside the front cover and Table 11-4.)

2. Refer to Principle 10 in chapter 2. Reread the part on adaptive mechanisms. How do the mechanisms involved in iron absorption relate to this principle?

   (Consider how a person's need for iron affects iron absorption.)

3. Assume you have been diagnosed as having iron-deficiency anemia. Your pharmacist suggests that you take your iron supplements between meals with orange or other citrus juice. Why would this recommendation be made?

   (Hint: What factors enhance iron absorption?)

4. The term *milk anemia* has been applied to iron deficiency that develops in young children who consume excessive amounts of whole milk. Explain why excessive milk consumption among young children could contribute to the development of iron deficiency.

   (Is milk included in the list of iron sources in Table 11-10?)

5. Zinc deficiency occurs among some people who consume adequate amounts of zinc from grain products. Suggest why zinc deficiency develops despite an adequate intake of zinc.

   (Remember phytates in whole grains?)

6. Would you expect individuals on very low salt diets to be at risk for developing iodine deficiency? State the rationale for your answer.

   (Hint: What is the source of most dietary iodine?)

7. Read the labels on cans of sauerkraut, peas, dog food, tuna, pickles, and several other foods. Is salt listed as an ingredient? If yes, is it listed as iodized salt, or as including potassium iodide? Does it appear that canned foods containing salt regularly use iodized salt?

8. A once-popular weight-loss diet purported that iodine supplements would facilitate weight loss. What do you expect was the rationale (actually, an irrational rationale) for this?

   (Clue: What is the major function of thyroxine?)

NOTES

1. Concensus Development Panel, Osteoporosis, *Journal of the American Medical Association* 252 (1984): 799–802.

2. J. Forster, Kemps unveils high-calcium yogurt, *Minnesota Daily*, 30 April 1986, p. 4.

3. M. Schwartz, F. Anwah, and R. N. Levy, Variations in treatment of post-menopausal osteoporosis, *Clinical Orthopedics*, January–February 1985, pp. 180–184.

4. S. R. Cummings, J. L. Kelsey, et al., Epidemiology of osteoporosis and osteoporotic fractures, *Epidemiology Reviews* 7 (1985): 178–207.

5. H. Spencer and L. Kramer, NIH Consensus Conference: Osteoporosis, *Journal of Nutrition* 116 (1986): 316–319.

6. R. B. Sandler, C. W. Slemenda, et al., Postmenopausal bone density and milk consumption in childhood and adolescence, *American Journal of Clinical Nutrition* 42 (1985): 270–274.

7. Life Sciences Research Office, Report on effects of dietary factors on skeletal integrity in adults: Calcium, phosphorus, vitamin D, and protein (Bethesda, Md.: Federation of American Societies of Experimental Biology, 1981).

8. M. F. R. Sowers, R. B. Wallace, and J. H. Lemke, Correlates of mid-radius bone density among postmenopausal women: A community study, *American Journal of Clinical Nutrition* 41 (1985): 1045–1053.

9. R. Davies and S. Saha, Osteoporosis, *American Family Physician* 32 (1985): 107–114.

10. S. O. Welsh and R. M. Marston, Review of trends in food use in the United States, 1909–1980, *Journal of American Dietetic Association* 81 (1982): 120–125.

11. R. R. Recker, A. Bammi, et al., Calcium absorbability from milk products, an imitation milk, and calcium carbonate, *American Journal of Clinical Nutrition* 47 (1988): 93–95.

12. R. P. Heaney, C. M. Weaver, and R. R. Recker, Calcium absorbability from spinach, *American Journal of Clinical Nutrition* 47 (1988): 707–709.

13. A. A. Albanese, Effects of dietary calcium:phosphorus ratios on utilization of dietary calcium for bone synthesis in women 20–75 years of age, *Nutrition Reports International* 33 (1986): 879–891.

14. R. Marston and N. Raper, Nutrient content of the U.S. food supply, *National Food Review* 5 (1987): 27–33.

15. J. A. T. Pennington and H. N. Church, *Food Values of Portions Commonly Used*, 14th ed. (New York: Harper and Row, 1985).

16. R. P. Heaney, J. K. Gallagher, et al., Calcium nutrition and bone health in the elderly, *American Journal of Clinical Nutrition* 36 (1982): 986–1013.

17. S. Miller, "Questions and Answers" section of the *Journal of the American Medical Association* 257 (1987): 1810.

18. S. C. Hartz and J. Blumberg, Use of vitamin and mineral supplements by the elderly, *Clinical Nutrition* 5 (1986): 130–136.

19. D. A. McCarron, C. D. Morris, and C. Cole, Dietary calcium in human hypertension, *Science* 217 (1982): 267–269.

20. F. J. Kok, Dietary sodium, calcium, and potassium and blood pressure, *American Journal of Epidemiology* 123 (1986): 1043–1048.

21. Nationwide Food Consumption Survey, USDA Nutrition Monitoring Division (Washington, D.C.: U.S. Department of Agriculture, 1986).

22. L. Page and B. Friend, The changing United States diet, *BioScience* 28 (1978): 192–197.

23. H. Spencer, Minerals and mineral interactions in human beings, *Journal of the American Dietetic Association* 86 (1986): 864–867.

24. D. M. Hegstad, Calcium and phosphorus, in *Modern Nutrition in Health and Disease*, eds. R. S. Goodhart and M. E. Shils (Philadelphia: Lea and Febiger, 1973), 268–286.

25. R. Wilkinson, Absorption of calcium, phosphorus and magnesium, in *Calcium, phosphate, and magnesium metabolism*, ed. B. E. C. Nordin (New York: Churchill Livingstone, 1976), 36–112.

26. A. A. Albanese, Effects of dietary calcium:phosphorus ratios on utilization of dietary calcium for bone synthesis in women 20–75 years of age, *Nutrition Reports International* 33 (1986): 879–891.

27. Food and Nutrition Board, National Research Council, *Recommended Dietary Allowances*, 9th ed. (Washington, D.C.: National Academy of Sciences, 1980).

28. K. J. Morgan, G. L. Stampley, et al., Magnesium and calcium dietary intakes of the U.S. population, *Journal of the American College of Nutrition* 4 (1985): 195–206.

29. C. Berkelhammer and R. A. Bear, A clinical approach to common electrolyte problems: Hypomagnesemia, *Canadian Medical Association Journal* 132 (1985): 360–368.

30. E. B. Flink, Magnesium deficiency in human subjects: A personal historical perspective, *Journal of the American College of Nutrition* 4 (1985): 17–31.

31. R. A. Reinhart and N. A. Desbiens, Hypomagnesemia in patients entering the ICU, *Critical Care Medicine* 13 (1985): 506–507.

32. L. S. Goodman and A. Z. Gilman, *The pharmacological basis of therapeutics*, 3rd ed. (New York: Macmillan, 1965).

33. S. Hercberg and P. Galan, Assessment of iron deficiency in populations, *Revue D'Epidemiologie et de Sante Publique* (Paris) 33 (1985): 228–239.

34. H. S. White, Iron-hemoglobin, in *Nutrition and the Adult*, eds. R. B. Alfin-Slater and D. Kritchevsky (New York: Plenum Press, 1980), 287–312.

35. U.S. Interdepartmental Committee for National Defense, *Nutrition Survey of the Armed Forces* (Washington, D.C.: Department of Defense, Reports published between 1956–61).

36. C. U. Moore, Iron, in *Modern Nutrition in Health and Disease*, eds. R. S. Goodhart and M. E. Shils (Philadelphia: Lea and Febiger, 1973), 297–323.

37. J. D. Cook and M. Layrisse, Food iron absorption measured by an extrinsic tag, *Journal of Clinical Investigation* 51 (1972): 805–815.

38. E. R. Monsen, M. Hallberg, et al., Estimation of available dietary iron, *American Journal of Clinical Nutrition* 31 (1978): 134–141.

39. S. Seshadri, A. Shah, and S. Bhade, Haematologic response of anaemic preschool children to ascorbic acid supplementation, *Human Nutrition Applied Nutrition* 39 (1985): 151–154.

40. L. Hallberg, The role of vitamin C in improving the critical iron balance situation in women, *Internationale Zeitschrift fur Vitamin und Ernahrungsforschung* 27 (1985): 177–187.

41. E. R. Monsen and J. L. Balintfy, Calculating dietary iron bioavailability: Refinement and computerization, *Journal of the American Dietetic Association* 80 (1982): 307–311.

42. W. Mertz, Trace elements, *Contemporary Nutrition* 3 (1978): 1–2.

43. W. Mertz, Mineral elements: New perspectives, *Journal of the American Dietetic Association* 77 (1980): 258–263.

44. Life Sciences Research Office, Assessment of the iron nutritional status of the United States population based on data collected in the second National Health and Nutrition Examination Survey (NHANES II), 1976–80 (Bethesda, Md.: Federation of American Societies for Experimental Biology, 1984).

45. N. S. Scrimshaw, Nutrition and preventive medicine, in *Public Health and Preventive Medicine*, 12th ed., ed. J. M. Last (Norwalk, Conn.: Appleton-Century-Crofts, 1986), 1515–1542.

46. D. I. Evans, Cerebral function in iron deficiency: A review, *Child Care Health Development* 11 (1985): 105–112.

47. V. Herbert, Recommended dietary intake (RDI) of iron in humans, *American Journal of Clinical Nutrition* 45 (1987): 679–686. Other articles in this issue give more information about the RDIs for vitamins and minerals. The recommendations they discuss would have been the 1985 RDAs, had they been released.

48. National Research Council Subcommittee on Iron, Committee on Medical and Biological Effect of Environmental Pollutants, *Iron* (Washington, D.C.: Division of Medical Sciences, Assembly of Life Sciences, National Academy of Sciences, 1979).

49. R. G. Stevens, Y. Jones, M. S. Micozzi, and P. R. Taylor, Body iron stores and the risk of cancer, *New England Journal of Medicine* 319 (1988): 1047–1052.

50. A. M. Trinkoff and S. P. Baker, Poisoning hospitalizations and deaths from solids and liquids among children and teenagers, *American Journal of Public Health* 76 (1986): 657–660.

51. A. S. Prasad, Discovery and importance of zinc in human nutrition, *Federation Proceedings* 43 (1984): 2829–2834.

52. N. W. Solomons, D. L. Helitzer-Allen, and J. Villar, Zinc needs during pregnancy, *Clinical Nutrition* 5 (1986): 63–71.

53. L. N. Klevay, S. J. Reck, and D. F. Barcome, Evidence of dietary copper and zinc deficiencies, *Journal of the American Medical Association* 241 (1979): 1917–1918.

54. K. Y. Patterson, J. T. Holbrook, et al., Copper and manganese intake in balance for adults consuming self-selected diets, *American Journal of Clinical Nutrition* 40 (1984): 1397–1403.
55. J. M. Holden, W. R. Wolf, and W. Mertz, Zinc and copper in self-selected diets, *Journal of the American Dietetic Association* 75 (1979): 23–28.
56. W. Mertz, Mineral elements: New perspectives, *Journal of the American Dietetic Association* 77 (1980): 258–263.
57. Zinc deficiency rates are from the results of NHANES II (National Health and Nutrition Examination Survey, 1976–80), reported in A. S. Prasad, Clinical manifestations of zinc deficiency, *Annual Review of Nutrition* 5 (1985): 341–363.
58. *Consumer Report* 54 (January 1980).
59. H. H. Sandstead, The role of zinc in human health, in *Trace Substances in Environmental Health*, Vol. XII, ed. H. H. Hemphill (Columbia, Mo.: University of Missouri Press, 1978).
60. J. S. Goodwin, W. C. Hunt, et al., Relationship between zinc intake, physical activity, and blood levels of high-density lipoprotein cholesterol in a healthy elderly population, *Metabolism* 34 (1985): 519–523.
61. R. K. Chandra, Excessive intake of zinc impairs immune responses, *Journal of the American Medical Association* 252 (1984): 1443–1446.
62. P. S. Metha, S. J. Metha, and H. Vorherr, Congenital iodide goiter and hypothyroidism: A review, *Obstetrics and Gynecology* 38 (1983): 237–247.
63. R. B. Gillie, Endemic goiter, *Scientific American*, 1971, 93–101.
64. N. Kochupilla and M. M. Godbole, Iodisal oil injections in goiter prophylaxis, *NFI Bulletin* 7 (1986): 1–4.
65. W. Mertz, The essential trace elements, *Science* 213 (1981): 1332–1338.
66. W. Mertz, Trace elements, *Contemporary Nutrition* 3 (1978): 1–2.
67. Food and Nutrition Board, National Research Council, *Recommended Dietary Allowances*, 9th ed. (Washington, D.C.: National Academy of Sciences, 1980).
68. J. A. T. Pennington, B. E. Young, et al., Mineral content of foods and total diets: The selected minerals in foods survey, 1982–1984, *Journal of the American Dietetic Association* 86 (1986): 876–891.
69. R. B. Gillie, Endemic goiter, *Scientific American*, 1971, 93–101.
70. S. Nagataki, Effect of excessive quantities of iodide, in *Handbook of Physiology, III: Endocrinology* (Bethesda, Md.: American Physiological Society, 1974), 329–344.

CHAPTER 12

MINERALS II

The nine minerals presented in this chapter are listed under the headings *trace elements* and *electrolytes* in the RDA tables. Copper, manganese, fluoride, chromium, selenium, and molybdenum are categorized as trace elements because humans require very small amounts of them—less than 5 milligrams per day. The trace elements are found in very small amounts in foods.

Sodium, potassium, and chloride are needed in much greater amounts than the trace elements, and they occur in larger amounts in foods than do the trace elements. The provisional RDA ranges for these minerals extend as high as 1,875–5,625 milligrams (1.875–5.625 grams) in the case of potassium. These minerals are classified as electrolytes because they conduct an electrical current when they are dissolved in water. As you will read, sodium, potassium, and chloride perform many important functions in the body in addition to conducting electrical currents.

COPPER (Cu)

Cu *abbreviates* cuprum, *Latin for "copper."*

Much of what we know about the importance of copper to human nutrition stems from observations of the dramatic effects of copper deficiency and overdose in livestock. Pigs, lambs, and calves fed plants grown in copper-deficient soil develop gross bone abnormalities such as "swayback" and some of them die suddenly from nervous system malfunctions. Sheep that are regularly fed fodder containing excess copper accumulate copper in their livers. Oddly enough, no signs of copper toxicity appear in the sheep until the excess copper is for some reason released wholesale from the liver into the blood. This causes a massive breakdown in red blood cells and death. Such serious effects of copper imbalance in livestock as these prompted investigations into the roles of copper in human health.

Functions

Copper functions as an enzyme cofactor in hemoglobin and collagen formation.

The human body contains only 100 to 500 milligrams of copper—about 0.04 ounce. Though the amount of copper in the body is small, its role is important; copper serves as a cofactor for enzymes, including the enzymes in-

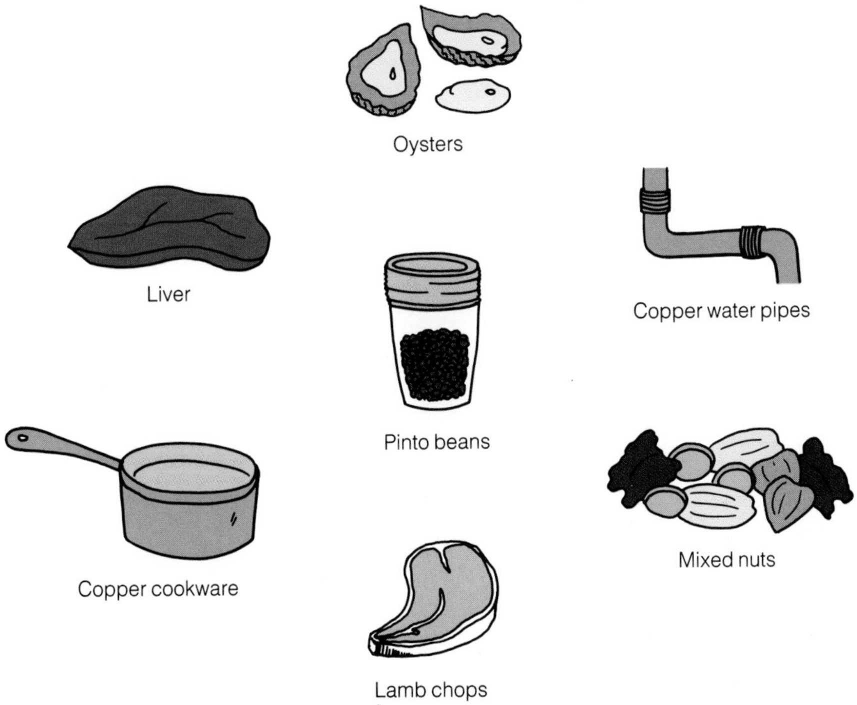

Sources of copper include a rather narrow assortment of foods and copper water pipes and cookware.

volved in hemoglobin and collagen formation. Copper is directly involved in reactions that incorporate iron into the structure of hemoglobin.

Sources

Milk, beef, chicken, and most types of fruits and vegetables commonly consumed in the U.S. are poor sources of copper. As shown in Table 12-1, only a few types of meat, nuts, and dried beans are considered good sources. Although most plants and animals require copper, they, like humans, do not contain very much of it nor store it in any quantity.

Copper water pipes and cookware also contribute to our copper intake. Hot water, especially, causes copper to leach from pipes and pans. These sources of copper may contribute significantly to our overall intake of copper, but the actual amount and whether it might be too much have not been determined.

Recommended Intake

The provisional adult RDA for copper is 2–3 mg. About 1.2 mg is needed each day to protect against a deficiency. Excluding the contribution of copper from water pipes and cookware, most people in the U.S. consume between 1 and 2 mg per day.[1]

Deficiency Severe copper deficiency causes anemia and reduced growth. It has been noted among young children suffering protein-calorie malnutrition and among critically ill adults. Mild deficiency may be common in the U.S., and it may contribute to increased blood cholesterol levels.[2] Because copper interacts with many other minerals in the body, specific symptoms of copper deficiency are difficult to pinpoint.

TABLE 12-1
Some food sources of copper

Food	Amount	Copper, mg*
Meats		
liver	3 oz	3.1
oysters	⅓ c	3.0
lamb	3 oz	0.7
pork	3 oz	0.3
white fish	3 oz	0.2
filberts	¼ c	0.4
walnuts	¼ c	0.4
pecans	¼ c	0.3
peanuts (Spanish)	¼ c	0.2
Legumes		
pinto beans (cooked)	½ c	0.4
white beans (canned)	½ c	0.3

*The provisional adult RDA is 2–3 mg.

Toxicity Copper overdose may be produced by regularly consuming 10 mg or more of the mineral per day. It also accompanies the rare genetic disorder called *Wilson's disease*, in which the person is not able to excrete copper. Consequently, it accumulates in tissues such as the liver, brain, and kidney and causes damage to them. Copper is rarely included in vitamin supplements, and cases of copper overdose are extremely rare.

MANGANESE (Mn)

Manganese's major function is as a cofactor to enzymes involved in energy metabolism.

Manganese is a cofactor of several enzymes involved in energy metabolism. It is widely distributed in foods, and it is assumed that most U.S. adults consume the provisional RDA of 2.5 to 5.0 mg. Deficiency and overdose of manganese are not problems, except for miners who are exposed to manganese dust each day. Manganese overdose among miners has been shown to produce liver damage, muscle spasms, and a monotone voice—due to the effects of excess manganese on the voice box.

The element fluorine (Fl) is an odorous, poisonous, greenish yellow gas consisting of single atoms of the element. Fluorides are nonpoisonous, solid compounds of fluorine and are the form of the mineral consumed in foods. (Note that fluoride *begins* flu-, *not* flo-.*)*

FLUORIDE (Fl)

Fluoride is best known for its importance in the prevention of tooth decay. About 50% of U.S. drinking water supplies are fluoridated, and sodium fluoride compounds are widely used in toothpastes and mouth rinses. The addition of fluoride to water, toothpastes, and mouth rinses has contributed

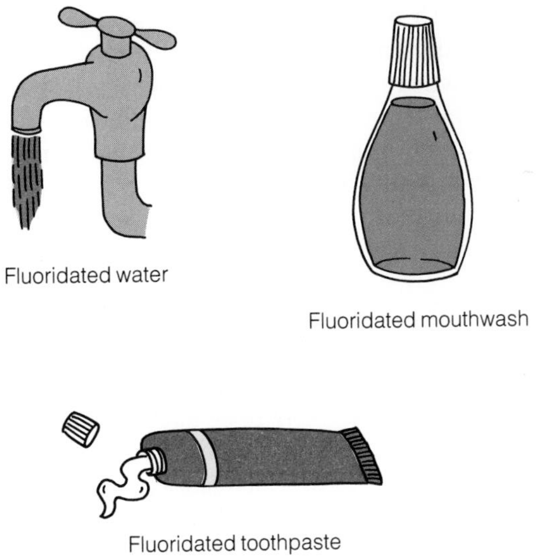

Sources of fluoride. Although milk, spinach, eggs, and some teas contain low amounts of fluoride, fluoridated water is our most important source.

to a very impressive reduction in the incidence of tooth decay in the U.S., Europe, and many other places in the world. Figure 12-1 shows the decline in the prevalence of tooth decay in the U.S. between the early 1950s and the 1980s.

Functions

Fluoride is considered to be an essential nutrient because of its beneficial effects on dental health. In the body, it is almost exclusively found in teeth and other bones where it is incorporated into their structure along with calcium, phosphorus, and other minerals. Fluoride has the overall effects of strengthening bones and helping teeth resist the decay caused by mouth bacteria.

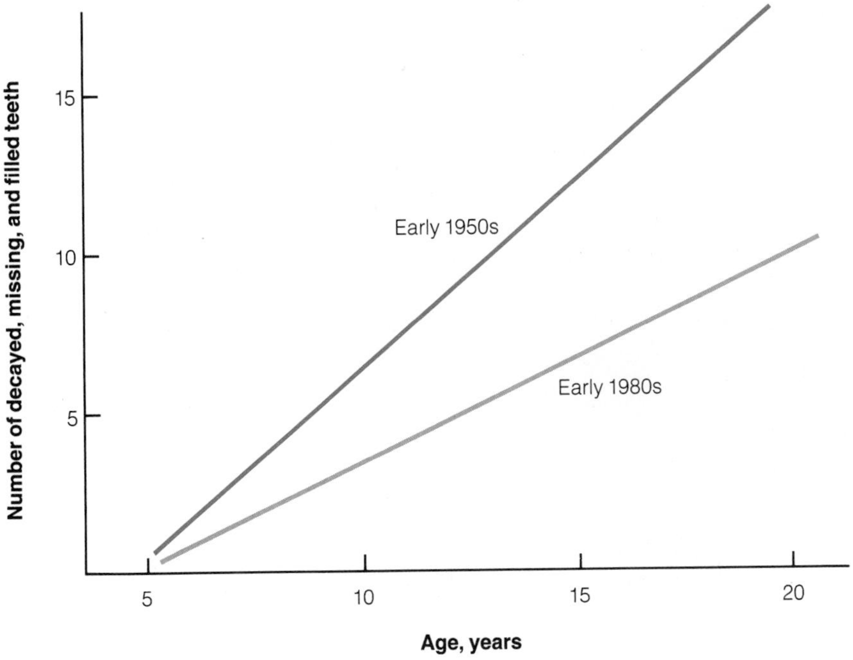

FIGURE 12-1
Decline in the prevalence of dental problems in the U.S.

The major function of fluoride in the body is its role in protecting against tooth decay.

Fluoride enters teeth both by exposure to fluoridated toothpaste and mouth rinses and through the fluoride content of blood that nourishes teeth. The teeth of children who regularly consume fluoridated water or use fluoridated toothpaste or mouth rinse contain more fluoride—and have 40% to 70% fewer cavities—than the teeth of people who do not have access to fluoride.[3,4] Adults benefit from fluoridated water, too.[3,5] Fluoride is also incorporated into adult teeth, although at a slower pace than in children. The total cost of water fluoridation in the U.S. is about 30 cents per person per year.

Although fluoridation has greatly reduced the incidence of tooth decay, it is still an important public health problem in the U.S. About half of the U.S. population does not have access to fluoridated water. (The map in Figure 12-2 shows where water is most likely to be fluoridated.) Some communities remain reluctant to fluoridate water supplies out of fear that fluoride may promote cancer and other diseases. Such fears are unfounded. Fluoridated water has not been shown to be even weakly related to the development of cancer, heart disease, birth defects, or other health problems.[6,7] Only trace amounts of fluoride are used to fluoridate water. Municipal water supplies contain 1 part fluoride per million parts of water—the equivalent of about 4 grains of salt per quart of water.

Water fluoridation is the least expensive and most effective way to prevent tooth decay, but other sources of fluoride are needed in areas where

FIGURE 12-2

Percentages of state populations with fluoridated water supply.

Alaska	80.5%	Maryland	98.6%	Rhode Island	90.9%
Connecticut	90.9%	Massachusetts	15.6%	Vermont	45.7%
Delaware	54.6%	New Hampshire	17.6%	District of Columbia	100.0%
Hawaii	13.3%	New Jersey	14.8%	Puerto Rico	93.7%

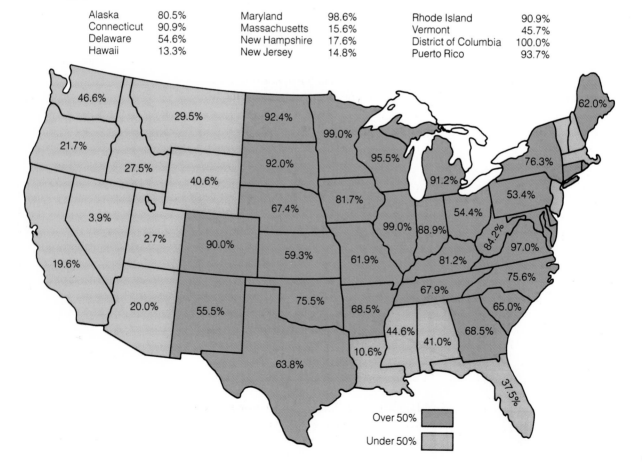

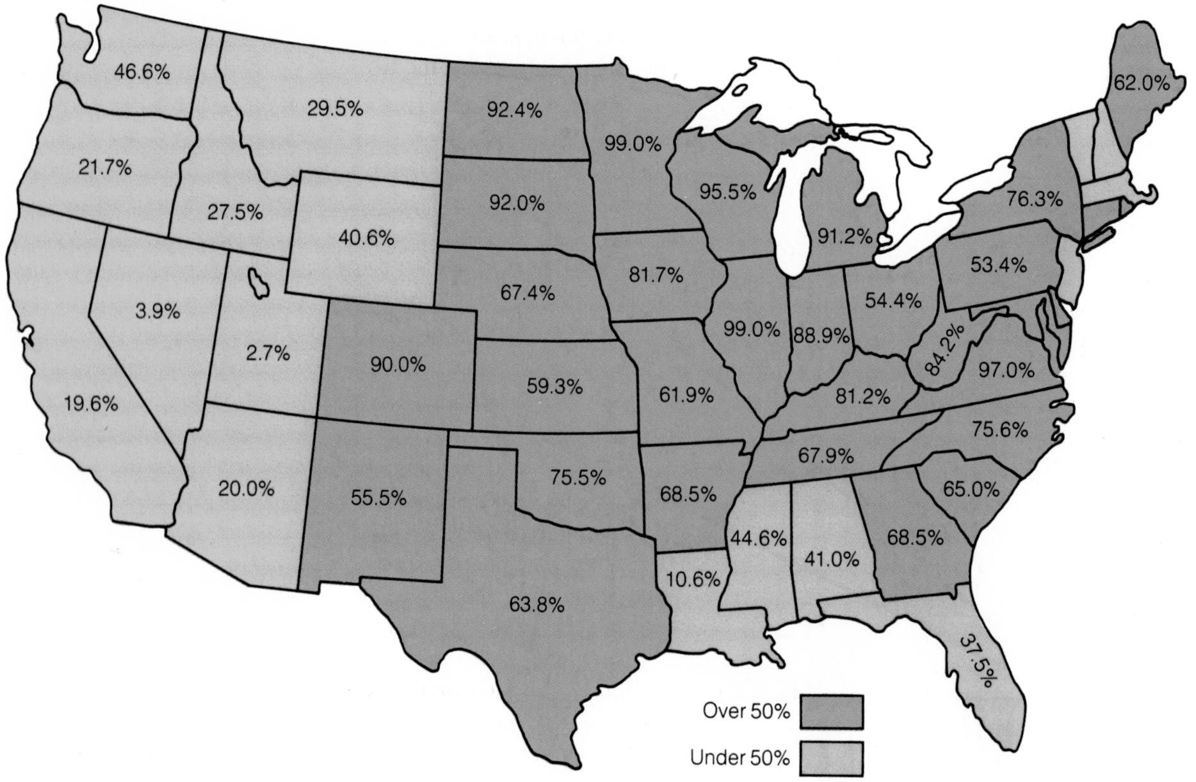

TABLE 12-2

Estimated fluoride intakes of people living in areas with and without fluoridated water[9]

	Average Fluoride Intake, mg/day
Fluoridated water supply	2.6
Nonfluoridated water supply	0.9

water is not fluoridated. Fluoride supplements and fluoridated toothpaste and mouth rinses have been used successfully to fill the "fluoridated-water gap." Regular use of fluoridated toothpaste or mouth rinse can decrease tooth decay in children by approximately 40%.[4] The English have successfully reduced the incidence of tooth decay by fortifying milk with fluoride.

Sources

Fluoridated water is our largest source of fluoride, and commercial products made with fluoridated water are the second. Milk, spinach, eggs, and some teas contain fluoride, but in very small quantities. There are no "excellent" food sources of this mineral. Consequently, our most important source of fluoride is fluoridated water.

Recommended Intake

Fluoride was recently added to the RDA tables. The provisional RDA for adults is 1.5 to 4.0 mg per day, the amount provided in 6 to 16 cups of fluoridated water. An intake of about 1.5 mg per day provides protection against the development of tooth decay.[8] Without fluoridated water, however, diets generally provide too little fluoride for full protection against decay; see Table 12-2.

fluorosis: Fluoride overdose characterized by discolored or "mottled" teeth in children. Fluorosis generally results from water supplies that contain over 1 part per million of fluoride.

Deficiency The only known effect of fluoride deficiency is the increased susceptibility to tooth decay. As much as half of the U.S. population may fail to consume the recommended level of fluoride.

Toxicity **Fluorosis**, the development of rusty-colored stains ("mottling") on the teeth, occurs among children in communities where the water supply is naturally high in fluoride (Figure 12-3). Mild fluorosis, which produces light staining of the teeth, occurs when children regularly consume water containing over 1 part per million (PPM) of fluoride. Severe fluorosis, which grossly discolors teeth, develops when long-term intakes of fluoride during childhood exceed 20 mg per day. Because the stains are part of the tooth structure, they are permanent. Adults do not develop mottled teeth as a result of fluorosis; it occurs only during tooth formation.

Mottled teeth may be unattractive, but they are highly resistant to decay. Aside from cosmetic concerns, fluorosis appears to have no undesirable effects.

Fluoride was once thought to help prevent osteoporosis. Recent evidence, however, suggests that above-average intakes of fluoride are not particularly effective in reducing the risk of osteoporosis.

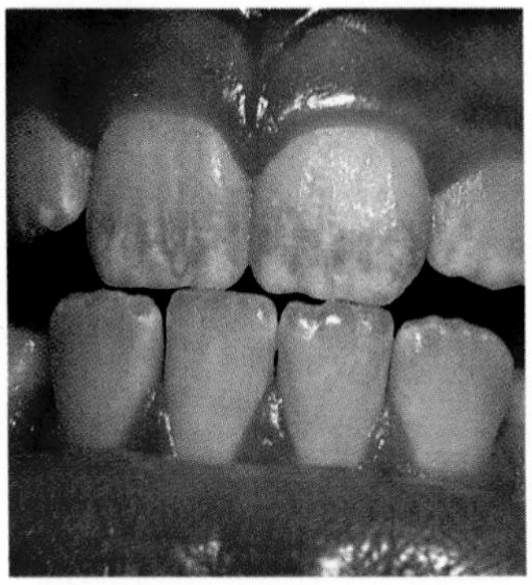

FIGURE 12-3
High levels of fluoride in drinking water cause mottling of children's teeth.

CHROMIUM (Cr)

Chromium is a very hard, corrosion-resistant metal used to make "chrome" platings on appliances, car parts, and tools. The name is derived from the German word for "color."

Chromium, like zinc, was thought to be a toxic substance and an environmental contaminant for many years. Eventually, a trial-and-error experiment identified it as essential to health. When researchers gave 40 test minerals to rats that had developed high blood glucose levels while on a limited diet, they found that only chromium was effective in bringing glucose levels back to normal.[10] This scientific "fishing expedition" led to the discoveries that chromium is essential to health and that it functions in glucose metabolism.

Functions

Major functions of chromium: as an enzyme cofactor for fat and cholesterol metabolism facilitates the action of insulin

The major function of chromium is as an enzyme cofactor; it is known to activate enzymes involved in fat and cholesterol metabolism. Its *most studied* function, however, is its role in glucose metabolism. Chromium appears to affect blood glucose levels by facilitating the binding of insulin to receptors located on cell membranes. When insulin receptors are occupied by insulin, blood glucose passes quickly into cells. An inadequate supply of chromium decreases the binding of insulin to its cell membrane receptors and causes blood glucose levels to increase such as happens in diabetes.

Chromium supplements have been used as a component of diabetes treatment. The supplements do not improve all cases of diabetes, but they are effective in reducing blood glucose levels to some extent among people who have chromium deficiency and people who develop diabetes late in life.[11]

Sources

Small amounts of chromium are found in meats, dairy products, whole grains, and herbs such as thyme and black pepper. Chromium also enters our food supply through chromium-contaminated soil and water.

Recommended Intake

The human body contains less than 6 mg of chromium, and only trace amounts are needed in the diet to protect against chromium deficiency. A provisional adult RDA was established in 1980 as 0.05 to 0.2 mg per day. Although minute, intakes of over 0.1 mg per day are difficult to obtain from typical U.S. diets. It is estimated that most people in the U.S. consume 0.05 to 0.1 mg of chromium per day.[12]

Deficiency The most prominent feature of chromium deficiency in humans is elevated blood glucose levels. Severe chromium deficiency produces a diabeteslike state. Low chromium intakes have also been related to elevated cholesterol levels and thus to the potential for increased risk of heart disease.[11]

Toxicity Chromium overdose rarely occurs in humans, but when it does it is generally related to consuming excessive levels of chromium in contaminated foods. A primary sign of chromium overdose is a disagreeable, metallic taste in the mouth. Other signs include diarrhea, cramping, and collapse. Chromium toxicity can be fatal.

■ ■ ■

SELENIUM (Se)

From selene, *Greek for "moon." One naturally occurring form of selenium has a gray color that resembles the color of the moon. Its acid is uniquely strong; selenic acid is the only acid known to be able to dissolve gold.*

Selenium was not identified as an essential nutrient until the early 1970s, and much remains unknown about its functions in human nutrition. Only one function of selenium is known with certainty: it is part of an enzyme that functions as an antioxidant. Roles of selenium in the development of **muscular dystrophy**, in sperm production, and in the body's response to infection have been proposed, but these functions are yet to be confirmed. The lack of research-based knowledge about the roles of selenium in human health has not kept it from being marketed by enterprising individuals, however. They have sold selenium supplements for curing cancer, heart disease, sexual problems, and poor eyesight and for preventing aging.

muscular dystrophy: A condition characterized by a wasting away and weakening of muscles.

Functions

Selenium functions as an antioxidant.

Selenium is a component of an enzyme that is found in every cell in the human body. This selenium-containing enzyme acts as an antioxidant in much the same way as does vitamin E. Both selenium and vitamin E repair damage to molecules and cell membranes caused by oxygen.

The antioxidant role of selenium and vitamin E is an excellent example of a nutrient–nutrient interaction. High vitamin-E intakes decrease the need for selenium, whereas adequate selenium intakes reduce the body's reliance on vitamin E for antioxidation reactions.

Selenium and Cancer Because selenium functions as an antioxidant, it has been suspected to play a role in cancer development. Research results clearly indicate a role of selenium in the development of cancer in laboratory animals, but the few studies involving humans have not produced clear-cut

Dietary sources of selenium.

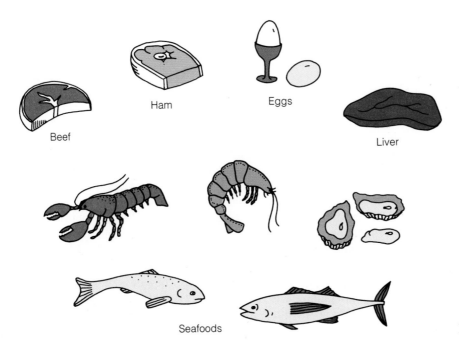

TABLE 12-3
Some food sources of selenium

Food	Amount	Selenium Content, mcg*
Seafood		
lobster	3 oz	66
tuna	3 oz	60
shrimp	3 oz	54
oysters	3 oz	48
fish	3 oz	40
Meats and Eggs		
liver	3 oz	56
egg	1 med.	37
ham	3 oz	29
beef	3 oz	22
bacon	3 oz	21
chicken	3 oz	18
lamb	3 oz	14
veal	3 oz	10

*The provisional adult RDA is 50–200 mcg.

results. It appears, however, that people who habitually consume approximately the RDA level of selenium from foods experience less cancer than those who consume less.[13] Selenium supplements have not been shown to reduce cancer, but a long-term study investigating the role of selenium pills in preventing cancer is underway. It is thought that adequate intakes of selenium may decrease a person's susceptibility to cancer by repairing oxidized molecules and thereby blocking the spread of cancer.[14]

Sources

Table 12-3 lists food sources of selenium, although the values given in the table may bear little resemblance to the actual selenium content of individual samples of the foods listed. This is because selenium content of meats and plants varies substantially depending on the availability of selenium in animal feeds, water, and soil (Figure 12-4). For example, the selenium in 3 ounces of beef has been found to range from 0.05 mg to 0.42 mg, whereas the amount in 3 ounces of tuna varies from 0.04 mg to 0.1 mg.[15] The selenium contents listed in Table 12-3 have been determined from foods obtained in the U.S. In countries such as Finland, where the water and soil contain very little selenium and the rates of cancer are high, selenium is added to fertilizers in order to increase the selenium content of foods.[14]

Meats are the best food sources of selenium; they generally contain far more selenium than plants. The reason for this is that the selenium in foods is attached to amino acids. Since meats contain more amino acids than do plants, more selenium becomes incorporated into meats.

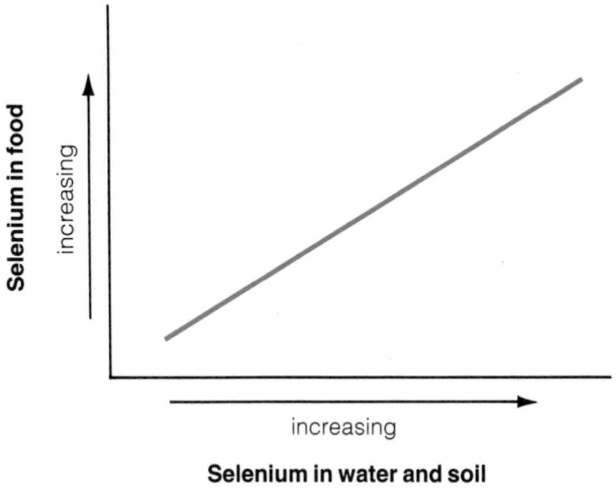

FIGURE 12-4
The selenium content of foods, particularly meats, reflects the selenium content of water and soil in the area where the food was produced.

Recommended Intake

The range of selenium intakes recommended for adults is 0.05 to 0.2 mg (50 to 200 mcg) per day. This wide range reflects the lack of detailed knowledge about selenium requirements and the effect of vitamin E intakes on the need for selenium. Most people who consume meat regularly are likely to receive adequate selenium.[16] It is estimated that at least 0.02 mg (20 mcg) per day is needed to prevent a deficiency.[17]

Deficiency Selenium deficiency has been associated with an increased risk of developing cancer and with a type of heart disease. Whereas selenium deficiency may be one of many factors that *contributes to* cancer development, it clearly *causes* a specific type of heart disease. A disease of the heart muscles directly linked to selenium deficiency has been identified among children living in parts of China where almost no selenium exists in the water or soil. Including selenium in the diets of these children has been shown to prevent the development of this disorder.[18]

Foods consumed by people in the U.S. come from many different parts of the country and the world, so the selenium content of our diets does not totally depend on local growing conditions. The selenium content of water and soil in western Oregon and in parts of the Midwest are known to be low, while the water and soil in the Great Plains area tend to be selenium-rich. Although there are selenium-rich and selenium-poor growing conditions in the U.S., genuine selenium deficiency almost never occurs here.

Toxicity Prior to 1970, selenium was thought of as a toxic substance, and one that was especially dangerous to livestock. We now know that selenium is both a toxic substance and an essential nutrient. The line between health and overdose depends upon the amount of selenium that is consumed.

Selenium toxicity is called **selenosis**. The symptoms of selenosis in cattle have been known for decades, but human symptoms were not well defined until a recent accident. A selenium supplement containing 25 to 30 mg of selenium per tablet reached the market due to a manufacturing error. Although intended to contain less than 0.2 mg, the tablet's dosage was sufficient to cause selenium toxicity. The first symptom observed was a garlic odor on the breath. Other signs of selenium overdose included hair and fingernail loss, discolored skin, gastrointestinal upset, weakness, and liver damage.[14]

selenosis: The selenium-toxicity disease.

Early signs of selenosis have been observed with daily intakes of 0.9 mg of selenium over a period of two years.[19] Because of the risks associated with selenium overdose, it is recommended that selenium supplements be used with caution and that they not exceed 0.2 mg per day.[14]

■ ■ ■

MOLYBDENUM (Mo)

Molybdenum's major function is as an enzyme cofactor in protein synthesis.

Molybdenum (mə lib′ də nəm) is needed by humans in very small amounts; the provisional adult RDA is 0.15–0.5 mg (15–50 mcg) per day. Although molybdenum is an essential cofactor for a number of enzymes involved in protein synthesis, dietary deficiencies or excesses of this mineral are currently regarded as unimportant in human nutrition.

■ ■ ■

SODIUM (Na)

Na *abbreviates the Latin word* natrium *for a sodium-containing compound widely used as a headache remedy in ancient Rome—what we know today as sodium bicarbonate (baking soda).*

On one hand, sodium is a gift from the sea; on the other, it is a hazard to health represented by the salt shaker. Sodium's life- and health-sustaining functions are frequently overshadowed by its effects on blood pressure when consumed in excess.

Extremely reactive, sodium occurs in nature combined with other elements. The most common chemical partner of sodium is chloride, and much

Processed foods and table salt are the leading sources of sodium in the U.S. diet.

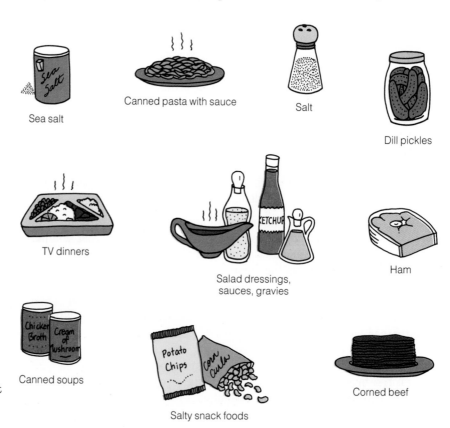

BOX 12-1

THE POWER OF SALT

There are six flavours, and of them all, salt is the greatest.
Sanskrit proverb, circa 800 B.C.

Throughout the ages, humans have gone to great lengths to get salt and maintain a supply of it. Now that salt is readily available and cheap, we are faced with the challenge of reducing our intakes to levels closer to those consumed when salt was scarce.

Due to the naturally low content of sodium in foods and the important roles of sodium in the body, humans appear to have evolved powerful mechanisms that promote sodium intake and conserve it once it is absorbed. Humans have a preference for the taste of salt, and it is the only identified nutrient for which humans develop an appetite in response to need.[20] A person could be seriously ill from scurvy, severely iron deficient, or suffer from pellagra, but still not seek out or spontaneously prefer foods that would cure the deficiency. Only sodium has built-in mechanisms that encourage consumption. Unfortunately, the body lacks mechanisms that decrease the appetite for salt when sufficient quantities have been consumed.[12,20]

The safeguards that encourage salt consumption likely developed in response to a shortage of sodium in the diets of early humans. The total dietary supply of sodium of our hunter–gatherer ancestors was derived from meats and plants and probably amounted to less than 2 grams per day. In contrast, people in industrialized, Western societies consume averages of 8 or more grams per day.[20] Obviously, these 40,000-year-old biological mechanisms do not serve us well today, when we can eat all the salt we want.

of the sodium present on this planet is in the form of sodium chloride—"table salt."[11] The oceans are far and away the leading source of sodium; they contain enough salt to cover the surface of the earth to a depth of more than 400 feet.

Although it is found in abundance in the oceans, humans have not always had access to enough salt to satisfy their taste for it. (Box 12-1 gives biological perspective to this discussion.) During times when there has not been enough salt to go around, wars have been fought over it. In such times, a pocketful of salt was as good as a pocketful of cash. (The word *salary* is derived from the Latin word *salarium*, "salt money.") Today, salt is widely available in most parts of the world, and the problem is that of limiting human intakes to levels that do not interfere with health.

Functions

Sodium's major function is the role it plays in maintaining the body's water balance.

Sodium appears directly above potassium in the periodic table (turn back to Figure 11-1), and the two work closely together in the body to maintain normal **water balance**. Nearly all of the body's supply of sodium is located in the blood and the fluid that surrounds cells, whereas potassium is located inside of cells (Figure 12-5). Cells can function normally when the amount of water outside them balances the amount inside them, and sodium and potassium help achieve that balance. Both sodium and potassium chemically

water balance: The ratio of the amount of water outside of cells to the amount inside of cells; this balance is needed for normal cell functioning.

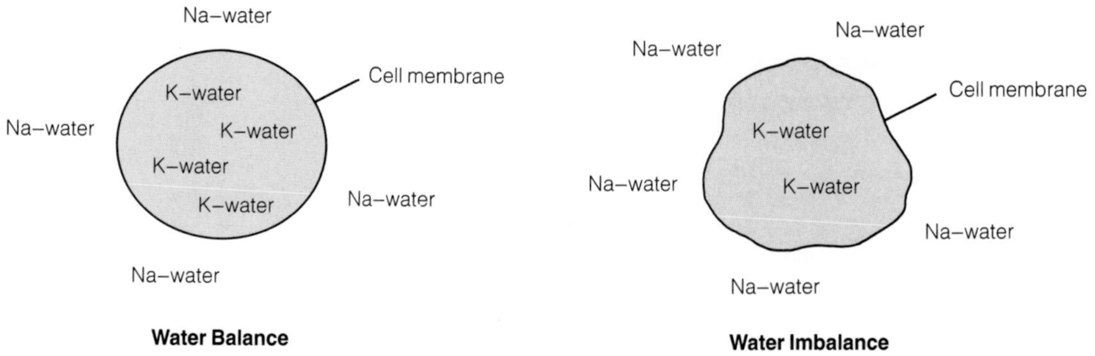

FIGURE 12-5 (left)
Schematic representation of the role of sodium (Na) and potassium (K) in maintaining water balance.

FIGURE 12-6 (right)
Water imbalance results from excessive levels of sodium outside of cells.

attract water, and under normal circumstances, each draws sufficient water to the outside or the inside of cells to maintain the necessary balance.

Water balance and cell functions are upset when there's an imbalance between the body's supplies of sodium and potassium. When the concentration of sodium outside the cells exceeds the concentration of potassium inside, the sodium on the outside draws water out of the cells (Figure 12-6). The shift in fluid balance leads to changes in the pressure of fluids inside and outside of cells, which can disrupt normal cell functions.

A number of adaptive mechanisms provide a degree of protection against the negative effects of an imbalance between sodium and potassium. The primary mechanisms are those that cause excessive blood levels of sodium to be excreted in the urine. Along with the sodium goes the rather large amount of water that the sodium chemically attracts. Thus, water is lost from the body when excessive amounts of sodium are consumed.

The loss of body water that accompanies high sodium intakes may have come to your attention. You have probably noticed that you become thirsty when you eat a large amount of salted potato chips or popcorn. The reason salty foods make you thirsty is that your body loses water when the high load of dietary sodium is excreted. The thirst signal tells you that you need water to replace what you have lost.

The loss of body water that accompanies ingestion of large amounts of salt explains why seawater neither quenches thirst nor satisfies the body's need for water. When a person drinks seawater, its high concentration of sodium causes more water to be excreted than is retained. Rather than increasing the body's supply of water, the ingestion of seawater increases a person's need for water.

In healthy people, the body's adaptive mechanisms provide a buffer against upsets in water balance due to high sodium intakes. It appears that many people are overwhelming the body's ability to cope with high sodium loads, however.

hypertension: A condition in which blood pressure is higher than normal; also referred to as *high blood pressure.*

High dietary intakes of sodium appear to play a critical role in the development of **hypertension**. Although the mechanisms by which excesses in dietary sodium lead to the elevation of blood pressure are not yet fully understood, it is suspected that they may be related to the function of sodium in maintaining water balance. A number of conditions in addition to dietary intake of sodium appear to influence the development of hypertension. They are discussed in the following subsection. Hypertension is generally defined as blood pressure levels that exceed 140/90 mm of mercury. (Box 12-2 explains how blood pressure is measured.)

BOX 12-2

MEASURING BLOOD PRESSURE

Blood, in order to continue to circulate through the body, must exist under pressure in the blood vessels. The amount of pressure exerted on the walls of blood vessels is greatest when pulses of blood are passing through them and least between pulses. Blood pressure measurement is a matter of learning the greatest and least amount of pressure existing in the blood vessels.

The first step in measuring blood pressure is to cut off the circulation of blood in the person's arm by tightening a cuff around the upper arm. The chest piece of a stethoscope is then gently pressed against the skin over an artery just below the cuff. Then the tension exerted by the cuff is gradually decreased so that the blood can begin to flow. When the pressure of the pulses of blood is the same as the pressure exerted by the cuff, the sound of initial pulses can be heard through the stethoscope, and the person taking the measurement records the corresponding pressure. The first and highest blood pressure reading is the *systolic blood pressure*. As the cuff is loosened further, the sound of the blood pulsing through the artery lessens and the sound of the blood beginning to flow between pulses can be heard. The pressure at which nonpulsing blood begins to flow is called the *diastolic blood pressure*.

A typical normal adult blood pressure is a systolic pressure of 110 and a diastolic pressure of 70 (a blood pressure of 110/70 mm of mercury). Several blood-pressure measurements are needed to confirm hypertension.

A Closer Look at Hypertension

Excess of salty flavor hardens the pulse.
—circa 1000 B.C.[21]

High salt intakes have been thought to cause high blood pressure for more than 2,000 years. It has only been in the past 50 years, however, that the relationship between blood pressure and sodium intake has been documented.

Hypertension is considered a major public health problem in the U.S. and other countries where salt intakes tend to be high. Although not considered a disease by itself, the presence of hypertension substantially increases the risk that a person will develop heart disease or kidney failure or will experience a heart attack or stroke. Hypertension occurs in 24% of U.S. adults and is more likely to develop as people become older.[23] About 75% of all cases of hypertension are classified as mild.

Although a common, health-threatening disorder, little is known about what causes hypertension. Of all the cases of hypertension that occur, only 5% can be linked directly to a cause. It's not yet clear what causes the other 95% of cases. People who have hypertension for which no cause has been identified are said to have **essential hypertension**. Because this type of hypertension represents 95% of the cases, it is the "hypertension" we speak of in this book. A number of potential causes of hypertension have been identified, and dietary factors appear to be among the most important. Of the dietary factors, the link between sodium intake and hypertension is the strongest.[22–24]

essential hypertension: Hypertension of no known cause; also called *primary* or *idiopathic hypertension*, it accounts for over 95% of all cases of hypertension.

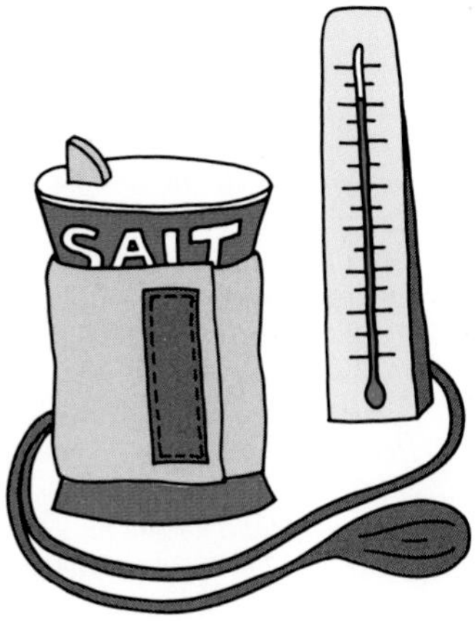

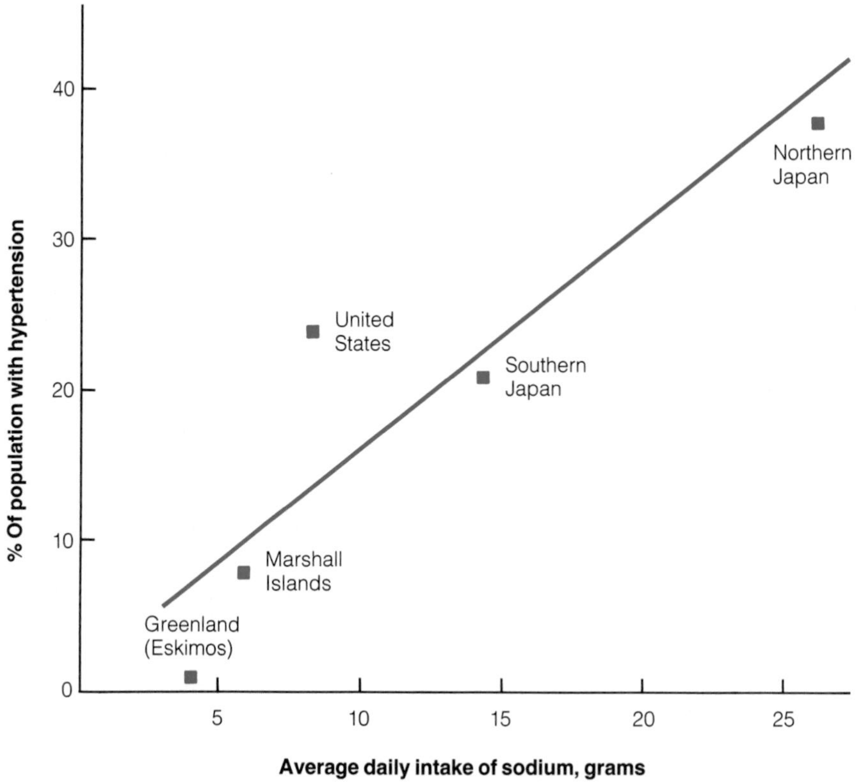

FIGURE 12-7
Relationship between average daily sodium intake and the incidence of hypertension within populations.

Several lines of evidence strongly indicate that high-sodium diets are a leading factor in the development of hypertension. Foremost among the evidence is the finding that the incidence of hypertension tends to increase within a population as the average daily intake of salt increases (Figure 12-7). People living in societies where salt intake is low, such as those of the Greenland Eskimos, African Pygmies, and Australian Aborigines, experience very little hypertension. They do tend to develop hypertension, however, when they switch to a high-salt diet.[24]

The Effects of Salt Restriction on Hypertension Low-sodium diets tend to reduce blood pressure among people with hypertension, and they may also help to maintain normal blood pressure levels among healthy people.[25] Mild hypertension—the diagnosis in about 75% of the cases of hypertension—can generally be lowered to normal by a diet that contains approximately 2 grams of sodium a day in normal-weight adults.[23] That amount of sodium roughly corresponds to 1 teaspoon of salt a day. A 2-gram-sodium diet can be achieved by avoiding processed foods and foods with added salt such as salty snacks, smoked meats, pickled foods, and convenience dinners and by not adding salt in food preparation or at the table.

To achieve a moderate-salt diet:
- *Eat fresh or frozen, unprocessed or lightly processed foods.*
- *Limit intake of salty snacks, canned soups, cured and smoked meats, processed cheese, and bottled sauces.*
- *Remove the salt shaker from the table.*
- *Read food labels. (You may be surprised to discover how many foods have added salt.)*

Moderate-salt diets that exclude processed foods offer an important fringe benefit: they tend to be high in potassium. High potassium intakes appear to protect against the blood pressure increases that accompany high-sodium diets.[26] Processing generally reduces the potassium content of foods and increases the sodium content by the addition of salt. Two examples of how processing foods changes their sodium and potassium content are given in Figure 12-8. The changes can be rather striking. Potassium is

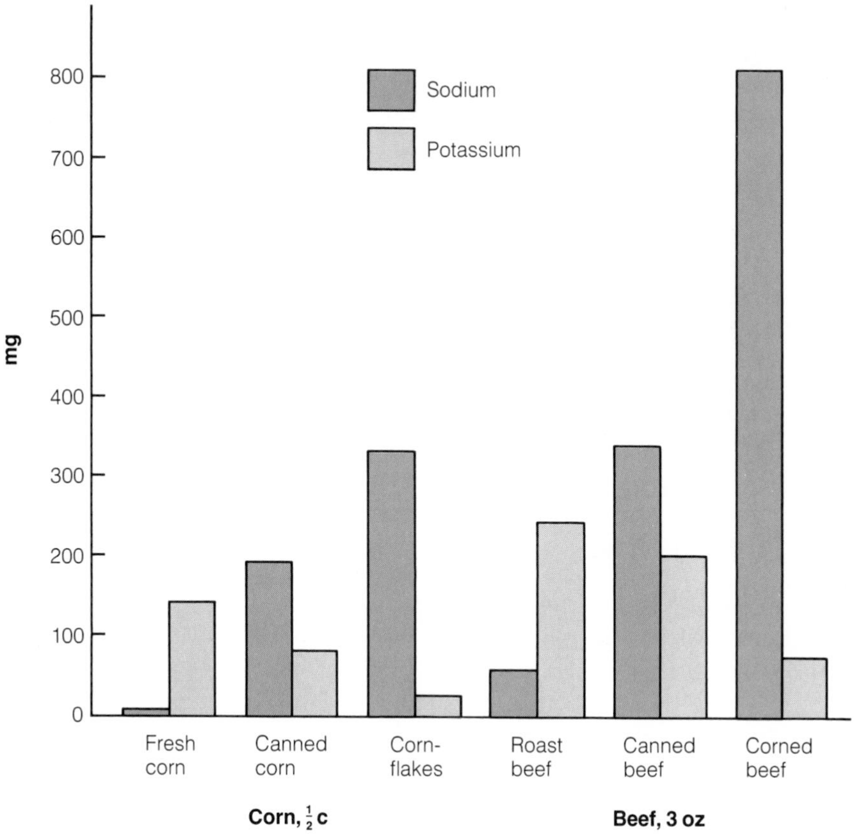

FIGURE 12-8
Effect of processing on the sodium and potassium content of corn and beef products.

lost from grains when the potassium-rich bran is removed, and it leaches out of foods when they are heated or stored in liquids.

People on moderate-salt diets often replace processed foods with fresh and unprocessed foods that contain more potassium than sodium. You can get a notion of how the inclusion or exclusion of processed and salty foods affects dietary intakes of sodium and potassium by studying the two menus presented in Table 12-4. The amount of sodium in the high-salt menu about equals the average U.S. intake when determined before salt is added to foods at the table. The high-salt menu contains three-and-a-half times the sodium and one-fourth the potassium of the moderate-salt menu. As shown in the graph at the bottom of the table, the moderate-salt menu contains more potassium than sodium—a combination that may help to lower blood pressure in people with hypertension.

Many people find moderate-sodium diets difficult to stick to initially because they miss the taste of salt. People who continue with the diet for two months, however, often find that it gets easier. After getting used to a moderate-salt diet, low amounts of salt taste "saltier" to them than before and they tend to prefer less-salty foods.[28]

Drugs that Lower Blood Pressure Since dietary changes may be difficult for some people to achieve, why put them through the trouble? Why not just use antihypertension drugs? Perhaps this thought occurred to you while you were reading about the human preference for salt. These are good questions, and they have good answers. Antihypertension drugs affect the

TABLE 12-4

Comparison of sodium and potassium content of two menus (not including any salt that is added at the table)

High-Salt Menu	Moderate-Salt Menu
Breakfast	Breakfast
orange juice, 6 oz	orange juice, 6 oz
egg sandwich, 1 (egg, Canadian bacon,* American cheese, and butter on English muffin)	egg, 1
coffee, 1 c	whole-wheat toast, 2 slices
	margarine, 2 t
	coffee, 1 c
Lunch	Lunch
hot dog,* 1, on bun	hamburger, 3 oz, on bun
catsup,* 1 T	sliced tomatoes, ½ c
dill pickle,* ¼	coleslaw, ½ c
potato chips,* 1 oz	milk, 1 c
milk, 1 c	
Dinner	Dinner
tomato soup,* 1 c	lettuce salad, 1½ c with 2 T Italian dressing*
meat loaf,* 3 oz	pork chop, 3 oz
scalloped potatoes, ½ c	baked potato, 1 med.
gravy,* ¼ c	green beans, frozen, ½ c
peas (canned), ½ c	milk, 1 c
milk, 1 c	

continued

body in ways other than reducing blood pressure. Their side-effects include raising blood cholesterol levels and decreasing potassium levels. The elevated cholesterol levels increase the risk of heart disease among people already at risk because of their hypertension. Potassium losses caused by some of the antihypertension drugs increase the risk of potassium deficiency, a potentially fatal disorder.[29,30] In contrast, moderate salt diets effectively reduce blood pressure in people with mild hypertension and do not appear to pose any risk to health.

Whereas simply reducing sodium intake is recommended for people with mild hypertension, antihypertension drugs plus dietary sodium reduction and weight loss if needed are the accepted treatments for moderate and severe cases of hypertension.[23,33]

Other Factors Related to the Development of Hypertension Hypertension appears to be a disorder that can have many causes. In addition to the effects of sodium and potassium, at least three other nutrients and such factors as smoking, high stress level, low physical activity level, obesity, and alcohol intake may contribute to its development. The three other nutrients that have been related to hypertension are calcium, magnesium,

TABLE 12-4, *continued*

High-Salt Menu	Moderate-Salt Menu
Snack	**Snack**
American cheese,* 1 oz	peanuts (unsalted), ¼ c
saltine crackers,* 4	apple, 1 med.
tea, 1 c	tea, 1 c

Analysis

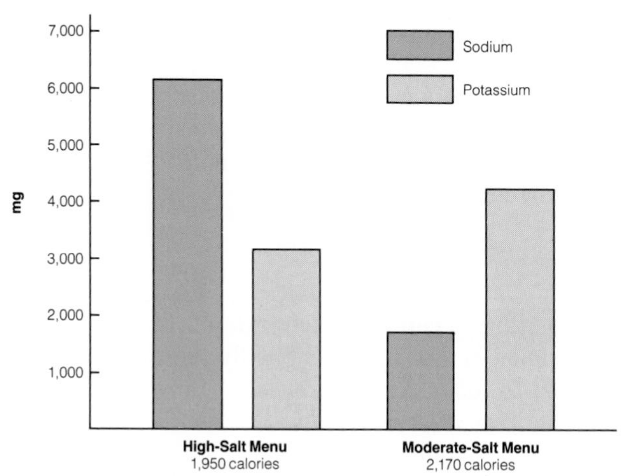

*A main contributor to the sodium level of the menu.

and polyunsaturated fats. Dietary intakes of each of these may play a role in the development of hypertension, but they appear to exert a less important effect on blood pressure than does either sodium or potassium.[32] People who quit smoking, reduce their day-to-day level of stress, and increase their physical activity level reduce their risk of developing hypertension.[27]

Obesity is clearly related to hypertension, and the risk of becoming hypertensive increases as body weight increases.[27] In contrast to underweight and normal-weight individuals, people who are obese benefit little from reductions in dietary sodium intake. For them, weight loss is the best antihypertension "medicine." Even small amounts of weight loss generally reduce blood pressure in obese people with hypertension.[25,33] Weight loss in the range of 16 pounds has been shown to produce a larger decrease in blood pressure than antihypertension drugs.[34]

Excessive alcohol consumption has also been related to hypertension. Alcohol intakes that habitually exceed two drinks per day are associated with above-average blood pressure levels. Blood pressure generally returns to normal among heavy drinkers when they reduce their intake to 2 or fewer drinks per day.[23]

Factors that appear to influence the development of hypertension:
- *sodium intake*
- *potassium intake*
- *smoking*
- *stress*
- *physical inactivity*
- *alcohol intake*
- *calcium intake(?)*
- *obesity*
- *magnesium intake(?)*
- *polyunsaturated fat intake(?)*

TABLE 12-5
Major sources of sodium in the U.S. diet

Source	Percentage of Total Sodium Intake
naturally occurring in foods	10
added during processing	60
salt added during cooking or at the table	30

Prevention of Hypertension Reducing salt intake is mainly regarded as a treatment for hypertension, but it may also help to prevent it, especially among people who have a parent with hypertension.[22,35] Moderate salt intakes beginning in early childhood and the maintenance of normal weight may be the most effective means of reducing the incidence of hypertension in the U.S.[23,36] Not smoking, being physically active, and consuming alcoholic beverages only in moderation would also contribute to reduced incidence of hypertension.

Sources

Very few foods naturally contain much sodium. In fact, only about 10% of the sodium consumed in the U.S. is originally present in food (Table 12-5).[37] The rest is added to foods during processing, preparation, and at the table.[31] The sodium level of the average U.S. diet would be that of a highly restricted sodium diet (similar to that of our hunter–gatherer ancestors) if salt were not added to our foods. Based on weight, only simple sugars are more commonly added to foods than is salt. (Box 12-3 explains some reasons for salt being added to processed foods.)

Food sources of sodium are listed in Table 12-6. Note in the table that most of the "rich" sources of sodium are "miscellaneous" foods, those that cannot be neatly assigned to a particular food category. Among the richest sources are table salt and sea salt (Box 12-4), smoked and canned foods, sauces, and salty snacks.

TABLE 12-6
Food sources of sodium

Food	Amount	Sodium, mg*
Miscellaneous		
salt	1 t	2,132
dill pickles	1 (4½ oz)	1,930
sea salt	1 t	1,716
chicken broth	1 c	1,571
ravioli, canned	1 c	1,065
spaghetti with sauce, canned	1 c	955

TABLE 12-6, *continued*

Food	Amount	Sodium, mg*
Miscellaneous, *cont.*		
baking soda	1 t	821
beef broth	1 c	782
gravy	¼ c	720
Italian dressing	2 T	720
pretzels	5 (1 oz)	500
green olives	5	465
pizza w/cheese	1 wedge	455
soy sauce	1 t	444
cheese twists	1 c	329
bacon	3 slices	303
French dressing	2 T	220
potato chips	10 pieces	200
catsup	1 T	155
Meats		
corned beef	3 oz	808
ham	3 oz	800
canned fish	3 oz	735
meat loaf	3 oz	555
sausage	3 oz	483
hot dogs	1	477
smoked fish	3 oz	444
bologna	1 oz	370
Milk and Milk Products		
cream soup	1 c	1,070
cottage cheese	½ c	455
American cheese	1 oz	405
cheese spread	1 oz	274
Parmesan cheese	1 oz	247
Gouda cheese	1 oz	232
cheddar cheese	1 oz	175
skim milk	1 c	125
milk, whole	1 c	120
Grain Products		
bran flakes	1 c	363
cornflakes	1 c	325
croissant	1 med.	270
bagel	1	260
English muffin	1	203
white bread	1 slice	130
whole-wheat bread	1 slice	130
saltine crackers	4 squares	125

*The provisional RDA for adults is 1,100–3,300 mg.

TABLE 12-7

Some low-sodium fruits and vegetables that are also good sources of potassium

Food	Amount	Sodium, mg	Potassium, mg
Fruits			
banana	1 med.	1	440
blueberries	½ c	1	60
cherries	½ c	1	130
grapefruit	½	1	130
peach	1 med.	1	200
strawberries	⅔ c	1	165
pear	1 med.	3	215
Vegetables			
corn	½ c	1	135
green beans	½ c	2	95
tomato	1 med.	4	300
cucumber	½ med.	4	125
potato	1 med.	5	780
cauliflower	½ c	5	150
broccoli	½ c	8	205
green pepper	½ c	10	155
lettuce	1½ c	10	160

Perhaps equally as important to know about as high-sodium foods are those that contain low amounts of sodium. Table 12-7 lists a number of very low sodium fruits and vegetables, all of which are also good sources of potassium. These foods are examples of good food choices for people with hypertension and for those at risk of developing hypertension because it runs in their family.

Recommended Intake

The average person in the U.S. consumes at least 6,690 mg (6.69 grams) of sodium from food each day and adds another 2,000 mg (2.0 g) to food at the table.[38] The provisional RDA for adults is 1,100 to 3,300 mg per day. Hu-

BOX 12-3

WHY IS SO MUCH SALT ADDED TO FOODS?

Salt is added to foods for several reasons. First, and perhaps most importantly, people tend to like the taste of salt. Salt also enhances the texture of many processed foods, such as bakery products,[37] and helps to protect foods from spoiling. Salt is used in the making of cheese, for example, because it draws fluid away from the solids contained in milk, thus helping to solidify the cheese. Although salt is added to many foods for taste appeal, it also functions in other ways that make it a mainstay of the food manufacturing industry.

BOX 12-4

IS SEA SALT A BETTER CHOICE THAN TABLE SALT?

Many people are attracted to sea salt and use it in preference to table salt, and many restaurants are offering it as an option to table salt. The general feeling is that it contains less sodium and more essential minerals than table salt.

As shown in the bar graph, sea salt contains somewhat less sodium and magnesium and slightly more calcium and potassium than table salt. Neither kind of salt is pure sodium chloride; both provide other essential minerals in addition to sodium. The high amount of sodium per teaspoon of each type of salt makes it hard to press the case for mineral advantages of sea salt.

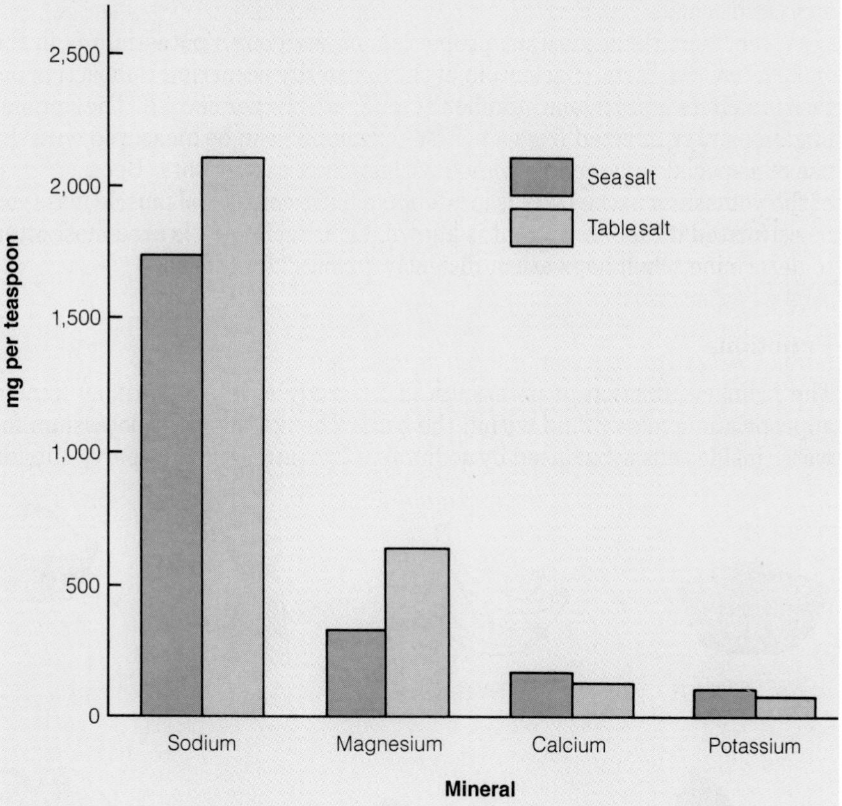

Comparison of the mineral content of one teaspoon of sea salt and one teaspoon of table salt.

mans actually need only 500 mg of sodium per day to maintain normal functioning, but intakes up to 3,300 mg per day do not appear to increase the risk of developing hypertension.[12]

Deficiency Most cases of sodium deficiency are caused by problems that increase sodium loss, such as diarrhea, vomiting, and some kidney disorders. Heavy sweating also can cause sodium deficiency if the lost sodium is not replaced by foods or fluids. A person with sodium deficiency feels very weak and shaky. These symptoms disappear within seconds after salt or another source of sodium is consumed.

Toxicity The primary consequence of excessive sodium intake appears to be hypertension, which is discussed earlier in this section.

■ ■ ■

POTASSIUM (K)

The symbol K abbreviates kalium, *Arabic for "potash." Potassium was first isolated from potash, a compound of potassium and carbon. Potash is extracted from wood ashes and has been used for centuries as a plant fertilizer.*

Potassium is a silvery white mineral with a brilliant shine. Free potassium is highly reactive and is widely used in the manufacture of explosives, detonators, and fireworks.

Potassium is found in all cells, but most of the body's 4½-ounce supply is located inside muscle cells. Very little potassium is found in fat and bone cells, or in the blood or fluid that surrounds cells. The potassium inside cells serves as the ionic counterpart of sodium, the principle ion in the fluid that surrounds cells.

A very small but constant proportion of the body's potassium is in the radioactive ^{40}K form. Each atom of this naturally occurring radioactive potassium emits a particular number of gamma rays per second. The number of gamma rays emitted from a person (or animal) can be measured with the use of a special compartment lined with gamma-ray sensors. Because most of the potassium in the body is located in muscle cells, total muscle mass can be estimated if the ^{40}K content is known. (This technique is used most often to determine when hogs are sufficiently "meaty" for market.)

Functions

Functions of potassium:
maintenance of fluid balance
conduction of nerve impulses and muscle contractions

The primary function of potassium in the body is its role in maintaining appropriate levels of fluid within the cells. The attraction of potassium for water inside cells is balanced by sodium's water-attracting property outside

Some dietary sources of potassium.

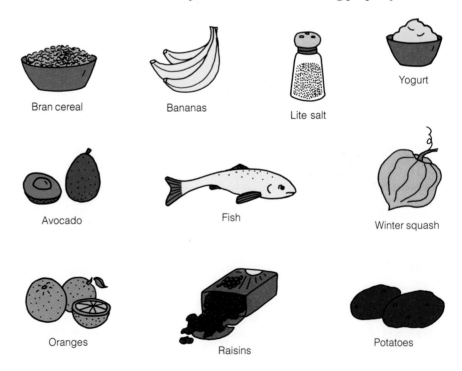

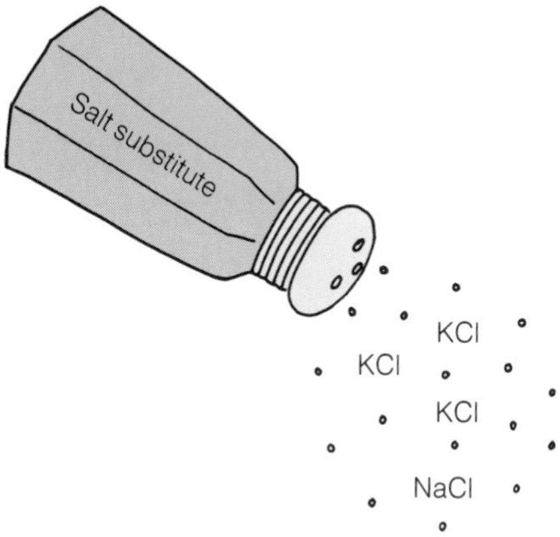

Salt substitutes are a source of potassium, some of them providing 200 mg with each "shake."

of the cells. The amount of fluid inside of cells and the amount outside the cells is kept in balance by the constant shifting of potassium and sodium across cell membranes.

Similar to calcium, potassium also functions in the conduction of nerve impulses and muscle contractions. The rapid cycling of potassium from the inside of cells to the outside and back again generates electrical impulses that stimulate specific cell activities.

Sources

Food sources of potassium are listed in Table 12-8. As you can see in the table, the single best source of potassium is potatoes. Most vegetables and fruits are good sources of potassium, but it is widely distributed in many foods.

A relatively new source of dietary potassium is gaining popularity in the U.S.—salt substitutes. Many salt substitutes provide about 200 mg of potassium with every shake.[30] Some low-sodium salts are produced by replacing the sodium in "sodium" chloride with potassium.

Recommended Intake

The average U.S. intake of potassium falls at the low end of the provisional RDA range of 1,875–5,625 mg per day.[39] Humans can adjust metabolically to a wide range of potassium intakes, and neither deficiency nor overdose has been found to be related to diet among healthy individuals. Deficiencies do occur, however, in conjunction with certain disease states and drugs, and overdoses have resulted from the overzealous use of potassium supplements.

Deficiency Potassium deficiency due to excessive losses of body potassium occurs rather frequently. Most cases of potassium deficiency are related to the use of certain diuretics ("water pills") used to control high blood pressure.[30,41] Over 100 million prescriptions for diuretics are written each year.[41] Potassium supplements or instructions for eating a high-potassium diet are generally given along with prescriptions for diuretics that can cause excessive losses of body potassium. Prolonged bouts of vomiting and diarrhea also can lead to potassium loss and a deficiency state. The most noticeable effects of low blood potassium levels are weakness and irregular heart beats.[42]

TABLE 12-8
Food sources of potassium

Food	Amount	Potassium, mg*
Vegetables		
potato	1 med.	780
winter squash	½ c	327
tomato	1 med.	300
celery	1 stalk	270
carrots	1 med.	245
broccoli	½ c	205
Fruits		
avocado	½ med.	680
banana	1 med.	440
orange juice	6 oz	375
raisins	¼ c	370
watermelon	2 c	315
prunes	4 large	300
Meats		
fish	3 oz	500
hamburger	3 oz	480
lamb	3 oz	382
pork	3 oz	335
chicken	3 oz	208
Grains		
Bran Buds®	1 c	1,080
Bran Flakes®	1 c	248
raisin bran	1 c	242
wheat flakes	1 c	96
Milk and Milk Products		
yogurt	1 c	531
skim milk	1 c	400
whole milk	1 c	370
Other		
salt substitutes	1 t	1,300–2,378

*The provisional RDA for adults is 1,875–5,625 mg.

Toxicity Excessive amounts of supplemental potassium are highly toxic and can cause death due to heart failure. An oral dose of 18 grams can make the heart stop beating. (Typically, 0.5 to 2 grams is prescribed to replace the potassium loss due to diuretic use.)

CHLORIDE

Chloride was added to the RDA tables in 1980. It is widely distributed throughout body fluids and functions in the maintenance of fluid balance and in digestion. Chloride is primarily found in the fluid that surrounds cells and in hydrochloric acid, a secretion of the stomach that aids digestion.

Major functions of chloride: maintenance of fluid balance as component of hydrochloric acid

Table salt is the primary dietary source of chloride. The body is able to adapt to wide fluctuations in chloride intake, and dietary deficiencies and overdoses occur only very rarely. Chloride deficiency most commonly develops from the excessive loss of stomach juices that accompanies severe vomiting or diarrhea. A mass deficiency affecting hundreds of infants occurred in 1979, however, when chloride was accidentally omitted from a commercial infant formula.

COMING UP IN CHAPTER 13

On tap in the next chapter is water. Water performs a variety of functions in the body, many of which are related to the utilization of the energy nutrients, vitamins, and minerals.

REVIEW QUESTIONS

1. The major source of fluoride in the U.S. is ____________.
2. Fluoride is considered an essential nutrient because of its role in ____________.
3. The most prominent feature of chromium deficiency in humans is ____________.
4. State one thing you know about molybdenum.
5. Selenium's primary role is as a(n) ____________.
6. Why does the content of selenium in food vary widely?
7. What are the two major approaches for treating mild hypertension?
8. What is the leading source of sodium in the U.S. diet?
9. What types of foods naturally contain much more potassium than sodium?
10. Low potassium and high sodium intakes have been related to the development of ____________.
11. True or false: Even mild cases of copper deficiency are rare in the U.S.

Answers

1. Fluoridated water.
2. Protecting teeth from decay.
3. Elevated blood glucose.
4. The provisional adult RDA for molybdenum is 0.15–0.5 mg; it's an essential cofactor for a number of enzymes involved in protein synthesis; dietary deficiencies and excesses are regarded as unimportant.

5. Antioxidant.
6. Because the selenium content of food depends on soil or water content, which varies a good deal from region to region.
7. Reduced-sodium diets (about 2 grams per day) and weight loss if overweight.
8. Processed foods.
9. Fruits and vegetables.
10. Hypertension.
11. False. Mild cases of copper deficiency may be common.

PUTTING NUTRITION KNOWLEDGE TO WORK

1. Table salt is 40% sodium and 60% chloride by weight. If you used one teaspoon of salt (weight 4 grams) on your food in one day, would that cause you to exceed the provisional RDA for sodium that day?
2. In previous chapters, you have examined your food intake by food groups and the "Dietary Guidelines for Americans." At this time, your instructor may ask you to analyze the nutrient composition of your diet using a computer program. To do this takes some planning and time. Completion of that assignment will require recording three days of food and beverage intake, including two weekdays and one weekend day. Select days that represent your *usual* intake. Be sure to record the amount of everything you eat and drink as well as a full description of the foods and beverages. Instructions and a form for recording your food intake are provided in Appendix G and in the manual that accompanies the DAS™ program.

NOTES

1. S. O. Welsh and R. M. Marston, Review of trends in food use in the United States, 1909 to 1980, *Journal of the American Dietetic Association* 81 (1982): 120–125.

2. I. M. Klevay, Hypercholesterolemia in rats produced by an increase of the ratio of zinc to copper ingested, *American Journal of Clinical Nutrition* 26 (1973): 1060–1068.

3. O. H. Leverett, Fluorides and the changing prevalence of dental caries, *Science* 217 (1982): 26–30.

4. K. H. Lu, O. J. Yen, et al., The effect of a fluoride dentifrice containing an anticalculus agent on dental caries in children, *Journal of Dentistry of Children* 52 (1985): 449–451.

5. V. L. Richmond, Thirty years of fluoridation: A review, *American Journal of Clinical Nutrition* 41 (1985): 129–138.

6. D. R. Collier, Fluoride: An essential element for good dental health, *Contemporary Nutrition* 4 (1979): 1–2. The article reviews documentation of the safety of fluoridation.

7. G. S. Leske, L. W. Ripa, et al., Dental public health, in *Review of Public Health*, eds. L. Breslow et al. (Palo Alto, Calif.: Annual Reviews, Inc., 1986).

8. National Research Council, *Fluorides* (Washington, D.C.: National Academy of Sciences, 1971).

9. V. L. Richmond, Thirty years of fluoridation: A review, *American Journal of Clinical Nutrition* 41 (1985): 129–138.

10. Is chromium essential for humans? *Nutrition Reviews* 46 (1988): 17–20.

11. S. K. Czarneck and D. Kritchevsky, Trace elements, in *Nutrition and the Adult,* eds. R. E. Alfin-Slater and D. Kritchevsky (New York: Plenum Press, 1980), 334–335.
12. Food and Nutrition Board, National Research Council, *Recommended Dietary Allowances*, 9th ed. (Washington, D.C.: National Academy of Sciences, 1980).
13. W. C. Willett, B. F. Polk, et al., Prediagnostic serum selenium and the risk of cancer, *Lancet* 2 (1983): 130–134.
14. L. C. Clark, The epidemiology of selenium and cancer, *Federation Proceedings* 44 (1985): 2584–2589.
15. A. Schubert, J. M. Holden, and W. R. Wolf, Selenium content of a core group of foods based on critical evaluation of published analytical data, *Journal of the American Dietetic Association* 87 (1987): 285–295.
16. M. A. Dubick and R. B. Rucker, Dietary supplements and health aids: A critical evaluation, *Journal of Nutrition Education* 15 (1983): 47–53.
17. X. M. Luo, H. J. Wei, et al., Selenium intake and metabolic balance of ten men from a low-selenium area of China, *American Journal of Clinical Nutrition* 42 (1985): 31–37.
18. O. A. Levander and R. F. Burke, Report on the 1986 ASPEN Research Workshop on selenium in clinical nutrition, *Journal of Parenteral and Enteral Nutrition* 10 (1986): 545–549.
19. G. Yang, S. Wang, et al., Edemic selenium intoxication of humans in China, *American Journal of Clinical Nutrition* 37 (1983): 872–881.
20. D. A. Denton, The hunger for salt. An anthropological, physiological, and medical analysis (Berlin: Springer–Verlag, 1982), 427–435.
21. *The Yellow Emperor's Classic of Internal Medicine*, circa 1000 B.C.
22. F. Skrabal, L. Hamberger, and E. Cerny, Salt sensitivity in normotensives with, and salt resistance in normotensives without heredity of hypertension, *Scandinavian Journal of Clinical Laboratory Investigation* (supplement) 176 (1985): 47–57.
23. N. M. Kaplan, Dietary aspects of the treatment of hypertension, *Annual Review of Public Health* 7 (1986): 503–519.
24. L. B. Page, Nutritional determinants of hypertension, in *Nutrition and the Killer Diseases*, ed. M. Winick (New York: John Wiley and Sons, 1981), 113–126.
25. H. G. Langford, M. D. Blaufox, et al., Dietary therapy slows the return of hypertension after stopping prolonged medication, *Journal of the American Medical Association* 253 (1985): 657–664.
26. G. Meneely and H. D. Battarbee, Sodium and potassium, in *Present Knowledge in Nutrition*, 4th ed. (Washington, D.C.: The Nutrition Foundation, 1976).
27. N. M. Kaplan, Dietary aspects of the treatment of hypertension, in *Annual Review of Public Health*, eds. L. Breslow et al. (Palo Alto, Calif.: Annual Reviews, Inc., 1986), 503–519.
28. G. K. Beauchamp, M. Bertine, and K. Engelman, Modification of salt taste, *Annals of Internal Medicine* 48 (1983): 763–769.
29. P. A. Hessel, Hypertension in white South African miners, *South African Medical Journal* 68 (1985): 229–232.
30. R. P. Russell, Potassium supplementation, potassium-retaining diuretics, and hazards of hyperkalemia, *Clinical Nutrition* 6 (1987): 70–75.
31. G. A. McGregor, Dietary sodium and potassium intake and blood pressure, *Lancet* i (1983): 750–753.
32. R. L. Weinsier and D. Norris, Recent developments in the etiology and treatment of hypertension: Dietary calcium, fat, and magnesium, *American Journal of Clinical Nutrition* 42 (1985): 1331–1338.
33. A. Rissanen, P. Pietinen, et al., Treatment of hypertension in obese patients: Efficacy and feasibility of weight and salt reduction programs, *Acta Medica Scandinavica* 218 (1985): 149–156.
34. S. W. MacMahon, G. J. MacDonald, et al., A randomized controlled trial of weight reduction and metoprolol in the treatment of hypertension in young overweight patients, *Clinical Experimental Pharmacology and Physiology* 12 (1985): 267–271.

35. M. C. Houston, Sodium and hypertension: A review, *Archives of Internal Medicine* 14 (1986): 179–185.

36. Salt intake and eating patterns of infants and children in relation to blood pressure, *Pediatrics* 53 (1974): 115–121.

37. S. C. Crocco, The role of sodium in food processing, *Journal of the American Dietetic Association* 80 (1982): 36–39.

38. F. R. Shank, Y. K. Park, et al., Perspective of the Food and Drug Administration on dietary sodium, *Journal of the American Dietetic Association* 80 (1982): 29–35.

39. D. R. Fischer, K. J. Morgan, and M. E. Zabik, Cholesterol, saturated fatty acids, polyunsaturated fatty acids, sodium, and potassium intakes of the United States population, *Journal of the American College of Nutrition* 4 (1985): 207–224.

40. E. B. Flink, Nutritional aspects of potassium metabolism, in *Potassium: Its Biological Significance*, ed. R. Whang (Boca Raton, Fla.: CRC Press, 1988), 37–44.

41. P. K. Whelton and M. J. Klag, Venticular ectopy, diuretics, and hypokalemia, *Clinical Nutrition* 6 (1987): 59–64.

42. R. E. Cronin and J. P. Knochel, The consequences of potassium deficiency, in *Acid–Base and Potassium Homeostasis*, ed. B. M. Brenner (New York: Churchill Livingstone, 1978), 205–231.

CHAPTER 13

WATER

Water differs from other nutrients in several respects. It is a liquid; our need for it is measured in cups, not in grams or milligrams; and if a person does not consume it, death comes quickly—usually within six days. Water is the largest single component of our diets as well as of our bodies, but despite its importance, it is often "the forgotten nutrient."

The importance of water to human nutrition is frequently taken for granted or overlooked—to the extent that it may not be recognized as an essential nutrient. Water qualifies in all respects as an essential nutrient: it is required for growth, development, and health; it performs specific, required functions in the body; and deficiency and toxicity signs develop when too little or too much of it is consumed.

Water is an essential nutrient.

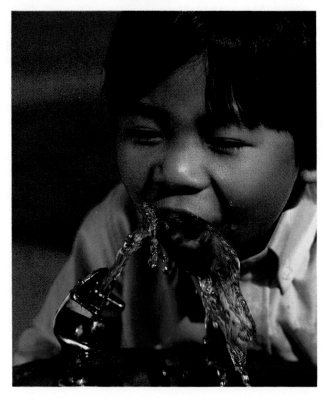

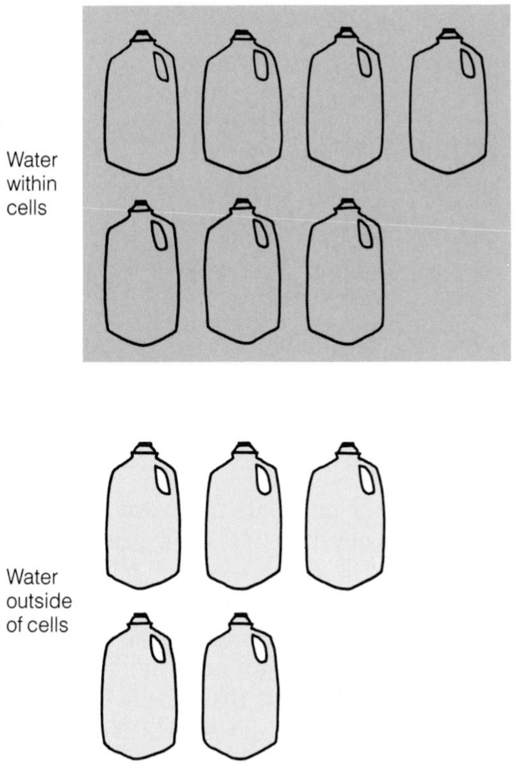

FIGURE 13-1
The body of a 140-pound person contains about 12 gallons of water—approximately 7 gallons within the cells, and 5 gallons in fluids outside the cells.

The human body is made up of 70% to 75% water. Most of the water—60% of the total—is located within the body's cells, and the rest is outside of cells in body fluids (Figure 13-1). The water composition of cells ranges from a high of 70% in muscles to a low of 10% in bone cells. Even fat cells are 30% water. Body water located outside of cells is mainly the water present in blood, lymph, digestive juices, the fluid that surrounds cells, and urine. Most of these body fluids are about 80% water.

FUNCTIONS OF WATER IN THE BODY

The physical and chemical properties of water make it the most basic essential substance for all forms of life. Water is the medium in which chemical reactions take place, it helps maintain ideal pH levels of body fluids, and it plays important roles in energy formation. Water is also important in the transport of nutrients and waste products. Furthermore, water is a critical component of the body's cooling system. (See Table 13-1.)

Medium for Chemical Reactions

Chemical reactions that take place in the body occur within a fluid environment. Water is needed to supply the fluid.

Maintenance of Acid–Base Balance

Whereas some of the chemical reactions that occur in the body require acidic fluids to proceed normally, other reactions require a neutral or basic fluid

TABLE 13-1
Functions of water in the body

Provides a medium for metabolic reactions
Helps body maintain proper acid–base balance
Participates in energy formation
Transports gases, nutrients, metabolic waste products, and other substances
Helps regulate body temperature

environment. Water, by separating into hydrogen ions (H^+) and hydroxide (OH^-) ions, can change the acidity or basicity (that is, pH) of a fluid and thereby help to maintain optimal fluid pH levels.

Energy Formation

Water is an end product of many metabolic reactions, including those involved in energy formation. The amount of water produced each day as a result of energy formation totals about a cup in physically inactive adults. The water produced by energy metabolism explains why people continue to form urine even when they have not consumed water. It also explains why the amount of urine people excrete in the morning exceeds the amount of water they consumed the night before. Energy metabolism goes on throughout the night, causing water to accumulate in the bladder.

Nutrient and Waste Product Transport

Water is the medium of transport for nutrients throughout the body. All gases, nutrients, and other substances found in blood, digestive juices, and urine are water-soluble, or made to be so. Fats and fat-soluble vitamins, which are not soluble in water by themselves, become attached to carriers that make them soluble in water. Water also carries the waste products of cellular metabolism away from the cells and out of the body in urine.

Regulation of Temperature

Another function of water is acting as the body's cooling system. The water content of blood "collects" heat generated by metabolic reactions and delivers it to the network of tiny blood vessels just beneath the surface of the skin. The heat-containing water passes through the walls of the blood vessels to the surface of the skin. Once exposed to air, the water evaporates and releases its heat, thus cooling the body. Water that escapes through the lungs when we exhale also helps to cool the body, but the amount of heat lost through the lungs is much less than the amount lost through the skin. The amount of heat that is lost through the skin and lungs is regulated by mechanisms that detect internal body temperature and control the amount of water released by the blood vessels.

The body's cooling system operates most efficiently when the air surrounding the body is low in humidity. Humid air contains a good deal of moisture and thus cannot "hold" much more; it is already partially saturated. This limits the amount of water that can evaporate from the skin.

This explains why people feel warmer and "stickier" on humid days than on equally warm but dry days.

The amount of water required for maintaining a normal body temperature increases dramatically when exercise or physical work is performed in a very warm environment. One runner studied during a "Death Valley cross" lost 30 pounds of water in the 55-mile, 17-hour race. During the race, the runner drank sufficient fluids to replace his water losses and took salt supplements to replace the sodium he lost. If he had not replaced his fluid losses, he surely would have experienced **heat cramps** or **heat exhaustion**.

heat cramps: Muscle spasms caused by a deficiency of water and sodium in the body resulting from prolonged physical exertion in a hot environment.

heat exhaustion: A condition marked by weakness, dizziness, nausea, and profuse sweating resulting from excessive exposure to heat; also called *heat prostration* and *heat collapse*.

heatstroke: A condition characterized by cessation of sweating, extremely high body temperature, and collapse resulting from prolonged exposure to high temperature; called *sunstroke* if caused by direct exposure to the sun.

Heat Cramps Heat cramps are muscle spasms caused by a deficiency of water and sodium in the body. They are most likely to occur when people perform heavy physical work in hot, humid environments and do not drink sufficient water or other fluids to replace those that are lost. Drinking fruit juices, sport drinks, and other beverages that contain sodium may also help to relieve the muscle cramps.

Heat Exhaustion Heat exhaustion (or *heat collapse* or *heat prostration*) results from excessive exposure to heat and a corresponding drop in the body's fluid and sodium content. A person suffering heat exhaustion feels weak, dizzy, and nauseated. The face becomes pale, and the skin feels cool and clammy. Both heat cramps and heat exhaustion are usually alleviated quickly if the person moves to a cool place, drinks ample fluids, and replaces sodium losses.

Heat exhaustion differs substantially from **heatstroke**, a much less common but more serious condition. Body temperature–regulating mechanisms break down in cases of heatstroke, causing the body temperature to exceed 105° F. Other symptoms of heatstroke include cessation of sweating and physical collapse.

SOURCES OF THE BODY'S WATER

The body gets water through beverages, foods, and energy metabolism. On the average, an adult receives about 6 cups per day by drinking water and other beverages, 4 cups from food, and 1 cup as a result of energy metabolism. Most beverages are more than 85% water, and fruits and vegetables are 75% to 90% water. Meats, depending upon their type and how they are cooked, are 50% to 70% water. Figure 13-2 shows the water composition of some common beverages and foods. Although it is nearly impossible to meet the body's total water need with foods, the water composition of foods makes important contributions to our total daily intakes.

An important new source of water in the U.S. diet is the wide assortment of "gourmet" bottled waters now sold in most supermarkets. In the 1960s, the drinking of "fine waters" became fashionable in France. Natives and tourists alike sat at sidewalk cafes for hours sipping their Perrier, chilled and served with thin slices of lemon. Since then the popularity of bottled waters has skyrocketed in many Western countries. "Mineral," "spring," and "seltzer" waters have sold very well in the U.S. (See Box 13-1.)

The trend toward consuming bottled waters is a healthy one. Bottled waters contain no sugar, they are generally low in sodium, and most of them

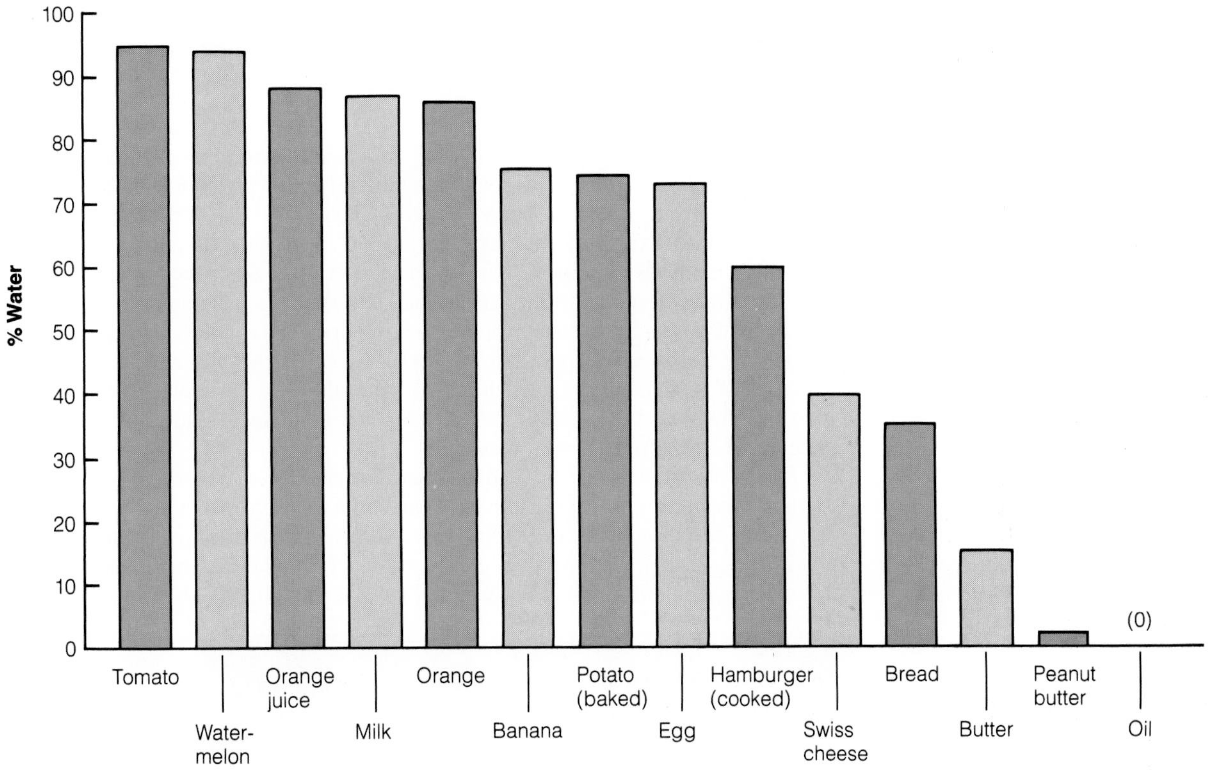

FIGURE 13-2
Water composition of selected foods.

contain no additives other than natural flavors. Furthermore, they quench thirst better than their major competitor, soft drinks.

"Hard" and "Soft" Water

Water can be classified by whether it is "hard" or "soft." Hard water generally comes from underground wells and characteristically contains calcium, magnesium, and iron. The mineral content of hard water interacts with the minerals in soap and detergents, inhibiting the chemical reactions that cause a lather to form and cleaning to occur. You know your water supply is hard if you must use a lot of soap to produce a good lather, if mineral deposits form in your teakettle or bathtub, and if your clothes become grayish after repeated washings. Hard water is made "soft" by water conditioners that replace the calcium, magnesium, and iron in it with sodium. Sodium does not interfere with the chemical actions of soap, and it does not precipitate out of water and leave deposits. Unfortunately, the sodium content of "softened" very hard water can contribute to an excessively high dietary sodium intake and the risk of developing hypertension.[1] Because of the sodium content of softened water, it is customary not to condition the kitchen water that is used for cooking and drinking.

The Earth's Supply of Water

Water covers about three-fourths of the earth's surface, but only about 3% of it is drinkable. Nearly 97% of the total supply is salt water. Only a fourth of the total fresh water supply is available for human use; three-fourths is

BOX 13-1

BOTTLED WATERS

Have you ever wondered what the differences are among "mineral," "spring," and "seltzer" water? True mineral water is taken from underground reservoirs that are lodged between layers of rocks. The water has dissolved some of the minerals in the rocks and, as a result, contains a higher amount of minerals than most sources of surface water. Spring water is taken from freshwater springs that form pools or streams on the surface of the earth. It may be mineralized or not depending upon the conditions present in the spring. Seltzers are sparkling waters that are naturally or artificially carbonated. Most seltzers are made bubbly by the addition of pressurized carbon dioxide. The gas stays in the water as long as it is under pressure, but exits quickly when the pressure is released.

A type of water that is not sold in supermarkets is *pure* water. All types of naturally occurring water contain gases and minerals. Even distilled water is not 100% pure water. In order for water to become truly pure, it must be distilled about 42 times. Water is considered pure when it no longer conducts electricity. It is quite likely that you will never drink pure H_2O.

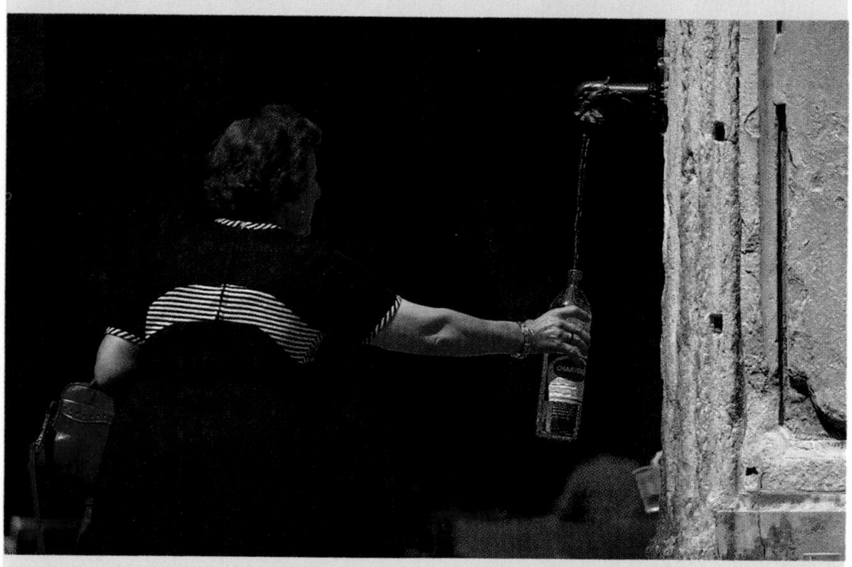

Many Europeans regularly visit the source of their favorite mineral water, bottles in hand. Aix les Bains, France.

located in polar and glacier ice. Although fresh water is abundant in most of North America, this is not the case in some parts of the world. (See Box 13-2.) Nonetheless, there is increasing concern about the adequacy, quality, and safety of the water supply in many parts of the United States.

THE BODY'S REQUIREMENT FOR WATER

Physically inactive adults living in moderate climates need about 10 cups of water each day to replace the water they lose in urine, perspiration, stools, and exhaled air. For individuals in other circumstances, the requirement for water is met when the amount ingested equals the amount lost. People who are physically active, who live in hot climates, or who have illnesses that produce vomiting, diarrhea, or fever need to consume more than 10 cups each day to replace their losses.

Consuming 10 cups of water per day from beverages and foods does not take a lot of advance planning. Table 13-2 presents an example menu and its water content. The menu provides enough water for healthy adults who do not experience above-average water losses. People who live in hot climates or who are physically active will need more than the 10 cups of water this menu provides.

Water Deficiency

Nature has equipped humans with very sensitive mechanisms that trigger thirst when the body's water supply is running low and the water balance is jeopardized. The failure to replace water losses results in increased concentrations of sodium and other mineral ions, which disrupts the body's water balance. Thirst signals the body's need for water to dilute the minerals and re-establish water balance. (Do you remember the explanation of why drinking sea water increases the body's need for water? The failure of sea water to meet the body's water needs is an excellent example of a high mineral load causing a need for water and thirst.)

TABLE 13-2
Water composition of an example one-day menu

Food	Water Content	
	Percentage	Ounces
Breakfast		
orange juice, 6 oz	88	5
cornflakes, 1 c	4	—
milk, 1 c	87	7
toast, 2 slices	35	1
margarine, 2 t	16	—
coffee, 2 c	98	16
Lunch		
chili, 2 c	72	12
crackers, 1 oz	3	—
orange, 1 med.	86	3
milk, 1 c	87	7
Dinner		
vegetable soup, 1 c	84	7
pork chop, 3 oz	46	1
applesauce, 1 c	89	7
corn, ½ c	76	3
ice cream ¾ c	63	4
milk, 1 c	87	7
Total water		80 oz (10 c)

BOX 13-2

WATER: THE MOST IMPORTANT NATURAL RESOURCE

Most people in the U.S. have the luxury of being able to take for granted an abundant supply of water. This may not be true in the future, and for people in many parts of the world, it has never been the case. Many rural communities in developing countries have very limited access to water and must rely on a central watering spot for all their water needs. This watering place may be shared by livestock and is used for washing clothes and bathing. Consequently, it is not uncommon for such sources of water to become contaminated with bacteria that cause local epidemics of infectious diseases.

Water is sufficiently scarce in some parts of the USSR that drinking water dispensers are coin-operated. Fresh water is so highly prized in sections of the arid Middle East that decorative outdoor fountains are status symbols of the wealthy class. Drinking water is sampled, judged, and celebrated in the Middle East just as ceremoniously as fine wines are in France.

Although water is still generally abundant in North America, growing numbers of people are concerned about the quality and safety of the water supply. The detection of hydrocarbons, chloroform, radioisotopes, and asbestos fibers in drinking water in parts of Canada and the U.S. has focused attention on the potential health effects of contaminated water. The list of chemicals that have been found in samples of drinking water in the U.S. includes 64 that are suspected of promoting cancer.[2] It is not yet clear if environmentally contaminated water causes cancer in humans. It *is* clear, however, that action needs to be taken to clean up the water supply in certain areas, even before complete information on the health effects of the contaminants becomes available.

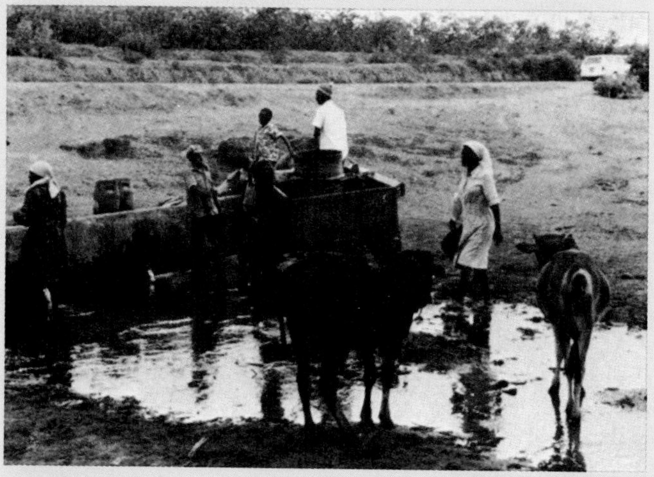

The central water supply of a Kenyan community. The water is shared by humans and livestock, and is transported to homes in buckets or large drums.

Built-in mechanisms that initiate thirst protect most people from consuming too little water and thus from becoming **dehydrated**. People who perform heavy physical work in hot environments, however, sometimes become dehydrated even though they drink in response to thirst. For such people with very great water needs, the thirst mechanism may not ensure

dehydration: A condition that occurs when water excretion exceeds water intake.

Marathon runners replace their fluid losses during the race—often without missing a step

sufficient intakes of fluids; thirst may be satisfied before the body's need for water is. It is recommended that physical laborers and athletes drink more fluids than indicated by their thirst signals during periods of prolonged physical exertion in hot environments.

Other Causes of Dehydration Prolonged bouts of vomiting, diarrhea, or fever can produce a substantial loss of water and dehydration, especially among young children. Protein intake and alcohol consumption also are related to the development of dehydration, because both increase urine production. If protein or alcohol is consumed in high amounts the intake of water should be increased. This is the reason people on high-protein diets are advised to drink lots of water. The increased water loss that accompanies alcohol consumption explains why many people feel tremendously thirsty after overindulging in the spirits.

causes of dehydration:
failure to consume sufficient water to replace losses
heavy physical activity in hot environments
high salt, protein, or alcohol intake; vomiting, diarrhea, fever

Symptoms of Dehydration Dehydrated people feel very sick. They are physically weak, nauseated, and dizzy and they may be unable to move. The ingestion of fluids produces quick recovery in all but the most serious cases of dehydration. However, if it is not resolved, dehydration can lead to kidney failure and death.

Water Overdose

It may seem strange, but people do overdose on water. **Water intoxication** occurs when people consume more water than can be readily excreted, or when the body's supply of essential minerals is too low to maintain a normal water balance. In some cases, this is caused by drugs and diseases that decrease the concentration of minerals in body fluids. Without the required minerals, water cannot be excreted. Excessive water in body fluids and cells interferes with the normal activities of the mineral ions and, thus, of the metabolic reactions.

water intoxication: A condition that occurs when water intake exceeds water losses. Water intoxication can result from consuming too much water or from drugs and diseases that decrease the concentration of minerals in body fluids.

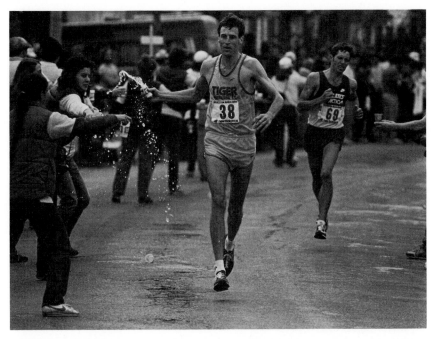

Edema (swelling), dizziness, vomiting, convulsions, and ultimately coma can be caused by water intoxication. Deaths from overdoses of water have been reported, but the overdoses have been short-term intakes measured by the bucket, not by the cup.

■ ■ ■

COMING UP IN PART THREE

Starting with chapter 14, our focus changes from the individual nutrients to the roles the nutrients play in promoting and maintaining health throughout life. We will return to many of the principles and issues we've discussed in the first 13 chapters as they relate to nutrition and the life course.

■ ■ ■

REVIEW QUESTIONS

1. Cite three characteristics that qualify water as an essential nutrient.
2. True or false? The human body contains about the same proportion of water as an egg.
3. What percentage of fat tissue is water?
4. True or false? More of the body's water is located inside of cells than outside of cells.
5. List five functions of water.

Answers

1. Water is required for growth and health; it performs specific, required functions in the body, and deficiency and toxicity signs develop when we consume too little or too much of it.
2. True. The human body is 70% to 75% water, and an egg is 74%.
3. 30%.
4. True. For a person who weighs 140 pounds, there are about 7 gallons inside of cells, and 5 gallons outside of cells.
5. See Table 13-1.

■ ■ ■

PUTTING NUTRITION KNOWLEDGE TO WORK

1. Assume that you have been lost in a hot desert and have endured a 100°F temperature for 24 hours. You are on the verge of dehydration. Alas! You come upon an oasis and a restaurant. Which of these fluids (available at the oasis restaurant) would rehydrate your body most efficiently and why: water, beer, or cola?

   (Answer: Water. This issue was addressed in chapter 3, too. The alcohol content of beer and the sugar in the cola would reduce the amount of water available to your body from the beverages.)

2. How many cups of water or other fluids do you usually drink each day, less than 5, 5 to 10, or more than 10 cups?

(Answer: You may have a hard time answering this question, especially if you sip water from drinking fountains. However, assuming you meet some of your need for water from foods and do not require more than 10 cups of water because of heavy physical activity or a hot climate, an intake of water and other fluids of between 5 and 10 cups per day should satisfy your need for water.)

■ ■ ■

NOTES

1. J. C. Hunt, Sodium intake and hypertension: A cause for concern, *Annals of Internal Medicine* 98 (1983): 724–728.
2. D. T. Wigle, Contaminants in drinking water and cancer risks in Canadian cities, *Canadian Journal of Public Health* 77 (1986): 335–342.

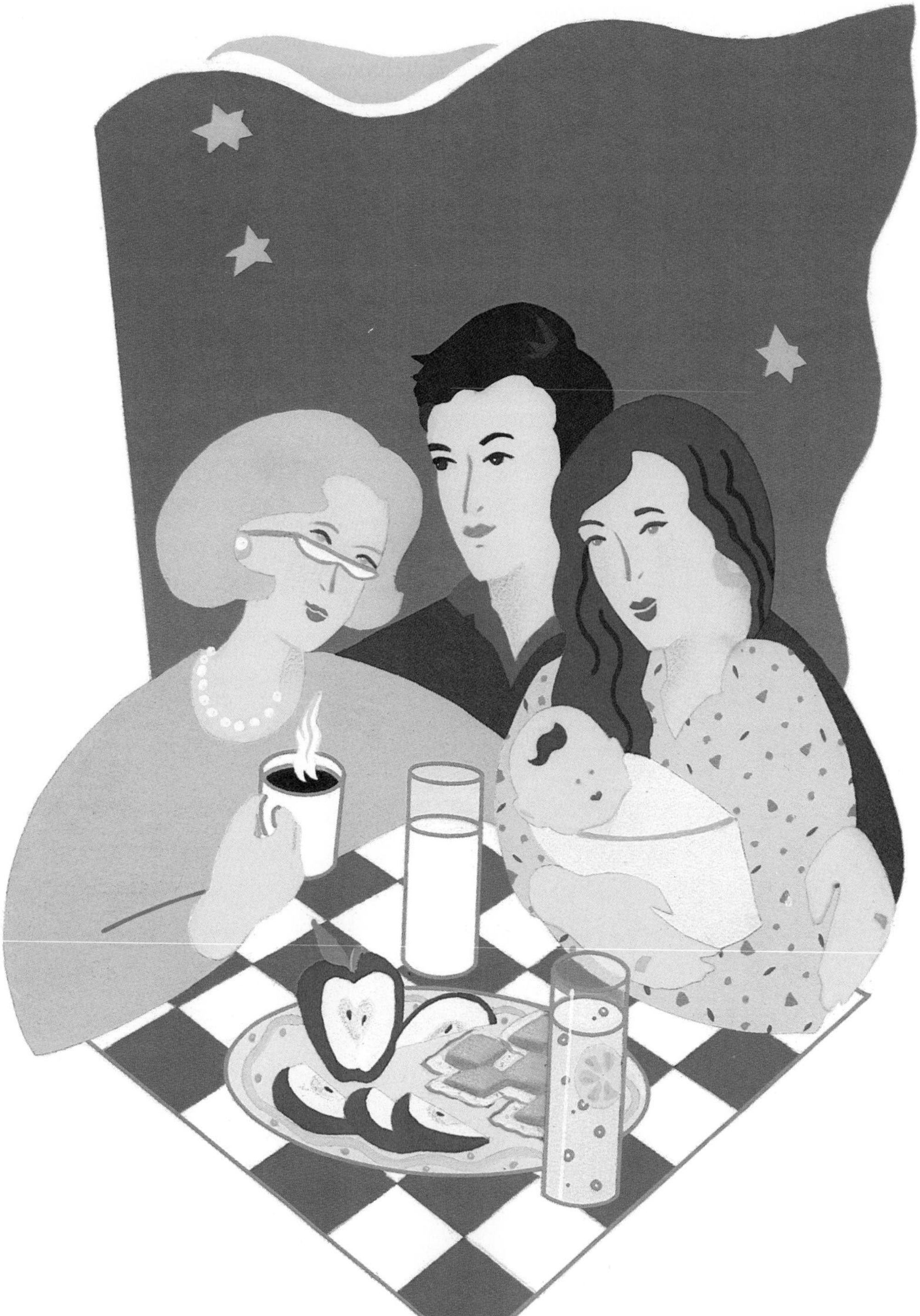

PART THREE

NUTRITION AND THE LIFE COURSE

CHAPTER 14

NUTRITION AND REPRODUCTION

fertility: The biological ability to conceive and maintain a pregnancy.

The influence of nutrition on reproduction is broad. It begins long before conception, because nutrition affects **fertility**, the biological ability to conceive and maintain a pregnancy. Nutrition also affects a woman's health during pregnancy and her ability to breast-feed her baby. A mother's nutrition *directly* influences the health, growth, and development of her child. There is no phase of the life cycle in which good nutrition pays a larger return for investment than the phase in which a new life is created.

NUTRITION AND FERTILITY

Female Fertility

menses: (from Latin *menses*, "monthly") Periodic uterine bleeding accompanied by a shedding of the endometrium (the lining of the uterus). On average, it occurs every 27 to 28 days and lasts 4 to 5 days. Also called *menstruation*.

infertility: Biological inability to conceive or to maintain a pregnancy.

> *To bring on the* **menses**, *recover the flesh by giving a woman puddings, roast meats, a good wine, fresh air, and sun.*
>
> Fertility advice, 1847[1]

It has long been suspected that nutrition plays a role in fertility, but research results to support the suspected relationships between nutrition and the biological ability to bear children did not become available until the 1940s. About 20% of married couples in the United States are **infertile**—unable to produce their own children—and some of them are infertile due to poor nutrition. Infertility is a problem of great importance and it is thought to have many different causes. Almost all of the cases that are related to nutrition can be corrected.

Some of the earliest evidence of a relationship between nutrition and fertility came from studies undertaken during World War II in Russia, the Netherlands, and Japan.[2–5] Famines occurred in those areas due to war-induced food shortages. The dietary intakes of people in Leningrad (Russia) and Japan went from marginally adequate to very inadequate during the war. People in the Netherlands (Holland), however, had enjoyed a high

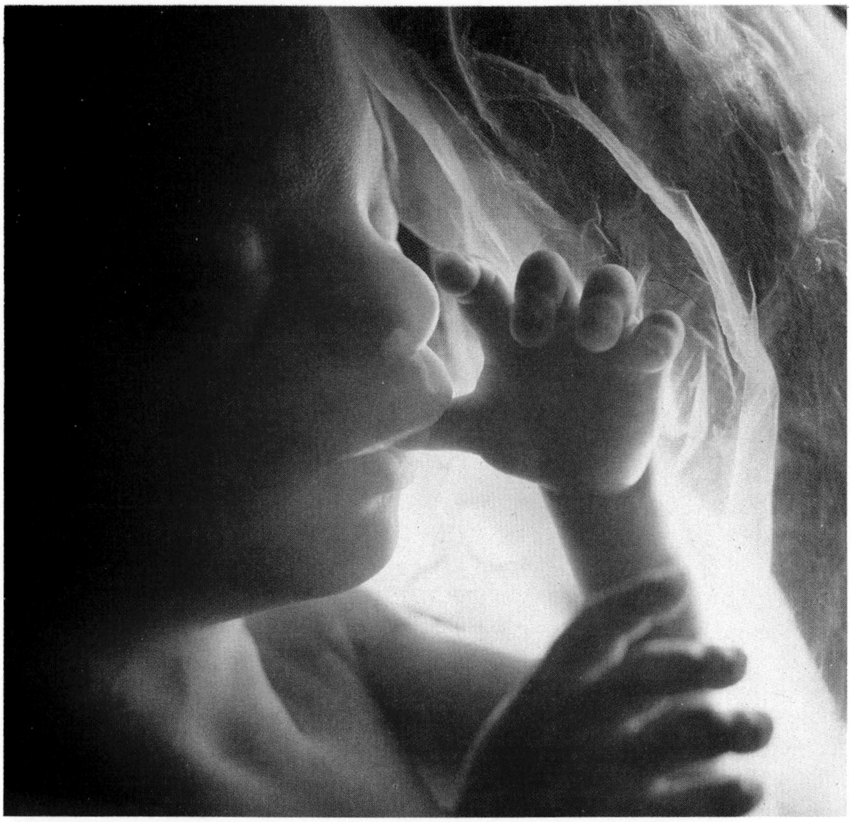

Eighteen-week-old fetus. By this time the fetus is about 7 inches long, and the sucking reflex has developed.

standard of living before the food shortages occurred and they were generally well-nourished when the famine began. The diets of the three groups studied were equally poor during the food shortage. In each area, the most common effect of the famine was a dramatic drop in fertility. In the Netherlands, half the women of childbearing age became infertile due to temporary loss of menses, and the birthrate fell by 53% during the period of food shortage. Nonetheless, menses and fertility were re-established among most Dutch women within six months after the famine ended. The return of normal fertility levels was slower in Leningrad and Japan, because the famine had lasted longer there and the women's nutritional status before the famine had been poorer in those two areas.[2–5]

Body fat content has been shown to be related to fertility. The loss of body fat that accompanies famines may explain the drop in fertility during the wartime famines.

Body Fat and Infertility Both inadequate and excessive levels of body fat have been found to be related to the development of infertility.[6–10] The effect appears to be due to the influence of body fat on estrogen production. This sex hormone is produced in fat stores as well as in the ovaries. Low levels of body fat tend to reduce the amount of estrogen that is produced, whereas high body-fat stores increase it.[9] Estrogen plays a leading role in maintaining normal **menstrual cycles**, such that when estrogen levels are unusually low or high, the cycles become abnormal or disappear until the levels return to normal. Figure 14-1 illustrates the proposed relationships between body fat level and fertility. Infertility due to abnormally low levels

menstrual cycle: The interval between the start of one menses and the beginning of the next.

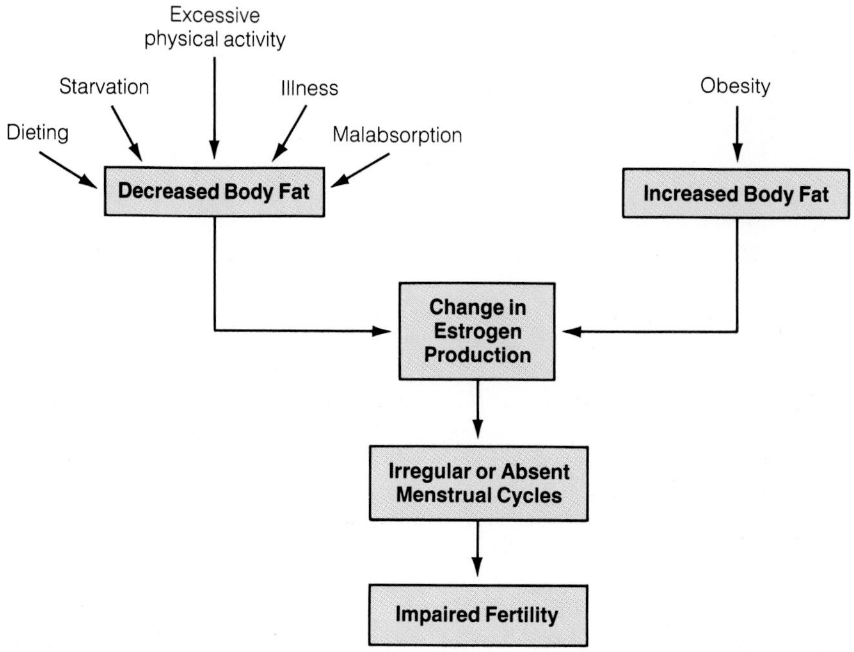

FIGURE 14-1
Proposed effects of low and high levels of body fat on fertility.

of body fat may account for 25% to 35% of all cases occurring in U.S. women.[9] Because fertility is interrupted only when a woman is very obese, obesity is probably a much less frequent cause of infertility than is underweight.

Females at highest risk for becoming infertile due to low levels of body fat are athletes,[11] females with anorexia nervosa,[6] and women who become thin while using oral contraceptive pills.[12] Menstrual periods may be absent in up to 50% of competitive runners, 44% of ballet dancers, 25% of noncompetitive runners, and 12% of swimmers and cyclists.[13] Because the cessation of menstrual cycles is characteristic of anorexia nervosa, females with this eating disorder are highly likely to be infertile.

It has been observed that some athletes intentionally maintain their weight at a level that prevents menstrual periods because the cramping, swelling, and other side effects of periods may interfere with their performance. Unfortunately, female athletes who "lose" their menstrual periods because of low body fat content may be compromising their bone health. Estrogen performs many functions in the body in addition to its role in maintaining normal menstrual cycles. One of these other functions is facilitating the deposition of calcium into bone; when estrogen levels are low, less calcium is deposited into bone. This effect can be particularly important if it occurs before the age of 30, when peak bone mass is accumulating. Bone density and peak bone mass may be decreased in female athletes who have low body-fat content, and this would predispose them to osteoporosis later in life.[14,15] Simple weight gain restores menstrual cycles and fertility in most women experiencing body-fat-related infertility.

Civilization is also thought to have an effect on body composition and fertility. Development that brings sedentary life styles and a reliable food supply can affect the body composition and fertility of entire populations. An example of just how rapidly changes in fertility can occur is given in Box 14-1.

BOX 14-1

FERTILITY SHIFTS AMONG THE !KUNG

One striking example of the influence of body composition on fertility is seen in the !Kung tribesmen of Botswana, in southern Africa.[16,17] Until recently, most of the !Kung lived as hunter–gatherers. As hunter–gatherers, their food supply and body weight fluctuated sharply from season to season.

The average age of the onset of menstrual cycles among female hunter–gatherers is 15.5 years, about 3 years beyond the average age of menarche of females in Western countries. Although girls marry at about age 15, the average age at first birth is 19.5 years. Conception rates are highest among these !Kung during the time of the year when nutrition is favorable and body weight highest. Infants born to hunter–gatherer !Kung women are breast-fed on demand for 3 to 4 years. The combination of the long period of breast feeding, periods of feast and famine, and a physically active lifestyle is thought to produce deficits in body fat stores that lead to periodic infertility.

In recent years, many of the !Kung have settled in farming communities, and few nomadic hunter–gatherers remain. Lifestyle in the farming communities is vastly different from the hunting–gathering lifestyle, and the change has affected fertility and birthrates. !Kung who farm do not ordinarily experience feast and famine cycles; they are heavier and taller; the females begin menses earlier and they have more children than their hunter–gatherer counterparts. It is believed that these changes in fertility can be partly explained by increases in body fat composition.[16,17]

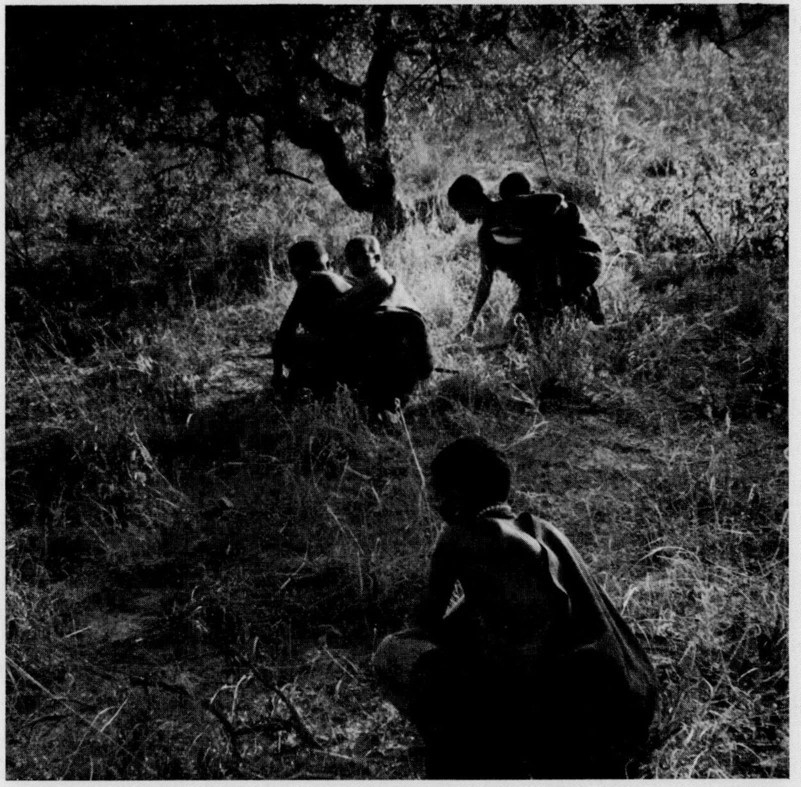

!Kung women gathering foods for their families' meals. Living off the land keeps these women physically active and lean.

Carotenemia and Infertility Excessive intakes of carotene-rich vegetables have been found to be associated with the development of reversible infertility. In one study, a number of infertile women were all found to have the habit of snacking on carrots or dried green-pepper flakes throughout the day. All were diagnosed as having carotenemia (in addition to being infertile). Normal menses returned in all of the women when they stopped snacking on those foods.[18]

Vitamin C, Vegan Diets, and Infertility Infertility has been reported in women who regularly consume megadoses of vitamin-C supplements and in women who are vegans.[19–21] It is not clear why vitamin C would produce this effect, but fertility has returned when the high-dosage supplements are stopped. It has been suggested that infertility among vegans may result from high intakes of estrogen-containing vegetables, from the possibility that a higher-than-normal excretion of estrogen may accompany high-fiber diets, or from vegans' lower levels of body fat.

Male Fertility

Much of what we know about the influence of nutrition on fertility in males comes from the starvation studies that were conducted on volunteers during the 1940s.[22] The first sign of impaired fertility observed in the starving men was a loss of sexual drive. Sperm motility decreased as weight loss progressed, and sperm production ceased entirely when weight loss exceeded 25% of normal body weight. When the men regained the weight, their libidos and their sperm motility and production returned to normal. It has been suggested that loss of body fat in men may affect fertility by altering sex hormone levels just as it appears to do in women.[23]

Relationships among undernutrition, zinc deficiency, and sexual maturation have been identified in males.[24] Chronic undernutrition and weight loss during **puberty** delays growth and sexual maturation in males. Moderate levels of zinc deficiency may delay puberty among adolescent males, and severe deficiency has been associated with impaired development of sex organs.

puberty: The stage in life during which humans become biologically capable of reproduction.

Although there is more to learn about nutrition and fertility relationships in males, it is prudent to consider the possibility that malnutrition in men may be responsible for infertility.

Oral Contraceptives and Nutrition

Whereas infertility is a problem for one out of five couples, fertility control may be an issue for the remaining four out of five. Controlling fertility also has implications for nutritional health.

Much of the clamor about the side effects of oral contraceptive pills has diminished since the introduction of the low-dose, estrogen–progesterone combination pill in 1975.[25] Use of the earlier pills was associated with a number of nutrition problems ranging from weight gain to vitamin B_6 deficiency. Today's oral contraceptives appear to be much safer than earlier ones, although some nutritional side effects remain.

The new generation of low-dose pills have been found to slightly increase blood glucose and triglyceride levels and the need for vitamin B_6 and folic acid (Figure 14-2).[26–28] The side effects of oral contraceptives occur with

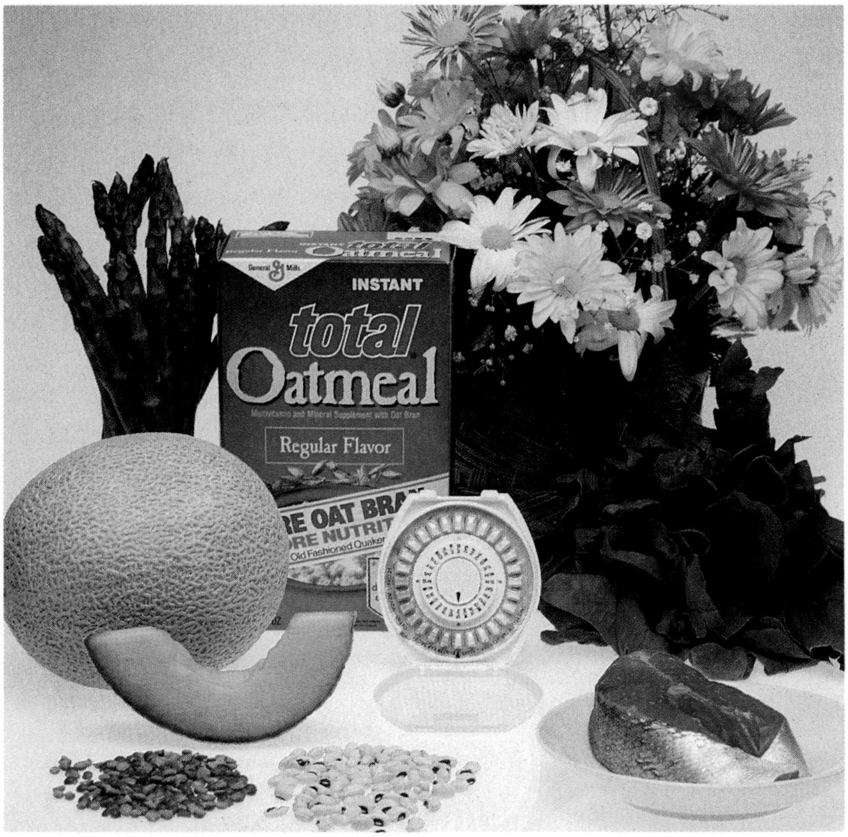

■
FIGURE 14-2
Women who use low-dosage oral contraceptive pills need to consume adequate food sources of vitamin B_6 and folic acid. These foods include liver, fish, leafy green vegetables, legumes, fruits, and oatmeal.

greater frequency among women who consume marginally adequate diets and those who take the pill continuously for five years and longer. A deficiency of vitamin B_6 may account for the depression that some women experience while using the pill. One group of researchers found that a supplement containing 10 mg of B_6 taken for 7 days during a menstrual cycle relieved depression in women who developed low B_6 levels while taking oral contraceptive pills.[28] The increased need for folic acid during pill use may put some women at risk of developing folic-acid deficiency if they become pregnant shortly after they stop using the pill. It is advised that women delay pregnancy until about six months after using oral contraceptive pills. This interval allows the woman's body to make up for deficits in vitamin B_6 and folic acid that may have occurred while taking the pill.[27]

Oral contraceptives are a very popular method of birth control. Approximately 19% of U.S. females aged 15 to 44 years (8.7 million females) use them.[29] They are effective in preventing pregnancy because they block the release of an egg from a woman's ovary during the menstrual cycle. They are not for everyone, however. Use of oral contraceptive pills is not recommended for women who are over 35 years of age, women who have diabetes, or women who are heavy smokers, since these conditions exaggerate the potentially negative side effects of oral contraceptives on blood glucose, cholesterol, and triglyceride levels.[30] All things considered, use of oral contraceptive pills poses fewer health risks than does pregnancy.[30] It is one of a very few highly effective forms of birth control for people who wish to delay pregnancy.

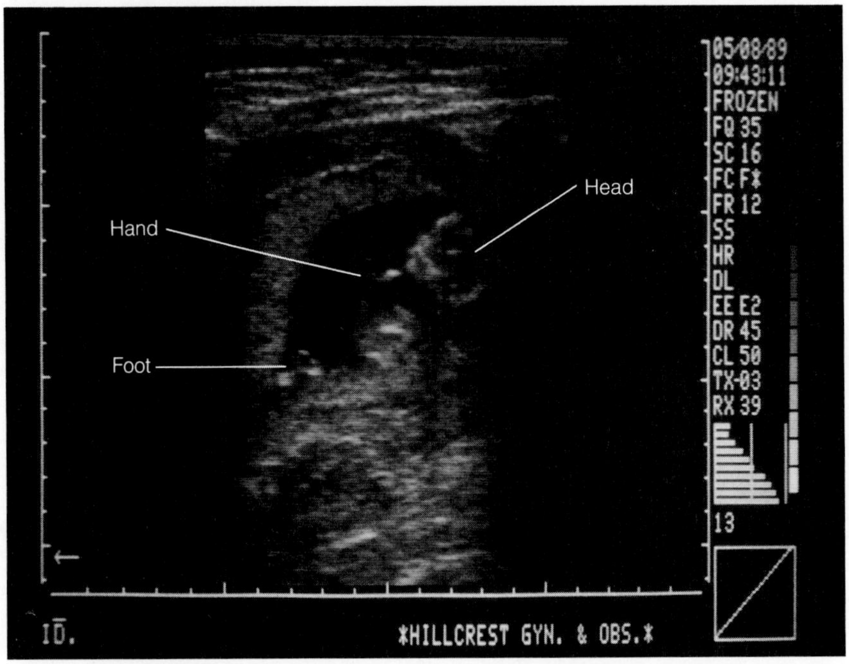

Ultrasound image of a 13½-week-old fetus.

NUTRITION AND PREGNANCY

Simply stated, the biological changes that occur with pregnancy are profound. How well they proceed largely determines how healthy the mother and the infant will be. Many factors affect how smoothly the pregnancy goes and how healthy the infant is at birth, but none of the factors is more important than nutrition.

The World War II studies that shed light on nutrition and fertility also demonstrated some effects of nutrition during pregnancy on infant health. Total calorie intake among pregnant women in Leningrad and the Netherlands averaged 1,100 calories per day during the food shortage. Average protein intake was about 30 grams per day—less than half the RDA for pregnant adult women—and it consisted primarily of low-quality proteins. The period of food shortage lasted only eight months in the Netherlands but for two years in Leningrad. The effects of the food shortage were also more profound in Leningrad because it was imposed on women who were marginally nourished in the first place. The impact of the food shortage on infant health in Leningrad included increased rates of **preterm** births, **low birth weight**, and **stillborn** births. In the Netherlands, the primary effect of the food shortage was a drop in birth weight.

Other information about nutrition and reproductive health was generated during World War II from studies in England. Due to a special food-rationing program, the dietary intakes of pregnant women improved during the war. The improvement in diets was associated with the birth of babies that were larger and healthier than babies born before the war. Furthermore, the rates of preterm birth and infant death declined during the period of special food rationing. Birth outcomes worsened, however, after the special food-rationing program ended.

preterm: Infants born at or before 37 weeks of pregnancy. Infants born between 38 and 42 weeks of pregnancy are considered to be "term."

low birth weight: Birth weight below 5½ pounds.

stillborn: Infant that is not alive when delivered.

Three important conclusions can be drawn from the World War II studies:

1. Nutrition prior to pregnancy affects infant health.
2. Poor nutrition has a greater, negative influence on infant health if it exists both before and during pregnancy.
3. Improvement in nutrition during pregnancy has a beneficial effect on infant health.

These conclusions have influenced public-health nutrition policies in the United States. Knowledge gained from these natural experiments was used to support the establishment of the Supplemental Food Program for Women, Infants, and Children. Generally referred to as "WIC," this public health program is available in every state in the nation. (Box 14-2 presents information about this successful public health program.)

Other indicators of nutritional status are known to influence infant health. Two of the most important are the mother's prepregnancy weight for height (*weight status*) and weight gain during pregnancy. Both influence infant health because of their effect on birth weight, and infant birth weight is known to be closely related to infant health. Small infants, especially those weighing less than 5½ pounds, are at least 12 times more likely to die or to have lasting health problems than are infants who weigh about 8 pounds at birth.[38,39] The average birth weight of infants born in the United States is 7½ pounds, and 7% of babies are classified as low birth weight. Women who enter pregnancy underweight or who fail to gain a certain minimum of weight during pregnancy are much more likely to deliver low-birth-weight infants than are women who are of normal weight or above and gain an appropriate amount of weight.[40]

Contrary to popular belief, the father's height has very little relationship to an infant's size at birth.[41] The size of an infant at birth is primarily determined by maternal, not paternal, factors.

Optimal Weight Gain during Pregnancy

There is no specific amount of weight gain during pregnancy that's right for everyone. How much a woman should gain depends on her weight status before pregnancy. Normal-weight women tend to deliver infants of optimal birth weight if they gain between 30 and 35 pounds. On average, higher prenatal weight gains among underweight women and lower gains among women who are overweight or obese correspond to the delivery of infants with the healthiest birth weights.[40,42,43] Maternal weight gains associated with delivery of infants of optimal birth weight are presented in the graph in Figure 14-3.

Two other factors are important to consider within this topic: the rate of weight gain and the quality of the diet that produces the weight gain. Weight gain should be gradual and should continue in an upward direction even for women who enter pregnancy overweight or obese. All guidelines assume that weight gain is achieved by eating high-quality diets.

Hunger and food intake fluctuate widely during pregnancy, and increases in food intake usually do not produce the smooth rate of maternal weight gain shown in weight gain graphs such as Figure 14-3. There are spurts in food intake and in weight gain.

Hunger, food intake, and weight gain generally are greatest in the second trimester. The calorie and nutrient stores that develop as a result of the increased food intake are used to support the high rate of fetal growth that

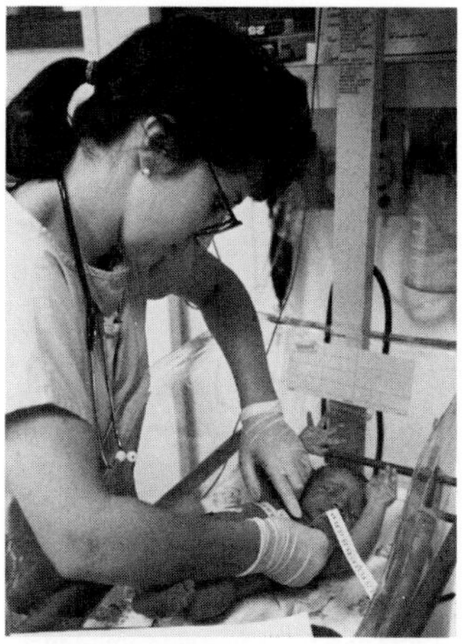

A nurse records a newborn's vital statistics.

FIGURE 14-3
Maternal weight gains during pregnancy that are associated with the birth of healthy-sized infants.[40,42]

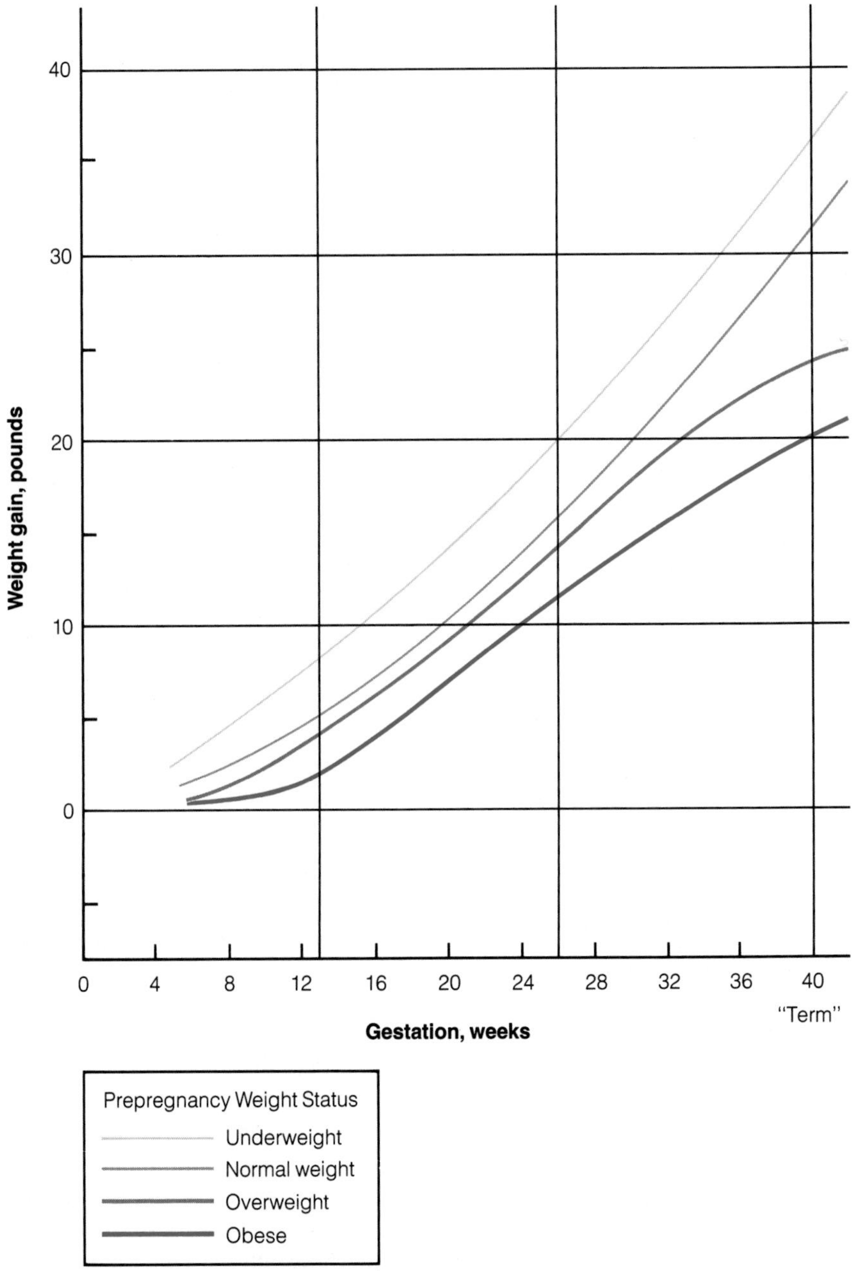

fetus: A baby in the womb from the eighth week of pregnancy until birth. Before then, it is referred to as an *embryo*.

uterus: The womb; a pear-shaped, muscular organ for containing the fetus during pregnancy.

amniotic fluid: Fluid that surrounds the fetus in the uterus. It and the fetus are contained in a thick membrane called the *amniotic sac*.

occurs in the last trimester. Thus, peak hunger, food intake, and rate of weight gain precede the time of the largest gains in fetal weight.[45]

Components of Weight Gain During the eighteenth and nineteenth centuries, it was thought that since an infant weighs only about seven pounds at birth, women do not need to gain much more than that amount. It was assumed that the only tissue that grew during pregnancy was the **fetus.** Now it is known that that is not the case. Fetal growth is accompanied by marked increases in maternal blood volume, fat stores, and breast and **uterus** size. The accumulation of **amniotic fluid** (the water that surrounds the fetus in the uterus), the increase in the volume of fluid that exists outside of cells, and the **placenta** also account for weight gain during pregnancy. Broken down into individual components, a gain of 30 pounds during pregnancy would be distributed approximately as shown in Table 14-1. At full term, an eight-pound infant accounts for only about 28% of the mother's total weight gain.

It does not appear that women whose weight gains are close to the recommended levels are more likely to become obese or to experience complications of pregnancy than are women who gain less.[43] On average, a new mother loses 15 pounds within the first week, and weight loss generally continues for several months after delivery.[43,44]

Nutritional Needs during Pregnancy

Pregnant women need more calories and essential nutrients than other women need. Consuming enough of each is important, but calories and the nutrients protein, folic acid, vitamin B_6, calcium, iron, zinc, and water are of paramount concern.

According to the RDAs, pregnant women need at least 15% more calories and 15% to 100% more of the nutrients than do nonpregnant women (Figure 14-4). The relatively high requirements for many nutrients mean that pregnant women should increase their intake of nutrient-dense foods more than they increase their consumption of calorie-rich foods.

Calories The need for additional calories in pregnancy increases from about 150 additional calories per day during the first three months (the first

TABLE 14-1

Components of weight gain during pregnancy, based on full-term eight-pound infant

	Pounds
Fetus	8
Uterus	2
Placenta	1½
Blood	4½
Amniotic fluid	2
Breast tissue	1
Tissue fluid	2½
Fat stores	8½
Total weight gain	30

placenta: The organ that connects the fetus with the mother's uterus and through which nutrients pass from the mother to the fetus.

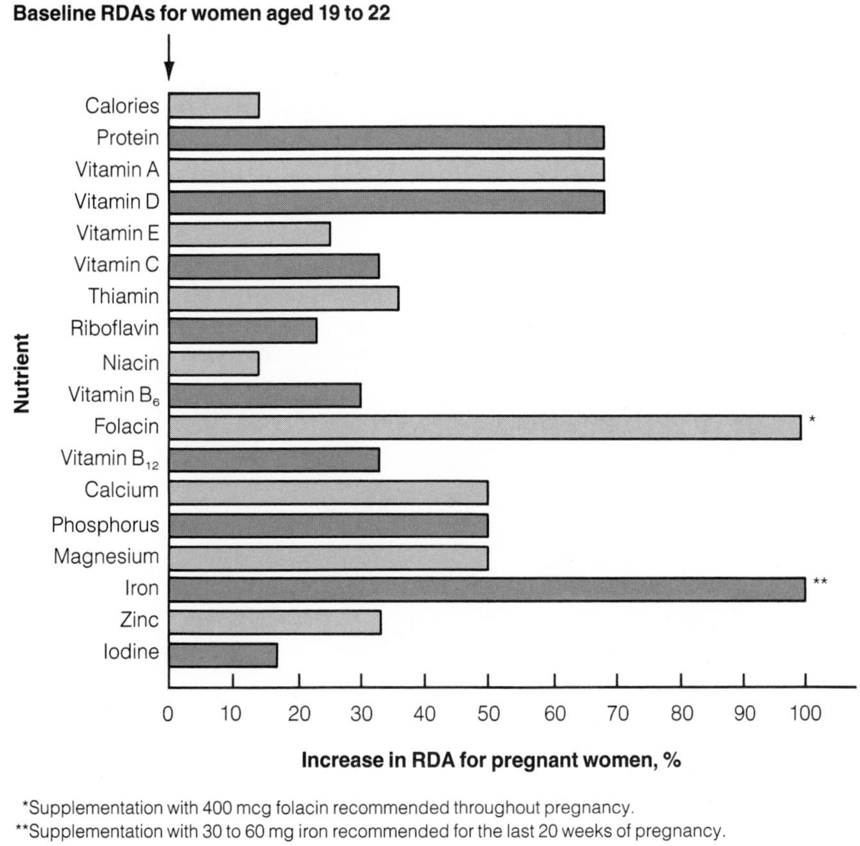

FIGURE 14-4

Percentage increases in RDAs for pregnant women aged 19 to 22 years.

BOX 14-2

WIC WORKS

The infant death rate in the United States is higher than those in many other industrialized countries. In 1987, for example, the U.S. ranked 19th among developed nations in infant death rate.[31] The primary reason infants are more likely to die in the U.S. than in places such as Sweden, Norway, Japan, Hong Kong, and England is the higher proportion of low-birth-weight infants born here. About 7% of the infants born in the U.S. are low-birth-weight, compared with only 3% to 4% in Sweden and Norway—countries with lower infant death rates.[32]

A number of factors are associated with the birth of low-birth-weight infants, and poor nutrition ranks high among them. The WIC program was enacted in 1974 to help reduce the incidence of low birth weight and to improve maternal and child health by providing nutrition education and food supplements. The program has proven to be effective and has grown in funding each year.

Pregnant women and children up to the age of 5 who live in poverty and are assessed as being at risk of poor nutrition are generally eligible for the program. Poor nutrition is defined as the presence of a condition such as underweight, iron deficiency, or inadequate diet. Once enrolled in WIC, pregnant and breast-feeding women and their children receive an assessment of their nutritional status, nutrition education, and coupons for foods to supplement their existing diets. Only such nutrient-dense foods as milk, infant formula, eggs, beans, cheese, peanut butter, and fruit juices are provided by the WIC program.

WIC works. Women who enroll in WIC during pregnancy are less likely to deliver low-birth-weight infants and to experience iron deficiency than are women who are eligible but do not participate.[33,34] Participation in WIC has also been shown to improve diet quality and to prevent iron deficiency in infants and young children.[35,36]

More information about the program can be obtained from your state or local public health department.

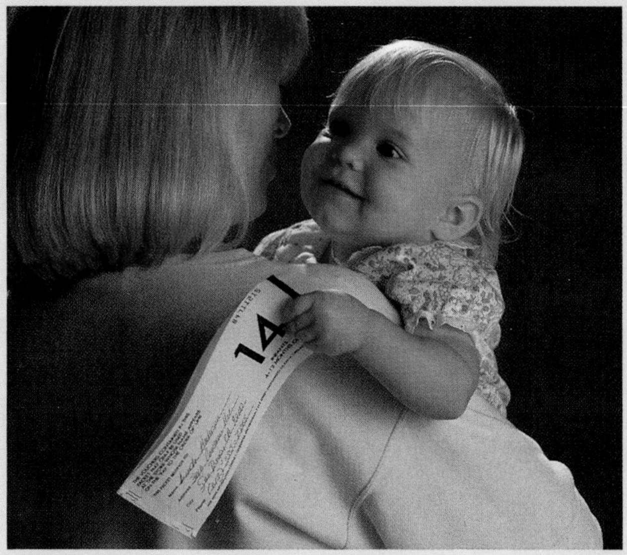

TABLE 14-2
Effects of low-calorie diets during pregnancy

Reduced availability of dietary protein for maternal and fetal protein tissue construction
Reduced availability of energy for fetal growth
Reduced supply of vitamins and minerals

trimester) to about 350 additional calories per day in the last six months (the second and third trimesters).[48] These are average figures. Women entering pregnancy underweight will need more calories than this, and those entering overweight will need fewer. In addition, physically active pregnant women require higher caloric intakes than these averages. It is generally easier and more accurate to monitor the adequacy of caloric intake by tracking weight gain than by counting calories.

Diets that provide fewer than about 1,800 calories per day are considered "low-calorie" during pregnancy. Such diets can present several problems for a growing fetus (Table 14-2). The first has to do with the availability of protein for fetal growth and tissue formation. Without enough calories to meet a pregnant woman's need for energy, dietary protein is diverted from use in tissue construction to use in energy formation. The requirement for energy is the body's first priority; only when the mother's energy needs are met can dietary protein be used for the mother's and the baby's tissue growth and maintenance needs. This principle applies throughout all phases of life but is particularly relevant to pregnancy when protein tissue formation is extensive. The second problem is that low-calorie diets do not supply enough energy to meet the needs for normal fetal growth. This increases the probability of low birth weight.[45] Thirdly, diets that fail to supply enough calories generally provide inadequate amounts of essential nutrients as well. This situation can leave the fetus with a short supply of vitamins and minerals and interfere with normal growth and development.[46,47]

The ill effects of low-calorie diets during pregnancy on fetal growth and development are most pronounced when the restriction continues throughout the pregnancy. Infants born under this circumstance may be permanently delayed in growth and intellectual development.[47] If low-calorie intakes are the exception rather than the routine, it is not likely that permanent damage to the infant will result; adaptive mechanisms help the fetus withstand fluctuations in maternal food intake. Ideally, the pregnant woman eats regular meals and snacks and avoids even short periods of fasting and weight loss.

Protein The protein content of a woman's body increases by about two pounds during pregnancy. About half of this increase is in the build-up of the mother's uterus, breasts, and blood supply; the other half is deposited in fetal tissues.[44] Protein intakes below the RDA (for pregnant adult women) of 74 grams have been associated with the birth of smaller than average infants.[48]

A number of studies have shown that infants born to women who consumed about 90 grams of protein daily during pregnancy tend to be healthier than infants born to women who have consumed less than that.[49–51]

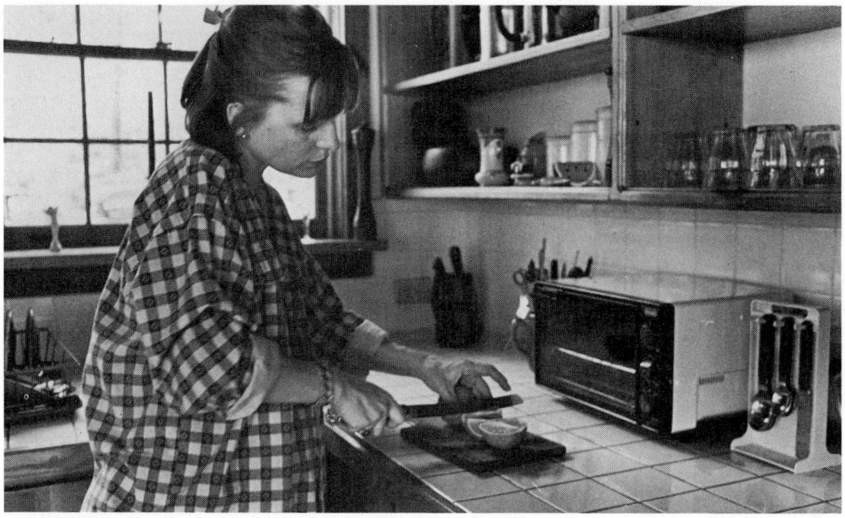

The quality and quantity of foods consumed during pregnancy influence the weight gain and health of both mother and baby.

Whether pregnant women in the U.S. should be encouraged to consume 90 grams of protein, rather than 74, is a matter of controversy. Most U.S. women consume between 70 and 90 grams of protein per day during pregnancy.[48]

Folic Acid Folic acid has been considered an important nutrient for pregnant women ever since the discovery that low folic acid intakes may cause fetal malformations and growth retardation.[48] The link between folic-acid deficiency and abnormal fetal growth and development is the role of folic acid in protein tissue construction: folic acid is a key coenzyme required for the normal production of most of the proteins formed within the body. Dietary deficiencies of folic acid have been closely associated with the development of spinal cord abnormalities such as spina bifida.[52,53]

The increased requirement for folic acid is often not met by the diets of pregnant women. Folic acid supplements of about 400 mcg per day (0.4 mg) throughout the pregnancy are recommended.[48]

Vitamin B_6 Vitamin B_6 is of concern during pregnancy not because of the likelihood of a dietary deficiency, but because it is often used to treat "morning sickness," the nausea and vomiting that many women experience in pregnancy. The nausea and vomiting are related to hormonal changes and they commonly occur only during the first trimester. For a small proportion of women, this "sickness" becomes a serious problem because it lasts longer than three months and produces dehydration, which can threaten the health of both the mother and baby. The morning sickness most typical in pregnancy, however, does not appear to be harmful to the pregnancy (although it may be a major inconvenience to the women).[54]

Daily doses of vitamin B_6 in the range of 5 to 10 mg relieve nausea and vomiting in some, but not all, women. Since vitamin-B_6 deficiency has not been shown to be related to the development of this condition, the relief it sometimes provides is due to a "drug effect" rather than to the normal functions of B_6 in the body. Nausea and vomiting during pregnancy that are severe and last beyond the first trimester requires close medical supervision and generally the intravenous administration of fluids to correct dehydration.

Calcium Calcium used to support the mineralization of bones in the fetus is supplied by the mother's diet and, if needed, by the calcium contained in the long bones of the mother's body. The fetus gets as much calcium as she or he needs even if the mother's diet contains little of it. The reason is that blood levels of calcium are tightly controlled and very stable. Calcium is drawn from the mother's bones if needed to maintain a constant blood level of calcium. Consequently, the fetus has access to as much calcium as needed. Calcium uptake by the fetus is especially high during the last trimester, when the fetus's bones are mineralizing.

Pregnant women who regularly consume low-calcium diets lose calcium from their bones during pregnancy.[47] Because any calcium losses are from the long bones, not from the teeth, the old saying "for every baby a tooth" has no basis in fact. Several studies have shown that teeth do not demineralize as a result of low-calcium diets during pregnancy.[45]

Iron Iron deficiency is the most common nutrient deficiency in pregnant women in the U.S.[48] It develops when a woman enters pregnancy with low iron stores and fails to consume enough iron during her pregnancy. Iron requirements increase during pregnancy due to increases in hemoglobin production and due to the storage of iron by the fetus.

Short of eating liver at least twice a day, it is virtually impossible for a pregnant woman to get enough iron from foods. Consequently, 30 to 60 mg of supplemental iron per day is recommended for the second half of pregnancy.[48] Women who do not take supplemental iron are more likely to develop iron deficiency and to deliver infants that are small and at risk of developing iron deficiency in their first year than are women who do take supplements.[47,55]

Concern has recently developed over the amount of supplemental iron that is prescribed for pregnant women. Experts are questioning whether too much is being passed out.[56] Rather than the recommended 30 to 60 mg during the second half of pregnancy, many health care professionals routinely recommend the use of much greater amounts (over 200 mg per day in some cases) throughout pregnancy. (Box 14-3 deals with this controversy.)

BOX 14-3

ARE PREGNANT WOMEN RECEIVING TOO MUCH IRON?

Knowledge of the importance of iron to maternal and infant health appears to have led some health professionals to overreact and routinely prescribe iron in amounts that are too high. It is not uncommon for pregnant women to be given supplements that provide well over the 30 to 60 mg of iron recommended daily. Excessive amounts of supplemental iron are poorly absorbed and can produce heartburn, gas, and constipation.[47] (Rather than cope with these side effects, it is suspected that many women simply quit taking their iron supplements.) Furthermore, doses of iron above 100 mg per day decrease zinc absorption and may lead to zinc deficiency.[56]

A panel of experts agreed in 1987 that 30 mg of iron per day is sufficient to meet the needs of most women during pregnancy.[57]

Ten or more cups of fluid each day are recommended during pregnancy.

Zinc An additional 5 mg of zinc per day is recommended during pregnancy. This extra amount is primarily used to support protein tissue formation in the mother and fetus. Since the RDA for nonpregnant women is 15 mg, the total recommended daily intake of zinc for pregnant women amounts to 20 mg. On average, however, pregnant women in the U.S. consume only about 8 mg of zinc per day.[58] Although this amount is sufficient to prevent serious zinc deficiency, marginal deficiencies of zinc may be quite common in pregnancy. High-dose iron supplements may contribute to the development of a zinc deficiency, since zinc absorption is diminished when high levels of iron are present in the gut. Zinc deficiency during pregnancy has been associated with abnormally long labors and with delivery of small and malformed infants.[59]

One important way of reducing the risk of zinc deficiency during pregnancy is limiting iron supplements to 30 mg per day.[56] Another is to eat at least three servings of meats and meat alternates per day. Supplementing pregnant women with zinc, however, is not currently recommended. Only folic acid and iron are formally recommended for supplementation during pregnancy.

Water Water requirements increase substantially during pregnancy. A pregnant woman needs more water because of increases in blood volume and in the amount of water used to maintain body temperature. She also needs additional water for diluting the fetal waste products that flow into her blood and are excreted in her urine. It is widely suspected that many pregnant woman may fail to drink enough water. It is generally advised that women stay well hydrated during pregnancy and that special attention be paid to fluid intake by women living in hot climates. For most women, a daily intake of 10 cups of fluids is sufficient.

Translating Nutrient Needs into a Good Diet

Regardless of the pregnant woman's age, and whether she is a vegetarian or not, her diet should contain:

1. Sufficient calories for adequate weight gain
2. A variety of foods from each food group
3. Regular meals and snacks
4. Sufficient dietary fiber (about 30 grams per day)
5. Ten or more cups of fluid each day
6. Salt to taste
7. No alcoholic beverages

Planning the diet around the basic food groups is the most straightforward approach to meeting nutrient needs for pregnancy. The guidelines are similar to those for nonpregnant adult women. See Table 14-3. The differences are an additional serving of milk or milk product and an additional serving of meat or meat alternate. Consuming only the minimum number of servings from each food group does not provide the needed calories. Additional servings of foods within the groups and from the "miscellaneous" category are needed for the calories they provide.

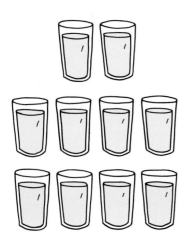

TABLE 14-3
Food group recommendations for pregnant women

Food Group	Minimum Number of Servings per Day
Breads and cereals	4
Vegetables and fruits	(4)
vitamin A-rich	1
vitamin C-rich	1
other	2
Milk and milk products	3
Meats or alternates	3
Miscellaneous	based on caloric need

Note: For additional information on foods contained in the groups and standard serving sizes, refer to Table 2-6.

Myths regarding Diet during Pregnancy

Although a good deal is known about dietary practices that foster maternal and infant health, numerous myths still exist. The problem with myths is that they misdirect dietary guidance. This can end up causing harm to mothers and infants. We discuss four common myths here.

Myth #1: The fetus is a parasite. It is a common misconception that the fetus is a parasite, drawing whatever it needs from the mother. The fetus is not a true parasite, because—with few exceptions—the fetus can get nutrients from the mother only if the mother has obtained them in sufficient quantity from her diet. In addition, the fetus has access to optimal levels of most nutrients only if they are available in amounts above and beyond the mother's own need for them.[45] This situation makes sense in terms of survival of the species, since more is lost if the woman's health is compromised than if the fetus's is; a woman can reproduce again. By meeting a pregnant woman's needs first, Nature protects the reproducer.

Rather striking evidence that the fetus is not a parasite has come from studies that have identified nutrient deficiencies in newborns that their mothers do not show.[47,60] Infants born to women with inadequate intakes of thiamin, iodine, folic acid, or zinc, for example, are more likely to develop the respective deficiency signs than are the mothers. By the same token, infants born to women who consume excessive levels of supplements are more likely to suffer harmful effects than are the mothers.[61,62] Also, underweight women who consume too few calories during pregnancy gain weight themselves at the expense of the fetus.[63]

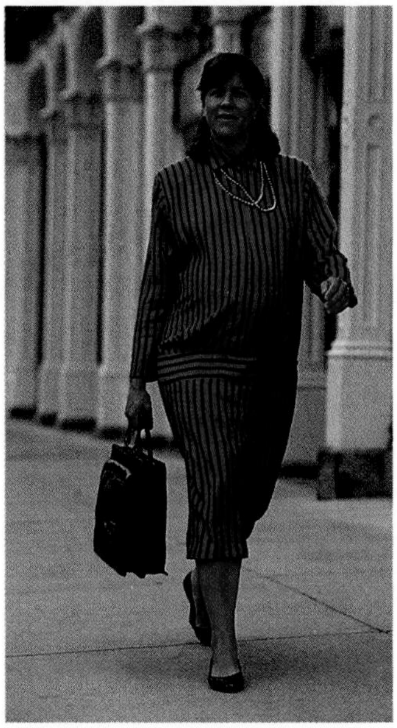

A lot of old myths about pregnancy are falling by the wayside.

Myth #2: Women's "maternal instincts" lead them to select healthy foods during pregnancy. There is no evidence that pregnant women are biologically drawn to a healthy diet. They may be more conscientious about "eating right" because they are pregnant, however.

Changes in food preferences and in the way certain foods taste and smell during pregnancy have been documented, but there is no evidence that these changes are instinctive or that they rectify poor diets.[64–66] It may be that the changes in food preferences that commonly occur during pregnancy are responsible for the myth that pregnant women will instinctively eat well.

Myth #3: Weight gain should be restricted during pregnancy in order to make delivery easier and to prevent toxemia. These commonly held notions have been around for a long time. Feelings about weight gain, difficult labors, and **toxemia** are so strong among women, doctors, and nurses that these myths have been difficult to dispel.

toxemia: Condition characterized by abnormally high blood pressure and extensive swelling throughout the body. Women who develop toxemia during pregnancy are at high risk of delivering a small infant early. The condition is now referred to as *pregnancy-induced hypertension* (*PIH*).

The general recommendation to restrict weight gain during pregnancy appears to have begun in the 1700s, when it was found that women whose pelvises had not grown to the normal size because of childhood rickets were better able to deliver babies that were small.[67] Rickets was common in industrialized cities in the 1700s because the smoke-filled air reduced vitamin-D production in the skin and the people's diets were deficient in vitamin D. Many women who had had rickets as children had contracted pelvises, which made delivery of full-term, normal-weight babies difficult. To partially overcome this problem, the physicians of the day recommended very low food and fluid intakes in the last half of pregnancy. The treatment worked; babies were smaller and easier to deliver. Of course, the treatment also compromised the infants' birth weight and health. Many of these small infants developed slowly, became sick, or died within the first year of life. Now that rickets is rare in the U.S. and Caesarian deliveries are a safe option for most women, the practice of limiting the growth of the baby to make it fit through a small pelvic opening should be abandoned.[68]

A related myth is that excessive weight gain causes toxemia of pregnancy—a disorder characterized by extensive swelling and high blood pressure. Toxemia occurs in 2% to 7% of first pregnancies and can cause convulsions in the mother and seriously jeopardize the health of the fetus. The cause of toxemia is not yet known. Rather than *causing* toxemia, however, large weight gains *result* from the swelling produced by toxemia.[69]

Myth #4: Salt intake should be restricted during pregnancy to prevent the development of hypertension. Hypertension during pregnancy is a potentially serious condition for both mother and baby. The seriousness of the disorder has lent a sense of urgency to the efforts to prevent it. Because salt restriction may decrease high blood pressure in nonpregnant adults, it has been reasoned that salt restriction also would help prevent hypertension during pregnancy. Results of a number of studies, however, have shown that the hypertension that develops in pregnancy is not related to high salt intakes.[70–72] In fact, salt-restricted diets tend to aggravate rather than decrease the problem of hypertension during pregnancy.[70] Thus, women should not be advised to restrict their salt intake during pregnancy unless they enter pregnancy with a form of hypertension that is lowered by a low-salt diet.

OTHER CONSIDERATIONS REGARDING NUTRITION DURING PREGNANCY

Alcohol and Pregnancy

As early as the 1800s, maternal consumption of alcohol during pregnancy was said to cause the birth of "sickly" infants. The ill effects of alcohol on babies were not fully acknowledged, however, until the 1970s, when several research reports were published that described a condition called *fetal alcohol syndrome*. Women who drank heavily or frequently binged on alcohol during pregnancy were found to be at high risk of delivering infants with specific malformaties and retarded physical and mental development.[73,74] The effect of maternal alcohol intake on the fetus was found to worsen with increasing alcohol intake. Heavy drinking in the first half of pregnancy was closely associated with the birth of malformed, small, mentally impaired infants. When excessive drinking had occurred only in the second half of the pregnancy, infants were less likely to be malformed, but they were still likely to be small and to suffer abnormal mental development. It was noted that these conditions are lasting; they cannot be corrected with special treatment, and the child does not outgrow them.

No amount of alcohol has been found to be absolutely safe during pregnancy. When only an occasional drink is consumed, however, the adverse effects of alcohol on fetal development appear to be small and rare. To exclude the possibility of even small impairments in fetal growth and development, it is recommended that women do not drink alcohol during pregnancy.[75]

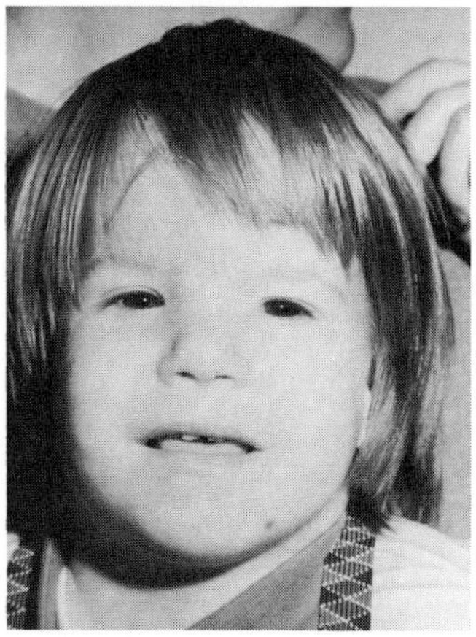

Children born with fetal alcohol syndrome have characteristic facial features.

Pica

Pica is defined as the regular consumption of nonfood substances. It is not uncommon for pregnant women (and children) to habitually consume such things as clay or laundry starch. Scientists know very little about the reason for this practice. Some evidence suggests that it may be related to iron deficiency, but the evidence is far from solid—and the substances typically consumed do not provide the body with iron.

pica: The regular ingestion of a nonfood substance, such as laundry starch, clay, or dirt; most commonly occurs during pregnancy and childhood.

It has been estimated that 28% of Southern blacks and 12% of whites regularly ingest clay during pregnancy. The estimates for laundry starch are 41% for Southern blacks and 10% for whites.[76] It is not known why some pregnant women eat these nonfood substances, but the women report that these items taste good to them.[77] Even the smell of the type of clay eaten by women with this type of pica is appealing to the women; they describe the

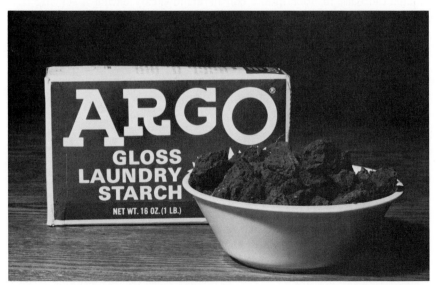

Many pregnant women who experience pica eat clay or laundry starch.

smell as "sweet and delicious." Pica seems less odd to people who have heard personal reports about how wonderful these substances taste from women who have experienced pica.

Although pica seems satisfying to the women who practice it, regular ingestion of clay or laundry starch can cause problems. Clay may contain bacteria and other harmful substances and it may reduce the amount of minerals absorbed from foods. Also, it may cause intestinal obstructions that must be surgically removed. Laundry starch may contain contaminants, since it is not manufactured for consumption as a food. The body digests and absorbs laundry starch just as it does other sources of starch. Laundry starch can become a significant source of "empty calories."[76]

Shifts in Food Preferences

An interesting and common effect of pregnancy that was mentioned in the discussion of myths is changing food preferences. Food preferences have been noted to change in 76% of pregnant women. Foods such as fish, beef, fried foods, alcoholic beverages, diet soft drinks, and coffee are often reported to taste or smell unpleasant during pregnancy; whereas ice cream, chocolate, salty snacks, milk, and fruit are reported to taste better.[65,66,79] Pregnant women are also less sensitive to the taste of salt; they prefer stronger salt solutions than they do after pregnancy.[64]

Present evidence indicates that shifts in salt preference may be related to changes in estrogen levels that occur during pregnancy. Nonpregnant monkeys that are given estrogen have been found to develop a preference for stronger salt solutions.[80] The increased preference observed among pregnant women for nutritious foods such as milk and fruit may be related to their desire to "eat well" during pregnancy.[79]

Constipation Constipation is a problem for many women during pregnancy. It appears to result from hormonal changes. It can be alleviated to some extent by including 10 additional grams of dietary fiber in the daily diet, for a total of about 30 grams.[81]

This increase in fiber intake can be achieved by eating a serving of a complete-bran cereal or by adding 2 tablespoons of bran to cooked cereal, yogurt, or other food. The level of bran in the diet should be increased gradually to avoid the gas, cramps, and diarrhea that sometimes occur when fiber intake is increased precipitously. Remember that water intake needs to be increased when fiber intake is increased. Fiber does not help to prevent constipation if fluid intake is low.

Overuse of Vitamin and Mineral Supplements

Only recently has concern about the effects of excessive levels of particular vitamins and minerals on the developing fetus become widespread. Before the present boom in the popularity of supplements, women very rarely took sufficient amounts of specific nutrients to cause noticeable problems in babies. Vitamin and mineral supplements were generally regarded as harmless. We now know that they are not always harmless.

Overdose reactions have been observed in pregnant women and newborns to 6 vitamins and 3 minerals: vitamins B_{12}, C, B_6, A, D, and E and iron, zinc, and iodine.[82] Amounts that have been associated with harmful effects start at two to three times the RDA. As we have said, a fetus is generally much more susceptible to the ill effects of vitamin and mineral overdoses than is a pregnant woman; this is primarily because of the small size and the rapid growth and development of the fetus. Overdoses of vitamin and mineral supplements produce the most serious threats to infant health when they occur early in pregnancy, when the fetus's organs are developing.[82]

Water-Soluble Vitamins "Rebound" deficiencies have been observed in infants whose mothers have taken excessive amounts of vitamin B_{12}, vitamin C, and vitamin B_6 in pregnancy. The excretion mechanisms that rid the fetus of the high levels of these vitamins appear to continue after birth, even though large amounts of the vitamins are no longer being received. Consequently, the newborns excrete too much of the vitamins and they develop deficiencies within a few days after birth. Infants can be protected from the effects of rebound vitamin deficiencies if they are supplemented with the particular vitamin and then gradually weaned from it.[47,83]

Other problems have also been associated with the overuse of water-soluble vitamins. Very high intakes of vitamin B_6, for example, have been related to infant malformations.[82]

Fat-Soluble Vitamins As little as 25,000 IU of vitamin A taken daily in the early months of pregnancy has been associated with central nervous system and bone abnormalities in newborns.[84] The increasingly popular use of vitamin-A-like compounds for the treatment of acne, wrinkles, and other skin conditions has led to new warnings about their use by women who are, or may become, pregnant.

Daily doses of supplemental vitamin D at levels five times the RDA (2,000 IU) have been associated with the birth of infants who are mentally retarded and have heart abnormalities.[83] There is also evidence to indicate that megadoses of vitamin E may result in spontaneous abortions—the early, unexpected loss of a fetus.[82]

Minerals Iron, zinc, and iodine supplements during pregnancy can also be hazardous.[82] Iron overdose primarily affects the pregnant woman by causing gastrointestinal upsets. The fetus does not receive excessive levels of iron, because high amounts are not usually absorbed by the mother's intestinal tract. Zinc supplements that deliver in the neighborhood of 100 mg per day (five times the RDA) provide excessive levels of zinc to the fetus. Zinc overdoses in pregnancy have been shown to be related to preterm delivery. The consequences of iodine overdose in pregnancy include the development of goiter and mental retardation in infants.

The effects of vitamin and mineral overdoses on pregnant women and infants are summarized in Table 14-4.

The ingestion of high amounts of supplemental vitamins and minerals by healthy pregnant women has never been found to improve maternal or infant health. All of the problems resulting from overdose could be prevented if women took no more than the RDA levels for vitamins and minerals during pregnancy. With the exception of folic acid and iron, pregnant women can, and should, get the nutrients they need from a balanced diet.

TABLE 14-4

Effects of vitamin and mineral overdoses on pregnant women and infants

Vitamin/Mineral	Overdose Effect
Water-Soluble Vitamins	
vitamin B_{12}	newborn rebound deficiency
vitamin C	newborn rebound deficiency
vitamin B_6	newborn rebound deficiency, malformations
Fat-Soluble Vitamins	
vitamin A	malformations of the infant's central nervous system and bones
vitamin D	infant mental retardation and heart abnormalities
vitamin E	spontaneous abortion
Minerals	
iron	maternal gastrointestinal upsets
zinc	preterm delivery
iodine	infant goiter and mental retardation

Teenage Pregnancy

Each day about 1,300 babies are born to teenagers in the United States.[85] Overall, the pregnancy rate is down for girls between the ages of 15 and 19, but it is up for girls below the age of 15. The major problems related to teenage pregnancy are the high incidence of health problems in the babies and the impact of the pregnancy and parenthood on the mother's educational and economic future. Few teenagers are psychologically and economically prepared to succeed in securing a healthy future for themselves while being the primary source of support for one or more children.[86]

It was once thought that the greater number of complications accompanying teenage pregnancies and the higher rates of low birth weight, illness, and death for babies born to teenage mothers were due to the mothers' biological immaturity. It was thought that these problems stemmed from the fact that the mother had not completed her growth and was thus not biologically prepared for pregnancy. It now appears that the most important factor is the day-to-day health practices of the mother.[87] Regardless of their age, teenage mothers who have healthy lifestyles—those who generally consume balanced diets, gain the recommended amount of weight during pregnancy, and do not smoke or use drugs—tend to be healthier and to remain healthier during pregnancy than other teenage mothers.[88] The infants of healthy teenage girls also tend to be healthy.[89,90] Poor nutritional practices—including frequent dieting, meal skipping, imbalanced diets, and inadequate weight gain during pregnancy—are more strongly associated with complications during pregnancy and poor infant outcomes than is the mother's age.[88–90]

The RDAs for pregnant teens are higher in general than those for pregnant adults. This is because teenage mothers need calories and nutrients for their own growth during and after the pregnancy.[90]

BREAST FEEDING

Food is the first enjoyment of life.
—Lin Yutang

A woman's capacity to nourish a growing infant does not end at birth; it continues in the form of breast feeding. Breast milk from healthy, well-nourished women is ideally suited for infant nutrition and health. It provides the calories and nutrients infants need *plus* regular doses of "preventive medicine." Unlike commercial formula or cow's milk, breast milk contains substances that help protect infants from infectious diseases and allergies.

Breast feeding is undergoing a resurgence of popularity in the U.S. (Figure 14-5). Before 1900, nearly every mother breast-fed her infant. By 1920, however, evaporated milk and commercial infant formulas had become widely available, and for a time they were considered to be better for infants than breast milk. Rates of breast feeding fell sharply from 1920 to 1955, but then rose sharply when the post World War II "baby boomers" began having families. Many of the breast-feeding mothers of the 1970s felt a bit like pioneers, not having been breast-fed as infants or having seen a relative or other role model breast-feed. Indeed, they were the leaders of a return to breast feeding. In 1985 it was estimated that 60% of women were

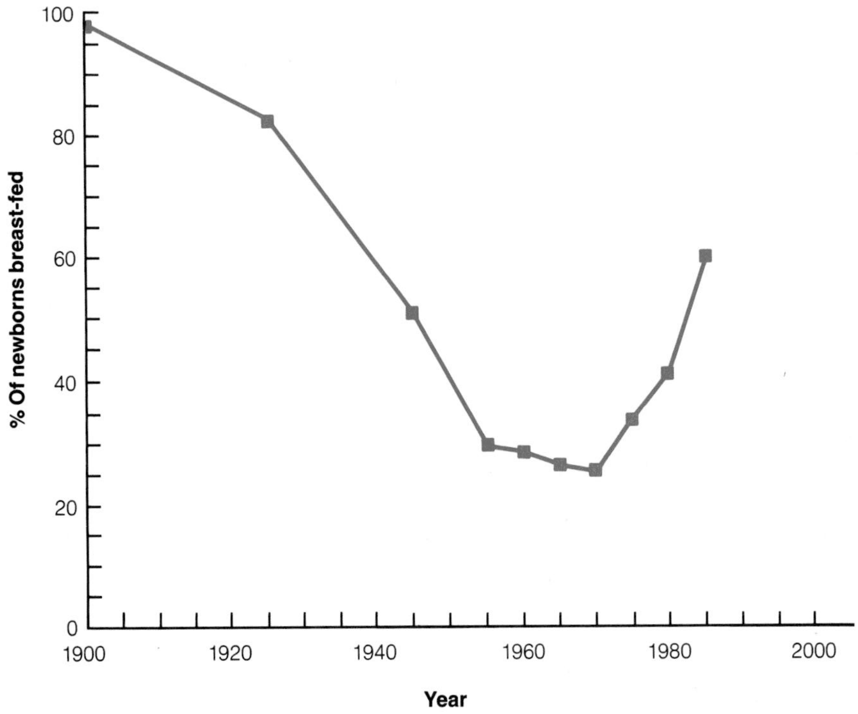

FIGURE 14-5
Percentage of breast-fed newborns in the U.S., 1900 to 1985.

breast-feeding their infants after delivery.[91] Due to the proportion of new mothers that are employed outside the home, it is expected that the incidence of breast feeding will remain at 60% through 1990.[91]

The trend toward higher rates of breast feeding is a healthy one. Although commercial infant formulas are an acceptable alternative to breast milk for mothers who cannot or do not want to breast-feed, they are different. The nutrient composition of well-nourished women's breast milk remains the standard for infant nutrient requirements. Infant formulas can be designed to approximate the nutrient composition of breast milk, but since the nutrient composition of breast milk varies with the maternal diet, and because not all of the components of breast milk have been identified or duplicated in formulas, breast milk and commercial formulas cannot be considered the same. No infant formula can duplicate the nutrient composition, digestibility, taste, or protective properties of breast milk. Additionally, no commercial formula can be as convenient, sterile, or continuously available at the ideal temperature as breast milk.

Comparison of Breast Milk, Commercial Infant Formula, and Cow's Milk

Every species of mammal produces a milk that best meets the specific needs of its offspring. The nutrient composition of milks varies because each species has particular nutrient needs influenced by its rate of growth, body composition and structure, and digestive and metabolic capabilities. Consequently, the milk of one species is not ideally suited to the needs of other species. Compared with other mammal species, human infants are born with immature digestive tracts and grow slowly. Thus, human milk contains less protein and minerals and more carbohydrate than do the milks of cattle, goats, rats, and others (Table 14-5). The young of each mammal species are born with the specific abilities to digest, absorb, and metabolize the milk of the species.

Because most commercial infant formulas are made from cow's milk, we will compare cow's-milk infant formula with human milk. You can get an idea of how cow's milk is modified in the production of commercial infant formula by reviewing the information in Table 14-6.

Protein The proteins in cow's milk do not contain the same levels or ratios of essential amino acids as breast milk proteins, and they are not as easily

TABLE 14-5

Comparison of milk composition and infant growth rate for selected mammals

	Composition of Milk, % of volume				Days Required to Double Birth Weight
	Fat	Protein	Carbohydrate	Minerals	
Cattle	3.7	3.4	4.8	0.7	47
Goats	4.5	2.9	4.1	0.8	19
Rats	15.0	12.0	3.0	2.0	6

■
TABLE 14-6

Average content of calories and selected nutrients in eight ounces of breast milk, commercial infant formula, and cow's milk[93,94]

	Breast Milk[1]	Commercial Infant Formula[2]	Cow's Milk
Calories	166	169	160
Carbohydrates, g	16	18	12
Protein, g	3	4	8
Fat, g	10	9	9
Cholesterol, mg	35	3	35
Calcium, mg	71	122	295
Sodium, mg	36	60	122
Iron, mg	0.1	0.4 to 3	0.1
Zinc, mg	0.4	1.2	0.9
Vitamin C, mg	12	13	4
Vitamin A, IU	600	600	341
Vitamin D, IU	5	96	102

[1]Breast milk composition represents average levels from well-nourished mothers.
[2]There are many brands of commercially prepared infant formulas and they vary somewhat in composition. A popular brand of infant formula that is available with and without iron fortification was used for this comparison.

digested by humans. To compensate for the shortage of certain essential amino acids in cow's milk, commercial formulas are fortified with several amino acids. The digestibility of cow's-milk protein is improved by partially breaking it down during the manufacture of formula.

Fat Breast milk, commercial formulas, and cow's milk all contain about the same amount of fat, but the types of fat in them are different. The fat in breast milk consists primarily of short- and medium-length chains of fatty acids, which are easily digested by humans. It contains a high amount of the essential fatty acid linoleic acid, as well as appreciable amounts of EPA, an omega-3 fatty acid.[92] (EPA is the fish-oil fatty acid of notoriety.) Linoleic acid provides approximately 15% of the total calories in breast milk but only 2% to 5% of the total calories in commercial formulas and cow's milk. Formulas provide far more long-chained, polyunsaturated fatty acids than does breast milk, because the butter fat in cow's milk is replaced with vegetable oils during processing. (Box 14-4 reports a concern about the polyunsaturated-fat content of infant formulas, and infants.)

Notice in Table 14-6 that the cholesterol content of breast milk is greater than that of formula. The cholesterol in breast milk serves several important purposes. It is used in the formation of cells of the infant's rapidly developing nervous system and is the chemical precursor of vitamin D formed in skin exposed to sunlight. It appears that the relatively high cholesterol content of breast milk does not place an infant at risk of developing heart disease later in life and that it is more beneficial than harmful.[95] A current question is whether cholesterol should be added to infant formulas.

Carbohydrate Nearly all of the carbohydrate in breast milk is in the form of lactose, whereas a commercial formula may contain lactose, sucrose, or another type of simple sugar. As the advantages of lactose have

BOX 14-4

POLYUNSATURATED INFANTS?

The use of vegetable oils as the source of fat in infant formulas has led to the notion that we are rearing a generation of "polyunsaturated infants." The type of fat in a person's body fat stores is strongly influenced by the type of fat consumed in the diet. The full implications of this situation are not understood, but it is known that a person's requirement for vitamin E increases with increasing intakes of polyunsaturated fats.

become clearer, the use of lactose rather than sucrose in formulas has increased. Lactose serves as a source of galactose, a simple sugar that is needed for the formation of brain cells. Lactose also increases the absorption of calcium and helps decrease the growth of certain disease-causing bacteria in the gut.

Vitamins With the exception of vitamin D, the vitamin content of cow's milk is adjusted during formula manufacture to bring the levels into line with the amounts normally found in breast milk. Breast milk, like cow's milk, naturally contains a low amount of vitamin D. (It has been suggested that the reason for this is that the babies of our early ancestors got enough of the vitamin from exposure to sunshine.[96]) Infants that are exposed to sunshine for about 30 minutes a week while wearing only their diapers do not require a dietary source of vitamin D. If clothed but not wearing a hat, infants' need for vitamin D can be met with two hours of sun exposure per week.[97] Infants that do not get this amount of sunshine should receive a vitamin D supplement.[98]

Minerals Calves grow rapidly and build a large amount of bone early in life. Consequently, they need several times the amount of minerals such as calcium and phosphorus as infants do (refer to Table 14-5 again). Because high mineral loads can cause dehydration in infants, some of the calcium, phosphorus, and sodium in cow's milk is removed during the production of infant formulas. Other minerals—iron and zinc, for example—are added to compensate for their lower level of absorption from formula than from breast milk. In breast milk, iron and zinc are attached to proteins that allow them to be easily absorbed. Because of this, relatively small amounts of these minerals are sufficient in breast milk. For infants born with adequate stores of iron, the iron content of breast milk is sufficient to prevent iron deficiency for at least the first 6 to 9 months of life.[99]

Low amounts of fluoride, a nutrient of concern for tooth formation and protection against decay, are found in breast milk. Although the amounts remain low even when breast-feeding women drink fluoridated water or take fluoride supplements, the teeth of their infants tend to be more resistant to decay than the teeth of formula-fed infants.[100] The difference is due to substances in breast milk that destroy decay-causing bacteria.[100] Fluoride supplements are not recommended for breast-feeding mothers or their infants. Formula-fed infants, infants no longer being breast-fed, and infants not being given fluoridated water after breast feeding stops may benefit from fluoride supplements.[100] Fluoride supplements are available only by prescription.

Taste Another difference between breast milk and commercial infant formula is that of taste. Although infants appear to find the taste of both foods highly acceptable, breast milk is sweeter than cow's milk. The preference for sweet-tasting foods with which human infants are born is not shared by calves—or by puppies, kittens, and the young of many other animals.

The composition of breast milk varies according to what the mother has eaten and from the beginning to the end of a feeding. These changes in composition alter the taste of the milk. Consequently, breast-fed infants are exposed to a broader range of tastes than formula-fed infants. The implications of this difference to infant health and nutrition are not known, although speculations about early taste experiences and later food preferences abound.

Health-Promoting Components of Breast Milk

Disease Resistance Breast milk "immunizes" infants against certain infectious diseases, and it may confer some protection against the development of cancer of the lymph system[101] and of insulin-dependent diabetes during childhood.[102] Protection against infectious diseases is particularly important in developing countries, where the purchase of formula represents a financial hardship and where refrigeration and medical care are lacking. The quality of the water used to dilute infant formulas is also a problem in some locales. When the water used to dilute formulas is contaminated with bacteria and other toxins, infants get a dose of them with every swallow. (Recall the central watering hole discussed and pictured in chapter 13.) These infants are exposed to a high level of disease-causing agents and at the same time are more vulnerable to disease because they do not receive the infection-protective substances of breast milk.

Breast-fed infants tend to get sick less often than do bottle-fed infants, even in economically developed countries; see Table 14-7. The data in the table are from a study in the U.S. There would be an even larger margin of safety associated with breast feeding if data from studies in developing countries were shown.

The substances in breast milk that are responsible for disease prevention are **antibodies**. Antibodies are proteins that an organism (the mother in

antibodies: Substances the body produces that can destroy certain types of bacteria and viruses, thereby protecting the body against disruptions and diseases caused by them. Immunizations protect against specific infectious diseases by supplying the body with antibodies that ward off invading germs.

TABLE 14-7
Significant episodes of infant illness by method of feeding

	Method of Feeding, % of infants	
Illness	Breast Milk	Formula/Other
Ear infections	3.7	9.1
Lower-respiratory illness	1.1	5.6
Diarrhea, vomiting	3.5	6.9
Hospital admissions	1.0	3.0
Average number of episodes of illness per infant	8.2	21.1

Source of data: Cunningham, 1979.

BOX 14-5

BREAST FEEDING AND AIDS

Breast feeding is regarded as a key factor in promoting infant health, especially in developing countries where infectious diseases are common. Nonetheless, if AIDS is found to be transmitted by breast milk, the already high levels of infectious disease in infants in these countries will increase, because more infants will have to be bottle-fed.

AIDS has infected 13 times as many males as females in the U.S., but that is not the case in some countries that have relatively high rates of AIDS-infected people.[109] In parts of Central Africa, for example, an equal proportion of females and males are infected. Up to 10% of pregnant women in that region have the AIDS virus, and it is estimated that 8% of infants are born with it.[109] Although it is clear that the AIDS virus can be passed from mother to infant during pregnancy, it has not been established that the virus is transmitted through breast milk. It may be that the milk of women who have the AIDS virus contains antibodies against it and therefore that breast milk may help protect infants against AIDS.

This lack of knowledge constitutes a huge dilemma for public health officials: if AIDS is not transmitted by breast milk, or if breast milk confers immunity against AIDS, then breast feeding should be strongly promoted. If breast feeding transmits the disease, then formula feeding should be promoted, even though the practice would lead to increased infant deaths due to infectious diseases.

It appears that not all infants (or adults, for that matter) who are infected with the virus develop AIDS. It is estimated that 20% to 30% of infected people will develop the syndrome within five years, and none can be expected to survive the disease.[109]

this case) produces in response to exposure to **antigens**—disease-causing bacteria, viruses, and other substances. The more infectious-disease antigens to which a woman is exposed, the broader the protection conveyed to her baby through breast milk.[103] Antibodies in breast milk can confer protection against diseases such as polio, "the flu," respiratory-tract infections, ear infections, meningitis, and gastrointestinal-tract infections.[104,105] Antibodies secreted into breast milk have been concentrated and effectively used to prevent diarrhea in infants and adults exposed to a strain of bacteria that causes diarrhea.[106]

Infants continue to receive **immunity** against a number of infectious diseases as long as breast feeding continues. Whether breast milk from AIDS-infected mothers protects infants against this infectious disease or exposes them to it is a critically important question that is not yet answered. (Discussion of this issue continues in Box 14-5.)

antigens: Bacteria, viruses, and other "foreign" proteins that enter the body and interfere with normal body processes. The presence of antigens prompts the body to produce antibodies, which attempt to destroy the antigens. The body's ability to produce antibodies varies with the type and amount of the antigen, the person's nutritional status, and other factors.

immunity: Resistance to a disease generally conferred by the presence of specific antibodies that destroy disease-generating bacteria and viruses.

Breast milk helps protect infants from:
- *polio*
- *influenza*
- *respiratory-tract infections*
- *ear infections*
- *meningitis*
- *gastrointestinal-tract infections*

Allergies Breast-fed infants are far less likely than formula-fed infants to develop allergies. Up to 7% of infants may be allergic to cow's-milk formula, whereas allergic reactions to breast milk are very rare—probably less than 1%.[107] Once an infant develops an allergy to cow's milk, he or she is at high risk of becoming allergic to other types of food.[108] Many infants who are allergic to cow's milk, egg white, and/or wheat grow poorly because they develop severe diarrhea and other problems when they consume these foods. They also experience other illnesses more often than do infants who do not have food allergies.

Infants born to parents who experienced food allergies early in life are at risk of developing allergies, too. Breast-feeding these infants holds a particular advantage in that it may prevent or postpone the development of food allergies. Although breast feeding does not protect all infants from developing allergies, it may be the ounce of prevention that is worth a pound of cure. Most infants "outgrow" food allergies by the time they are two years old.[107] By then, their gastrointestinal tracts have matured sufficiently to overcome the adverse effects of the offending substances in foods.

Advantages and Disadvantages of Breast Feeding for Mothers

Advantages Breast feeding offers advantages to mothers as well as to infants. Breast feeding causes the release of **oxytocin**, a hormone that stimulates the muscles of the uterus to contract. Contraction of the uterus helps stop the bleeding caused by the detachment of the placenta from the wall of the uterus during delivery. (This effect of breast feeding is quite noticeable. During the first few days after delivery, women can feel their uterus contract while they are breast-feeding.)

oxytocin: The hormone that causes the release of hind milk from the milk-producing cells in the breast. Oxytocin release is stimulated by nursing an infant and in some cases by the woman's psychological response to a baby's cry or thoughts about breast feeding.

Breast feeding may help women return to their prepregnancy weight over time. About 800 calories are used to produce an average infant's daily intake of breast milk during the first three months.[110] Consequently, a breast-feeding mother expends about 800 additional calories per day.

Another advantage of breast feeding is a reduced risk of developing breast cancer later in life. The longer a woman breast-feeds, the less likely she is to develop breast cancer. Also, the risk of developing breast cancer decreases as the number of infants breast-fed increases.[111]

Disadvantages Breast feeding is not best for everyone. Although at least 96% of women are biologically capable of breast feeding, not all women are psychologically able to do it successfully.[112] Many women who feel socially pressured into breast feeding, for example, find that their attempts fail. Breast feeding can also fail if the mother does not receive social and emotional support for her decision to breast-feed. Women who are exposed to high levels of stress and women who suffer depression or other psychological disorders also may be unable to breast-feed successfully.[112] Infant growth and development can be delayed or permanently retarded if breast feeding is continued when it does not go well and infants fail to get enough to eat.

Although breast feeding is a very natural process, problems are not unusual, and generally they can be overcome with supportive guidance. The importance of the early establishment of successful breast feeding has led to the policy in many European countries of not allowing mothers to leave the hospital with their babies until breast feeding is going well. The usual practice in some African countries is to relieve a breast-feeding mother's work load so that she can devote nearly full time to feeding and caring for her young infant. A relative may move in with the family and take over household chores, or the mother and baby may live with her parents for a time. As a cultural practice, supporting new mothers by relieving them of family and household responsibilities does not appear to be nearly as common in the U.S. as in other parts of the world.

Breast feeding limits the participation of fathers in feeding their infants and intensifies the mother's responsibility and commitment. Since most infants eat every three or four hours around the clock during the first month or so, breast-feeding mothers can become exhausted. These disadvantages can be overcome to an extent if the mother *expresses* her milk—releases it from the breast by hand or with the aid of a special pump—and stores it for later use. This allows the father or a babysitter to give the baby feedings of expressed milk from a bottle.

How expressed breast milk is stored is important. It should be placed in a clean, air-tight container and either frozen or refrigerated. Breast milk stays fresh for at least a month if it is solidly frozen, and it holds up well in a refrigerator for two days. The anti-infection components of breast milk help it stay fresh when stored; bacteria that enter breast milk multiply much more slowly than the bacteria that contaminate formulas.[113]

How Breast Feeding Works

The mother's body prepares for breast feeding during pregnancy. Fat is deposited in breast tissue, and networks of blood vessels and nerves infiltrate the breasts. Ducts that will channel milk from the milk-producing cells forward to the nipple—the milk-collection ducts—also mature. (See Figure 14-6.)

Hormonal changes that occur at delivery signal milk production to begin. Because delivery, not length of pregnancy, initiates milk production, breast milk is available for infants born prematurely.

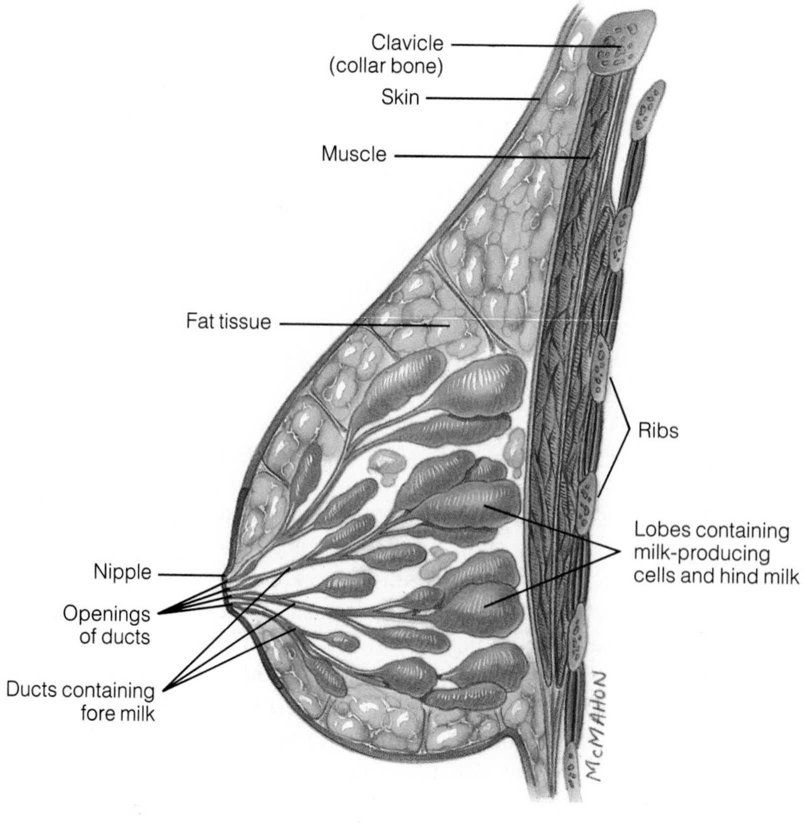

FIGURE 14-6

Cross section of the breast. The blood vessels and nerves that infiltrate the breast tissue are not shown.

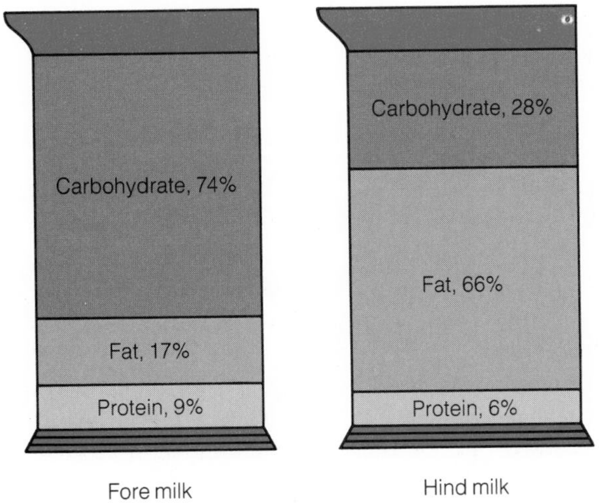

FIGURE 14-7
Comparison of the fat and protein content of fore milk and hind milk. Because of its higher fat content, hind milk better satisfies infants' hunger than does fore milk.

The breast milk produced during the first three days or so after delivery is different from the milk produced later. Called **colostrum**, this early milk contains higher levels of protein, minerals, and antibodies than does "mature" milk.[114] The "extra" infection-fighting antibodies help newborns remain healthy during the transition from a germ-free environment to a germ-filled one. Colostrum looks different from mature milk, too; it is thicker and has a yellowish color.

Mature milk is comprised of about one-third **fore milk** and two-thirds **hind milk**. Before a feeding, fore milk is present in the milk-collection ducts that lead from the milk-producing cells to the nipple and is thus available to the infant first. It contains less fat and protein, and therefore fewer calories, than hind milk (Figure 14-7). Hind milk is produced and stored in the milk-producing cells and is not initially available to the infant. It is released ("let down") by oxytocin, the hormone that also signals the uterus to contract after delivery. Oxytocin causes the milk-producing cells to contract and thereby release the hind milk. This process is commonly referred to as the **let-down reflex**, and it is so powerful that milk is actually ejected from the breast. The let-down reflex gives the infant access to the fat-rich milk stored in the milk-producing cells. If the hind milk is not released, the infant will not receive sufficient nourishment and will soon be hungry again. If this continues, the infant will be hungry most of the time, and may grow and develop poorly. These consequences are discussed because a number of conditions can interfere with the release of oxytocin during breast feeding. The failure of the let-down reflex is a major cause of breast-feeding failure.

colostrum: The milk produced during the first few days after delivery. It contains more antibodies, protein, and certain minerals than mature milk, milk that is produced later. It is thicker than mature milk and has a yellowish color.

fore milk: Milk that accumulates in the milk-collection ducts of the breast. It makes up about one-third of the total amount of milk available to an infant during a normal feeding.

hind milk: Milk that is stored in the milk-producing cells of the breast. It is released by hormonal stimulation about a minute after sucking begins and makes up about two-thirds of the total amount of milk available to an infant during a normal feeding.

let-down reflex: The release of the hind milk. It is stimulated by the hormone oxytocin, which causes the milk-producing cells to contract.

The Let-Down Reflex The let-down reflex is unique as a physiological process in that it can be initiated by either physical or psychological stimuli. Normally, the let-down reflex is triggered when the mother feels the infant sucking at her nipple. It can also occur when the mother hears her infant cry in hunger or when the thought "it's time for a feeding" enters her mind. The physical or psychological stimulus signals a part of the mother's brain to release oxytocin into the bloodstream. When the oxytocin reaches the milk-producing cells, they contract and "let down" milk. Oxytocin is normally released within a minute after breast feeding starts. During the first few weeks of breast feeding, and sometimes longer, the mother may feel the let-down reflex as a tingling sensation in the nipples.

The let-down reflex in breast-feeding women can be initiated by:
- *nursing an infant*
- *psychological stimuli*

It can be inhibited by:
- *stress*
- *pain*
- *anxiety*

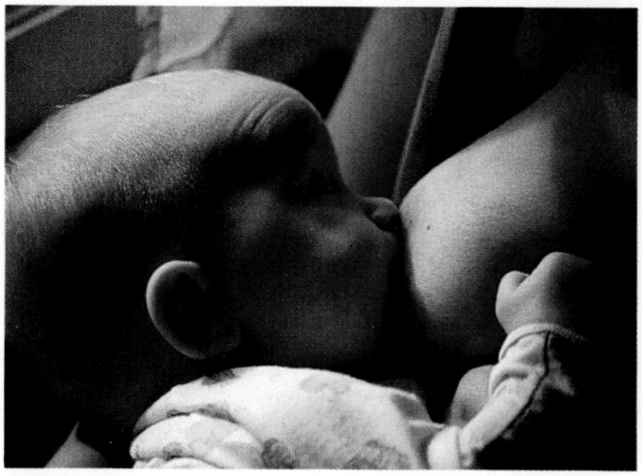
(a)

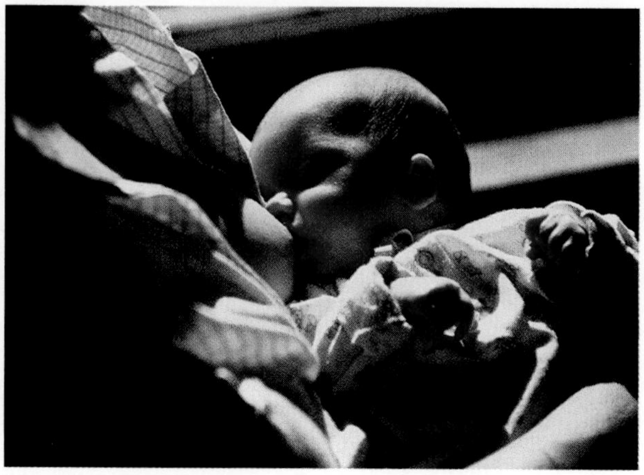
(b)

FIGURE 14-8
(a) A hungry baby feeds with intensity—and clenched fists. (b) The baby loses interest in food when he or she feels full, and the hands become relaxed.

Certain physical and psychological stimuli can prevent the let-down reflex from occurring. Stress, pain, anxiety, and other distractions can block the release of oxytocin. If the mother is distracted by pain or if she is pressured for time, for example, the let-down reflex may not occur—and the infant will not get enough to eat. If this happens often enough, the mother may think she does not have enough milk for her baby and may decide to switch to bottle feeding.

rooting reflex: Instinctive movement of an infant's mouth to the nipple when his or her face touches a breast.

The Rooting Reflex Humans, like other mammals, are born with a **rooting reflex**. When an infant's face touches the mother's breast, he or she instinctively "roots around" for the nipple. Once the nipple is felt, the hungry infant places her or his mouth around it and begins to suck vigorously. If the flow of milk is not limited, the infant will feed until he or she is full and then lose interest in eating. A hungry infant feeds with enormous intensity. (It has been said that minor surgery could be performed painlessly on an actively breast-feeding infant.)

Infants demonstrate that they are hungry in a number of ways: they move their head toward a breast if they are being held, they act irritable, and they cry. They also demonstrate it (and not that they simply want to suck on something or that they are agitated because they need a diaper change or are tired) by the way they start to feed. Hungry infants start to feed with intensity and with their fists tightly clenched. They gradually loosen their fists as their hunger is satisfied, and their hands are fully relaxed and open when they have had enough to eat.[116] See Figure 14-8.

prolactin: The hormone that initiates milk production. Its release is stimulated by an infant's sucking and the emptying of milk from the breasts.

Memory aid: Prolactin is the milk-producing hormone (whereas oxytocin is the milk-releasing hormone).

Breast-Milk Production While an infant is consuming one meal, she or he is "ordering" the next one. The pressure produced inside of the breast by the infant's sucking and the emptying of the breasts during a feeding cause the hormone **prolactin** to be released from special cells in the brain. Prolactin stimulates the production of milk so that as much milk is produced for the next feeding as the infant consumes. It generally takes about two hours for the milk-producing cells to produce sufficient milk for the next feeding.[115] An important exception to this occurs when an infant enters a growth spurt.

Growth Spurts: Resetting the Dial on Breast-Milk Production Like children and adolescents, infants grow in spurts, not at a constant rate. In preparation for a growth spurt, hunger increases and the demand for milk may double. The increased food intake causes a gain in weight, which in turn is followed by an increase in height (Figure 14-9).

Growth spurts occur frequently between an infant's third and seventh week of life, but less often after that.[117] The initial increase in hunger associated with a growth spurt makes it take longer to produce a refill in milk supply. Instead of two hours, up to 24 hours may be needed for the supply of breast milk to catch up with the infant's increased need for it. This means that for about a day, the infant will want to feed often and may not be completely satisfied. Although the mother may spend much of her day (and night) breast-feeding an infant who is entering a growth spurt, she may feel that she does not "have enough milk" to satisfy the baby and will give the baby a bottle. Because breast-milk production is determined by how much and how often an infant feeds, supplementary bottle feedings lead to a decrease in milk production. With less breast milk available, the mother's feeling that she has too little breast milk is strengthened. Some women stop breast-feeding because of these longer-than-usual delays in producing enough milk to satisfy their growing infants' need for food.

It is very rare that a breast-feeding woman cannot produce enough milk. As long as an infant is allowed to breast-feed as often as desired, milk production will catch up with the baby's need.

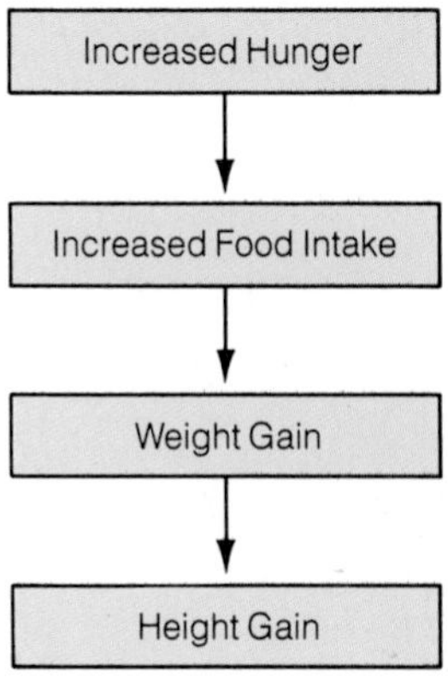

FIGURE 14-9
Sequence of a growth spurt.

How Long Should Breast Feeding Continue? No one knows what length of breast feeding is ideal in terms of infant health. It has been observed over time, however, that women in most cultures breast-feed for 6 months to 2 years.[112] Milk-producing animals such as cats, dogs, mice, and rats tend to breast-feed for about the same length of time as their gestation (pregnancy). The gestation period for rats, for example, is about 21 days, and rats breast-feed their young for approximately 21 days. Whether 9

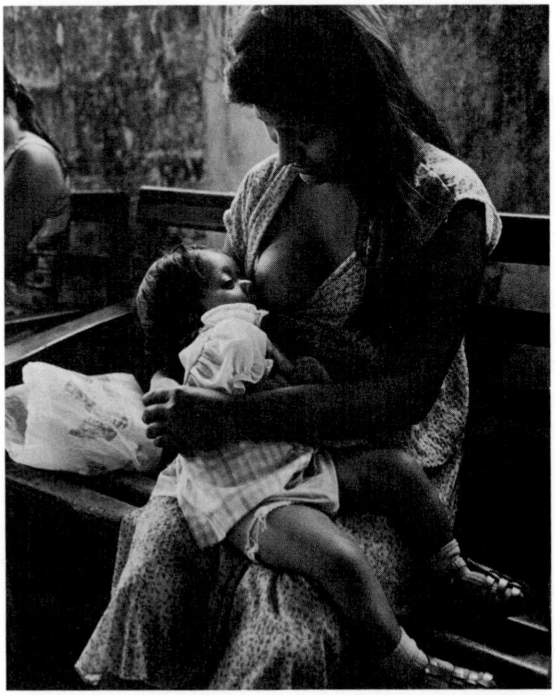

An Ecuadoran woman and her daughter. Mothers in most of the world's cultures breast-feed for 6 months to 2 years.

months is the ideal breast-feeding period for humans is debatable. The current recommendation of the American Academy of Pediatrics, however, is that breast feeding continue for 6 months.[100] Few breast-feeding mothers continue it that long, and setting a goal to breast-feed longer than 6 months (such as for the recommended 9 months) may represent too drastic a change for now. The desired duration of breast feeding is likely longer in economically developing countries where infectious diseases and malnutrition are common.

As long as an infant feeds at the breast, breast-milk production continues. Milk production decreases when the intervals between feedings lengthen and when the breasts are not completely emptied in feedings. It ceases altogether when the infant stops breast-feeding.

NUTRITION FOR BREAST-FEEDING WOMEN

Breast-feeding women need an adequate and balanced diet in order to replenish their bodies' nutrient stores, maintain their health, and produce sufficient milk for their babies. After using diet and nutrient stores to support fetal growth for 9 months, these women continue to supply all of the energy and nutrients their infants need through breast feeding. However, their babies are larger then, and they require greater amounts of energy and most nutrients than they did before they were born.

Calorie and Nutrient Needs

The RDA for calories is about 25% higher for breast-feeding women than for other women. (See Figure 14-10.) The actual increase in caloric need is higher than the RDA; it's around 40%. Energy supplied from fat stores that normally accumulate during pregnancy contribute to meeting energy needs during breast feeding, so not all of the calories must come from the mother's diet. The RDA calls for increasing caloric intake by 500 calories per day. An additional 300 calories are needed to support breast feeding (recall that the average is 800 calories during the first 3 months), but this energy is assumed to be provided by maternal fat stores.

The average increases in nutrient allowances for breast feeding are generally higher than the increases for pregnancy. (Compare Figures 14-4 and 14-10.) As during pregnancy, proportionately higher amounts of nutrients than calories are required, which indicates the need for a nutrient-dense diet. As you can see in Figure 14-10, the increases in nutrient RDAs for breast feeding vary. The needs for vitamins D and C and zinc increase the most. The impressive increases in the RDAs for these nutrients are related to infants' needs for them for bone and tissue formation. Calcium, phosphorus, magnesium, and vitamin A are all involved in bone formation, and those RDAs show 50% increases.

Concern has been expressed about the possibility that breast feeding may weaken a woman's bones if she fails to get enough calcium and other bone-building minerals in her diet, and it appears that this concern has some basis in fact. Breast-feeding women, especially those below 30 years of age who have not achieved peak bone density, may lose minerals from their

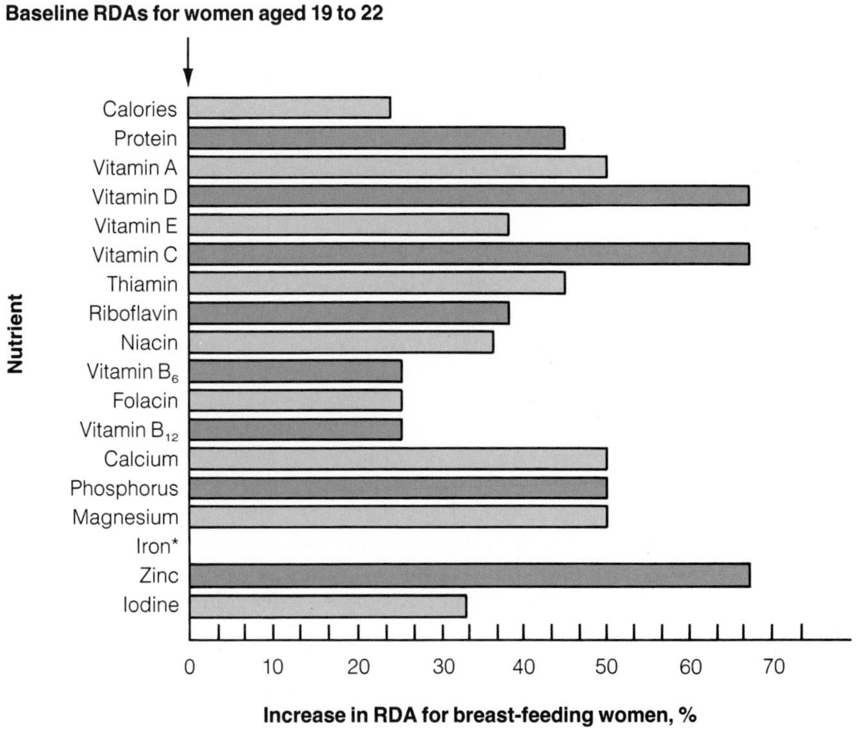

*Dietary iron needs do not increase during breast feeding, but it is recommended that prenatal iron supplements of 30 to 60 mg per day be continued for 2 to 3 months after delivery to replenish stores.

FIGURE 14-10
Percentage increases in RDAs for breast-feeding women aged 19 to 22 years.

bones if they consume a low-calcium diet during breast feeding.[118] Breast-feeding four or more children while consuming a low-calcium diet may increase the risk that a woman will develop osteoporosis later in life.[118]

With the exception of iron, the RDAs for vitamins and minerals increase by at least 25% during breast feeding. The RDA for iron is not increased because of the savings in iron that occurs with breast feeding. A woman who breast-feeds generally does not resume menstrual periods until the infant consumes most of his or her calories from foods other than breast milk. The resulting iron savings reduces the breast-feeding woman's need for dietary iron.

Dietary Recommendations for Breast-Feeding Women

The calories and nutrients needed by the breast-feeding woman can be obtained from a varied diet that includes foods from each of the basic food groups. The recommended numbers of servings from each food group are shown in Table 14-8. Compared with the recommendations for pregnancy (Table 14-3), breast-feeding women are advised to consume an additional serving of a vitamin C-rich fruit or vegetable and an additional serving of milk or a milk product.

Increases in hunger and food intake that accompany breast feeding generally take care of meeting caloric needs. If the diet includes at least the recommended minimal number of servings from each food group and sufficient calories, the breast-feeding woman is helping to assure herself and her infant adequate diets. Failure to consume enough calories from food can

TABLE 14-8

Food group recommendations for breast-feeding women

Food Group	Minimum Number of Servings per Day
Breads and cereals	4
Vegetables and fruits	(5)
vitamin A-rich	1
vitamin C-rich	2
other	2
Milk and milk products	4
Meats or alternates	3
Miscellaneous	based on caloric need

Note: For additional information on foods contained in the groups and what standard serving sizes are, refer to Table 2-6.

decrease milk production. Weight loss that exceeds 1½ pounds per week—even in women with a good supply of fat stores—can reduce the amount of milk women produce.[119]

Effects of Maternal Diet on Breast-Milk Composition Milk-producing cells in the breast are supplied with the raw materials they need to manufacture milk from the mother's blood. For a number of substances, what ends up in the mother's blood reflects what she has consumed, so that the composition of breast milk varies with the maternal diet. For other substances, the amount that enters breast milk is regulated within the milk-producing cells; the levels of these substances remain fairly constant regardless of maternal diet.

Milk-producing cells enforce "quality-control" processes on the amount of carbohydrate, protein, fat, and minerals (including calcium, sodium, potassium, iron, and fluoride) in breast milk. They also regulate the amount of milk produced when the maternal caloric intake is low. Rather than the energy content of milk being diluted in response to a low-calorie diet, the volume of milk is decreased.[120,121]

The amount of carbohydrate, protein, and fat in breast milk varies only slightly in response to maternal diet, but the type of fat present can vary substantially.[122] (See Table 14-9.) If a woman consumes more vegetable oils than animal fats, her breast milk will contain a high proportion of unsaturated fats. If she fasts, her milk will contain the type of fat present in her fat stores.

The vitamin content of breast milk corresponds more closely to maternal intake than is the case for the energy nutrients.[123,124] The amounts of thiamin and vitamins C and B_{12} in breast milk, for example, vary with the types of food and supplements that the mother ingests. Thiamin deficiency (beriberi) and vitamin-B_{12} deficiency (pernicious anemia) have been diagnosed in infants breast-fed by mothers deficient in those vitamins.[124]

The amounts of several minerals in breast milk also are influenced by what the mother eats. It is clear that the amounts of zinc and iodine in breast milk reflect the mother's diet.[124,125] Infants who fail to get sufficient zinc and iodine grow and develop slowly.

TABLE 14-9
Relationship of maternal diet to breast milk

Breast-Milk Components Affected by Maternal Diet	Breast-Milk Components *Not* Affected by Maternal Diet
total amount of milk	total amounts of carbohydrate, protein, and fat
type of fat	calcium
most vitamins	sodium
zinc	potassium
iodine	iron
	fluoride

In many respects, a mother's diet and the supplements she takes affect the nutrient content of her breast milk and may influence her infant's growth and development. Consequently, what and how much a woman eats while she is breast-feeding are important to her infant's health as well as her own. Eating an adequate and balanced diet—relying on foods rather than supplements to meet vitamin and mineral needs—is the best way to achieve good nutrition during breast feeding.

Other Substances that Enter Breast Milk As explained in chapter 2, foods contain many substances in addition to nutrients, and other substances enter the body through drugs, medications, and other ingested nonfood substances. All of these substances may end up in breast milk.

When a breast-feeding woman drinks coffee, her infant receives a small dose of caffeine. Breast-fed infants of women who are heavy coffee drinkers (10 or more cups per day) may develop "caffeine jitters."[126] Alcohol also is transferred from a woman's body to breast milk.[127] Oddly enough, however, beer or wine is sometimes recommended to breast-feeding women to help them relax before feeding periods. Although one or two alcohol-containing beverages per day appear to pose no harm to the breast-fed infant, heavy drinking during breast feeding (6 or more standard-size drinks per day) exposes infants to levels of alcohol that may harm their development. The development of the brain and nervous system of infants born to chronic, heavy drinkers appears to be retarded.[128] If breast-feeding women were to take the advice to relax with a beer before each breast feeding, they would qualify as "heavy drinkers" because infants eat every 3 to 4 hours during their first few months.

The composition of breast milk can be affected by maternal:
- *diet*
- *calorie reserves*
- *vitamin/mineral supplement use*
- *drug and alcohol intake*
- *exposure to environmental contaminants*

Almost any drug or toxin that enters the mother's blood will end up in her breast milk.[124] Environmental contaminants such as DDT, chlordane, PCB, and PBBs, for example, are transferred into breast milk. Many environmental contaminants are fat-soluble, and if they are ingested they may be stored in a woman's fat tissues. When the fat stores are later broken down for use in breast milk, the contaminants stored in the fat will enter her milk. The ingestion of fish from contaminated waters in Lake Ontario and Lake Michigan has been directly linked to abnormally high levels of PCB in breast milk.[129,130] Infants exposed to PCBs can develop rashes, digestive upsets, and nervous-system problems.[124]

Infants are much smaller than women, and it takes a smaller dose of caffeine, alcohol, drugs, or environmental contaminants to have an effect on them than on an adult. Whereas breast-feeding mothers may show no adverse effects from these substances, their infants may.

Breast-feeding women are advised to limit their consumption of regular coffee to 4 or fewer cups a day and to limit alcohol consumption to no more than 2 drinks daily. Drugs or medications should be taken only on the advice of a physician, and fish from contaminated lakes should not be consumed.

Other Cautions Some infants may be sensitive to components of certain foods a mother consumes that are transferred into breast milk. Peanut butter, chocolate, egg whites, and nuts contain substances that enter breast milk and cause some infants to develop a rash, wheezing, or a runny nose. Onions and foods from the cabbage family such as cabbage, broccoli, and brussels sprouts also are suspected to cause adverse reactions in breast-fed infants. Although causing no distress to the mother, these foods may give some infants pronounced cases of gas and cramps.

Why some infants are sensitive to certain components of the foods in their mothers' diets is not known, and many of the conclusions drawn about the relationships are based on hear-say because the appropriate studies have not been done. The general advice for breast-feeding women is to first experiment with small amounts of the potentially offending foods to see if the infant is sensitive. If the infant does not appear to be, these foods do not need to be omitted from the diet.

COMING UP IN CHAPTER 15

Chapter 15 highlights the relationships between nutrition and growth, mental development, and health. It covers the important areas of food preference and habit formation, the effect of the psychological environment on nutrition and growth, and the nutrient needs of infants, children, and adolescents. Relationships between diet during childhood and chronic disease development later in life also are discussed.

REVIEW QUESTIONS

1. List three ways in which disruptions in nutritional status are related to infertility.
2. Body fat content likely affects fertility because of its influence on the body's production of ____________.
3. The need for which two vitamins is increased by the use of oral contraceptive pills?
4. Studies undertaken in Russia, the Netherlands (Holland), and England during World War II led to at least three important conclusions about the influence of nutrition on reproduction. State the three conclusions discussed in the chapter.

5. What is the main goal of the WIC program, and what does the program provide?
6. Name two maternal nutrition factors that influence infant birth weight.
7. What range of maternal weight gain during pregnancy for women entering pregnancy normal weight is associated with the birth of infants of optimal weight and health?
8. True or false? A woman's need for calories increases by a greater percentage during pregnancy than does her need for protein and most vitamins and minerals.
9. What are two problems associated with the consumption of low-calorie diets during pregnancy?
10. Dietary deficiency of which vitamin is associated with the birth of infants with spinal cord abnormalities?
11. ____________ deficiency is the most common nutrient deficiency among pregnant women in the U.S.
12. A deficiency of zinc during pregnancy has been associated with the birth of ____________ infants.
13. How much alcohol is considered a "safe" amount during pregnancy?
14. True or false? Shifts in food preferences rarely occur in healthy women during pregnancy.
15. Name five vitamins that if taken in high amounts during pregnancy may adversely affect the health of the fetus or newborn.
16. List five characteristics of a good diet for pregnant women.
17. What vitamin and mineral supplements are recommended for pregnancy?
18. Fill in the "Minimum Number of Servings per Day" columns with the food group recommendations for pregnant and breast-feeding women:

	Minimum Number of Servings per Day	
Food Group	Pregnant Women	Breast-Feeding Women
Breads and cereals		
Vegetables and fruits		
vitamin A-rich		
vitamin C-rich		
other		
Milk and milk products		
Meats or alternates		

19. The caloric and nutrient content of infant formulas is modeled on the composition of ____________.
20. Cite five differences in the compositions of breast milk and infant formula.
21. What is the main component of breast milk that protects infants from infectious diseases?
22. Cite two health benefits of breast-feeding to the mother.
23. True or false? Almost all women are biologically able to breast-feed.
24. How do colostrum, mature milk, fore milk, and hind milk differ?

25. What is the let-down reflex?
26. Which hormone triggers the let-down reflex, and which triggers milk production?
27. The composition of breast milk is affected by a variety of factors. Name five.
28. List three nutrient components of breast milk whose amounts vary according to the maternal diet, and three components whose amounts do not vary substantially.

Answers

1. Low and high body fat content, carotenemia, regular megadoses of vitamin C, vegan diets, and in males, zinc deficiency.
2. Estrogen.
3. Vitamin B_6 and folic acid.
4. They are listed in the Nutrition and Fertility section.
5. The main goal of the WIC program is to improve the health of pregnant women, infants, and young children; it provides nutrition education and food supplements.
6. Prepregnancy weight status and weight gain during pregnancy.
7. 30 to 35 pounds.
8. False. Although pregnant women need more calories, their needs for protein, vitamins, and minerals increase by a higher percentage. This is why a nutrient-dense diet is recommended during pregnancy.
9. The use of protein as a source of energy; reduced fetal growth; inadequate intakes of vitamins and minerals needed for fetal growth and development.
10. Folic acid.
11. Iron.
12. Small, malformed.
13. None. It is recommended that pregnant women do not drink alcohol-containing beverages during pregnancy.
14. False. They commonly occur among healthy pregnant women and are considered normal.
15. High amounts of vitamins B_{12}, C, and B_6 have been associated with the development of "rebound" deficiencies in infants; high amounts of vitamins A and D have been associated with the development of a variety of abnormalities in newborns.
16. Seven characteristics are listed in the subsection, Translating Nutrient Needs into a Good Diet.
17. Folic acid (400 mcg per day throughout the pregnancy) and iron (30–60 mg per day in the last half of pregnancy).
18. See Tables 14-3 and 14-8.
19. Human milk.
20. Refer to the subsection, Comparison of Breast Milk, Commercial Infant Formula, and Cow's Milk.

21. Antibodies.
22. Tightened uterine muscles and less uterine bleeding after delivery, increased caloric expenditure after pregnancy, reduced risk of developing breast cancer later in life.
23. True.
24. Many of the differences are made clear by the margin definitions.
25. The release of the hind milk by oxytocin.
26. Oxytocin stimulates the let-down reflex, and prolactin triggers milk production.
27. The breast-feeding woman's diet, caloric reserves, vitamin and mineral supplement use, drug and alcohol intake, and exposure to environmental contaminants.
28. Nutrients in breast milk that vary with the maternal diet: type of fat, most vitamins, zinc, and iodine. Nutrients that do not vary substantially: amount of carbohydrate, protein, fat, calcium, sodium, potassium, iron, and fluoride.

■ ■ ■

PUTTING NUTRITION KNOWLEDGE TO WORK

1. How would you respond if someone asked you what you think about this statement? A fetus takes the nutrients it needs from the mother. Therefore, it matters little what a woman eats during pregnancy.

   (*Myth #1 addresses this issue.*)

2. Assume Penny enters pregnancy underweight and gains a total of 12 pounds during pregnancy. How might these factors affect the size and health of the infant?

   (*Penny is at risk of delivering a low-birth-weight infant because she entered pregnancy underweight and because her weight gain was sufficiently low to reduce fetal growth. Low-birth-weight babies are at increased risk of developing a number of short- and long-term health problems.*)

3. Say you have a friend who is restricting her weight gain during her pregnancy because she thinks it will make her delivery easier. What facts may your friend have failed to consider when she decided to do this?

   (*Refer to the subsections on optimal weight gain and calories and to Myth #3.*)

4. Jane had been breast-feeding her son for about a month when she suddenly became concerned that her milk supply wasn't sufficient to satisfy him. What is the most likely explanation for her concern?

   (*Hint: Remember "hunger periods"?*)

5. Table 14-10 lists U.S. infant mortality rates by region and state. Find the rate for your home state. Compare it with the rates for the entire country and for the five states closest to your home state. Which state has the highest, and which the lowest infant mortality rate? Speculate about the reasons the rates vary by state. The table is on the next page.

TABLE 14-10

Provisional 1987 U.S. infant mortality rates per 1,000 live births

Region/State	Infant Mortality Rate*	Region/State	Infant Mortality Rate*
New England	7.6	North Carolina	11.4
Maine	6.4	South Carolina	12.9
New Hampshire	7.2	Georgia	12.2
Vermont	9.1	Florida	10.7
Massachusetts	7.8	East South Central	11.5
Rhode Island	8.3	Kentucky	8.0
Connecticut	7.3	Tennessee	12.4
Middle Atlantic	10.2	Alabama	12.7
New York	10.7	Mississippi	12.6
New Jersey	8.0	West South Central	9.6
Pennsylvania	10.9	Arkansas	8.6
East North Central	10.2	Louisiana	11.7
Ohio	9.3	Oklahoma	9.8
Indiana	9.9	Texas	9.2
Illinois	11.3	Mountain	8.8
Michigan	10.8	Montana	7.5
Wisconsin	8.8	Idaho	7.8
West North Central	9.8	Wyoming	5.5
Minnesota	8.7	Colorado	10.3
Iowa	7.9	New Mexico	6.9
Missouri	12.3	Arizona	8.8
North Dakota	8.8	Utah	9.8
South Dakota	10.1	Nevada	9.1
Nebraska	9.9	Pacific	9.2
Kansas	8.5	Washington	9.1
South Atlantic	11.2	Oregon	9.7
Delaware	9.1	California	9.2
Maryland	9.8	Alaska	9.6
District of Columbia	20.3	Hawaii	9.8
Virginia	9.8	**United States**	**10.4**
West Virginia	9.1		

*National Center for Health Statistics data.

NOTES

1. J. M. Duncan, *Fecundity, Fertility, and Sterility and Applied Topics*, 2nd ed. (Edinburgh: Adam and Charles Black, 1871).

2. Z. Stein, M. Susser, et al., *Famine and Human Development: The Dutch Hunger, Winter of 1944–45* (New York: Oxford University Press, 1975).

3. A. N. Antonov, Children born during the siege of Leningrad in 1942, *Journal of Pediatrics* 30 (1947): 250–259.

4. C. A. Smith, Effects of maternal undernutrition upon the newborn infant in Holland, *Journal of Pediatrics* 30 (1947): 229–243, and C. A. Smith, The effect of wartime starvation in Holland upon pregnancy and its product, *American Journal of Obstetrics and Gynecology* 53 (1947): 599–608.

5. P. Gruenwald, H. Funakawa, et al., Influence of environmental factors on foetal growth in man, *Lancet* i (1967): 1026–1028.

6. H. Fries, Secondary amenorrhea, self-induced weight reduction, and anorexia nervosa, *Acta Psychiatrica Scandinavica* (supplement) 248 (1974): 5–45.
7. R. E. Frisch, Food intake, fatness, and reproductive ability, in *Anorexia Nervosa*, ed. R. Vigerky (New York: Raven Press, 1977), 149–161.
8. A. J. Hartz, P. N. Barboriak, et al., The association of obesity with infertility and related menstrual abnormalities in women, *International Journal of Obesity* 3 (1979): 57–63.
9. Z. M. van der Spy, Nutrition and reproduction, *Clinical Obstetrics and Gynaecology* 12 (1985): 579–604.
10. R. E. Frisch, Body fat, puberty, and fertility, *Biology Review* 59 (1984): 161–188.
11. E. R. Baker, Menstrual dysfunction and hormonal status in athletic women: A review, *Fertility and Sterility* 36 (1981): 691–696.
12. H. Fries and S. J. Nillius, Dieting, anorexia nervosa, and amenorrhea after oral contraceptive treatment, *Acta Psychiatrica Scandinavica* 49 (1973): 669.
13. E. M. Nelson, E. C. Fisher, et al., Diet and bone status in amenorrheic runners, *American Journal of Clinical Nutrition* 43 (1986): 910–916.
14. M. Martin, Health issues, women, and physical exercise, in *Nutrition and Physical Exercise* (Washington, D.C.: U.S. Department of Health and Human Services, 1984), 16–21.
15. M. Parrish, Exercising to the bone: Is there a connection between athletic amenorrhea and bone loss? *Women's Sports*, 25 April 1983.
16. G. B. Kolata, !Kung hunter–gatherers. Feminism, diet, and birth control, *Science* 185 (1974): 932–934.
17. L. A. van der Walt, E. N. Wilmsen, and T. Jenkins, Unusual sex hormone patterns among desert-dwelling hunter–gatherers, *Journal of Clinical Endocrinology Metabolism* 46 (1978): 658–662.
18. E. Kemmann, S. A. Pasquale, and R. Skaf, Amenorrhea associated with carotenemia, *Journal of the American Medical Association* 249 (1983): 926–929.
19. P. B. Hill, L. Garbaczewski, et al., Gonadotropin release and meat consumption in vegetarian women, *American Journal of Clinical Nutrition* 43 (1986): 37–41.
20. S. M. Brooks, C. F. Sanborn, et al., Diet in athletic amenorrhea (letter), *Lancet* i (1984): 559.
21. *Proceedings of the International Conference on Vitamin C*, New York Academy of Sciences, New York City, October 8–10, 1986.
22. A. Keys, Human starvation and its consequences, *Journal of the American Dietetic Association* 22 (1946): 582–587.
23. K. P. Brownell, S. N. Steen, and J. H. Wilmore, Weight-regulation practices in athletes: Analysis of metabolic and health effects, *Medicine and Science in Sports and Exercise* 19 (1987): 546–556.
24. A. S. Prasad, Clinical manifestations of zinc deficiency, *Annual Review of Nutrition* 5 (1985): 341–363.
25. M. Hansen, R. Hatcher, et al., Update on oral contraceptives, *Journal of Reproductive Medicine* 30 (1985): 691–713.
26. D. P. Rose, R. Strong, et al., Erythrocyte aminotransferase activities in women using oral contraceptives and the effect of vitamin-B_6 supplementation, *American Journal of Clinical Nutrition* 26 (1973): 48–52.
27. A. Shojania, R. Hornady, and P. Barnes, The effect of oral contraceptives on blood platelet metabolism, *American Journal of Obstetrics and Gynecology* 111 (1982): 782–791.
28. M. S. Bamji, K. Prema, et al., Vitamin supplements to Indian women using low-dosage oral contraceptives, *Contraception* 32 (1985): 405–416.
29. R. Russell-Briefel, T. Ezzati, and J. Perlman, Prevalence and trends in oral contraceptive use in premenopausal females ages 12–54 years, United States, 1976–80, *American Journal of Public Health* 75 (1985): 1173–1176.
30. J. D. Forrest, The public and the pill: Is the pill making a comeback? *American Journal of Public Health* 75 (1985): 1131–1132.
31. M. E. Wegman, Annual review of vital statistics—1987, *Pediatrics* 82 (1988): 817–827.

32. L. S. Bakketeig, J. H. Hoffman, and A. R. T. Oakley, Perinatal mortality, in *Perinatal Epidemiology*, ed. M. B. Bracken (New York: Oxford University Press, 1984).

33. J. Metcoff, P. Costiloe, et al., Effect of food supplementation (WIC) during pregnancy on birth weight, *American Journal of Clinical Nutrition* 41 (1985): 933–947.

34. J. W. Stockbauer, Evaluation of the Missouri WIC program: Prenatal components, *Journal of the American Dietetic Association* 86 (1986): 61–67.

35. J. E. Brown and P. Tieman, Effect of income level and WIC on the energy and key-nutrient intake of preschool children, *Journal of the American Dietetic Association* 86 (1986): 1189–1191.

36. V. Miller, S. Swaney, and A. Deinard, Impact of the WIC program on the iron status of infants, *Pediatrics* 75 (1985): 100–105.

37. L. L. Birch, S. I. Zimmerman, and H. Hind, The influence of social-affective context in the formation of children's food preferences, *Child Development* 51 (1980): 856–861.

38. M. C. McCormick, The contribution of low birth weight to infant mortality and childhood morbidity, *New England Journal of Medicine* 312 (1985): 82–90.

39. R. L. Williams, R. K. Creasy, et al., Fetal growth and perinatal viability in California, *Obstetrics and Gynecology* 59 (1982): 624–632.

40. J. E. Brown, K. W. Berdan, et al., Prenatal weight gains related to the birth of healthy-sized infants to low-income women, *Journal of the American Dietetic Association* 86 (1986): 1679–1683.

41. D. W. Smith, *Growth and Its Disorders* (Philadelphia: W. B. Saunders Co., 1979).

42. J. E. Brown, B. Abrams, et al., Conclusions of an expert panel on prenatal weight gain, *Public Health Reports* (1990).

43. J. E. Brown, Weight gain during pregnancy: What is optimal? *Clinical Nutrition* 7 (1988): 181–190.

44. F. E. Hytten and L. Leitch, *The Physiology of Human Pregnancy*, 2nd ed. (Oxford: Blackwell Scientific Publications, 1971).

45. P. Rosso and C. Cramoy, Nutrition in pregnancy, in *Nutrition, Pre- and Postnatal Development*, ed. M. Winick (New York: Plenum Press, 1979), 133–228.

46. W. Doyle, M. A. Crawford, et al., Dietary survey during pregnancy in a low socioeconomic group, *Human Nutrition Applied Nutrition* 36A (1982): 95–106.

47. M. Winick, *Nutrition and pregnancy* (White Plains, N.Y.: March of Dimes Birth Defects Foundation, 1986).

48. *Recommended Dietary Allowances*, 9th ed., Food and Nutrition Board, National Research Council (Washington, D.C.: National Academy of Sciences, 1980).

49. B. S. Burke, V. V. Harding, and H. C. Stuart, Nutrition studies during pregnancy, IV: Relation of protein content of mother's diet during pregnancy to birth length, birth weight, and condition of the infant at birth, *Journal of Pediatrics* 23 (1943): 506–515.

50. A. C. Higgins, E. W. Crampton, and J. E. Moxley, Nutrition and the outcome of pregnancy, *Proceedings of the Fourth International Congress of Endocrinology* 273 (1972): 1071–1077.

51. C. Phillipps and N. E. Johnson, The impact of quality of diet and other factors on birth weight of infants, *American Journal of Clinical Nutrition* 30 (1977): 215–225.

52. K. M. Laurence, Prevention of neural tube defects by improvement in maternal diet and preconceptional folic acid supplementation, *Progress in Clinical Biological Research* 163B (1985): 383–388.

53. N. C. Nevin, The role of periconceptual vitamin supplementation in the prevention of neural tube defect, *Progress in Clinical Biological Research* 163B (1985): 396–398.

54. F. O. Tierson, C. L. Olsen, and E. B. Hook, Nausea and vomiting of pregnancy and association with pregnancy outcome, *American Journal of Obstetrics and Gynecology* 155 (1986): 1017–1022.

55. P. N. Singla, V. K. Gupta, and K. N. Agarwal, Storage iron in human foetal organs, *Acta Paediatrica Scandinavica* 74 (1985): 701–706.

56. V. Herbert, Recommended dietary intake (RDI) of iron in humans, *American Journal of Clinical Nutrition* 45 (1987): 679–686.

57. J. Reece, P. R. Donovan, and A. Y. Pellett, Iron supplementation in pregnancy: Testing a new clinic protocol, *Journal of the American Dietetic Association* 87 (1987): 1682–1683. See also reference no. 56.

58. L. J. Taper, J. T. Oliva, and S. J. Ritchey, Zinc and copper retention during pregnancy: The adequacy of prenatal diets with and without supplementation, *American Journal of Clinical Nutrition* 41 (1985): 1184–1192.

59. J. Apgar, Zinc and reproduction, *Annual Review of Nutrition* 5 (1985): 43–68.

60. J. Warkany, Production of congenital malformations by dietary measures, *Journal of the American Medical Association* 168 (1958): 2020–2023.

61. D. R. Miller and K. C. Hayes, Vitamin excess and toxicity, in *Nutritional Toxicology*, ed. J. N. Hathcock (New York: Academic Press, 1982), 81–133.

62. W. A. Cochrane, Overnutrition in prenatal and neonatal life: A problem? *Canadian Medical Association Journal* 93 (1965): 893–899.

63. W. T. Tompkins, D. G. Wiehl, and R. M. Mitchell, The underweight patient as an increased obstetric hazard, *American Journal of Obstetrics and Gynecology* 69 (1955): 114–123.

64. J. E. Brown and R. B. Tomas, Taste changes during pregnancy, *American Journal of Clinical Nutrition* 43 (1986): 414–418.

65. R. E. Little, F. A. Schultz, and W. Mandell, Drinking during pregnancy, *Journal of Studies on Alcohol* 37 (1976): 375–379.

66. E. B. Hook, Dietary cravings and aversions during pregnancy, *American Journal of Clinical Nutrition* 31 (1978): 1355–1362.

67. L. Prochownik, Uber ernahrungscuren inder schwangerschaft, *Therapy Monat* 15 (1901): 446.

68. N. J. Eastman and E. C. Jackson, Weight relationships in pregnancy: I. The bearing of maternal weight gain and prepregnancy weight on birth weight in full-term pregnancies, *Obstetrics and Gynecology Survey* 23 (1968): 1003–1025.

69. *Maternal Nutrition and the Course and Outcome of Pregnancy* (Washington, D.C.: National Academy of Sciences, 1970).

70. R. L. Pike and H. A. Smiciklas, A reappraisal of sodium restriction during pregnancy, *International Journal of Gynaecology and Obstetrics* 10 (1972): 1–8.

71. R. de Alvarez and E. K. Smith, The influence of dietary sodium uptake on water, electrolyte, and nitrogen balance in pregnancy toxaemia: A metabolic study, *American Journal of Obstetrics and Gynecology* 72 (1956): 562–588.

72. M. Robinson, Salt in pregnancy, *Lancet* i (1958): 178–181.

73. K. L. Jones, Pattern of malformation in offspring of chronic alcoholic mothers, *Lancet* i (1973): 1267–1271.

74. H. L. Rosett, L. Weiner, and K. C. Edelin, Treatment experience with pregnant problem drinkers, *Journal of the American Medical Association* 249 (1983): 2029–2033.

75. H. J. Osofsky, Relationships between nutrition during pregnancy and subsequent infant and child development, *Obstetrics and Gynecology Survey* 30 (1975): 227–241.

76. *Alternative Dietary Practices and Nutritional Abuses in Pregnancy*, Committee on Nutrition of the Mother and Preschool Child (Washington, D.C.: National Academy Press, 1982).

77. R. B. Sayetta, Pica: An overview, *Journal of Family Practice* 33 (1986): 181–185.

78. J. E. Brown and R. Tomas, Taste and food preference changes in pregnancy (abstract), *American Public Health Association Annual Meeting Program*, 1986.

79. F. D. Tierson, C. L. Olsen, and E. B. Hook, Influence of food cravings and aversions on diet in pregnancy, *Ecology of Food and Nutrition* 17 (1985): 117–129.

80. D. A. Denton, The hunger for salt: An anthropological, physiological and medical analysis (Berlin: Springer-Verlag, 1982), 427–435.

81. A. S. Anderson and M. J. Wichelow, Constipation during pregnancy: Dietary fibre intake and the effect of fibre supplementation, *Human Nutrition and Applied Nutrition* 39 (1985): 202–207.

82. B. Worthington-Roberts, The role of nutrition in pregnancy course and outcome, *Journal of Environmental Pathology, Toxicology, and Oncology* 5 (1985): 1–80.

83. W. A. Cochrane, Overnutrition in prenatal and neonatal life: A problem? *Canadian Medical Association Journal* 93 (1965): 893–899.

84. *Surgeon General's Report on Nutrition and Health*, Public Health Service, DHHS publication no. (PHS) 88-50210, 1988, 557–559.

85. *Nutrition and Adolescent Pregnancy*, Joint project of March of Dimes Birth Defect Foundation and U.S. Departments of Health and Human Services and Agriculture (Washington, D.C.: National MCH Clearinghouse, 1986).

86. S. B. Friedman and S. Phillips, Psychosocial risk to mother and child as a consequence of adolescent pregnancy, *Seminars in Perinatology* 5 (1981): 33–37.

87. B. S. Zuckerman, D. K. Walker, and D. A. Frank, Adolescent pregnancy: Behavioral determinants of outcome, *Journal of Pediatrics* 105 (1984): 857–863.

88. G. B. Forbes, Pregnancy in the teenager: Biologic aspects, *Birth Defects* 17 (1981): 85–90.

89. S. M. Garn, Characteristics of the mother and child in teenage pregnancy, *American Journal of Diseases of Children* 137 (1983): 365–368.

90. A. C. Sukanick, K. D. Rogers, and H. M. McDonald, Physical maturity and outcome of pregnancy in primiparas younger than 16 years of age, *Pediatrics* 78 (1986): 31–36.

91. G. Martinez and F. W. Krieger, 1984 milk-feeding patterns in the United States, *Pediatrics* 76 (1985): 1004–1008, and G. Martinez, personal communication (1988).

92. W. E. M. Lands, Renewed questions about polyunsaturated fatty acids, *Nutrition Reviews* 44 (1986): 189–195.

93. G. H. Anderson, S. A. Atkinson, and M. H. Bryan, Energy and macronutrient content of human milk during early lactation from mothers giving birth prematurely and at term, *American Journal of Clinical Nutrition* 34 (1981): 258–265.

94. S. J. Fomon, *Infant Nutrition*, 2nd ed. (Philadelphia: W. B. Saunders, 1974). See also *Pediatric Nutrition Handbook*, 2nd ed. (Elk Grove Village, Ill.: American Academy of Pediatrics, 1985).

95. C. C. Roy and N. Galeano, Childhood antecedents of adult degeneration disease, *Pediatric Clinics of North America* 32 (1985): 517–533.

96. L. Cosgrove and A. Dietrich, Nutritional rickets in breast-fed infants, *Journal of Family Practice* 2 (1985): 205–209.

97. B. L. Specker, B. Valanis, et al., Sunshine exposure and serum 25-hydroxyvitamin D concentration in exclusively breast-fed infants, *Journal of Pediatrics* 107 (1985): 372–376. See also B. L. Specker, R. C. Tsang, and B. W. Hollis, Effect of race and diet on human milk vitamin D and 25-hydroxyvitamin D, *American Journal of Diseases of Children* 139 (1985): 1134–1137.

98. B. L. Specker and R. C. Tsang, Cyclical serum 25-hydroxyvitamin D concentrations paralleling sunshine exposure in exclusively breast-fed infants, *Journal of Pediatrics* 110 (1987): 744.

99. U. M. Saarinen, Need for iron supplementation in infants on prolonged breast feeding, *Journal of Pediatrics* 93 (1978): 177–180.

100. The use of whole cow's milk in infancy, American Academy of Pediatrics, Committee on Nutrition, *Pediatrics* 72 (1983): 253–255.

101. Reported in M. K. Davis, D. A. Savitz, and B. I. Graubard, Infant feeding and childhood cancer, *Lancet* i (1988): 365–368.

102. E. J. Mayer, R. F. Hamman, et al., Reduced risk of insulin-dependent diabetes mellitus (IDDM) among breast-fed children: A case-control study, *Diabetes* (in press).

103. L. A. Hansen, S. Ahlstedt, et al., Protective factors in milk and the development of the immune system, *Pediatrics* 75 (supplement) (1985): 172–176.

104. A. S. Cunningham, Breast feeding and health, *Journal of Pediatrics* 4 (1987): 658–659.

105. N. F. Sheard and W. A. Walker, The role of breast milk in the development of the gastrointestinal tract, *Nutrition Reviews* 46 (1988): 1–8.

106. C. O. Tacket, G. Losonsky, et al., Protection by milk immunoglobulin concentrate against oral challenge with enterotoxigenic *Escherichia coli, New England Journal of Medicine* 318 (1988): 1240–1243.

107. T. Fourchard, Development of food allergies with special reference to cow's milk allergy, *Pediatrics* 75 (supplement) (1985): 177–181.

108. A. J. Cant, Diet and the prevention of childhood allergic disease, *Human Nutrition and Applied Nutrition* 38 (1984): 455–468.

109. T. C. Quinn, The global epidemiology of the acquired immunodeficiency syndrome, in *Report of the Surgeon General's Workshop on Children with HIV Infection and Their Families*, U.S. Department of Health and Human Services, DHHS publication no. HRS-D-MC-87-1, 1987.

110. E. R. Buskirk and J. Mendez, Energy: Caloric requirements, in *Nutrition and the Adult*, R. B. Alfin-Slater and D. Kritchevsky (New York: Plenum Press, 1980), 49–95.

111. M. K. Davis, D. A. Savitz, and B. I. Graubard, Infant feeding and childhood cancer, *Lancet* i (1988): 365–368.

112. A. P. Simopoulos and G. D. Grave, Factors associated with the choice and duration of infant-feeding practices, *Pediatrics* 74 (supplement) (1984): 603–614.

113. W. B. Pittard, D. M. Anderson, et al., Bacteriostatic qualities of human milk, *Journal of Pediatrics* 107 (1985): 240–243.

114. A. M. Thomson and F. E. Hytten, Psychophysiological aspects of human lactation, in *Infant and Child Feeding* (New York: Academic Press, 1981), 37–46.

115. R. A. Lawrence, *Breastfeeding: A Guide for the Medical Profession* (St. Louis: C. V. Mosby, 1980).

116. L. J. Roberts, *Nutrition Work with Children* (Chicago: The University of Chicago Press, 1930).

117. R. M. English, Breast-milk production and energy exchange in human lactation, *British Journal of Nutrition* 53 (1985): 459–466.

118. G. M. Wardlaw and A. M. Pike, The effect of lactation on peak adult shaft and ultradistal forearm bone mass in women, *American Journal of Clinical Nutrition* 44 (1986): 2836. For information on adolescents, see G. M. Chan, P. Slater, et al., Bone mineral status of lactating mothers of different ages, *American Journal of Obstetrics and Gynecology* 144 (1982): 438–441.

119. M. A. Strode, K. G. Dewey, and B. Lonnerdal, Effects of short-term caloric restriction on lactational performance of well-nourished women, *Acta Paediatrica Scandinavica* 75 (1986): 222–229.

120. D. B. Jelliffe and E. F. P. Jelliffe, The volume and composition of human milk in poorly nourished communities: A review, *American Journal of Clinical Nutrition* 31 (1978): 492–515.

121. R. R. Ereman, B. Lonnerdal, and K. G. Dewey, Maternal sodium intake does not affect postprandial sodium concentration in human milk, *Journal of Nutrition* 117 (1987): 1154–1157.

122. J. E. Chappell, M. T. Clandinin, and C. Kearney-Volpe, Trans fatty acids in human milk lipids: Influence of maternal diet and weight loss, *American Journal of Clinical Nutrition* 42 (1985): 49–56.

123. B. W. Hollis, W. B. Pittard, and T. A. Reinhardt, Relationships among vitamin D, 25-hydroxyvitamin D, and vitamin D-binding protein concentrations in the plasma and milk of human subjects, *Journal of Clinical Endocrinology and Metabolism* 62 (1986): 41–44.

124. S. A. Miller and J. G. Chopra, Problems with human milk and infant formulas, *Pediatrics* 74 (supplement) (1984): 639–647.

125. I. Krieger, B. E. Alpern, and S. C. Cunnane, Transient neonatal zinc deficiency, *American Journal of Clinical Nutrition* 43 (1986): 955–958.

126. B. Watkinson and P. A. Fried, Maternal caffeine use before, during, and after pregnancy and effects upon offspring, *Neurobehavioral Toxicology and Teratology* 7 (1985): 9–17.

127. J. E. Ryu, Caffeine in human milk and in serum of breast-fed infants, *Developmental Pharmacology Therapy* 8 (1985): 329–337.
128. B. Worthington-Roberts, personal communication, April 1988.
129. R. P. Whalen, Statement before the Subcommittee on Health and Scientific Research, Committee on Human Resources, U.S. Senate, June 8, 1977.
130. P. M. Schwartz, S. W. Jacobson, et al., Lake Michigan fish consumption as a source of polychlorinated biphenyls in human cord serum, maternal serum, and milk, *American Journal of Public Health* 73 (1983): 293–296.

CHAPTER 15

NUTRITION FOR GROWTH AND DEVELOPMENT

The first twenty years of a human life span are the time of **growth** and **development**. These are complex processes that require the right combination of inborn traits and **environmental conditions** to proceed normally. How well they proceed can determine a person's health and performance throughout life.

Infants, children, and **adolescents** are growing and developing physically and mentally. This makes nutrition an important consideration during these stages of life. The diets of infants, children, and adolescents directly affect the progress of growth and development.

This chapter examines the relationship of nutrition to growth, mental development, and health. It discusses the important areas of food preference and habit formation, the relationship of the psychological environment to nutrition and growth, and the normal nutrient needs of infants, children, and adolescents. Relationships between nutrition during childhood and chronic disease development later in life are also discussed.

growth: An increase in size due to increases in the number of cells and the sizes of cells.

development: The processes involved in enhancing the capabilities of a human; the maturation of humans to more advanced and complex stages of functioning. (The brain *grows* in size, whereas the ability to reason *develops*.)

environmental conditions: Physical, economic, psychosocial, and dietary factors that determine the circumstances under which people live.

infancy: Birth to 1 year of age.
childhood: 1 to 11 years of age.
adolescence: 12 to 18 years of age.

NUTRITION AND GROWTH

A definite program has been adopted in our state for instruction to public schools in health and in sanitation. It will begin when the child first enters school and will continue through the high school. It will apply to every child in school. It will include daily health inspection of each pupil and will be under the direction of the teacher. It will establish a physical rating for every child on admission to school and will give school credit for health improvement as well as for mental progress. . . . Attention will be given to the correction of defects found, and special emphasis will be placed on the need of keeping well. The teacher in charge will be held responsible for the success of the work in her room.

—W. A. Howe, New York State, 1921

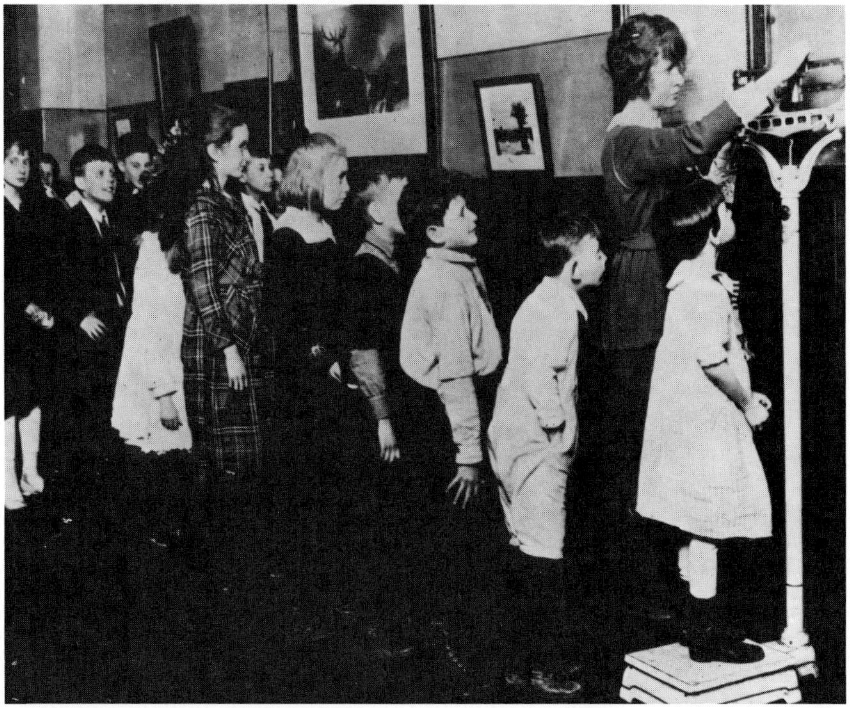
An elementary school teacher measures her students' growth, circa 1920.

The progress of children's growth has long served as a primary measure of the health status of a society's children. Worldwide, the number-one determinant of how well children grow is the availability of ample supplies of the right assortment of foods.[1] As the growth status of a society's children changes, so does the profile of the children's health problems. In general, as growth improves, so does health.[1]

During the first week or two of life, most infants lose 5% to 10% of their birth weight in adjusting to the new surroundings and food supply. After that, the newborn grows fast. Most infants double their birth weight in 4 months and triple it in the first year. In the first year of life, an infant increases in length by 50%. (If this growth rate were to continue, a 10-year-old would be as tall as a ten-story building and weigh more than 221 tons!) After infancy, a child's growth rate declines, and it remains fairly low until the adolescent growth spurt begins. Between the ages of 2 and 10, a child normally gains an average of 4 to 7 pounds and adds 2 to 3 inches in height a year.

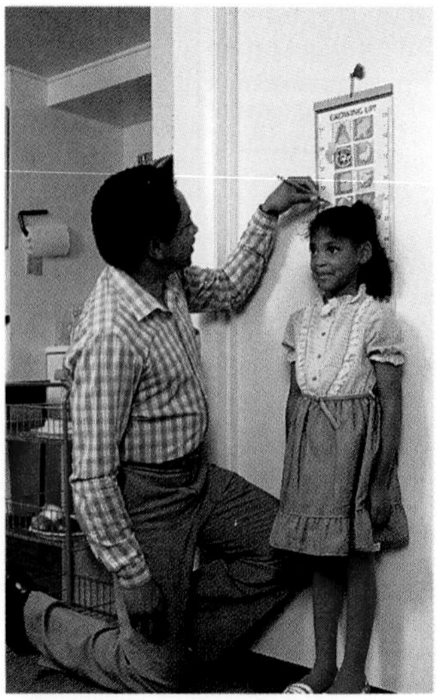
Recording growth progress is a delightful ritual for many families.

Growth picks up rapidly upon the arrival of the adolescent growth spurt. (See Figure 15-1.) Between the ages of 11 and 15, for girls, or 12 and 17, for boys, children normally gain 20% to 25% of their adult height, 50% of their adult weight, and 45% of their total bone mass. The size of organs such as the liver, heart, lungs, and kidneys also increases dramatically during adolescence. During the peak year of growth, girls gain an average of 20 pounds and boys, 22 pounds.[2] Increases in appetite, food intake, and nutrient requirements closely parallel the spurts in growth that occur throughout the growing years.

A big question in the back of many parents' minds is how tall their children will become. Ultimate height is very difficult to predict with any precision, as Box 15-1 explains. In general, children of genetically short parents

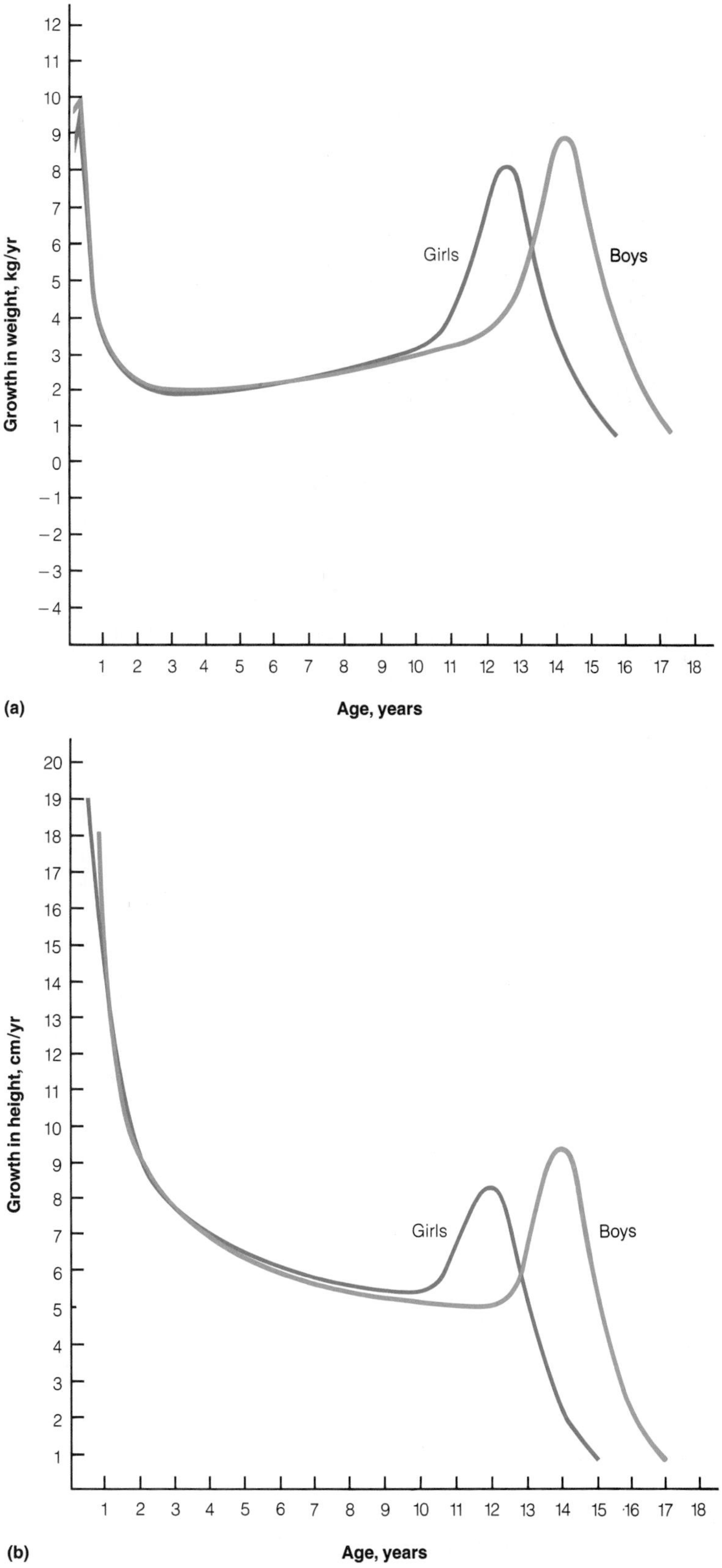

FIGURE 15-1
Average yearly growth in (*a*) weight and (*b*) height for girls and boys.

BOX 15-1

DETERMINANTS OF ULTIMATE HEIGHT

Individuals appear to have a genetically determined maximum height that cannot be predicted by any tests or procedures currently available. Whether a person achieves his or her potential height is mainly determined by environmental conditions, the most important of which is nutrition. It appears that children who receive adequate diets and remain healthy throughout their growing years achieve their potential height, and that no "superdiets," supplements, or anything else will increase height beyond the increments related to adequate diets.

Most people's adult height is somewhere between their parents' heights. Of course, if the mother's or father's growth was compromised by poor nutrition or another condition, their well-nourished, healthy child may grow to be taller than either parent. This was clearly demonstrated in Japan after World War II. Japanese children born after the war, when food supplies were dramatically better, normally outgrew their parents in height.[3] Such increases in adult height from one generation to the next appear to be continuing in many developed countries.[4]

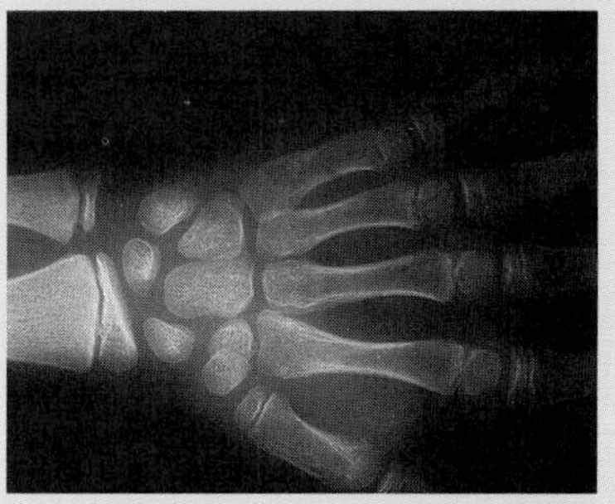

(a)

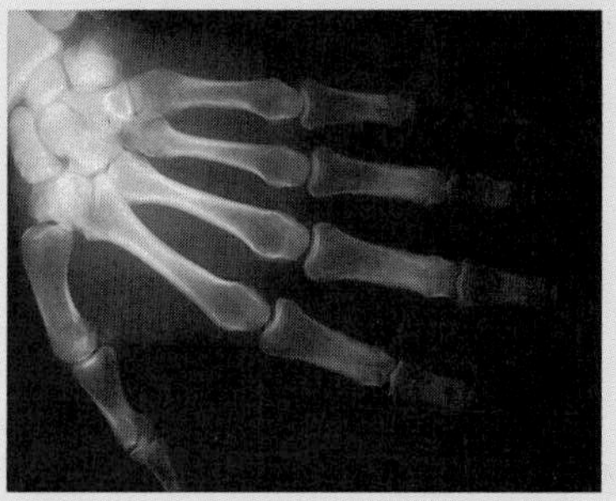

(b)

X rays of (*a*) a child's hand and (*b*) an adult's hand.

Rate of growth in the early years of life is only weakly predictive of eventual height. Length and weight at birth and rate of growth in the first year of life do not appear to predict subsequent growth.[5]

How tall a person will be can only be determined after the fact. Adult height is usually achieved by the age of 18 for boys who are shorter than average and by the age of 23 or 24 for boys who are taller than average. Girls destined to be shorter than average tend to achieve their maximum height by the age of 16, whereas tall girls may grow until they are 21. Thus, adult height is generally achieved between the ages of 18 and 24 for males, and 16 and 21 for females.[6]

How can it be determined if growth in height is completed? X-rays will show if the fibrous plates (the *epiphyses*, pronounced ē-pif′ə-sēs) that cover the ends of bones have become part of the bones. As long as the fibrous plate is separate from the end of the bone (*part a of the figure*), growth has not been completed. When the plate has fused with the end of the bone (*part b*), further growth is not possible.

tend to be short and those of genetically tall parents, tall, but there are many exceptions to this.

How Growth Proceeds

Growth results whenever cells in the body increase in number or in size. Cell multiplication takes place first, and it is followed by increases in the size of existing cells. Every organ and tissue in the body—including the brain, muscles, bone, and liver—has its own **critical period** for cell multiplication. The critical periods of growth for four tissues are shown in Figure 15-2. The critical period of cell multiplication in the brain is during fetal development and the first year after birth. Increases in brain size after the first year are mainly due to enlargement of existing cells.

critical period: Pertaining to growth, a specific interval of time during which the cells of a tissue or organ are programmed to multiply. If the supply of nutrients to cells is not adequate during a critical period of growth, cell division does not occur and the affected tissues or organs remain smaller than they would otherwise.

If the supply of nutrients needed to support cell multiplication is not available during a critical period for a particular tissue or organ, fewer than the normal number of cells will be formed. This constitutes a missed oppor-

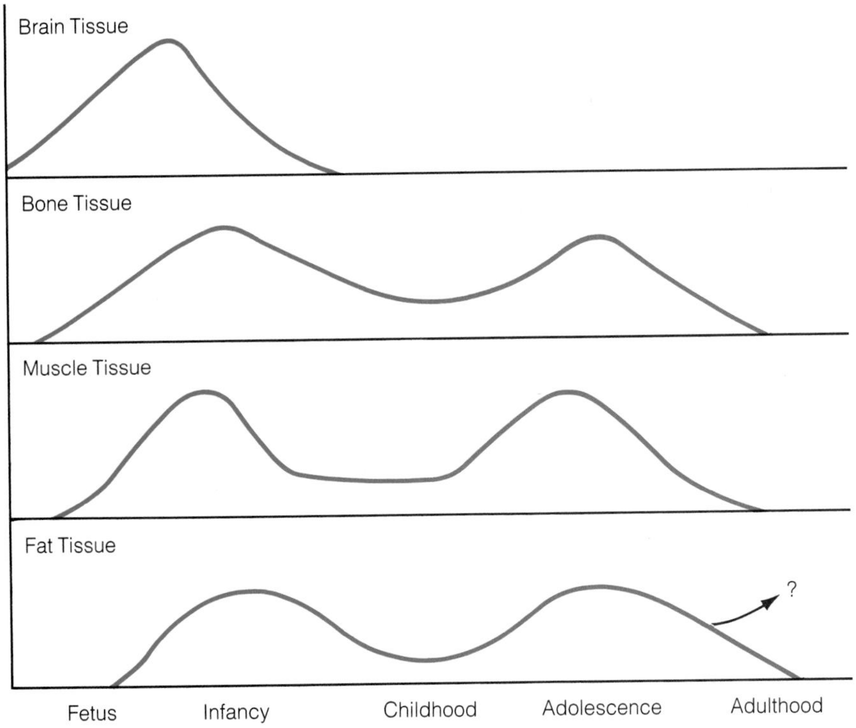

FIGURE 15-2
Critical periods of cell multiplication for selected body tissues. Fat cell numbers may increase during the adult years if additional fat storage sites are needed.

tunity for growth. Permanent setbacks in growth and development result when undernutrition exists throughout one or more critical periods of cell multiplication.

Unlike the critical periods for growth in the number of cells, growth in cell size can occur at various times. Growth in cell size is simply delayed if nutrient supplies are low, and the cells "catch up" later when nutrients become available. Undernutrition that occurs during the time that cells normally increase in size does not necessarily produce permanent reductions in cell growth or functioning. With "nutritional rehabilitation," children can generally catch up in growth in terms of the size of cells.

Nutrition and Mental Development

Malnutrition has the greatest impact on mental development when it is severe and occurs during the critical period for brain cell multiplication. For humans, this vulnerable period begins during pregnancy and ends after the first year of life. Impairment in mental development is less severe when malnutrition occurs only during pregnancy or only during infancy than if it occurs throughout both pregnancy and infancy.

Mental development is also greatly influenced by the social and psychological environment in which children are raised.[1] Because malnutrition is generally accompanied by both social and psychological deprivation, these factors often contribute jointly to poor mental development. For children in the U.S., poverty, neglect, psychological problems, and illnesses appear to be the main causes of undernutrition and poor mental development.[8] Recently, undernutrition of children of middle- and upper-class families

MIDDLE-CLASS MALNUTRITION

A new type of malnutrition has recently been identified in the U.S. It is undernutrition among infants and children from middle- and upper-income families, and it is associated with low-calorie, low-fat diets.[9] Some parents say that they implement this sort of diet to help their children form good lifelong eating habits and avoid obesity and heart disease. Nonetheless, parents' fear that their children will become obese appears to be the major motivation for restricting their children's food intake.

Limiting diets for the purpose of preventing obesity may also occur in about 2% of adolescents from middle- and upper-income families.[9] While not being anorexic or bulimic, adolescents may moderately and continually restrict their weight gain. Unlike people with anorexia nervosa or bulimia, the goal of these adolescents is not to *lose* weight, but to *avoid gaining* weight.

Failure to gain weight during periods of growth has an unavoidable consequence: it halts growth in height.[9,10] Because few adolescents want to be short, counseling is usually effective in getting them to eat more to allow growth in height to proceed.

The growth progress of a girl who decided to restrict her weight gain to avoid obesity is shown in the graph.[9] She started her diet at the age of ten and continued it until she was 16. When her adolescent growth spurt did not occur, she was referred to a medical specialist. After nutritional counseling, the teenager began eating normally and gained weight. As you can see in the graph, her growth in height followed her gain in weight. Not all teenagers treated for "growth failure" are able to respond to nutritional rehabilitation in this way. Increases in height are not possible if the bones have stopped growing.

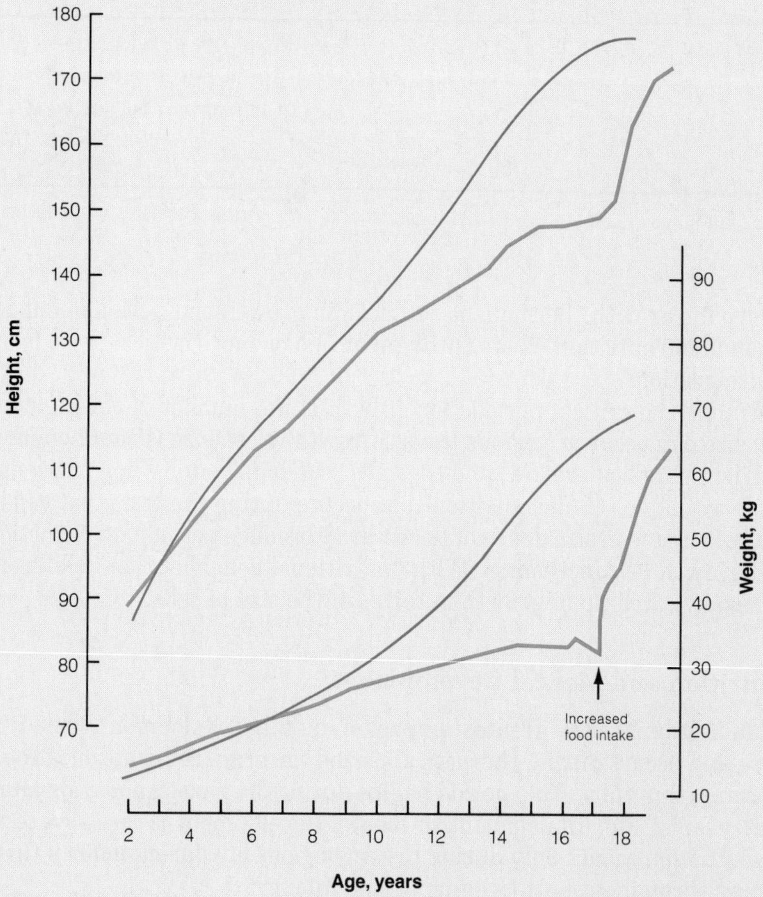

Example of how inadequate food intake can delay the adolescent growth spurt. Note that weight gain precedes height gain once food intake has been increased.

has also been reported, and it appears to be related to some parents' overzealous attempts to prevent obesity. (Box 15-2 gives more information about this new undernutrition.)

The adverse effects of malnutrition on mental development can be lessened to some extent if the child is placed in a stimulating and secure envi-

BOX 15-3

DIETARY SUPPLEMENTS AND I.Q.

The results of a recent, and controversial, study suggest that dietary supplements may improve the learning ability of children who are marginally malnourished.[13]

In the study, one group of school-aged children were given a vitamin and mineral supplement each day for eight months, and another group were given a placebo. Children who entered the study marginally malnourished attained higher scores on *written* intelligence tests after receiving the supplements, but they did no better on *oral* tests of intelligence. Test scores of children who entered the study well nourished did not change with supplementation.[13]

ronment and provided with a good diet. Malnourished infants and young children from economically developing countries adopted by U.S. couples have been found to exhibit better mental development than the children who have remained in the country of birth.[11] The difference is thought to be largely due to the higher level of intellectual stimulation and enrichment the adopted children receive. In a long-term food supplementation program in Guatemala that began with women during pregnancy and continued for the first few years of their children's lives, significant gains in learning ability and social behaviors were observed among supplemented children. They were able to command more attention from their parents, were happier, and more social than children who did not receive the food supplements.[12] It appears that the improved nutrition and health brought about by the supplementation may have enriched the children's social and psychological environment, too. Their fathers, though culturally unaccustomed to interacting much with very young children, showed a greater tendency to play with and pay attention to these alert, healthy infants.

The mental development benefits of correcting childhood undernutrition have led some people to wonder if giving normal children vitamin and mineral supplements might improve their learning ability. Although this possibility seems to stretch the conclusions of food supplement studies among undernourished children, it is an idea that has gained popularity. Box 15-3 reports the results of one study on this topic.

Body Composition and Proportion Change with Growth

Humans grow up and out, and their body composition and proportions change as growth progresses. Although generally measured by gains in pounds and inches, growth reflects changes in bone mass, in organ size, in body proportions, and in body composition of water, muscle, and fat. Infants' heads are very large in relation to the rest of their bodies, for example. Brain growth takes precedence over trunk and limb growth early in life, and the body eventually grows to "fit" the head (Table 15-1). A child's shape may normally progress from the shape of a loaf of bread to one that approaches that of a string bean within the first ten years of life.

Body composition also changes with age (Figure 15-3). Infants gain body fat rapidly during the first four months of life. As they grow and become more physically active, some of the fat is replaced by protein. Body fat

TABLE 15-1
Declining proportion of brain weight relative to body weight

Age	Brain Weight as % of Total Body Weight
2-month fetus	20
newborn	12
10 years	6
16 years	3

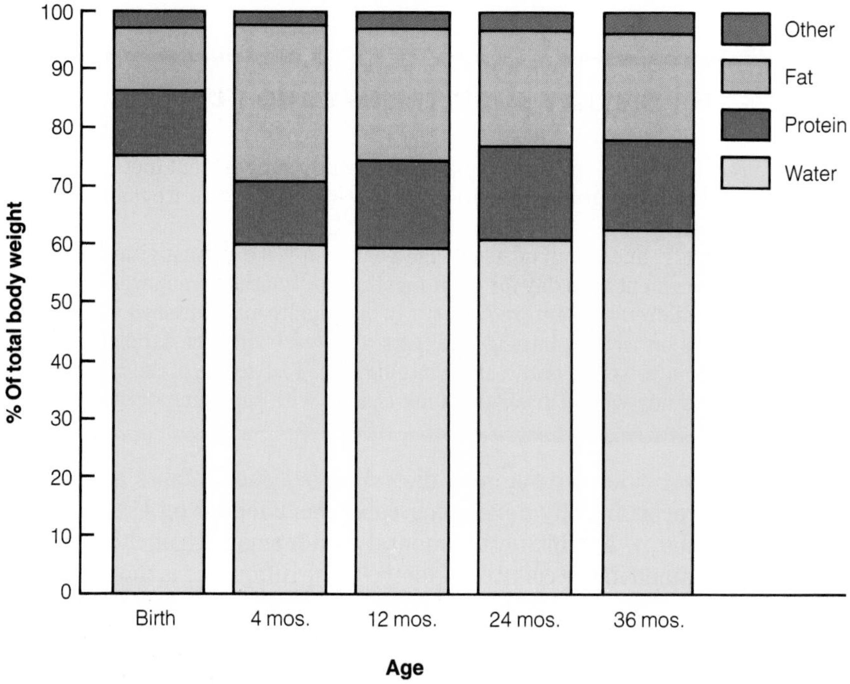

FIGURE 15-3
Body composition of infants and young children.

levels normally stay low until a year or two before the adolescent growth spurt begins. Both boys and girls tend to enter this growth spurt with about 18% of their total body weight as fat. Four years after the spurt, boys will have shed some fat (it will be down to about 15% of their body weight), and girls will have increased their body fat content to about 25%. Boys accumulate more muscle and bone tissue during the adolescent growth spurt than do girls. Due to the effects of the hormone testosterone, boys complete their growth spurt with about 50% more muscle tissue than do girls.

Monitoring Growth

Weight-for-length curves are used to identify underweight and overweight.

Length-for-age curves are used to identify growth stunting or probable long-term undernutrition.

Growth progress is a concern for parents, children, and health professionals. Measurements of weight and height are taken routinely during childhood check-ups, and the typical U.S. home has a "measuring wall" someplace. When measured accurately, gains in weight and height over time can be used to assess undernutrition, excessive body weight, and general health status. (Because of the importance of the results, weight and height should be measured accurately. Instructions are provided in Box 15-4.)

Standard growth charts, such as those in Figures 15-4 and 15-5, are available for tracking growth progress. The charts that plot weight for height are commonly used to assess underweight, normal weight, or overweight. Length-for-age charts are used to assess how a child's height corresponds to that of other children the same age. Children who fall below the 5th **percentile** in weight for length are generally classified as underweight; those whose measurements are between the 90th and 95th percentile, overweight; and children who exceed the 95th percentile, obese. Children whose measurements are below the 5th percentile in length for age are generally considered to be stunted in growth and to have experienced long-term undernutrition.

percentile: Point on a scale of 100 that represents the percentage of measurements equal to or below a particular measurement. For example, 15% of children have growth measurements that place them between the 75th and 90th percentiles on growth curves. If a child is at the 50th percentile, 50% of children are smaller than the child and 50% are bigger.

BOX 15-4

HOW TO MEASURE WEIGHT AND HEIGHT

WEIGHT

Body weight should be measured with a beam-balance scale (see figure) calibrated so that it reads zero when no weight is applied. (Many scales have a knob that can be used for calibration.) The scales should be placed on a flat, hard surface. Weight should be measured while a person is unclothed or wearing only lightweight clothing and no shoes.

HEIGHT

The most accurate way to determine height (short of laser technology) is by using a height-measuring board—or a nonstretch measuring tape attached firmly to a wall—and an angle board (see figure). Height should be measured without shoes, with the person's heels, buttocks, and shoulders touching the wall. To be certain that the head is in the right position, the person should look straight ahead. After the person is in position, the angle board should be placed so that one side is flat against the measuring tape mounted on the wall and the other side is resting on top of the head. (If you don't have an angle board, a two-inch-thick book will do.)

Measuring height by using a bar device attached to a beam-balance scale is a rather inaccurate method. This is the method commonly used in doctors' offices. If your height has never been measured by the process described here, find a helper and follow the directions.

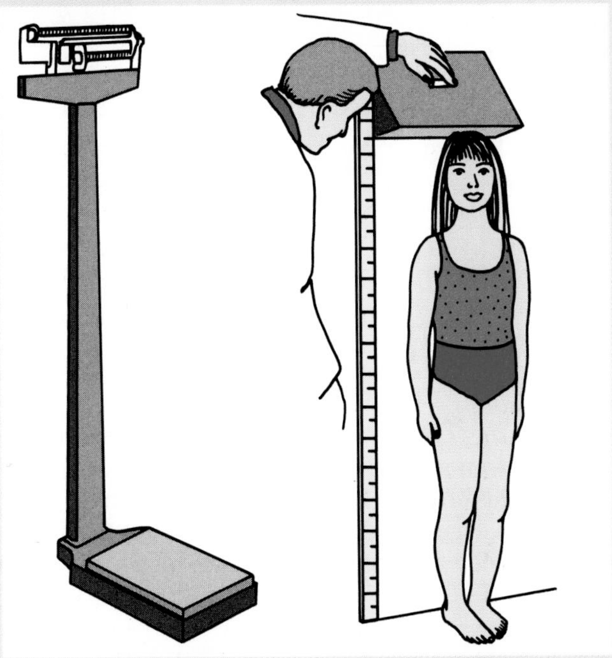

Beam-balance scale Height-measuring board

FIGURE 15-4*

Girls' weight-for-age growth chart, birth to 36 months.

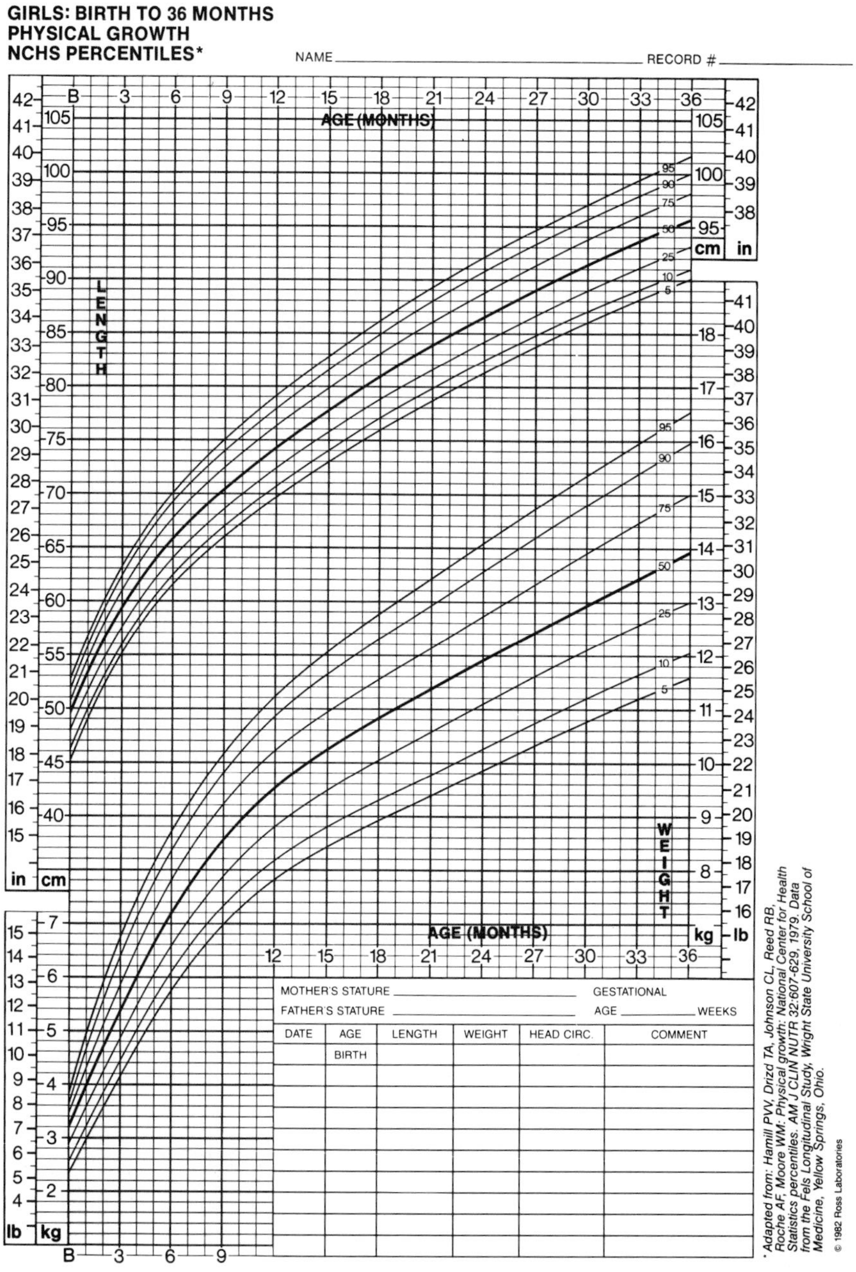

A drawback in using the growth charts to make these determinations is that particular children may be genetically short, big-boned, or otherwise not "average" in terms of age-related increases in weight or height. A child's growth may be quite normal and yet not appear so when plotted. Additional assessments are needed to verify the existence of any growth problems.

*To use the grids in Figures 15-4 and 15-5, move the right edge of a firm square of paper to the point corresponding to the child's age. Then move the square of paper up or down to align its top edge with the point corresponding to the child's weight. With the edges of the paper aligned with both measurements, mark the graph at the location of the top right corner of the square of paper.

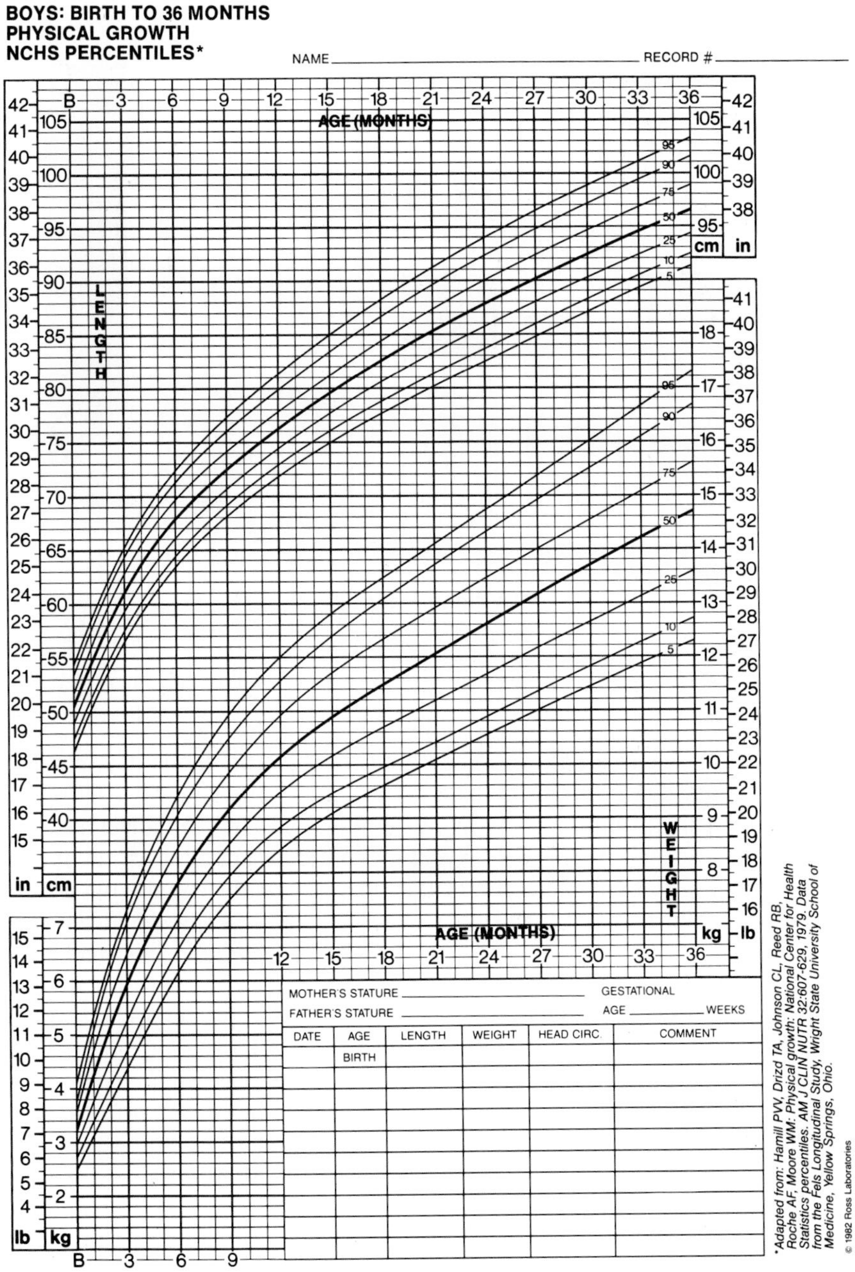

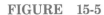

FIGURE 15-5

Boys' length-for-age growth chart, birth to 36 months.

Childhood Obesity

Childhood obesity is rapidly becoming a major public health concern in the U.S. Over the past 20 years, the incidence of obesity in children and adolescents has increased by about 50%. Approximately one in four children between the ages of 5 and 14 years weigh too much for their height.[14]

Obesity during childhood presents both physical and psychological problems. Children who are obese tend to have higher than average blood pressure and cholesterol levels,[14,15] and they are frequently targets of other children's teasing and ridicule.[16] The psychological implications of growing

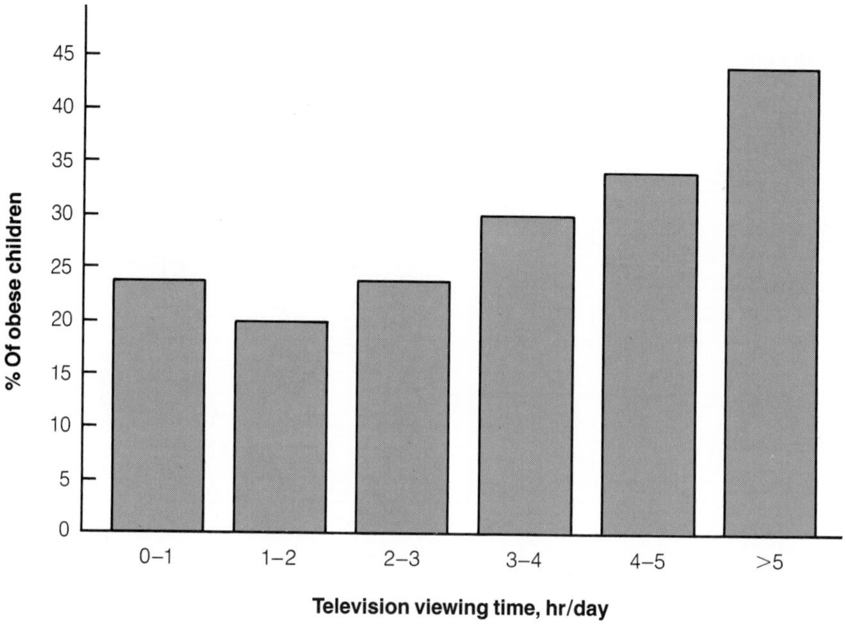

FIGURE 15-6
The likelihood of children becoming obese increases as the amount of TV they watch each day increases.

up obese likely have a greater impact on a child's health and sense of well-being than the physical problems that stem from the obese state.

Explanation for the Increase It appears that the underlying reason for the increase in obesity in children in the U.S. is not primarily related to increased food consumption. The average caloric intake of children has not changed significantly in the past 20 years, and it does not appear that obese children in general eat more than their normal-weight counterparts.[4,17] Some obese children have been shown to actually eat less than children who are not obese.[4] The major difference between obese and nonobese children is the level of physical activity.[4,17]

Obese children tend to be much less physically active than children of normal weight. Overall, physical activity levels of U.S. children are decreasing, and the decrease is partly related to an increase in the time they spend watching television. A statistical relationship has been found between the amount of time a child spends sitting in front of a television set and the child's likelihood of becoming obese (Figure 15-6).[18] Furthermore, while children are watching TV they are being exposed to many advertisements for foods that are not found in the tables that list the food sources of nutrients in Part Two of this book. Box 15-5 discusses the influence of television viewing on the foods children eat.

Prevention and Treatment The best way to prevent the development of obesity in children is also the best way to treat obesity: help the child to establish and enjoy a physically active lifestyle. Increasing children's regular level of physical activity, rather than counting calories, appears to be the best way to prevent and to reduce obesity.[4,23,24] For some children, the substitution of active play for television watching may go a long way toward preventing obesity.[18] Teaching children to eat for the right reasons—to satisfy hunger and the body's need for calories and nutrients—may also help children form eating habits that keep their body weights healthy.

BOX 15-5

CHILDREN'S TELEVISION VIEWING TIME AND DIET

On average, U.S. children spend more time watching television in a year than they do attending school.[19] Their average viewing time of 26 hours per week includes hundreds of commercials. During children's programming hours, the most heavily advertised product is food, and the food product advertised the most is presweetened breakfast cereal. After breakfast cereals come snacks and beverages—such items as potato chips, candy, soft drinks, and fruit-flavored beverages.[20]

It appears that children can be sold by the food advertisements. Studies show that children's television-viewing habits are correlated with the foods they request, with the foods their parents purchase, with their consumption of advertised foods, and with the amount of between-meal snacking they do.[21,22]

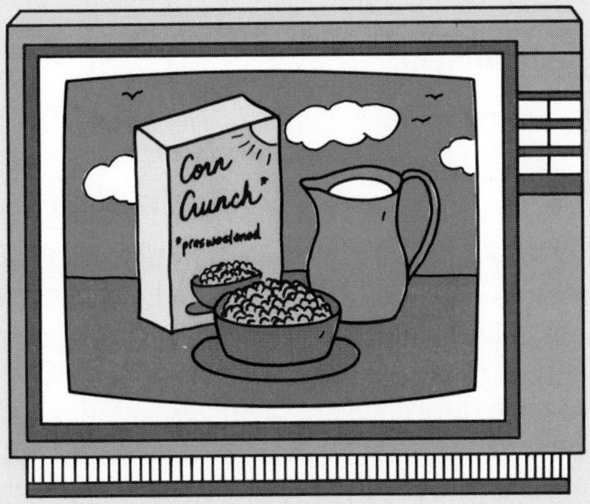

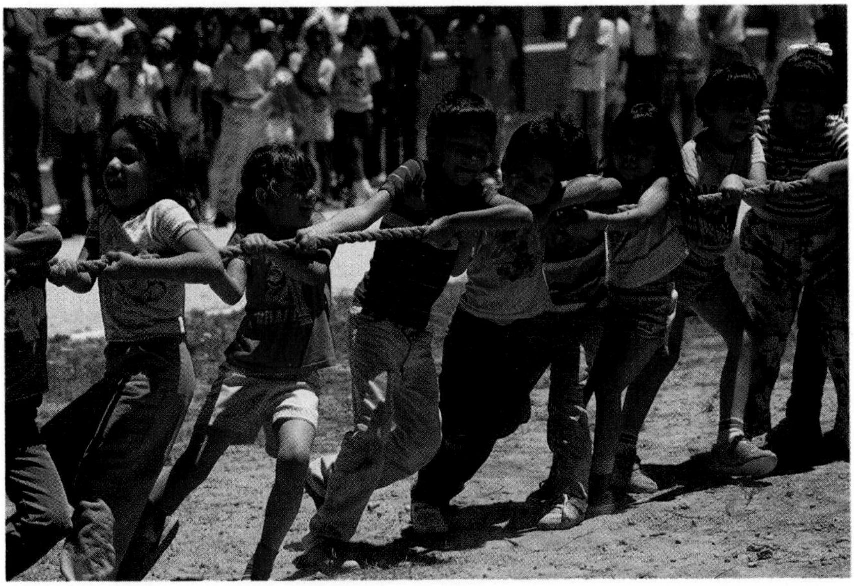

Physical activity is children's play—and it's good for their health.

There are other advantages of increasing children's physical activity levels. Regular physical activity increases a child's level of fitness, reduces blood pressure, and increases HDL-cholesterol levels (the "good" type of cholesterol).[25] In turn, these improvements may reduce the risk of developing heart disease and hypertension later in life.[25]

Do Fat Children Become Fat Adults? This very common question has no simple or satisfying answer. It appears that childhood overweight and obesity are only weakly predictive of those conditions in adulthood. Whether obesity continues into the adult years appears to be related primarily to the degree of the childhood obesity and to whether a physically inactive lifestyle is carried over from childhood to adulthood. Children who are very obese are more likely to be obese as adults than are children who are overweight or moderately obese.[26] Very obese children may form an abnormally large number of fat cells during growth, which may make it more difficult for the person to maintain an ideal weight.[27]

The Growth Environment

Better is a dinner of herbs where love is,
than a fatted ox and hatred with it.

—Proverbs, 15:17 (RSV)

Nutrition is clearly an important factor influencing growth progress. However, it is not the only factor that affects how well growth proceeds. The environment in which children are raised can have important effects on growth.

TLC is a vital growth-promoting factor for infants and children. The comfort, security, and sense of well-being that come with tender, loving care foster normal physical and mental growth and development. Infants in newborn intensive care units tend to eat and grow better if they are frequently cuddled than if they are handled only in the course of treatment.[28] Children hospitalized for growth failure tend to gain weight more quickly if dietary rehabilitation is accompanied by "TLC" than if it is not.[29] Even if a good diet is available to children, a poor social environment at mealtime can extinguish their appetites and reduce food intake and growth. (Box 15-6 may make you forever aware of the potential influence of social environment on growth in children.) Providing the calories and nutrients required for growth and development is an essential factor in the formula for rearing healthy infants and children. For best results, however, good diets should be accompanied by favorable environmental conditions, because these conditions may promote the many intricate, complex processes involved in growth and development.

FOOD PREFERENCES

Jack Spratt would eat no fat,
his wife would eat no lean . . .

Food preferences are another important influence on children's diets. Children learn about what a good diet is, and what foods they do and do not like through the social circumstances surrounding mealtimes and the offer-

BOX 15-6

SOCIAL ENVIRONMENT, DIET, AND GROWTH

In 1951, Dr. Ellie Widdowson, a highly respected nutritionist, reported some intriguing results from a study designed to assess the effects of dietary improvements on growth.[30] The study was conducted in two orphanages in Germany, each housing about 50 boys and girls. Funds available to the orphanages were limited, and rarely was enough food available to satisfy the children's hunger. The goal of the study was to determine if changes in growth took place after additional foods were made available to the children.

The usual rate of growth of the children was assessed while they received the standard diet over a six-month period. During the second six months, children in one of the orphanages received additional bread and jam and were given orange juice. Children in the other orphanage (the control group) continued to receive the standard menu. The growth of children in both orphanages was assessed throughout this six-month period.

Surprisingly, it was found that the children who received the extra food grew *less* than the children who continued to receive the standard diet. It was also noted that the growth rates of children at the two orphanages differed even before the dietary change was introduced. Obviously, something was counteracting the effects of the improved diet on growth.

As you can imagine, Dr. Widdowson scratched her head and asked "What happened?" Her question appeared to be answered when it was discovered that the social environment at the orphanage where the children grew well was much better than at the other orphanage. A stern matron who ruled her charges with "a rod of iron" administered the orphanage where growth was poorer. Children and staff in that orphanage lived in constant fear of her reprimands and criticisms. She used mealtimes to administer rebukes and would single out individual children for ridicule. By the time she had finished her mealtime tirades, the children would be upset and their appetites dampened. The matrons in charge of the orphanage where children grew better were described as bright, happy women who were genuinely fond of the children, and the children were fond of them.

By coincidence, the stern matron had been transferred from the orphanage where children failed to grow well to the other orphanage in the study at the start of the six-month period in which the children were given additional food. Her negative effects on the social environment—and the children's appetites—at the first orphanage were repeated at the second one. Even though the extra food was available, the children grew less under her rule than they had in the previous six months.

As harsh as this matron was, she had her favorites. When she was transferred to the second orphanage, she convinced authorities to allow her to take eight children along with her. She never scolded these children, and she praised them regularly. These children stood out from the others in that they grew better. On average, these eight children gained more than twice as much weight as the others did during the six-month period when extra food was available.

Although it is not clear if the social environment or the quantity of food consumed was responsible for the observed difference in growth rates, the study clearly showed that environment can play a key role in growth.

---

ing of food. The environment in which food is offered and received can have a lifelong impact on the maintenance of good eating habits. This is especially true in the first few years of life, which is when food preferences begin to form.

Have you ever met anyone who likes and dislikes exactly the same foods as you? Some people love raw fish and fish eggs, whereas other people find it hard just to think about eating those foods. Brussels sprouts may be your favorite vegetable or a vegetable that never reaches your plate. Certain people strongly prefer salad dressing over mayonnaise, margarine over butter, and pizza *with* anchovies. Food preferences are very individual.

In situations in which a variety of foods is readily available, food preferences strongly influence the foods that are consumed.[31] Food likes and dis-

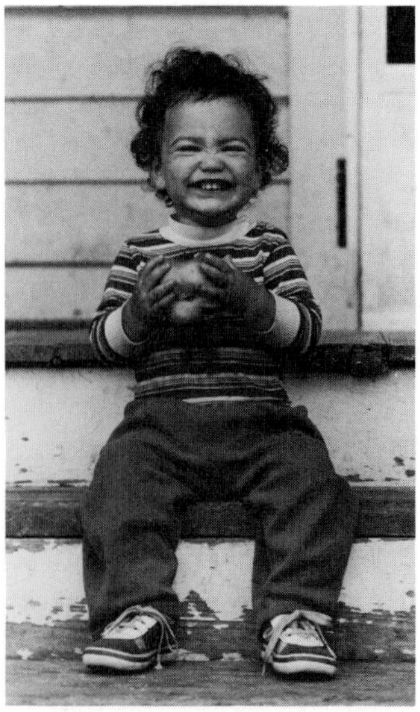

It appears that the critical time for the formation of food preferences is during the first few years of life.

likes can either lead to food choices that promote health or disease, or they may have absolutely no effect on a person's health. People can live without brussels sprouts, for example. The food likes and dislikes people develop can affect health negatively if they lead to diets that contain a limited variety of nutrient-dense foods. The regular consumption of foods that add up to a diet that is excessively high in fat, sodium, and sugar may place a child at risk of developing heart disease and hypertension later in life and dental problems at any age. Although food likes and dislikes change to some extent over time, it appears that the critical time for the formation of food preferences is in the first few years of life.[32]

How do food preferences form? Are they "shaped" by early learning experiences, or are they inborn and beyond anyone's control?

Basically, there are two theories about how food preferences develop, the "nature" theory and the "nurture" theory. The weight of the evidence available to date indicates that nurture, or learning experiences that take place during life, have more to do with food likes and dislikes than do inborn traits. Data that drive both of the theories are presented.

The Nature Theory

Scientists, health professionals, and others who take the nature point-of-view of food-preference development cite the inborn preference for sweet-tasting foods and the notion that children instinctively know what to eat as supportive evidence. However, children commonly form preferences for many foods that aren't sweet (foods such as hamburgers, potatoes, noodles, and milk, for example), so there must be more to food preferences than an attraction to sweetness. The notion that children instinctively know what to eat, and therefore if allowed to choose from a wide assortment of food would select and consume a well-balanced diet, is only a notion. (Box 15-7 tells the story of how this belief gained popularity.)

It is not known what sort of diet children would choose if they were given free choice of basic foods such as breads, meats, and vegetables *and* cookies, salty snack foods, candy, soft drinks, and the like (although many parents think they can predict the results of such an experiment). It is a difficult question for research studies to answer. It is unlikely that many parents would be willing to risk allowing their children to be given free access to what they consider "junk foods" for the weeks or months such a study would necessitate. Researchers may also hesitate to do such a study because of the potential negative effects on a young child's diet and food preferences.

The belief that young children instinctively know what to eat can be hazardous to a child's health. It may produce an overly relaxed attitude toward poor food habits and contribute to the development of health problems later in life. Informed parents should decide what types of food their child should be offered, but the decision about how much to eat should be left to the child.[33]

The Nurture Theory

Food likes and dislikes appear to be almost totally shaped by the environment in which children learn about food. Which foods children are offered,

DO YOUNG CHILDREN INSTINCTIVELY KNOW WHAT TO EAT?

The answer appears to be no. With the possible exception of an increased appetite for salt when the body's sodium levels are low, no evidence indicates that young children are drawn to foods that contain nutrients they need. Nonetheless, the notion that they do is still advanced in medical textbooks and other literature.[33] The belief that young children instinctively know what to eat became popular after publication of results of feeding experiments conducted by Dr. Clara Davis in the late 1920s. Oddly enough, Dr. Davis did not draw this conclusion; it was drawn for her by people who misinterpreted her results.

Clara Davis conducted her most often quoted feeding experiments with three infants aged 7 to 9 months who lived in an orphanage connected to a large hospital.[34] Three times a day, the infants were offered a tray of foods similar to the one in the photograph. Altogether, the infants were offered 32 types of food during three daily meals for at least six months. The meals consisted of fresh, unprocessed, unseasoned, and simply prepared basic foods. They included milk, beef, kidney, bone marrow, liver, brain, thymus, ocean fish, whole-wheat cereals, raw eggs, sea salt, 15 fresh fruits, and 10 fresh vegetables. No desserts, sugars, syrups, or sweetened foods were offered. The infants quickly formed preferences and narrowed their choices to 14 of the 32 foods offered. Vegetables were found to be the least-liked type of food, whereas milk, bone marrow, eggs, bananas, apples, oranges, and oatmeal were chosen frequently.

Davis found that the infants were able to digest the adult-type food without problems and that they ate enough to grow normally. She added a note of caution about how the results should be interpreted. She concluded that self-selection can have but doubtful value if the diet must be selected from inferior foods.[35]

The primary conclusions arising from her research were that young children should be offered only foods of the highest nutritional value and that a young child's appetite is the best indicator of how much food he or she needs. Both of these conclusions have withstood the test of time. It is indeed unfortunate that results Davis did not report and conclusions she did not draw are so commonly credited to her research.

An example of a meal offered to infants in the Clara Davis feeding experiment in the late 1920s.

the way they are offered, and how frequently a type of food is offered all influence whether particular foods will be liked or not.[31]

Infants are born with a tendency to be cautious about accepting new things, including foods.[36] They may need to get used to new foods in order to trust them. A new food may need to be offered on five or more occasions before a decision is made.[36] Sometimes children decide they like the food, and sometimes they really don't like it. It is not uncommon for infants and young children not to like strong-flavored vegetables, spicy foods, and mixed foods. Forcing a young child to eat foods she or he does not like can

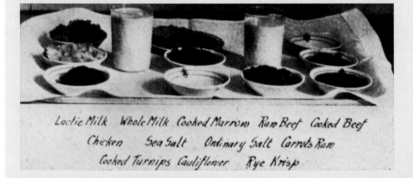

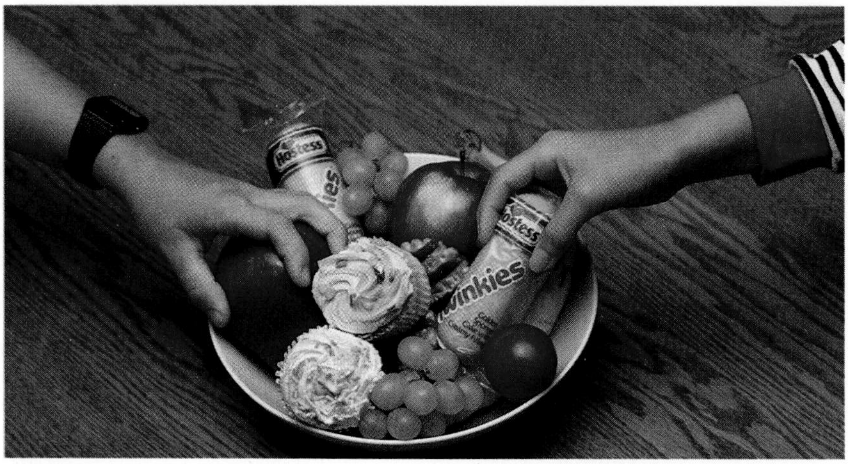

Children learn food preferences primarily from their environment.

produce lifelong, negative effects on food preferences and health, as Box 15-8 illustrates. When attempts to get a child to eat a particular food turn the dinner table into a battleground for control, nobody wins. Foods should be offered in an objective, nonthreatening way so that the child has a fair chance to try the food and make a decision about it.

INTERVIEWER: What was the worst advice your father ever gave you?
SALLY STRUTHERS: To clean my plate. My father grew up in the Depression, and he'd make my sister and me eat all our peas and carrots, or sit with them until they grew mold.

As the child's rate of growth declines, the intervals between meals lengthen and he or she shows less interest in food or eating. A seemingly sudden onset of a disinterest in food can make parents anxious. The anxiety can be magnified when the child reaches the age of about a year and a half. In addition to periods of disinterest in food, most children go on "food jags" from that age until about four. During a "food jag," a child may want the same food for meals and snacks for weeks to months at a time. These "jags" are normal and they generally correspond to periods of slow growth and disinterest in food.[38] Because children aren't eating as much as expected and tend to eat a limited variety of foods, parents may coax their children into eating more. As long as children grow normally and remain healthy, they are likely getting enough food and should be allowed to eat only as much as they want.

BOX 15-8

DISLIKE FOR VEGETABLES: A CASE STUDY

Bonnie, a 39-year-old woman confined to a wheel chair due to childhood polio, needed to lose 40 pounds so that the surgery she needed would be less risky to her health. She went to see a nutritionist for help in planning a weight-reduction diet. The counseling session started with a review of what Bonnie usually ate. After reviewing Bonnie's usual diet and noticing that it contained not a single vegetable, the nutritionist asked, "What about vegetables?"

"Vegetables?" Bonnie replied. "I haven't eaten them since I was a kid in the hospital. The staff was so concerned about my eating the vegetables served every day that they nagged at me until I choked them down. To this day, I can't stand them . . . no way!"

And to this day, she doesn't eat them.

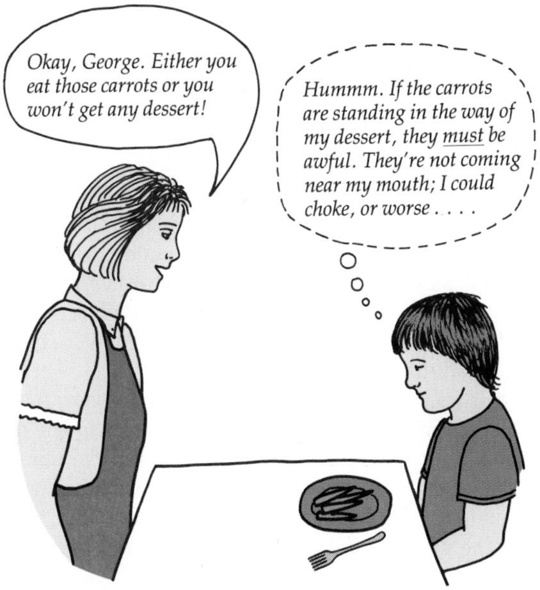

Children appear to have a major advantage over many adults in that they tend to eat only as much food as they need.[31] (One study that showed that children seem to have built-in "calorie counters" is summarized in Box 15-9.) Because only the child knows when she or he is hungry, and full, children should be allowed to decide how much food they need. This means that parents and child-care workers should be sensitive to the "I'm hungry" and "I'm full" cues that young children give during the first three years of life. The average age at which children become able to verbalize the fact that they are hungry is three.[39]

By the time children are three or four, a whole new universe of foods becomes available to them. By then they are tall and mobile enough to get their own food. When children start to receive allowances and can buy snacks in vending machines or stores, they have direct access to almost any

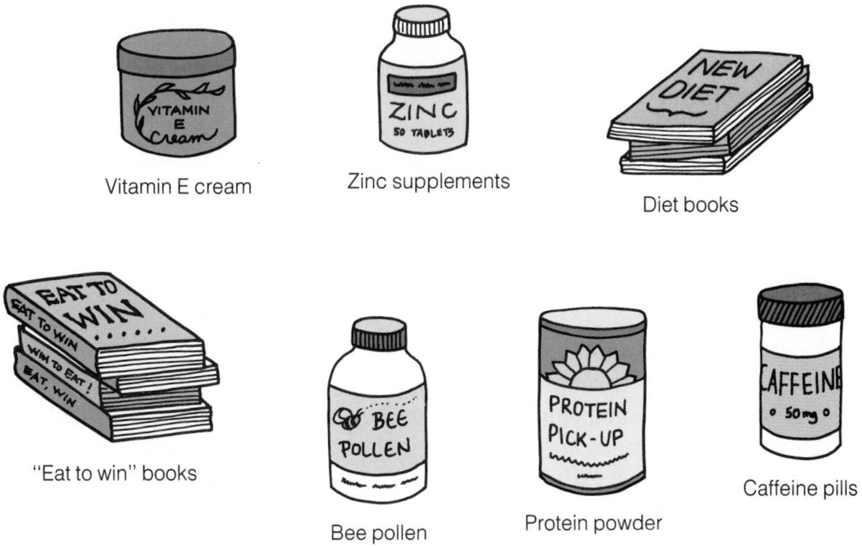

Lose-weight, get-stronger, gain-the-edge, look-better products appeal to many teenagers.

BOX 15-9

THE PUDDING STUDY

Visualize a day care center for preschoolers. It is lunchtime, and the children are seated around a large, round table. Today's lunch will be different from usual: it will start with pudding. Unknown to the children, each one will receive one of two kinds of pudding. Both puddings look the same and taste the same, but one has 150 calories and the other has 40 calories per serving. The amount of pudding consumed by the children will be secretly recorded, as will their consumption of the rest of the lunch. This experiment will be repeated on adults.

This experiment was conducted, and the results are very interesting. The children compensated almost perfectly for the calories in the different puddings by eating varying amounts of the other foods in the lunch. Those who were given the high-calorie pudding ate less than the children who were given the low-calorie pudding. On the other hand, the adults did not adjust their caloric intake as the children did. The adults appeared to modify their food intake according to cues not related to the caloric content of the foods. How the food tasted, the amount of food they were used to eating for lunch, and the amount of food offered influenced the adults' decisions about how much they ate.[36]

It was concluded from this study that young children have an internal "calorie counter" that regulates their food intake. Somewhere between the first few years of life and adulthood, the calorie-intake-regulating mechanisms may lose their adjustment or be overridden by other drives. External forces that influence how much food is consumed may come to override the internal processes that regulate meal-by-meal calorie intake.

type of food they can afford. Between the ages of 4 and 8, appetite and food intake gradually increase, and they do not fall off again until near the end of the adolescent growth spurt.

Patterns of food intake often change dramatically during adolescence, as do many other behavioral patterns. Adolescents have a lot of emotional and physical changes to go through. They have started the search for their individual identity and independence. They have also started the search for the bath soap, fashionable clothes, and the right hair-do. To the inconvenience of other people in the house who want to use the bathroom, physical appearance becomes a preoccupation. Because of the strong desire to look good, teenagers are targeted by companies selling products that promise weight loss, weight gain, clear complexions, and rippling muscles. Some of the products work, but many of them are absolutely useless and some are downright dangerous.

Teenagers may be too busy with school, sports, a part-time job, and friends to eat at regular mealtimes with the family. Although their appetites can be tremendous during periods of growth, teenagers may skip meals and make it through the day on snacks. The sheer volume of food consumed by many growing adolescents helps them to meet their need for nutrients, even if many foods of marginal nutritional value are consumed. Adolescents can generally feel vigorous and healthy even when they are accumulating diet-related risk factors that will influence disease development later in life.

HEALTH IMPLICATIONS OF FOOD INTAKE PATTERNS DURING THE GROWING YEARS

The usual diets of children and adolescents have an effect on their current and future health (Table 15-2). In the short-term, diets that provide inadequate amounts of calories, protein, iron, or zinc can lead to growth retardation. A lack of calories can produce underweight and an increased susceptibility to infectious diseases. Overweight or obesity may result when usual

TABLE 15-2

Nutritional risk factors for health problems of childhood and adolescence

Health Problem	Nutritional Risk Factors*
Childhood	
Growth retardation	inadequate calories, protein, iron, or zinc
Underweight	inadequate calories
Obesity	physical inactivity; excessive intake of calories
Dental decay	frequent consumption of sweets; inadequate fluoride intake
Iron-deficiency anemia	inadequate iron intake; inadequate intake of absorbable forms of iron
Allergies, intolerances	early exposure to cow's milk, wheat, egg white, citrus fruits, or certain other foods
Infection	undernutrition; vitamin-A deficiency; vitamin-C deficiency
Constipation	low fiber intake
Adolescence	
Underweight	inadequate calories
Delayed growth spurt	undernutrition
Obesity	physical inactivity; excessive intake of calories
Dental decay	frequent consumption of sweets; inadequate fluoride intake
Iron-deficiency anemia	inadequate iron intake; inadequate intake of absorbable forms of iron
Elevated serum cholesterol	excessive total fat, saturated fat, or cholesterol intake
Elevated blood pressure	obesity; physical inactivity; high-sodium diet

Source: Adapted from Brown, 1984.

*A nutritional risk factor is defined as a characteristic dietary pattern, or component of a pattern, that increases the likelihood that an individual will develop a particular disease or condition.

A NOTE OF CAUTION

Children are not miniature adults, and dietary recommendations for them must take into account their relatively high need for calories and nutrients for growth. Severe restrictions in calories and fat may reduce growth and lead to deficient intakes of protein, vitamins, and minerals. The results of overly restrictive diets during childhood are already apparent in the growing number of cases of "middle-class malnutrition" in the United States. It is clear that dietary recommendations intended to improve health can be taken too far.

physical activity levels are low. Constipation and recurring abdominal pain, a problem in 10% to 18% of school-aged children, appear to be directly related to low fiber intakes.[40] The health of adolescents can be compromised by underweight and obesity, as well as by high-sugar diets that promote tooth decay. Diets of children and adolescents that contain too little iron or iron that is not readily absorbed can develop iron-deficiency anemia.

In the long-term, the usual diets consumed by children and adolescents can affect their risk of developing certain chronic conditions, foremost of which are heart disease, hypertension, and osteoporosis.[41,42]

We now move on to discuss the relationships between the diets of youth and the development of specific health problems. The influence of calcium intake during the growing years on the risk of developing osteoporosis was presented in chapter 11. That content is not repeated here.

Iron Deficiency

Iron deficiency during childhood is generally due to iron intakes that fail to meet the body's need for iron. Recall from our discussion of iron in chapter 11 that the condition produced by iron deficiency is called iron-deficiency anemia.

Children experience an increased requirement for iron because their bodies' iron-containing cells increase in number during growth. Red blood cells, which contain the iron-loaded molecule hemoglobin, and muscle cells, which contain iron, increase in number and size as blood volume and muscle tissue grow. Females have a greater need for iron than do males after about the age of 12 or 13, because they need to replace iron lost in monthly menstrual periods.

Children and adolescents with iron-deficiency anemia generally have poor appetites, tire easily, and grow more slowly than do children whose iron levels are adequate.[43,44] Iron-deficiency anemia has also been associated with abnormally low levels of mental and physical performance and an increased susceptibility to certain illnesses.[44] These conditions are generally reversed when iron nutrition improves.[44]

The risk of developing iron-deficiency anemia is not evenly distributed across all ages during the growing years. It peaks between the ages of 1 and 2 and again during adolescence. Adolescent girls are at highest risk of developing anemia between the ages of 15 to 17 years. For boys, the age range of peak incidence is 12 to 14 years.[45] Teenagers that are physically very active—such as members of the track team—are at higher risk of develop-

TABLE 15-3

Age-related incidence of iron-deficiency anemia in U.S. children and adolescents[45,48]

Gender/Age Group	Percentage with Iron-Deficiency Anemia
Males and females 6 months to 5 years	2.9
Males 12 to 14 years	6.3
Females 15 to 17 years	4.6

ing iron-deficiency anemia than are inactive teens.[46,47] Iron deficiency among athletes has been referred to as *sports anemia*. It is likely due to a combination of inadequate iron intake plus a greater need for iron due to losses of iron from wear and tear on muscle and other tissues of the body. The rates of iron-deficiency anemia at various ages among U.S. children and adolescents are shown in Table 15-3.

The incidence of iron-deficiency anemia among infants and young children living in low-income households in the U.S. has declined steadily since 1975.[48] In that year, nearly 8% of infants and children between the ages of 6 months and 5 years were anemic. Ten years later, the rate had fallen to about 3%. Improved dietary iron intakes, such as those achieved by WIC-program participants, are largely responsible for the decline.[48,49] Because vitamin C improves iron absorption, higher intakes of this vitamin may also be related to the improved iron status of low-income children in the U.S.

Heart Disease and Hypertension

Heart disease and hypertension are regarded as pediatric problems, because their roots can become established in childhood and adolescence. Both heart disease and hypertension can take twenty or more years to develop, and they are seldom identified before the processes that lead to them are well underway. The usual diet of children and adolescents appears to affect when those processes begin.

Heart Disease A primary indicator of the risk of developing heart disease is elevated blood cholesterol, and children and adolescents' cholesterol levels vary with their dietary intake of fat and cholesterol.[42] Cholesterol levels of children in countries with high rates of heart disease (such as the U.S.) are higher than they are in countries where heart disease rates are low (such as Mexico); see Table 15-4. Plaque formation that leads to hardening of the arteries also appears to vary among populations according to usual dietary practices. (Plaque formation is one of the first signs of impending heart disease.) It tends to occur sooner in populations whose diets are high in animal fat and cholesterol. When animal-fat and cholesterol consumption levels decrease—a trend in U.S. diets over the past 30 years—plaque formation is postponed. This is supported by the fact that while 45% of American servicemen who died in Vietnam in the late 1960s had plaque-lined arteries, 77% of Korean Conflict servicemen examined in the 1950s showed plaque formation.[50,51]

TABLE 15-4

Typical blood cholesterol levels of children in two countries[42]

Country	Typical Childhood Cholesterol Level
U.S.A.	150–170 mg
Mexico	100 mg or less

TABLE 15-5

Comparison of average and recommended intakes of carbohydrate, protein, and fat calories and cholesterol by children 12 to 14 years of age[41,52]

	Percentage of Total Calories			
	Carbohydrate Calories	Protein Calories	Fat Calories	**Cholesterol, mg**
Average				
Females	48.0	14.7	37.3	371
Males	48.6	14.4	38.3	373
Recommended				
Females	50–55	10–15	30–35	300
Males	50–55	10–15	30–35	300

Reducing total fat and cholesterol intakes during childhood would appear to be an effective way to further reduce the incidence of heart disease in countries with high rates. To this end, goals have been established for optimal levels of fat and cholesterol intake for U.S. children. The American Heart Association recommends that the daily diets of children over two years of age provide 30% to 35% of total calories as fat and 300 mg or less of cholesterol. Carbohydrate intake (mainly complex carbohydrates) should be increased to 50% to 55% of the total calories, and protein intake should provide 10% to 15% of the total calories.[41] As shown in Table 15-5, only children's protein intakes tend to fall within the recommended ranges. In a study of 148 children aged 10 to 13 in Alabama, not one child's dietary intake was found to correspond to these goals.[53] The American Heart Association recommendations obviously are goals; they do not reflect current dietary practices of children in many parts of the U.S.

Diets that provide 30% to 35% of total calories as fat and less than 300 mg of cholesterol per day can generally be achieved if low- or reduced-fat dairy products are consumed and if intakes of fried foods and fatty meats are limited. An example menu that approximates the dietary goals set for children is given in Table 15-6. It is a menu that most children would find tasty, and it's the type of diet that would foster good lifetime eating habits.

Obesity and smoking also are risk factors for the progression of heart disease during the adolescent years.[54] Furthermore, the risk for developing heart disease as an adult is greater if heart disease "runs in the family." Diets that are low in fat and cholesterol are particularly important for children who have a parent that developed high cholesterol levels during childhood or as a young adult.

Hypertension High-sodium diets may increase blood pressure in children and adolescents who have a hypertensive parent.[41] Blood pressure also tends to increase with excessive body weight; this makes childhood obesity a risk for the development of hypertension.[41] U.S. children tend to consume far more sodium than is recommended.[55]

TABLE 15-6

A good menu for children 7 to 10 years of age

Breakfast

oatmeal, 1 c
brown sugar, 1 t
2% milk, ½ c
bran muffin, 1
margarine, 1 t
orange juice, ½ c

Snack

peanut butter, 2 T
whole-wheat bread, 1 slice
apple juice, ¾ c

Lunch

spaghetti with sauce, 1 c
whole-wheat bun, 1 oz
margarine, 1 t
plums, 2
2% milk, 1 c

Snack

chocolate-chip cookies, 2
orange juice, 1 c
banana, 1

Dinner

baked chicken (no skin), 2 oz
rice, 1 c
margarine, 1 t
carrot, raw, ¼
2% milk, ½ c
ice milk, ¾ c
 or ice cream cone, 1

Food Constituent Analysis

	Percentage of RDA	Percentage of Total Calories	Amount
Calories	91		2,180
Carbohydrate		60	335 g
Protein	232	13	79 g
Fat		27	69 g
Cholesterol			127 mg
Sucrose		(14)*	77 g
Dietary fiber			25 g
Calcium	149		1,190 mg
Zinc	89		8.9 mg
Iron	140		14 mg
Thiamin	125		1.5 mg
Riboflavin	150		2.1 mg
Niacin	125		20 mg
Vitamin C	227		102 mg

*Sucrose calories are included in the contribution of carbohydrates to total caloric intake. By itself, it contributes 14% of the total calories in the menu.

■ ■ ■

DIETARY REQUIREMENTS OF INFANTS, CHILDREN, AND ADOLESCENTS

Caloric and nutrient requirements per pound of body weight are greatest for the youngest humans (Figure 15-7). This is because infants and young children are growing rapidly and have high basal metabolic rates. (*A*

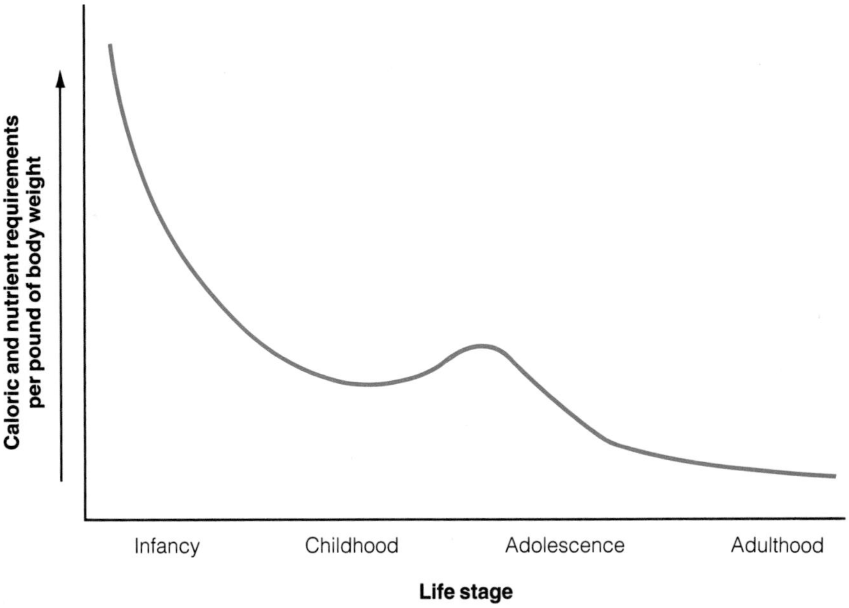

FIGURE 15-7
Changes in caloric and nutrient requirements per pound of body weight from infancy to adulthood.

reminder: Basal metabolic rate is the amount of energy needed for ongoing body processes such as maintenance of body temperature, blood circulation, breathing, and tissue construction and repair over a 24-hour period.) A 4-month-old infant, for example, requires approximately 52 calories per pound of body weight for growth, basal metabolism, and physical activity. A 30-year-old adult, on the other hand, needs only about 17 calories per pound of body weight to meet her or his total caloric need. Adults do not need calories for growth, and they require only about half as many calories as infants require per pound of body weight for basal metabolism.

An infant's relatively high need for calories is also apparent when we examine the level of food intake per pound of body weight required to meet caloric needs. A 15-pound 4-month-old whose sole source of food is breast milk or formula normally consumes nearly one-sixth of his or her body weight in milk per day. If a 154-pound adult were to consume one-sixth of his or her body weight in milk each day, the person would drink 3¼ gallons of it! Growth has a profound effect on caloric and nutrient requirements. Although the total amount of calories and nutrients a person needs increases with body size, the requirement per pound of body weight decreases.

The RDAs serve as the basic guide for identifying the amounts of calories and nutrients that diets should provide. They increase in a steplike fashion during the growing years (Figure 15-8). Other guides, such as the American Heart Association's dietary goals for children (shown previously in Table 15-5), indicate desirable levels of fat, protein, carbohydrate, and cholesterol intake. These guides are commonly used to identify the strengths and weaknesses of children's diets and to pinpoint dietary problems that may interfere with the growth and health status of children.

Evaluation of Typical Children's Diets

In general, the diets of U.S. children provide adequate levels of calories, protein, thiamin, riboflavin, niacin, vitamin B_{12}, phosphorus, and iodine. Less than 5% of children consume low amounts of these nutrients. Several

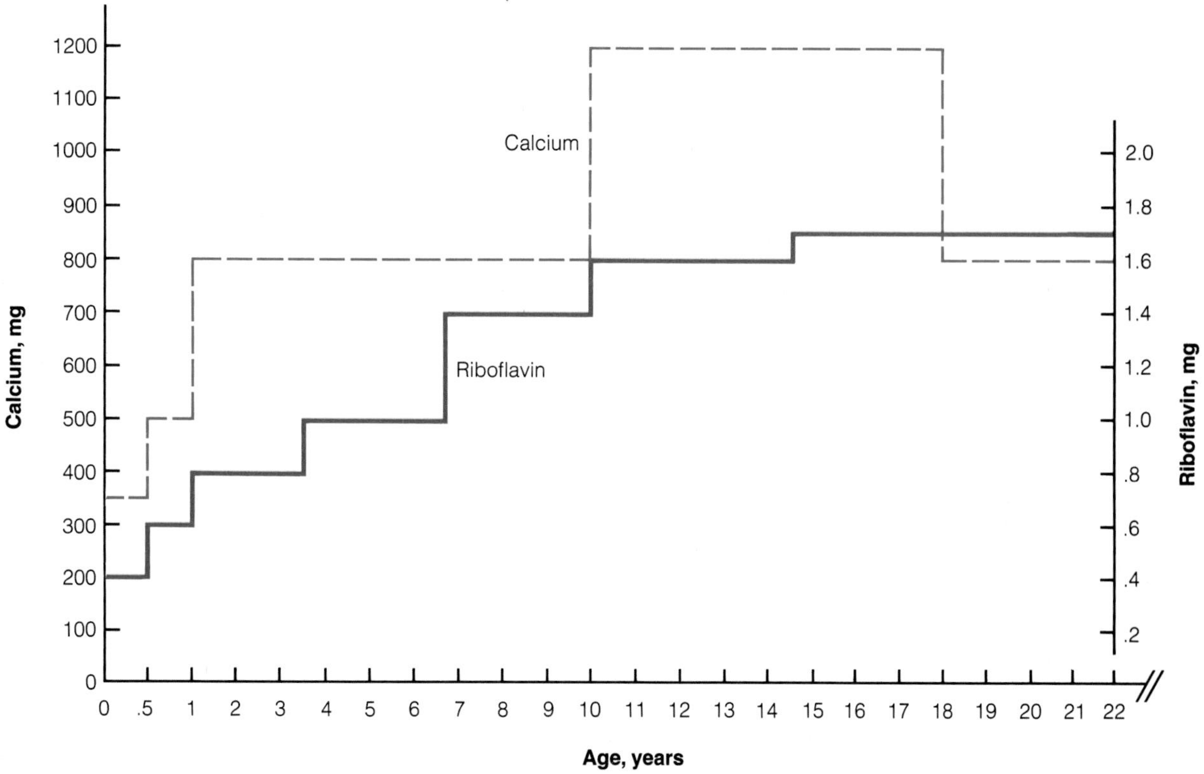

FIGURE 15-8
Examples of steplike increases in the RDAs for males from birth to age 22.

other nutrients have been found to be consumed in low amounts by children one to five years of age in the U.S.[56] Although those low levels do not automatically mean that a growth or health problem will develop, they do indicate problem areas that may compromise the growth and health of many young children. The nutrients identified as being in short supply in the diets of at least 10% of children are listed in Table 15-7. Because low intakes of dietary fiber also are common, fiber appears in the table.

TABLE 15-7
Percentage of U.S. children with low intakes of selected nutrients and dietary fiber[56]

Nutrient	Percentage of Children with Low Intake*
Vitamins	
vitamin C	11
folic acid	15
vitamin B_6	15
Minerals	
calcium	22
iron	53
zinc	46
magnesium	14
Dietary fiber	50

*Defined as less than 70% of the RDA.

TABLE 15-8

"Problem" nutrient–missing foods linkages

"Problem" Nutrient	Foods Missing from the Diet
Vitamin C	fruits and vegetables
Folic acid	fruits and vegetables
Iron	meats
Zinc	meats
Calcium	milk and milk products
Dietary fiber	whole-grain breads and cereals, fruits, and vegetables

Nutrients generally contained in adequate amounts in the diets of children 1 to 5 years old:
- *calories*
- *protein*
- *thiamin*
- *riboflavin*
- *niacin*
- *vitamin B_{12}*
- *phosphorus*
- *iodine*[56]

The strengths and weaknesses of adolescents' diets are generally thought to be similar to those of children's diets. Low calcium intakes, for example, have been found for 85% of adolescents.[55] Teens tend to consume about the same amount of calcium they consumed as infants, even though they need higher amounts.[55] A recent study conducted in Alabama found that 85% of teenagers had low folic-acid intake, and that 47% had deficient blood levels of this vitamin.[59]

The diets of U.S. children and adolescents tend to contain excessive levels of fat, cholesterol, sodium, and sugar.[58] These dietary excesses are as important to short-term and long-term health as inadequate nutrient intakes are.

Nutrient–Food Linkages

The nutrient inadequacies of children and adolescents in the U.S. can be traced to the lack of particular types of foods in the diet (Table 15-8). Low levels of vitamin C intake, for example, are commonly due to a lack of citrus fruits in the diet. When folacin (the "foliage" vitamin) intake is low, it usually indicates that the diet contains few fruits and vegetables.[59] The best food sources of iron and zinc are meats such as pork, beef, and poultry. Deficient intake most likely occurs when the average daily diet provides less than 2 ounces of meat.[57] (Most U.S. children consume more than this amount.) The failure to increase the number of servings of milk and milk products with age is the primary reason calcium intakes fall short of the RDAs.[60] Low dietary-fiber intakes are generally due to a lack of whole-grain breads and cereals or to a dietary shortage of fiber-rich fruits and vegetables.

DIETARY RECOMMENDATIONS FOR INFANTS, CHILDREN, AND ADOLESCENTS

The dietary recommendations for infants, children, and adolescents have changed substantially over the years, and they will continue to change as more is learned about how diet influences health during growth. Because a number of important questions about the effects of diet on the health of infants, children, and adolescents remain unanswered, the current dietary recommendations are somewhat controversial. For example, it is not known with certainty which solid foods should be given to infants or when they should be introduced. Neither are the age at which the fat or sodium content of a child's diet should become a health concern, and which children will benefit most from reduced-fat or reduced-sodium diets. Much remains to be learned about the role of modified diets during childhood and adolescence in preventing diseases that run in families. It may be that future dietary recommendations for children will vary depending on the results of tests that indicate which diseases a child has a genetic tendency to develop. A child with a genetic tendency for heart disease, for example, may benefit much more from early and long-term restriction of dietary fat than will a child who does not have that genetic tendency. Dietary recommendations for children in general—regardless of genetic background—will continue to be refined as the relationships between diet and growth, development, and health become better understood.

Current recommendations for good diets are based on available knowledge of the levels of calories and nutrients needed by infants, children, and adolescents, and on the results of studies that show relationships between particular characteristics of diets and health. Caloric and nutrient needs and diet–health relationships differ to some extent among infants, children, and adolescents. Consequently, dietary recommendations for these three stages of growth also differ.

Infants

Dietary recommendations for infants must address a number of special considerations:

1. Because infants grow and develop more rapidly than children and adolescents, they are more vulnerable to the effects of malnutrition. Consequently, there is less room for error when making dietary recommendations for infants.
2. Humans are born with the ability to suck and swallow in a series of coordinated mouth and tongue movements, but the abilities to chew and swallow foods and to digest many types of solid foods do not develop until four months or so after birth. Therefore, dietary recommendations for infants must take into account developmental readiness as well as the caloric and nutrient needs.
3. Infants are much more likely to develop food allergies and intolerances than are older children. Thus foods that may not be tolerated well must be excluded when formulating dietary recommendations for infants.
4. Infants receive only what they are fed. The selection of good diets for infants is totally in the hands of the people who feed them.

Because of these considerations, a special set of dietary recommendations is needed for infant feeding.

Current dietary recommendations for infants call for breast or formula feeding for the first six months of life. Infants should be fed "on demand"; that is, when they indicate they are hungry, rather than on a rigid schedule set by the clock.[61] In the first few months of life, most infants will get hungry every 3 to 4 hours.

Soft, solid foods should be added to an infant's diet of breast milk or infant formula between the ages of 4 and 6 months (Table 15-9).[62] The specific type of soft, solid food that should be offered first is rice cereal. It is

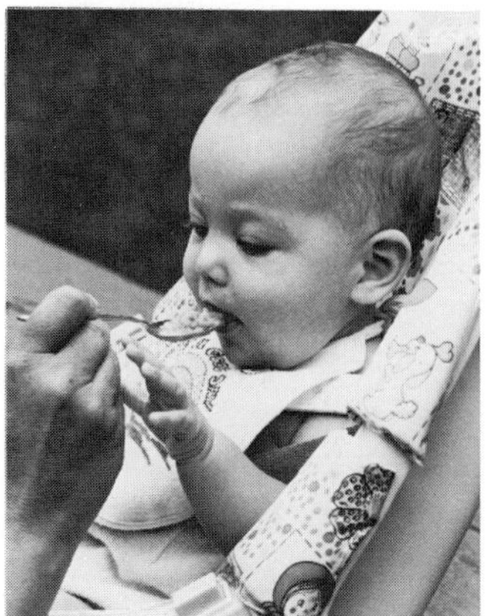

This infant eagerly accepts solid foods from a spoon.

TABLE 15-9
Infant feeding recommendations[62]

Breast-Fed Infants	Formula-Fed Infants
• Breast-feed for 6 months.	• Use infant formula for at least 6 months.
• Give vitamin D supplement if exposure to sunshine is limited.	• Give fluoride supplement if water supply is not fluoridated.
• Add iron-fortified cereal between 4 and 6 months.	• Add cereal between 4 and 6 months—iron-fortified if not using iron-fortified formula.
• Provide a variety of basic, soft, solid foods after 6 months.	• Provide a variety of basic, soft, solid foods after 6 months.

easily digested by infants of this age, and allergies to rice are extremely rare. It is recommended that iron-fortified rice cereal be given to all breast-fed infants and to bottle-fed infants that are not receiving iron-fortified formula. The iron provided by iron-fortified rice cereal or formula helps to restock the infant's iron stores, which have been drawn upon since birth. Infants between 4 and 6 months of age are also developmentally ready to chew and swallow foods. Wheat cereals should not be given to a child until after the first birthday, because they are more apt to cause allergic reactions.

Once it was thought that solid foods should be offered to infants within the first month of life. Although such young infants are unable to swallow much of the food offered (more of it ends up on their face and bib) or to digest completely what they do swallow, solid foods were thought to help the baby grow and sleep through the night. Giving solid foods before the age of 4 months does not accomplish either. Infants who receive solids early are no more likely to sleep through the night than are infants who start to receive solid foods between 4 and 6 months of age.[63] The age at which an infant begins to sleep for 6 or more hours during the night depends on other factors, including the infant's developmental level and how much he or she has slept during the day. Neither the infant nor the infant's mother or father is likely to get a full night's sleep for at least 4 months.

The recommendations for the timing and sequence of offering rice cereal and other solid foods to infants are shown in Table 15-10. It is generally recommended that solid foods prepared for infants consist of single, basic foods such as strained vegetables, fruits, or meats. Solid foods for infants can be purchased as commercial baby food or prepared at home. The home preparation of baby foods should be done carefully to avoid contamination and to achieve the right consistency of food. (Box 15-10 provides instructions.) New foods should be offered to infants one at a time. The new offerings should be separated by several days so that any allergic reactions to a food can be identified. Variety is key to achieving a healthy diet for infants in their second six months of life, and an assortment of basic foods should be given. (An example of how monotonous diets can cause problems appears in Box 15-11.)

■

TABLE 15-10

Introduction of "solid" foods to infants

Food	Age, months							
	4–6	7	8	9	10	11	12	13
Iron-fortified infant rice cereal	■	■	■	■	■	■	■	
Strained vegetables	■	■	■					
Strained fruits	■	■	■					
Toast, crackers		■	■	■	■	■	■	■
Strained meats		■	■	■	■	■	■	
Apple and grape juices		■	■	■	■	■	■	■
"Finger foods"*		■	■	■	■	■	■	■
Orange and grapefruit juices				■	■	■	■	
"Junior" (textured) vegetables				■	■	■	■	
Mashed soft, ripe fruits				■	■	■	■	
Mashed potatoes and pastas				■	■	■	■	
"Junior" meats				■	■	■	■	
Yogurt, cottage cheese, cheese					■	■	■	■
Cut up, mashed table foods							■	■

Note: Except for the introduction of iron-fortified infant rice cereal between 4 and 6 months of age, little evidence exists to support the timing of the introduction of other foods into an infant's diet. Consequently, these guidelines are tentative and general.

Foods such as egg white, wheat, and peanut butter that cause allergic reactions in some infants should not be introduced until after the age of one year. Cow's milk and cow's milk products should probably not be given to infants until at least 6 to 9 months of age. Honey should be avoided during the first 12 months as a precaution against the development of infantile botulism.

*"Finger foods" include well-cooked vegetables cut up into bite-size pieces, arrowroot biscuits, dry toast, Cheerios®, crackers, and ripe banana pieces. Raisins, nuts, frankfurter pieces, hard candy, and popcorn should not be given as finger foods.

Breast feeding should continue for at least 6 months and during the time the infant is receiving an increasing variety of solid foods. Infants appear to digest cow's milk without problem after the first 6 to 9 months of life.[62] Whole cow's milk, rather than reduced-fat milk, such as skim or 2% milk, is recommended for older infants and young children up to two years of age.[54] The use of reduced-fat milks is viewed as inappropriate for the first two years of life, because infants and young children need dietary fat for brain- and nerve-cell development. They may also need the higher level of calories provided by whole milk.

The textures of the foods offered to an infant should change as the infant gets older. The first solid foods should be strained and soft-to-soupy in consistency. After about 6 months of age, soft but lumpy foods should be given, because this helps them develop their chewing and swallowing skills. The introduction of foods of varying textures at about 7 months of age may also foster the normal development of processes involved in speech. Finger foods, such as well-cooked vegetables, infant biscuits (as well as the other foods listed in the footnote to Table 15-10), and commercially available "junior" baby foods are appropriate types of textured food. Infants eat small amounts at a time, but they get hungry often.

BOX 15-10

HOW TO MAKE BABY FOOD AT HOME

Equipment Needed: A blender or baby-food mill and a strainer.
Set-Up: Clean all utensils, equipment, and counter surfaces thoroughly. Wash hands with soap and water.

PREPARATION

Use fresh or frozen foods instead of canned if possible. Use basic foods that do not contain added sugar, salt, spices, margarine, butter, or other additives. After the infant is 7 months old, make the food a bit lumpy, but still soft.

Fruits

Use clean and ripe fruits. Remove all skin, seeds, and cores. Use only the pulp. Puree in blender or food mill thoroughly. (Cook hard fruits like apples first.) Mash if the fruit is soft enough.

Examples: Mashed bananas; applesauce; pureed apricots, pears, and peaches.

Vegetables

Clean thoroughly. Remove stems and any tough skin or seeds. Boil or steam until soft. Puree and serve lukewarm.

Examples: Pureed green beans, peas, squash, carrots, and potatoes.

Meats

Cook the meat thoroughly. Trim off fat, skin, and gristle. Blend or grind meat with enough water to make a puree (generally, ½ c water to 1 c cooked meat).

Examples: Pork, chicken, fish, beef, lamb, turkey.

Juices

Use frozen or bottled apple, cranberry, and grape juice. Reconstitute frozen juices according to directions on the container. Strain juice if needed. Avoid "fruit drinks."

STORAGE

Freeze extra servings in tightly covered ice-cube tray or other airtight container, *or* store tightly covered in refrigerator for no more than three days. Do not thaw and refreeze.

Discard any leftovers in the baby's dish. When the spoon used to feed the child contacts the food, bacteria is introduced that may cause the food to spoil while stored.

BOX 15-11

INFANTS NEED VARIETY, TOO

Seven-month-old twins were admitted to a hospital because of the presence of "bulges" on the top of their heads and because they frequently vomited and were irritable. An evaluation of the twins' usual diet revealed the cause of the problems. Concerned about the additives in commercial baby foods, their mother chose to prepare their food herself and she prepared only one type of food: pureed chicken liver. The twins had been eating the liver every day for four months. The long-term intake of 40,000 IUs of vitamin A provided by this diet caused the twins to develop vitamin-A toxicity.

Within months after the infants were taken off the chicken liver and given a variety of foods, their bone formation improved, they stopped vomiting, and their irritability disappeared. The follow-up on the infants was insufficient for determining if any long-term problems resulted from the vitamin-A overdose.[65]

By 9 months of age, infants are ready for mashed foods and some types of food that do not need special preparation such as yogurt, cottage cheese, and soft cheeses. Most infants have several teeth by this time, and they are able to bite into and chew soft foods.

Infants graduate to adult-type foods after the age of 12 months. Although most foods still need to be mashed or cut up into small pieces for them, one-year-olds are able to eat the same types of food as the rest of the family. They can feed themselves with a spoon and drink from a cup. They have come a long way in 12 months.

Vitamin and Mineral Supplements In the days when infant formula was made at home by adding corn syrup and water to evaporated cow's milk, dietary recommendations for infants included vitamin and mineral supplements. The evaporated-milk formula contained low levels of vitamins A, C, D, and E and too little iron. Now that infants are breast-fed or receive nutritionally complete infant formulas, there is no longer a need for supplements for all infants.

Two situations, however, call for the use of a specific vitamin or mineral supplement during infancy. One is the situation in which breast-fed infants fail to get direct exposure to sunshine and therefore need a vitamin-D supplement. The other recommendation applies to formula-fed infants. If the formula is not diluted at home with water that has been fluoridated, then fluoride drops should be given.

Foods to Avoid Not all foods can be considered "baby foods." Some foods should be omitted from an infant's diet because they are apt to cause allergic reactions or are too difficult for infants to chew into small pieces and swallow. Table 15-11 provides a master list of foods that should not be offered to infants.

Food Allergies and Intolerances **Food allergies** can seriously threaten infant health, but they are often misunderstood. Only a specific type of adverse reaction to food qualifies as an allergic reaction. Other types of adverse reactions to food are considered food intolerances. The difference between an allergy and a **food intolerance** is that the body's immune system

food allergy: The development of immune-system reactions in response to the presence of an offending food substance in the body. True allergies can be diagnosed by the abnormally high presence of antibodies in the blood following ingestion and absorption of an antigen—the offending component of food. Common food antigens include wheat gluten, egg-white protein, and cow's-milk protein.

food intolerance: Any adverse reaction caused by the consumption of food or a particular component of food that does not involve the body's immune system. Lactose intolerance, adverse reactions to monosodium glutamate (MSG), and the gas and intestinal cramps related to the consumption of dried beans, cabbage, cauliflower, and certain other vegetables are examples of food intolerances.

TABLE 15-11

Foods to avoid in the first year of life

Foods that May Cause Allergic Reactions	Foods that May Cause Other Problems	Foods that May Lead to Choking
cow's milk*	prune juice	raisins
soy protein	blueberries	hard candy
wheat products	corn	frankfurter pieces
egg white	coffee	popcorn
peanut butter	tea	nuts
nuts	honey	hard pieces of vegetables
		grapes

*Withhold through the first 6 to 9 months.

(disease-defense system) becomes involved only in allergic reactions. The immune system produces antibodies to neutralize the invading *antigen*—the offending component of food that has entered the body proper. While present in the body, antigens cause disruptions in normal cell functions that can result in diarrhea, hives, rashes, a runny nose, sneezing, wheezing, and irritated eyes. Adverse reactions to cow's milk protein, soy protein, the gluten component of wheat, and egg-white protein are appropriately termed "allergic" reactions. The vast majority of allergic reactions that occur among infants are due to the ingestion of one or more of these four substances. Peanut butter and nuts also cause allergic reactions in some infants.

Food intolerances can be caused by effects of certain components in food on digestive processes (such as lactose intolerance), or they can be due to direct effects of absorbed substances on cell functions. The diarrhea that some infants experience when they consume prune juice, blueberries, or corn are examples of food intolerances.

Once confirmed, food allergies should not be taken lightly. They can seriously affect a child's growth and health, and they may threaten life. Although most food allergies disappear or substantially diminish by the age of two, allergic reactions to foods can persist throughout a lifetime.[66] Many cases of food allergies can be prevented or postponed if cow's milk is not given to infants until the child is 6 months to a year old, and if soy protein, wheat, egg white, peanut butter, and nuts are not introduced into diets until after the first year.

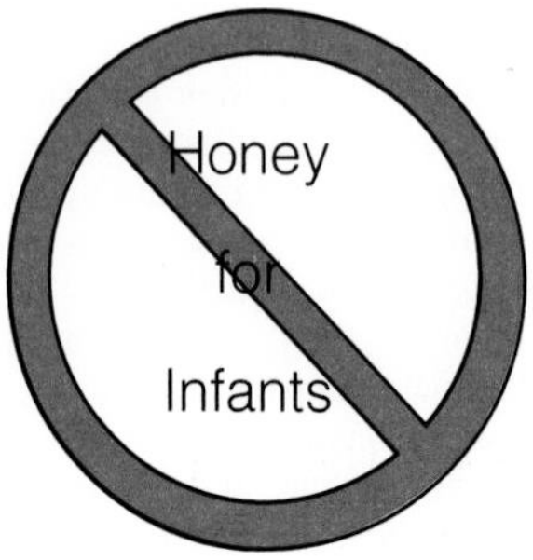

Other Problem Foods Honey is an example of a food that should not be given to infants, and there is a very good reason: bees may have contaminated it with *Clostridium botulinum* spores they picked up from plants or soil. The spores, which may produce toxins in the gastrointestinal tract, are not destroyed during the processing of honey. Consequently, the ingestion of honey by infants can lead to the development of botulism, a potentially fatal disease.[67] Infants become resistant to the toxin produced by *C. botulinum* spores with age. After the age of one, honey is considered safe for children.

Tea is not a basic food for infants, either. It is not recommended for infants because it decreases the absorption of iron from milk, grain products,

TABLE 15-12

Food-group recommendations for children and adolescents

Food Group	Minimum Number of Servings per Day: Children	Adolescents
Breads and cereals	4	4
Vegetables and fruits	(4)	(4)
vitamin A-rich	1	1
vitamin C-rich	1	1
other	2	2
Milk and milk products	3	4
Meats or alternates	2	2
Miscellaneous	based on caloric need	

and vegetables. The consumption of a cup of tea a day by 6- to 12-month-old infants has been shown to contribute to the development of iron deficiency.[64]

Infants should also not be given foods that they cannot chew into pieces before swallowing. Several hundred infants die each year from choking on foods. The two foods that are most likely to cause choking are hard candy and frankfurter pieces.[68]

Children and Adolescents

Good diets for children and adolescents can generally be achieved if the food-group recommendations shown in Table 15-12 are followed. The number of servings listed for each food group is a minimum standard. Additional servings from one or more of the food groups will often be required for meeting caloric needs. It should also be emphasized that recommended portion sizes vary by age. Obviously, preschool children (ages 1 to 4 years)

Snacks are a major part of most teenagers' diets.

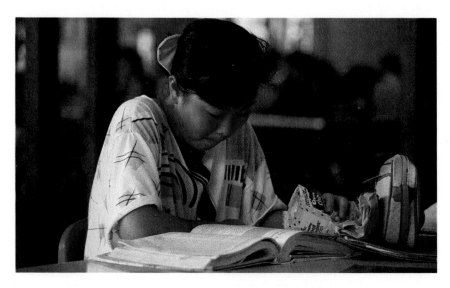

TABLE 15-13

Food serving sizes for preschool children

Food	Serving Size
Breads and Cereals	
bread	½ to 1 slice
cooked cereal	¼ to ½ c
dry cereal	½ c
spaghetti, macaroni, noodles, rice	¼ to ½ c
crackers	2 to 3
Vegetables and Fruits	
cooked vegetables	2 to 4 T
raw vegetables	several "chunks"
fruit	½
applesauce	4 T
juice	2 to 4 oz
Milk and Milk Products	
milk	3 to 4 oz
cheese	½ oz
yogurt	3 to 4 oz
Meat and Meat Alternates	
chicken, fish, beef	1 to 2 oz
egg	1
dried beans, cooked	¼ c
Miscellaneous	
desserts	¼ to ½ c
butter, margarine	½ t
bacon	1 slice

cannot eat as much at a time as older children and adolescents. The serving sizes intended for them are shown in Table 15-13.

The type of foods selected from the food groups is important. Whole-grain breads and cereals should be represented in diets; and boiled, broiled, and baked foods should be consumed more often than fried foods. Many of the foods sold in fast-food restaurants, for example, fit into the basic food groups. A hamburger on a bun contributes to the meat and meat alternates group and to the bread and cereals group. French fries could fit into the vegetable group. Nonetheless, the hamburger and fries are high in fat, and the bun is low in fiber. If these and other high-fat, low-fiber foods are commonly chosen, a diet can become out-of-balance. The analysis of the three days' intake of a 16-year-old girl who eats most of her meals and snacks at fast-food restaurants shown in Table 15-14 gives an idea of how a diet with an abundance of fast foods might rate nutritionally. Although adequate in calories, the diet is high in fat and low in dietary fiber and a number of vitamins

TABLE 15-14

Three days' intake reported by a 16-year-old girl who ate primarily at fast-food restaurants

Day 1	Day 2	Day 3
Breakfast		
Sausage Egg McMuffin®, 1		
Lunch	Lunch	Lunch
fried chicken, 4½ oz cola, 16 oz	cheeseburger, 1 potato chips, 5 oz cola, 16 oz	fried chicken, 5 oz cola, 12 oz
Snack	Snack	Snack
cola, 24 oz	cola, 24 oz	cola, 24 oz
Dinner	Dinner	Dinner
pizza with extra cheese, mushrooms, and Canadian bacon, 4 pieces cola, 12 oz	roast beef sandwich, 1 french fries, regular order cola, 12 oz	roast beef, 2 oz corn, 2 oz cola, 12 oz

Food Constituent Analysis

	Percentage of RDA	Percentage of Total Calories	Amount
Calories	102		2,150
Carbohydrate		50	270 g
Protein	152	13	70 g
Fat		37	90 g
Cholesterol			277 g
Sucrose		(28)*	150 g
Dietary fiber			4 g
Calcium	52		625 mg
Zinc	73		11 mg
Iron	83		15 mg
Thiamin	82		0.9 mg
Riboflavin	77		1.0 mg
Niacin	129		18 mg
Vitamin C	48		29 mg
Vitamin A	25		988 IU

*Sucrose calories are included in the contribution of carbohydrates to total caloric intake. By itself, however, sucrose contributes 28% of the total calories in this diet.

and minerals—especially in calcium and vitamins A and C.

Foods from the "miscellaneous" group that contribute mainly calories may be needed by children and teenagers. Although cakes, candy, cookies, potato chips, and so on are generally considered "sometimes" foods rather than "always" foods, they can serve as sources of needed calories for children and adolescents. Snacks also are an important source of calories in the

Good snack foods.

diets of children and teenagers. Good choices for snacks include:

yogurt	pears	grapes
cheese	melon	raisins
2% milk	bananas	carrots
ice milk	oranges	cucumbers
peanuts	apples	popcorn
peanut butter	apple juice	

■ ■ ■

OTHER TOPICS IN CHILD AND ADOLESCENT NUTRITION

Good diets are essential for good health in growing children, but they mean more than that to many people. Diets are the basis of several debates about the effect of food on health, behavior, and appearance. Two of the controversies are explored here: the relationship between diet and hyperactivity in children, and diet and complexion. Then, the chapter ends with a discussion of what can be thought of as the largest fast-food restaurant in the world. It's likely one you've eaten at a thousand or more times.

Diet and Hyperactivity in Children

Depending upon the criteria used to diagnose the disorder, between 1% and 25% of children are considered hyperactive.[69] The condition is characterized by a short attention span, a high level of physical activity, and impulsiveness.[69] The regular, high level of activity and the short attention span cause disruptions in the child's learning progress as well as in classroom and home environments. Children who are hyperactive are generally hard to manage and may frequently "test" the limits of patience of loving parents and busy teachers.

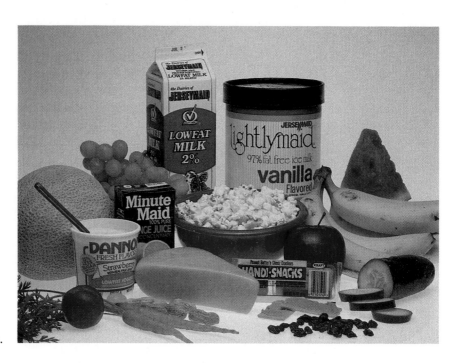

The only cure for hyperactivity appears to be age. Children tend to outgrow the condition as they pass through the teen years. However, their parents have probably gone to great lengths to get them to slow down and decrease disruptive behavior by then. Treatments for hyperactivity include behavioral modification counseling, psychotherapy, drugs, and dietary intervention, and none of these approaches is totally effective. The main drug used to control hyperactivity carries with it the side effects of decreased appetite and growth. (Interestingly enough, the main drug used to treat hyperactivity is a stimulant in adults, but has the opposite effect in hyperactive children.) Many parents prefer to treat the condition with dietary modification because they see it as safer than the regular use of a drug and as more effective than behavioral modification or psychotherapy.

Many types of special diets have been used to treat hyperactivity. In general, such diets attempt to eliminate foods that contain food dyes, artificial flavorings, and salicylates (pronounced sə-lis′ə-lāts). Salicylates are naturally occurring compounds in almonds, cucumbers, apples, tomatoes, and certain other fruits and vegetables. Because many commonly consumed foods contain these compounds, the dietary attempts to control hyperactivity demand a good deal of planning and preparation time.

Results of research on the effectiveness of dietary modifications for treating hyperactivity have generally shown that very few children benefit. For the few who do improve while on a special diet, it is not clear whether the improvement is due to the increased attention given to them or to the elimination of particular substances from their diet.[70] Concern has been expressed that the dietary modification approach may lead children to believe that their behavior is a direct result of the food they eat. ("Sorry, Mom. I didn't mean to break the lamp. It must have been that slice of tomato I ate. . . .") It has been suggested that special diets are warranted if they are healthful and if they appear to be effective for the individual child.[70]

Diet and Complexion

Acne can really ruin a good time for a teenager, and almost every teenager develops it. Pimples usually start to appear around the age of 12 to 13 in girls and 14 to 15 in boys. They do not appear to be caused by eating chocolate or by any form of dietary indiscretion.

The development of acne is a side effect of the hormonal changes that occur during sexual maturation. Acne formation starts about one-eighth inch below the skin. A budding pimple contains fatty acids that serve as a source of food for bacteria that enter through the skin. As the bacteria feed, they multiply and cause a local infection commonly called a *pimple*.

Because pimples develop below the surface of the skin, they cannot be washed away and cannot be prevented by good hygiene. They can be treated with creams containing benzoyl peroxide, antibiotics, or a combination of the two. Many over-the-counter acne creams contain benzoyl peroxide. Severe cases of acne are best treated by prescription drugs such as antibiotics and retinoic acid (a form of vitamin A). Accutane™ and Retin-A™ are two vitamin A–like drugs used to treat stubborn cases of acne. Although highly effective, these drugs can produce a number of side effects, including dry and itchy skin, fatigue, headaches, elevated cholesterol levels, and birth defects if taken shortly before or during early pregnancy.

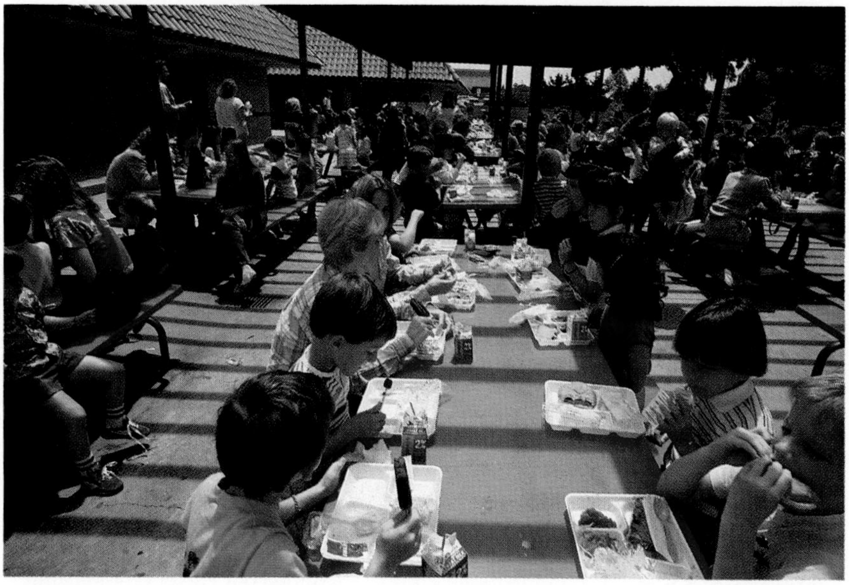

The School Lunch Program serves approximately 23 million meals every school day.[71] A child who eats school lunches from kindergarten through twelfth grade will have consumed nearly 2,000 of them by the time he or she graduates.

Therefore, their use is reserved for serious cases of acne, and they should not be used at all by women who may become pregnant. Dietary modifications do not appear to prevent or cure acne.

The School Lunch Program

The U.S. Department of Agriculture established the School Lunch Program in 1946 to help safeguard the health of children by providing nutritious meals and to promote the consumption of domestic agricultural products.[72] The need to improve child health was being felt at the time because many candidates for military service during World War II had to be rejected because of conditions related to malnutrition.[73] Also, the farm economy was depressed in the 1940s, and the School Lunch Program was viewed as a way to improve the financial and employment conditions in rural sections of the country.

It is a goal of the program to serve lunches that provide one-third of the RDAs of each student served. Children who participate in the program tend to have higher nutrient intakes at lunch—and for the day—than children who bring their lunches from home.[74,75] Although the level of nutrients provided in the lunches is a strong advantage of the program, concern has been expressed about the high levels of fat, sodium, and sugar and the low levels of fiber in the menus.[76] Recipes have been revised to address these problems, and more balanced school lunches are now being served.

In 1966 the School Breakfast Program was established to address the widespread problem of children coming to school hungry. Ten percent of the children who participate in the breakfast program are from low-income households.

An important provision of both the lunch program and the breakfast program is the availability of free and reduced-price meals. In 1989, children from families of four whose household income was less than about $15,000 a year were eligible for free meals. If the household income was less than approximately $20,000, the children were eligible for reduced-price meals.

School food programs are operated throughout the world. In economically developing countries as well as the U.S., providing meals at school is viewed as a way to increase children's ability to pay attention in class, to concentrate, and to learn. Teachers have long known that a child cannot learn "on an empty stomach"—that a child's body must be fed before his or her mind can be fed.

■ ■ ■

COMING UP IN CHAPTER 16

The need for good nutrition does not end when physical growth has been completed. Good nutrition continues to be important for promoting health and preventing disease through the adult years. The relationships between nutrition and health in men and women are examined next.

■ ■ ■

REVIEW QUESTIONS

1. Explain what is meant by "critical period" for growth.
2. When are the critical periods for brain growth in humans? For muscle growth?
3. Between the ages of 11 and 15 for females, and 12 to 17 for males, children normally gain ____% of their adult weight and ____% of their total bone mass.
4. True or false? Ultimate height is generally achieved two years after the onset of puberty for both females and males.
5. Which situation would have the greatest impact on the mental development of an infant?

   Situation 1: Maternal malnutrition during pregnancy only.

   Situation 2: Maternal malnutrition during pregnancy and infant malnutrition during the first 6 months of life.

   Situation 3: No maternal malnutrition during pregnancy, infant malnutrition during the first 6 months of life.
6. A child whose growth is stunted may have experienced __________.
7. What environmental factor is closely associated with the development of obesity during childhood?
8. Cite three factors associated with the development of food preferences in children.
9. True or false? A child who is forced to eat a certain food is likely to develop a lasting dislike for the food.
10. True or false? The average age at which children are able to verbalize the "I'm hungry" and "I'm full" feeling is two years.
11. List five ways the diets of children and adolescents influence their current health and five ways their diets can influence their future health.
12. Iron deficiency most commonly occurs among children between the ages of ____ and ____. For adolescents, iron deficiency most commonly occurs between the ages of ____ and ____ years for boys, and ____ and ____ years for girls.

13. List four nutrients that tend to be found in low amounts in the diets of children, and four that tend to be contained in excessive amounts.
14. Current recommendations call for breast or formula feeding for at least the first _____ months of life.
15. Solid foods such as rice cereal should be introduced into an infant's diet between the ages of _____ and _____ months.
16. True or false? Eating solid foods helps a young infant sleep through the night.
17. True or false? Infants should be fed on demand, rather than according to a strict time schedule.
18. True or false? The use of reduced-fat milk is not recommended for the first two years of life.
19. Are vitamin and mineral supplements recommended for all infants?
20. What is the major difference between a food allergy and a food intolerance?
21. List five good snacks for children. (*Good* means "nutrient-dense.")
22. As a goal, School Lunch Program menus are designed to provide _____ of the students' RDAs.

Answers

1. A critical period for growth is the interval of time during which cells of a tissue or organ are programmed to multiply. Growth by cell division occurs only during these preset time intervals.
2. See Figure 15-2.
3. 50%, 45%.
4. False. Females and males continue to gain height (although at a slow pace) well into their late teen years. Adult height is generally achieved between the ages of 16 and 21 for females, and between 18 and 24 years for males.
5. Situation 2.
6. Long-term undernutrition.
7. Physical inactivity.
8. The types of foods offered; how foods are offered (the mealtime environment and social meanings attached to foods); how frequently a food is offered. The inborn preference for sweet-tasting things also influences children's food preferences.
9. True.
10. False. According to the Denver Developmental Test, children don't normally reach that point until the age of 3.
11. Refer to Table 15-2.
12. 1 and 2, 12 and 14, 15 and 17.
13. Refer to the subsection, Evaluation of Typical Children's Diets.
14. 6.
15. 4 and 6.
16. False.
17. True.

18. True.
19. No, but some infants may benefit from vitamin D or fluoride supplements.
20. The body's immune system becomes involved only in *allergic* reactions.
21. Refer to the list in the subsection on dietary recommendations for children and adolescents.
22. One-third.

■ ■ ■

PUTTING NUTRITION KNOWLEDGE TO WORK

1. Assume Beth weighed 8 pounds 2 ounces at birth and grew normally in her first year of life. About how much would you expect her to weigh on her first birthday?

   (Hint: What's 3 times 8 pounds, 2 ounces?)

2. How tall are your mother and father? What height is at the middle of the range of their heights? How tall are you and any adult sisters and brothers you have? How near to the middle point between your parents' heights are you and your brothers and sisters?
3. At age 14, John decided he did not want to gain any more weight. His weight was normal for his height (5′5″) at the time, and he was able to hold himself at that weight until the age of 19. X-rays of John's bones on his 19th birthday showed that the epiphyses at the ends of his long bones had fused. Last week, shortly after his birthday, John decided that his lack of weight gain must be interfering with his growth in height and that he should gain some weight because he wants to become taller.

   If John eats well and gains weight, will he grow in height? What critical periods for growth were missed?

   (See Box 15-2 and Figure 15-2.)

4. Debra is 18 months old and weighs 26 pounds. What range of weight-for-age growth percentiles is she in? Refer to Figure 15-4.

   (Answer: Debra's weight for age is between the 75th and 90th growth percentiles.)

5. Consider Debra from question 4 again. Is she at risk of becoming an obese adult? Why or why not?

   (Answer: Debra is no more at risk than other children her age of becoming obese as an adult. Her weight for age does not classify her as overweight. In addition, the relationship between overweight early in life and subsequent obesity is a very weak one.)

6. When you were a child, were you forced to "clean up your plate," or not allowed to leave the table until you had eaten your vegetables, or not given dessert until you had eaten a particular food that was served to you? If so, what do you think was the logic behind the practice? Do those early experiences influence what you eat and how much you eat now? Also, in what ways did they influence your food attitudes and behaviors?
7. Thirty minutes after consuming 6 ounces of cow's milk, two tablespoons of rice cereal, and a tablespoon of applesauce, 6-month-old Todd develops diarrhea. Assume that the diarrhea was caused by one of these foods.

Which is the likely culprit? What type of reaction (a food intolerance or an allergy) likely caused this diarrhea?

(Hint: See Table 15-11 and the discussion of infant food allergies and intolerances.)

8. Fill in the minimum number of servings:

Food Group	Minimum Number of Servings per Day	
	Children	Adolescents
Breads and cereals		
Vegetables and fruits		
vitamin A-rich		
vitamin C-rich		
other		
Milk and milk products		
Meats or alternates		

(Refer to Table 15-12.)

9. Make up a one-day menu for a 5-year-old that includes the minimum number of servings from each food group. Then do the same thing for a teenager.

■ ■ ■

NOTES

1. H. H. Gifft, M. B. Washbon, and G. G. Harrison, *Nutrition, Behavior, and Change* (Englewood Cliffs, N.J.: Prentice-Hall, 1972). See also J. L. Sutphen, Growth as a measure of nutrition status, *Journal of Pediatric Gastroenterology and Nutrition* 4 (1985): 169–181.
2. H. V. Barnes, Physical growth and development during puberty, *Medical Clinics of North America* 59 (1975): 1305–1317.
3. S. Kondo, E. Takahashi, et al., Secular trends in height and weight of Japanese pupils, *Tohoku Journal of Experimental Medicine* 126 (1978): 203–213.
4. C. L. Shear, D. S. Freedman, et al., Secular trends of obesity in early life: The Bogalusa Heart Study, *American Journal of Public Health* 78 (1988): 75–77.
5. L. R. Shapiro, et al., Obesity prognosis: A longitudinal study of children from the age of 6 months to 9 years, *American Journal of Public Health* 74 (1984): 968–972.
6. A. F. Roche and G. H. Davila, Late-adolescent growth in stature, *Pediatrics* 50 (1972): 874–880.
7. M. Winick, Nutrition and cell growth, *Nutrition Reviews* 26 (1968): 195.
8. J. D. Lloyd-Still, I. Hurwitz, et al., Intellectual development after severe malnutrition in infancy, *Pediatrics* 54 (1974): 306–311.
9. F. Lifshitz, Nutrition and growth, *Clinical Nutrition* 4 (1985): 40–47.
10. M. T. Pugliese, M. Weyman-Dunn, et al., Parental health beliefs as a cause of nonorganic failure to thrive, *Pediatrics* 80 (1987): 175–182.
11. H. McKay, L. Sinisterra, et al., Improving cognitive ability in chronically deprived children, *Science* 20 (1978): 270–278.
12. D. E. Barrett and M. Radke-Yarrow, Effects of nutritional supplementation in children's responses to novel, frustrating, and competitive situations, *American Journal of Clinical Nutrition* 42 (1985): 102–120.
13. D. Benton and G. Roberts, Effect of vitamin and mineral supplementation on intelligence of a sample of schoolchildren, *Lancet* i (1988): 140–143.

14. S. L. Gortmaker, et al., Increasing pediatric obesity in the United States, *American Journal of Diseases of Childhood* 141 (1987): 535–540.

15. D. S. Freedman, G. L. Burke, et al., Relationship of changes in obesity to serum lipid and lipoprotein changes in childhood and adolescence, *Journal of the American Medical Association* 254 (1985): 515–520.

16. R. E. Patterson, J. T. Typpo, et al., Factors related to obesity in preschool children, *Journal of the American Dietetic Association* 86 (1986): 1376–1381.

17. L. R. Shapiro, et al., Obesity prognosis: A longitudinal study of children from the age of 6 months to 9 years, *American Journal of Public Health* 74 (1984): 968–972.

18. W. H. Dietz and S. L. Gortmaker, Do we fatten our children at the television set? Obesity and television viewing in children and adolescents, *Pediatrics* 75 (1985): 807–812.

19. *Neilsen Report on Television, 1985* (Chicago: A. C. Neilsen Co., 1985).

20. J. E. Brown, Graduate students examine TV advertisements for food, *Journal of Nutrition Education* 9 (1976): 120–122.

21. K. Clancey-Hepburn, A. A. Hickey, and G. Nevill, Children's behavior responses to TV food advertisements, *Journal of Nutrition Education* 6 (1974): 93–96.

22. J. P. Galst and M. A. White, The unhealthy persuader: The reinforcing value of television and children's purchase-influencing attempts at the supermarket, *Child Development* 47 (1976): 1089–1096.

23. S. B. Roberts, J. Savage, et al., Energy expenditure and intake in infants born to lean and overweight mothers, *New England Journal of Medicine* 318 (1988): 461–466.

24. L. H. Epstein, R. R. Wing, and A. Valoski, Childhood obesity, *Pediatric Clinics of North America* 32 (1985): 363–379.

25. R. R. Fripp, J. L. Hodgson, et al., Aerobic capacity, obesity, and atherosclerotic risk factors in male adolescents, *Pediatrics* 75 (1985): 813–818.

26. D. S. Freedman, et al., Persistence of juvenile-onset obesity over eight years: The Bogalusa Heart Study, *American Journal of Public Health* 77 (1987): 588–592.

27. J. Hirsch and J. L. Kaittle, Cellularity of obese and nonobese human adipose tissue, *Federation Proceedings* 29 (1970): 1516.

28. H. H. Gifft, M. B. Washbon, and G. G. Harrison, *Nutrition, Behavior, and Change* (Englewood Cliffs, N.J.: Prentice-Hall, 1972), 187–221.

29. H. N. Ricciuti, Adverse environmental and nutritional influences on mental development: A perspective, *Journal of the American Dietetic Association* 79 (1981): 115–120.

30. E. M. Widdowson, Mental contentment and physical growth, *Lancet* i (1951): 1316–1318.

31. L. L. Birch, The acquisition of food acceptance patterns in children, in *Eating Habits: Food Physiology and Learned Behavior*, eds. R. Boakes, D. Poppelewell, and D. Burton (Chichester, England: John Wiley, 1987). See also L. L. Birch, The role of experience in children's food acceptance patterns, *Journal of the American Dietetic Association* 39 (1988) (supplement): 5-36 to 5-40.

32. M. R. Kare and G. K. Beauchamp, The role of taste in the infant diet, *American Journal of Clinical Nutrition* 41 (1985) (supplement): 418–422.

33. M. Story and J. E. Brown, Do young children instinctively know what to eat? The studies of Clara Davis revisited, *New England Journal of Medicine* 316 (1987): 103–106.

34. C. M. Davis, Self-selection of diet by newly weaned infants, *American Journal of Diseases of Children* 36 (1928): 651–679.

35. C. M. Davis, Results of the self-selection of diets by young children, *Canadian Medical Association Journal* 41 (1939): 257–261.

36. L. L. Birch, Presentation at national conference on nutrition education research, Chicago, September 1986.

37. L. L. Birch, S. I. Zimmerman, and H. Hind, The influence of social-affective context in the formation of children's food preferences, *Child Development* 51 (1980): 856–861.

38. V. A. Beal, Dietary intake of individuals followed through infancy and childhood, *American Journal of Public Health* 51 (1961): 1107–1117.

39. W. K. Frankenburg and J. B. Dodds, The Denver Developmental Screening Test, *Journal of Pediatrics* 71 (1967): 181.

40. W. Feldman, P. McGrath, et al., The use of dietary fiber in the management of simple, childhood, idiopathic, recurrent abdominal pain: Results of a prospective, double-blind, randomized, controlled trial, *American Journal of the Diseases of Children* 139 (1985): 1216–1218.

41. C. C. Roy and N. Galeano, Childhood antecedents of adult degenerative disease, *Pediatric Clinics of North America* 32 (1985): 517–533.

42. Epidemiological section of conference on the health effects of blood lipids, Optimal distribution for populations, *Preventive Medicine* 8 (1979): 612–678.

43. M. A. Aukett, et al., Treatment with iron increases weight gain and psychomotor development, *Archives of Diseases of Children* 61 (1986): 849–857.

44. L. Chwang, A. G. Soemantri, and E. Pollitt, Iron supplementation and physical growth of rural Indonesian children, *American Journal of Clinical Nutrition* 47 (1988): 496–501.

45. P. R. Dallman, R. Yip, and C. Johnson, Prevalence and causes of anemia in the United States, 1976 to 1980, *American Journal of Clinical Nutrition* 39 (1984): 437–445.

46. H. J. Nickerson, M. Holubets, et al., Decreased iron stores in high-school female runners, *American Journal of the Diseases of Children* 139 (1985): 1115–1119.

47. R. T. Brown, S. M. McIntosh, et al., Iron status of adolescent female athletes, *Journal of Adolescent Health Care* 6 (1985): 349–352.

48. Declining anemia prevalence among children enrolled in public nutrition and health programs, selected states, 1975–85, *Journal of the American Medical Association* 256 (1986): 2165.

49. J. E. Brown, M. Serdula, et al., Ethnic group differences in nutritional status of low-income children, *American Journal of Clinical Nutrition* 44 (1986): 938–944.

50. J. J. McNamara, M. A. Molot, et al., Coronary artery disease in combat casualties in Vietnam, *Journal of the American Medical Association* 216 (1971): 1185–1187.

51. W. F. Enos, R. H. Holmes, and J. Beyer, Coronary disease among United States soldiers killed in action in Korea, *Journal of the American Medical Association* 152 (1953): 1090–1093.

52. P. O. Kwiterovich, Jr., and K. M. Salz, Pediatric aspects of the new diet–heart hypothesis, in *Infant and Child Feeding* (New York: Academic Press, 1981), 283–313.

53. R. P. Farris, J. L. Cresanta, et al., Dietary studies of children from a biracial population: Intakes of carbohydrate and fiber in 10- and 13-year-olds, *Journal of the American College of Nutrition* 4 (1985): 539–552.

54. American Academy of Pediatrics Committee on Nutrition, Prudent lifestyle for children: Dietary fat and cholesterol, *Pediatrics* 78 (1986): 521–525.

55. G. C. Frank, L. S. Webber, et al., Sodium, potassium, calcium, magnesium, and phosphorus intakes of infants and children: Bogalusa Heart Study, *Journal of the American Dietetic Association* 88 (1988): 801–807.

56. *Nationwide Food Consumption Survey*, Nutrition Monitoring Division, NFCS, CSF11 (Washington, D.C.: U.S. Department of Agriculture, 1988).

57. P. D. S. Vanderkooy and R. S. Gibson, Food consumption patterns of Canadian preschool children in relation to zinc and growth status, *American Journal of Clinical Nutrition* 45 (1987): 609–616.

58. Second National Health and Nutrition Examination Survey (NHANES II), 1976–1980, Centers for Disease Control and the National Center for Health Statistics (Washington, D.C.: Department of Health and Human Services, 1987).

59. A. J. Clark, S. Mossholder, and R. Gates, Folacin status of adolescent females, *American Journal of Clinical Nutrition* 46 (1987): 302–306.

60. R. Marston and N. Raper, Nutrient content of the U.S. food supply, *National Food Review* 5 (1987): 27–33.

61. A. M. Thomson and F. E. Hytten, Psychophysiological aspects of human lactation, in *Infant and Child Feeding* (New York: Academic Press, 1981), 37–46.

62. The use of whole cow's milk in infancy, *Pediatrics* 72 (1983): 253–255.

63. V. A. Beal, Termination of night feeding in infancy, *Journal of Pediatrics* 75 (1969): 690–692.

64. H. Merhav, Y. Amitai, et al., Tea drinking and microcytic anemia in infants, *American Journal of Clinical Nutrition* 41 (1985): 1210–1213.

65. Dietary vitamin A toxicity in infants, *Pediatrics* 65 (1980): 893.

66. S. A. Bock, Prospective appraisal of complaints of adverse reactions to foods in children during the first three years of life, *Pediatrics* 79 (1987): 683–688.

67. S. S. Arnon, T. F. Midura, et al., Honey and other environmental risk factors for infant botulism, *Journal of Pediatrics* 95 (1979): 331.

68. C. S. Harris, S. P. Baker, et al., Childhood asphyxiation by food: A national analysis and overview, *Journal of the American Medical Association* 251 (1984).

69. B. Bolsen, No agreement on diets for "hyperactive" kids, *Journal of the American Medical Association* 247 (1982): 948, 953, 956.

70. Defined diets and childhood hyperactivity: Consensus conference, *Journal of the American Medical Association* 248 (1982): 290–292.

71. *Participation in the National School Lunch Program*, Report to the Chairman of the Senate Committee on Agriculture, Nutrition, and Forestry (Gaithersburg, Md.: U.S. Government Accounting Office, 1985).

72. K. M. Maurer, The national evaluation of the school nutrition programs: Program impact on family food expenditures, *American Journal of Clinical Nutrition* 40 (1984): 448–453.

73. J. Mayer, Social responsibilities of nutritionists, *American Journal of Clinical Nutrition* 42 (1986): 714–717.

74. S. Hanes, J. Bermeersch, and S. Gale, The national evaluation of school nutrition programs: Program impact on dietary intake, *American Journal of Clinical Nutrition* 40 (1984): 390–413.

75. W. A. Johnson and J. R. Jensen, Influence of noon meal on nutrient intakes and meal patterns of selected fifth-grade children, *Journal of the American Dietetic Association* 84 (1984): 919–923.

76. *Nutrition Week*, 18 September 1986, 4–5.

CHAPTER ·16·

NUTRITION FOR ADULTHOOD

The health advantages of eating wisely continue on into adulthood. The focus on nutrition, however, changes from promoting growth and development to maintaining health. Good nutrition during the adult years helps to prevent and postpone the development of disease and helps to ensure a long, active, and healthy life.

People are generally considered "adults" when they reach the age of 18, regardless of whether they have stopped growing or not. Young adulthood is accompanied by major changes in lifestyle and responsibilities. People then have complete freedom to decide what to purchase, prepare, and eat. In addition, it is the phase in the life cycle when most people assume responsibility for the care and feeding of others.

Some people have their own definitions for age ranges. For example, "'Old' is any age beyond my own."

Four subgroups of adults have been defined: young, middle-aged, old, and very old adults. Age ranges have been arbitrarily assigned to each group: *young* adults are those between the ages of 18 and 35; *middle-aged*

The titles of popular books express the nutrition concerns of adults.

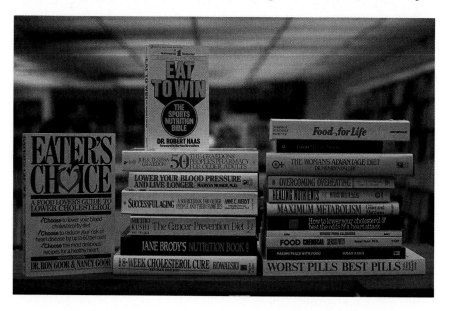

adults, those between 35 and 65; *old* adults, those between 65 and 80; and *very old* adults, those that are over 80 years of age. For adults of all ages, however, physical status is a far better indicator of health status than is age.

The cumulative effects of poor diets and other lifestyle factors on health tend to emerge during adulthood as specific disease states. One doctor states it this way: "After fifty, it's all fix, fix, fix!" As this chapter will explain, it may not have to be that way. Most health problems that occur with age are not inevitable results of aging; they are the result of disease processes that influence physical health.

A range of topics related to nutrition and health during the adult years is presented in this chapter. The importance of these topics is placed in perspective in the initial discussion of the aging of the U.S. population. Relationships among nutrition, health, and longevity are explored, and the characteristics of desirable diets for adults are presented. The topic of food safety is addressed, too, because it represents an important area of particular concern to adults. The chapter ends with some thought-provoking excerpts from a lecture on nutrition delivered by a renowned authority.

THE "GRAYING" OF AMERICA

Attention to the roles of nutrition in maintaining health during the adult years is increasing due to the growing proportion of old and very old adults in the U.S. Whereas only one-fourth of the U.S. population is 18 years old or younger, 12% are 65 years and older (Figure 16-1), and the age group of 74 to 85 years is now the most rapidly growing age segment in the U.S. These figures represent a dramatic shift from 1900, when only 4% of the U.S. population lived beyond the age of 65. It is estimated that by the year 2030, when the current generation of 25- to 34-year-olds enters the old-age range, 25% of the population will be 65 or older (Figure 16-2).[1] The number of people reaching the age of 100 also is growing rapidly.

In 1970, about 7,000 U.S. citizens had attained the age of 100. By 1985, the number had increased to about 25,000.

The "graying" of America can be seen in life-expectancy statistics. In 1900, the average life span of both males and females in the U.S. was about 47 years. Today it is 75 years, but there is a gender gap in life expectancy. Life expectancy for females is now about 78 years, and for males it is about

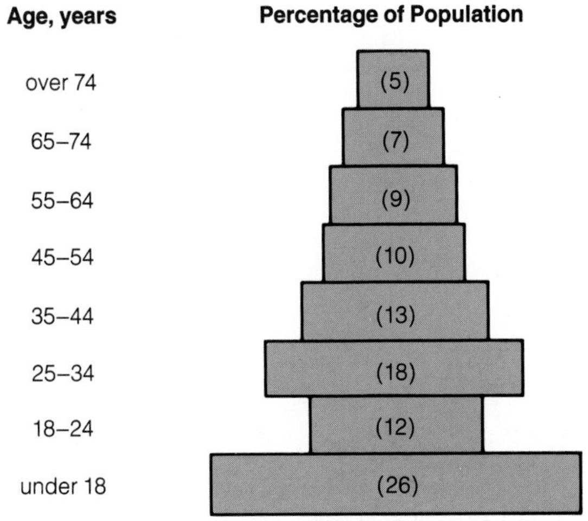

FIGURE 16-1
Age distribution of the U.S. population, 1980 census.

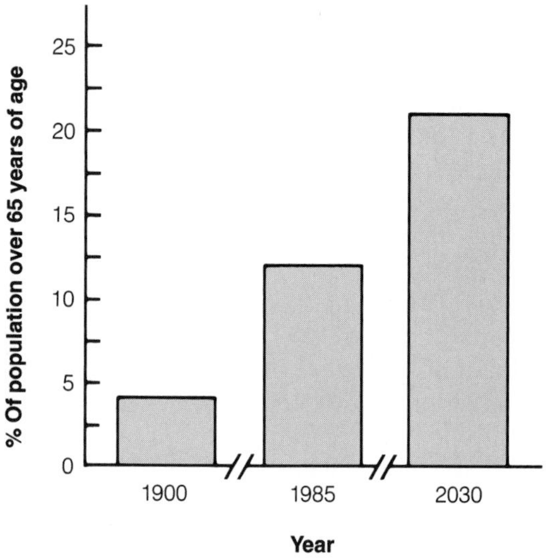

FIGURE 16-2
The "graying" of the U.S. population.

71 years. Females tend to outlive males in countries that enjoy relatively long life expectancies (Table 16-1). The gender difference in average life span in the U.S. appears to be largely related to behaviors. U.S. males tend to smoke more and consume more alcoholic beverages and to pay less attention to what they eat and seek medical care less often than do females.[2]

Factors affecting Life Expectancy

Most of the gains in life expectancy in the U.S. are attributable to improvements in infant health. In 1900, 1 out of 10 newborns died in the first year of life; today the proportion is 1 in 100. Infant health has improved primarily because of widespread advances in housing, nutrition, sanitation, and hygiene.[3,4] These environmental improvements led to the control of many infectious diseases that had caused most infant deaths. The provision of an inexpensive supply of uncontaminated milk in New York City, for example, played a major role in reducing the city's very high rate of infant deaths in

TABLE 16-1
Life expectancies in selected countries, 1986

Average Life Expectancy			
Females		Males	
Switzerland	80.8	Japan	74.8
Japan	80.7	Switzerland	73.8
Iceland	80.6	Iceland	73.8
Netherlands	79.8	Israel	73.1
Norway	79.8	Netherlands	73.0
Australia	79.0	Norway	72.8
United States	78.4	Australia	72.2
West Germany	78.1	West Germany	71.3
Hungary	73.3	United States	70.9

BOX 16-1

MILK DEPOTS

The first "milk depot" was opened in 1893 in New York City through the philanthropy of Nathan Straus, the owner of Macy's department store. By 1917, eight depots were open year-round and eighteen were open only during the summer, when milk tended to spoil more quickly. These depots served as the prototype for depots in 127 other cities in the United States and in many foreign countries. Activities such as this that help to control the spread of infectious diseases have a large impact on increasing life expectancy in a population.

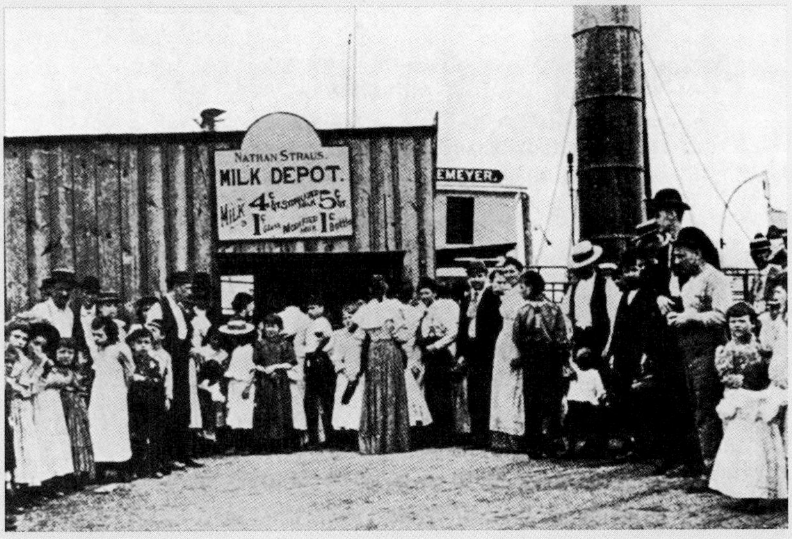

the early 1900s (Box 16-1). The consumption of milk containing bacteria that caused tuberculosis and other infectious diseases combined with undernutrition constituted a major threat to infant health.

The discovery and mass use of vaccines that prevented common infectious diseases such as pertussis ("whooping cough"), diphtheria, and tetanus contributed to reductions in infant and child deaths starting about 1930. Medical advances in treatments and surgery have improved the quality of life for many people but have added only a few years to life expectancy in the U.S.[4]

A person's genetic background has an effect on longevity, but it is relatively small in comparison with the effects of environmental factors. Life insurance company statistics reveal that children of long-lived parents have a greater life expectancy than do children of short-lived parents. The advantage amounts to an additional three years.[3] Since no one has the opportunity to select his or her parents, it is perhaps fortunate that environmental factors generally are more important than genetic background in determining life expectancy.

Heart disease, cancer, and stroke are the major causes of death in adults. They are diseases that are linked to lifestyles. Future gains in life expectancy and health will likely follow widespread changes in diet, smoking,

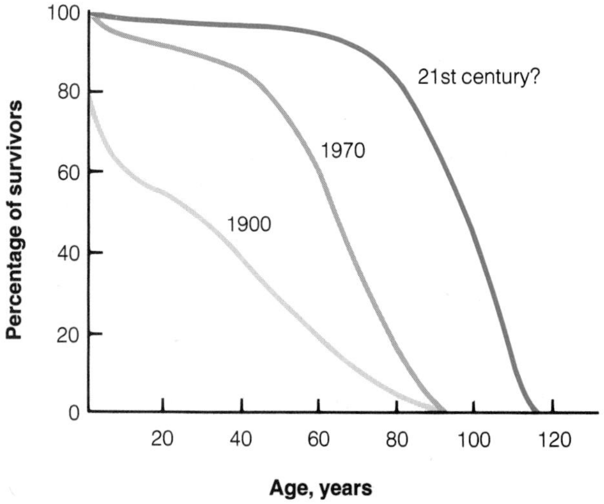

FIGURE 16-3
Survival curves for U.S. males in 1900 and 1970, and a projection for the next century.

physical activity, weight control, and other behaviors associated with the development of chronic diseases.[5] In the next century, normal life expectancy may increase to 85 to 110 years.[6] Figure 16-3 reports the increase in male life expectancy in the U.S. since 1900 and a projection for the future.

Health-enhancing changes in lifestyle habits are generally thought to be beneficial for both women and men, although the risk factors for disease development appear to vary by gender.[7,8] Some of the identified gender differences in heart disease risk factors are listed in Table 16-2. It is expected that more gender-based nutrition risk factors for chronic diseases will be identified.

"Pockets" of people in the world who appear to live well into very old age have been identified. Three of these populations have been studied to determine the secrets of long life. Some fascinating results of the studies are presented in Box 16-2.

Diet and Life Expectancy in Laboratory Animals

Dietary factors associated with longevity have been studied extensively in laboratory animals. Although the results of the studies are not directly applicable to humans, they provide insights into what some of the specific dietary factors of importance may be.

TABLE 16-2
Risk factors for heart disease by gender[7,8]

Risk Factors for Heart Disease	
Females	**Males**
diabetes	elevated blood cholesterol
hypertension	hypertension
obesity	smoking
smoking	family history of heart disease
family history of heart disease	

BOX 16-2

LIFESTYLES OF THE OLD AND HEALTHY

Three communities in the world have been identified where more than an expected number of people live to a very old age.[3,9] The people in the communities share a number of characteristics: (1) they live in isolated, mountainous areas and make their living farming, (2) they lead physically active lives and tend to be slightly underweight, and (3) they maintain close family ties. Many of the old people in these communities drink wine or other spirits, and some use tobacco. All have diets that consist primarily of foods grown on local farms.

The three communities studied are located in mountainous areas of Ecuador, the Soviet Union, and Pakistan. Life is reported to be tranquil and primitive. Throughout their lives, these peoples work hard physically as they farm the mountain slopes. They seem to play hard occasionally, too, at all-night feasts and parties. Reportedly, it is not uncommon for people to live 100 years or more and to remain healthy, physically active, and mentally alert. The oldest ages attained by people in the communities are reported to be 121 and 140 years for two men.[3]

One of the communities studied is Abkhazia on the eastern shore of the Black Sea in Soviet Georgia (see map). Many nationalities are represented among the Abkhazians, so no one set of genes pervades the population. There is a higher percentage of long-lived people in this mountainous area than on the coastal plain below it. People in Abkhazia are half as likely to have atherosclerosis ("hardening of the arteries," a precursor to heart attack or stroke) than are people who live below them on the coast.[3] Their diets consist of a variety of foods, and include meat, dairy products, vegetables in large amounts, breads, pastries, and some sweets. They also eat yogurt and other soured dairy products regularly. About 18% to 27% of the caloric intakes of the Abkhazians are from fat. Blood cholesterol levels tend to be low and not to increase with age. Their protein intake of 70 to 90 grams per day is ample.[3]

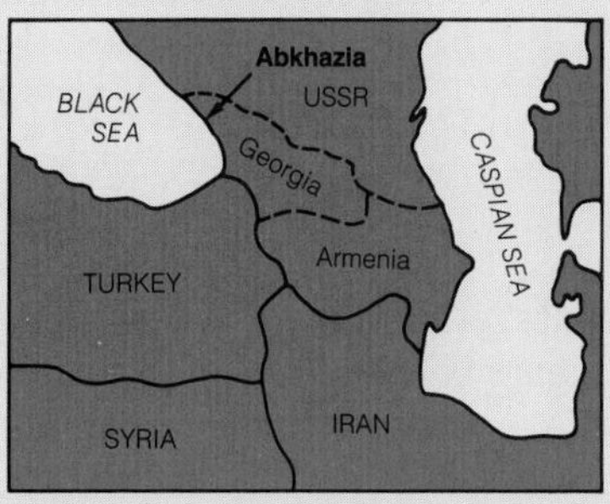

Studies of the genetic and lifestyle backgrounds of long-lived people in these communities have led researchers to conclude that vigorous physical activity, low-fat diets, and the prevention of overweight may be key factors of longevity.

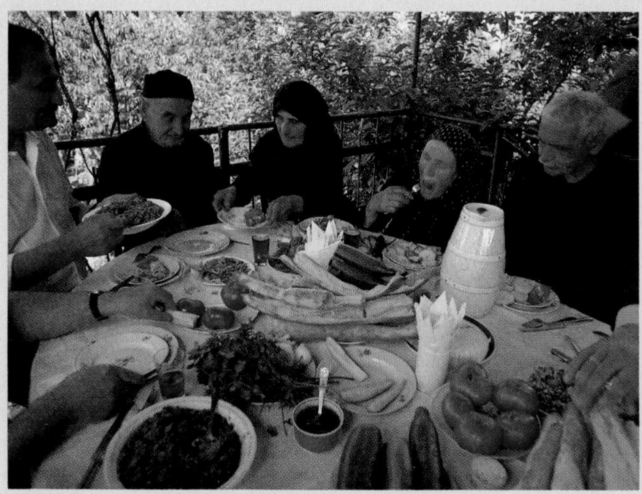

Abkhazian meals include many vegetables.

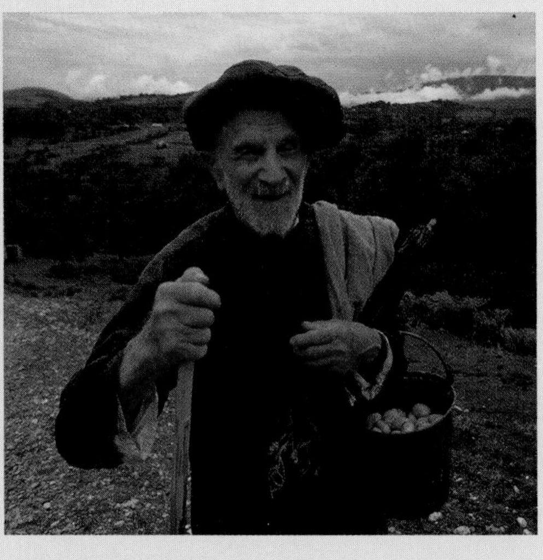

An Abkhazian centenarian harvests potatoes.

Underfeeding mice, rats, and other laboratory animals during pregnancy and early in life shortens life expectancy, whereas underfeeding mature animals appears to prolong life.[10,11] Feeding adult laboratory rats 70% of the amount of food normally eaten by adult rats is associated with a doubled life expectancy.[11] These results have been widely used to support the thinking that low-calorie diets and underweight prolong life. The effectiveness of low-calorie diets and underweight in prolonging *human* life have not been demonstrated, although it appears that people who are slightly underweight tend to live longer than people who are very underweight or overweight.[12]

There is more to the story about diet and longevity in laboratory animals. The main idea of the rest of the story is that diets that promote growth and development are different from the diets that appear to promote longevity.[10] Underfeeding young rats increases the rate of early death and causes growth stunting, impaired functional and behavioral development, and an increased susceptibility to certain types of disease.[11] Although underfed adult rats tend to live longer, it is not known if they live *better*. Are they more susceptible to diseases that do not lead to death? Do they exhibit the same level of strength and stamina as rats that are allowed to feed freely, or do they limit their activity to conserve their energy? It's hard to measure the quality of life of laboratory rats. As for humans, however, how well one lives may be as important as how long.

NUTRITION AND ADULT HEALTH

The centerpiece of attention in the area of nutrition and health during the adult years is the cumulative effects of diet on chronic, rather than infectious disease development. (Only one infectious disease in the U.S. is of mounting concern, and that disease is AIDS. Box 16-3 discusses some nutrition implications for AIDS treatment.) For the most part, relationships between nutrition and health in adults can be viewed as elongating chains that represent the accumulation of problems over time. Each link that is added to the chain increases the risk that a disease will develop. The presence of a disease can indicate that the "chain" has gotten "too long"—that the accumulation of problems is sufficient to interfere noticeably with the normal functions of cells and tissues.

It appears that the length of the "chain" can be shortened if dietary and other behaviors improve. It is clear, for example, that correcting obesity during the young adult or middle adult years helps to lengthen life expectancy.[12] It is also known that reducing saturated fat intake slows or halts the continued development of hardening of the arteries (atherosclerosis) in some people and that it may reduce the amount of plaque contained in the walls of arteries.[16] Maintaining an adequate level of calcium intake during the adult years may decrease bone loss and help prevent or postpone the development of osteoporosis.[17] The health status of adults is not necessarily "fixed" by age; it can change for the better or the worse, or it may not change at all.[18]

Since nutrition exerts its effects on chronic disease development over time, chronic diseases related to poor dietary habits are most likely to

emerge in older adults. The occurrence of diseases related to environmental factors such as smoking, physical inactivity, and obesity also increases among older people. In addition to the accumulation of the health effects of environmental exposures, people age biologically. The combined effects of poor diets, risky lifestyle behaviors, and biological aging may increase the rates of serious disease in adults. Nearly 80% of people 65 years and older have one or more chronic conditions.[19] How soon a disease develops largely depends on the intensity and duration of exposure to the environmental factors that contribute to it. These environmental factors also affect the progress of the biological aging processes.

Aging Is Not a Disease

Aging is a normal process, not a disease. Processes involved in normal aging do not cause diseases; rather they produce changes that make people more susceptible to diseases.[20,21] Biological processes related to normal aging that may contribute to disease development include reductions in muscle and bone mass, the development of fragile cell membranes, and changes in the levels of some hormones.[22] For a woman, aging brings the hormonal changes that accompany **menopause**, the cessation of her ability to reproduce.

menopause: The period of a woman's life when ability to reproduce stops. Menopause generally occurs around the age of 50 and is accompanied by changes in the level of sex hormones the body produces.

Secondary Malnutrition and Adult Health

Malnutrition may also influence the short-term health of adults, and it may or may not be related to dietary intake. Primary and secondary malnutrition were discussed in chapter 2 in the explanation of the eleven principles of

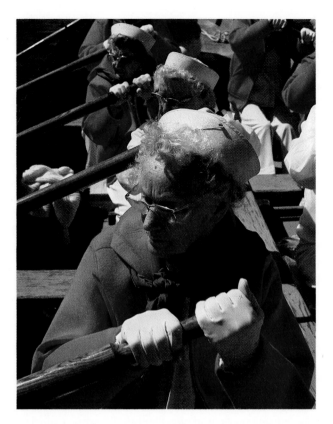

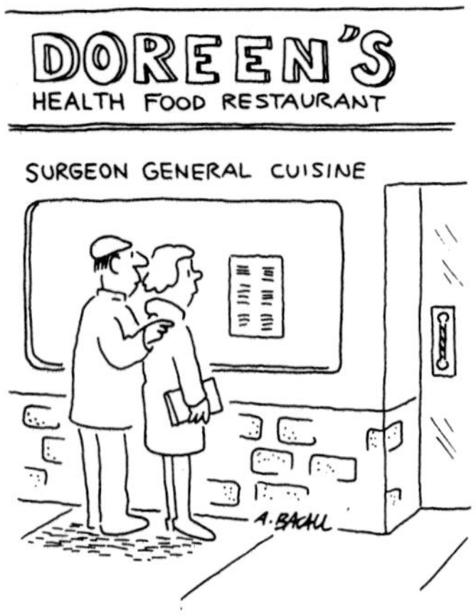
DOREEN'S
HEALTH FOOD RESTAURANT
SURGEON GENERAL CUISINE

From *The Wall Street Journal*—Permission, Cartoon Features Syndicate.

nutrition. Some common health problems of older adults such as obesity, heart disease, hypertension, certain types of cancer, and osteoporosis are thought to be directly related to people's usual diets. As such, they represent *primary malnutrition.*

Other nutritional problems result from *secondary malnutrition*—malnutrition that is not directly related to diet. Secondary malnutrition in older adults often results from illnesses and medications that interfere with nutrient absorption or utilization. Diuretics, for example, are used in treating hypertension and are the number-one drug prescribed to adults. They may cause potassium deficiency and elevated blood cholesterol levels.[23] Antibiotics given to treat infections and some anticancer drugs decrease the absorption and utilization of certain vitamins and minerals. Diseases of the gastrointestinal tract also can interfere with digestion and nutrient absorption. Secondary malnutrition is a common cause of nutrient deficiencies in older adults. Adequate dietary intakes through diets or supplements may not prevent nutrient deficiencies from developing in older adults with health problems because of secondary causes of malnutrition.[24]

NUTRIENT REQUIREMENTS DURING ADULTHOOD

The biologic processes and lifestyle changes that generally accompany aging affect the caloric and nutrient needs of adults. Caloric needs generally decrease with age during the adult years because of decreases in physical activity levels, muscle mass, and basal metabolic rates. Caloric intakes generally decline as well.[25,26] U.S. men and women over the age of 65 have respective average caloric intakes of 1,650 and 1,250 calories per day.[25,26] These levels would represent calorie-restricted diets in childhood or young adulthood. Caloric need, muscle mass, and basal metabolic rates remain higher, however, for men and women who are physically active.

While caloric needs decrease, the need for certain nutrients such as protein,[27] vitamin C,[28] vitamin D,[29] and calcium[30] may increase through the adult years. The increased need for protein appears to be a result of a decreased efficiency of protein utilization by the body.[27] Dietary requirements for vitamin C and calcium may increase due to the decrease in stomach acidity that often occurs with age. Decreased stomach acidity reduces the amounts of vitamin C and calcium that are absorbed from food or supplements.

Lactose intolerance also appears to occur more commonly as people age. The inability to digest the lactose in milk may cause many older adults to decrease their consumption of milk.[31] It is estimated that more than 80% of adult women and 50% of adult men fail to consume the RDA for calcium.[32]

Decreased consumption of milk also reduces vitamin D intake.[31] Since people over the age of 65 produce about half as much vitamin D in their skin as do younger adults from the same amount of exposure to sunshine, it is easier for older adults to become vitamin-D deficient when their intakes are inadequate.[29] It is estimated that 15% of the elderly may be vitamin-D deficient.[33]

Dietary fiber intake may also represent a problem area in adults. Although there is no RDA for fiber, it is generally thought that an intake of 25 grams per day helps prevent constipation and perhaps colon cancer in adults. The dietary fiber intake of U.S. adults tends to fall well below this amount.[1]

The RDAs for adults are primarily based on research with young adult males. Therefore, the RDAs for older adult males and all adult females are only rough estimates of adequate nutrient intake levels. Much remains to be learned about optimal nutrient intake levels for adults of all ages. The nutrient needs of older Americans are receiving more attention as the baby boom becomes the "senior boom" and as more attention is paid to improving the health of the elderly.

Good Diets for Adults

The RDAs and "Dietary Guidelines for Americans" serve as the standards for judging the adequacy of adults' diets. The best diet for adults appears to be one that contains a wide variety of basic foods and provides 30% of total calories from fat, 15% of calories from protein, and 55% of calories from carbohydrates, mainly complex carbohydrates.[1] Furthermore, unsaturated fats from vegetable sources should be the primary type of fat in the diet, and cholesterol intake should be kept below 300 mg per day. A balanced and adequate diet can be obtained by judiciously selecting at least the minimum number of foods from the basic food groups; see Table 16-3. It is important to select *judiciously* because not all foods within the respective food groups are equally desirable. Food choices should emphasize the low-fat, -cholesterol, and -sodium and the high-fiber members of the food groups. Once the minimum numbers of servings from each food group are in the diet, remaining caloric needs can be met by adding servings from the various groups.

Altering food habits in favor of healthy diets appears to be common among adults of all ages. A study of 100 women and men over the age of 60 found that 100% had made some change in their food choices in the recent past. The changes had been for health, taste, convenience, and social reasons.[34] Clearly, a person's food choices and intake levels (as well as preferences) change throughout life, and the changes can be for the better.

TABLE 16-3
Food group recommendations for adults*

Food Group	Minimum Number of Servings per Day
Breads and cereals	4
Vegetables and fruits	(4)
vitamin A-rich	1
vitamin B-rich	1
other	2
Milk and milk products	2–4**
Meats or alternates	2
Miscellaneous	Based on caloric need

*For additional information on the foods contained in each food group and standard serving sizes, refer to Table 2-6.
**Women may benefit from more than 2 servings of milk and milk products. Four servings of low-fat milk and milk products per day may foster bone health.

Box 16-3

NUTRITION AND AIDS

Black plague, typhoid fever, typhus, small pox, tuberculosis, syphilis—epidemics of deadly diseases have been a fact of life for humans throughout history. Most epidemics of infectious diseases have been conquered when their spread has been brought under control through improved sanitation, nutrition, vaccines, and medical treatments. There is one infectious disease that is yet to be conquered. It is AIDS (acquired immunodeficiency syndrome). Only recognized and labeled as a disease syndrome in 1981, AIDS has already reached epidemic proportions in the U.S., Haiti, Central Africa, and other countries. The Centers for Disease Control in Atlanta, Georgia, predict that more than 300,000 cases of AIDS will exist in the U.S. in 1991. Many more people than that, perhaps two million, will be infected with the human immunodeficiency virus (HIV) and at risk of developing AIDS. About 72% of U.S. victims of the disease are homosexual males, and about 20% are intravenous drug users. Most of the remainder of the victims are persons who have received blood transfusions, heterosexual partners of drug users, and babies born to infected mothers.

AIDS is not one disease; it represents a collection of different diseases. People with AIDS develop a number of diseases because of the underlying problem characteristic of all cases of AIDS: the loss of a key component of the body's immune system. HIV, the virus that initiates AIDS, attacks and destroys cells involved in protecting the body from various diseases. Without this key component of the body's immune system in place, infectious diseases and certain types of cancer are able to spread freely. They spread faster than they can be controlled by current medical treatments.

Certain drugs and treatments may prolong the lives and decrease the suffering of AIDS victims, but a vaccine or other type of cure for AIDS is yet to be discovered. It is estimated that if the epidemic is not controlled, the cost of caring for AIDS patients in the U.S. will be 14 billion dollars per year in 1991. No country can afford such a cost. The hope for the control of AIDS lies in its prevention. That's where nutrition may come in.

It has been observed that not all people who test positive for HIV develop AIDS. Why this is so is not known, but the answer is very important if AIDS is to be controlled worldwide. Nutrients play essential roles in the function of the immune system, and differences in nutritional status may represent an important factor in resistance to AIDS. Zinc deficiency and protein–calorie malnutrition are known to produce a reversible form of an immunodeficiency disease that is less severe but otherwise much like AIDS.[13] Zinc supplements appear to improve immune-system functions in AIDS patients.[14] Adequate calories and protein may support the body's ability to control the spread of infection and improve a patient's level of comfort and strength.[15] Although very low blood levels of zinc and protein–calorie malnutrition occur with AIDS, it is not clear if they are involved in its development.[13]

Nutritional therapy is a key component in the treatment of AIDS. Infected individuals who avoid losing weight rapidly appear to respond better to medical treatments and therefore may live longer than patients who are undernourished. Because the appetites of people with AIDS are generally poor, and because the diarrhea that often accompanies AIDS reduces nutrient absorption, maintaining adequate levels of nutrients is difficult. The three-day food record shown in the table

Nutrition Programs for Older Adults

Many older adults find it difficult to prepare and consume well-balanced meals, and their health may suffer because of it. Many elderly people live alone, no longer drive, and are no longer able to shop for or prepare foods. Some of these elderly people become stuck in the rut of "tea and toast" diets.

Recognition of the problems faced by many older persons in purchasing food and preparing good meals led to the establishment of the Nutrition Program for Older Americans in 1973. The purpose of the program is to help keep seniors—defined as people aged 60 and over for this program—healthy and independent by providing them with complete, nutritious meals at their homes or at congregate dining sites. Services provided by the represents the diet of an AIDS patient who, under the guidance of a registered dietitian, was making an effort to gain weight and improve his nutritional status. Although 5′10″ tall, this 35-year-old male weighed only 90 pounds and was in a state of protein–calorie malnutrition. He was thin before he developed AIDS, weighing only 135 pounds. His intake of 1,350 calories per day was low, but not low enough to account for the large amount of weight he had lost. Additionally, his protein intake was adequate for a healthy male. The malabsorption of nutrients and the increased caloric and protein needs that result from infections and fever contributed to his poor nutritional status.

Much more may be known about the role of nutrition in preventing and treating AIDS by the time you read this. Knowledge is expanding rapidly, but there is still a great deal to learn about AIDS.

Three-day food record of the AIDS patient

Day 1	Day 2	Day 3
raisin bran, 1 oz	scrambled egg, 1	toast, 1 slice
Ensure®, 1 c*	sausage links, 2	cream cheese, 1 T
cheese, ½ oz	toast, 1 slice	jam, 1 t
crackers, 4	margarine, 1 t	tuna–noodle casserole, ¼ c
banana bread, 2 slices	chicken, 1½ oz	sirloin steak, 4 oz
margarine, 1 t	corn, ½ c	baked potato, 1
fruit cocktail, ¾ c	coleslaw, ¾ c	mixed vegetables, ½ c
beef stew, 1½ c	beets, ½ c	whole-wheat bread, 1 slice
green salad, 1½ c	potatoes, ½ c	butter, 1 t
cream pie, 1 slice	ice cream bar, 1	Ensure, 1 c
		cookies, 4

Food Constituent Analysis

	Amount	Percentage of RDA
Calories	1,350	50
Protein	52 g	93
Zinc	10 mg	67

Most other nutrients were contained in low amounts due to the low caloric intake.

*Ensure is a commercially available, nutrient-dense food product used for nutritional rehabilitation.

program include home-delivery of meals (often called "Meals on Wheels" or "Mobile Meals") and congregate meals in community settings such as churches and schools. Together with the Food Stamp Program, home-delivered meals and congregate dining serve more than two million older U.S. adults each year.

Vitamin and Mineral Supplements

Adults in general tend to be heavy users of vitamin and mineral supplements, although it is observed that the adults who least need them are most likely to take them.[35] About 45% of adult men and 55% of women take at least one vitamin or mineral supplement at least occasionally.[35] The use of

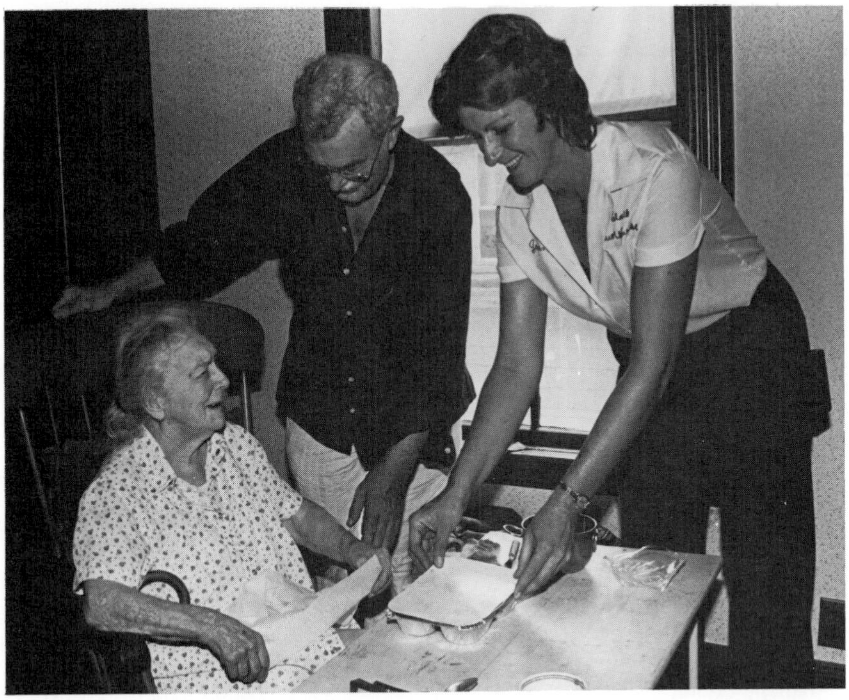

A Meals on Wheels delivery.

megadoses of supplements is of most concern because of the toxicity diseases that can result and because they may be used inappropriately to treat diseases. Because regular use of vitamin and mineral supplements can be expensive, it causes a financial strain for some elderly persons who have little money.

FOOD SAFETY

food poisoning: An imprecise term for an illness resulting from ingestion of foods containing a harmful substance such as bacteria, a bacterial toxin, a poisonous insecticide, or a toxic material such as mercury or lead.

Concern for the safety of the food supply ranks high on the list of nutrition concerns of adults. The primary concern with regard to food safety is avoiding **food poisoning**. It is estimated that two million cases of food poisoning occur in the U.S. each year and that many more cases go undiagnosed. (Some illnesses such as stomach flu are mislabeled as food poisoning.)

Bacterial Infections

Food poisoning is generally thought of as what happens when you eat "spoiled" food. Ingesting food that has been contaminated with bacteria causes an upset stomach, vomiting, and/or diarrhea. The effects can be serious if they occur in adults who already have digestive-system problems or who are in frail health.

Most cases of food poisoning caused by eating spoiled foods can be prevented by handling and storing food properly and by paying attention to expiration dates printed on food labels. Foods are most likely to become contaminated after they have been removed from their packaging and handled. Handling foods with clean hands and utensils on clean surfaces reduces the amount of bacteria that come in contact with the food.

Some types of food spoil more quickly than do others, so particular care needs to be taken when handling and storing them. Dairy products such as milk and cheese may spoil in about a week if they are contaminated with germs from the air or hands. For example, if you hold cheese in its wrapper when you take it out of the refrigerator to cut a slice, it is not as likely to spoil as if you take it completely out of its packaging and hold it in your hands. The same is true for other foods that spoil easily.

If a food smells or looks unusual, it should not be eaten. The general rule that "when in doubt, throw it out" should be applied. One of the most effective ways to prevent foods from spoiling is to store, prepare, and serve them at the proper temperatures; see Figure 16-4. Few types of bacteria grow at temperatures above 170°F or below 40°F. When foods are "held" before serving, hot foods should be kept hot, and cold foods cold. Freezing foods

Two key food safety tips:
When in doubt, throw it out.
Serve hot foods hot and cold foods cold.

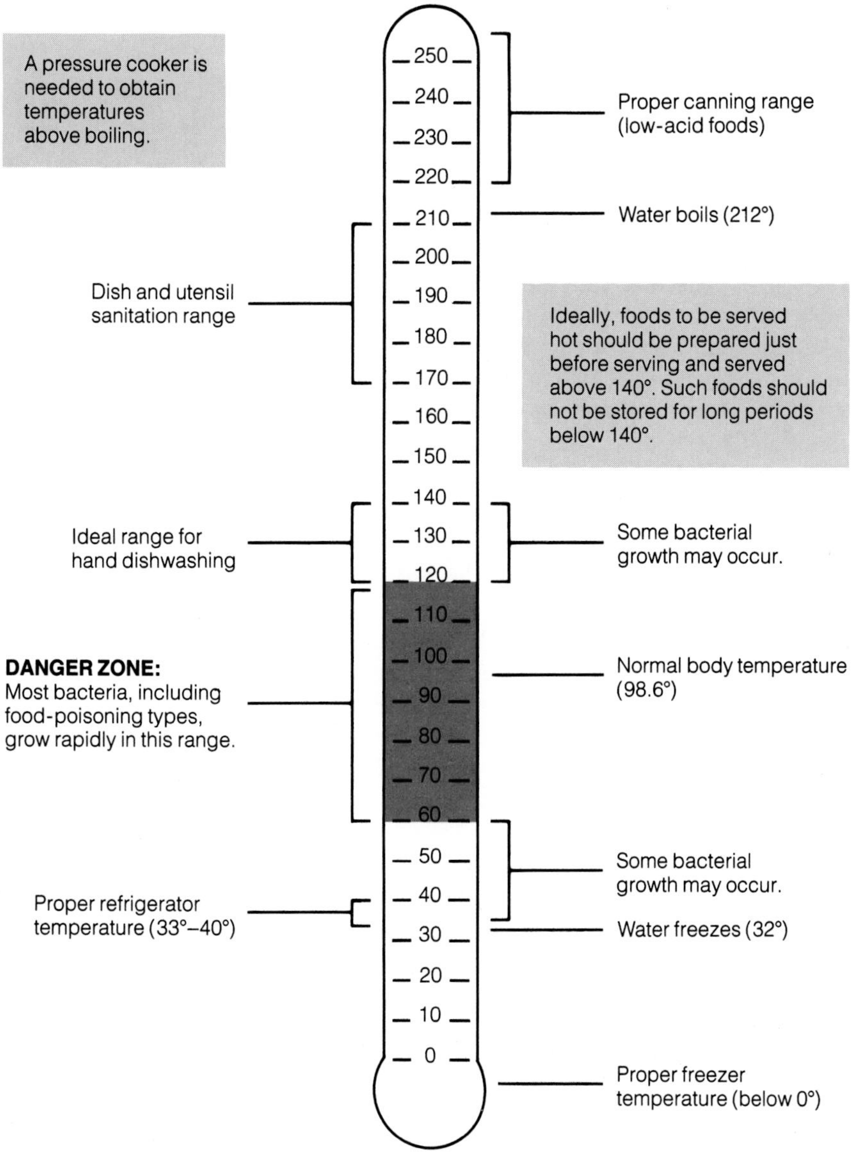
A pressure cooker is needed to obtain temperatures above boiling.
250
240
230
220
210
200
190
180
170
160
150
140
130
120
110
100
90
80
70
60
50
40
30
20
10
0
Proper canning range (low-acid foods)
Water boils (212°)
Dish and utensil sanitation range
Ideally, foods to be served hot should be prepared just before serving and served above 140°. Such foods should not be stored for long periods below 140°.
Ideal range for hand dishwashing
Some bacterial growth may occur.
DANGER ZONE: Most bacteria, including food-poisoning types, grow rapidly in this range.
Normal body temperature (98.6°)
Some bacterial growth may occur.
Proper refrigerator temperature (33°–40°)
Water freezes (32°)
Proper freezer temperature (below 0°)

FIGURE 16-4
Temperature guide for safe food; all temperatures °F.

halts the growth of bacteria that commonly contaminate foods. Once foods are thawed, however, bacterial growth may resume, and foods can become contaminated while they are thawing.

The range of temperature most conducive to bacterial growth is 60°F to 120°F. Because the room temperature of most homes is comfortably within this range, foods that tend to spoil should not be stored outside of the refrigerator or freezer or left out longer than necessary.

Commercially canned foods are generally heated to the point where all bacteria are killed after the can is sealed. Consequently, canned foods are sterile, and most can be safely stored unopened for years. Canned foods spoil if the can develops a pinhole leak or if errors made during the canning process allowed bacteria to enter the food. An indication of spoilage is a bulging of the top of the can caused by a buildup of pressure inside the can. The buildup of pressure may have resulted from bacteria that cause botulism, and the food should not be used.

An Example: Salmonella Poisoning Eating foods that are contaminated with salmonella bacteria can lead to serious health problems. Salmonella poisoning is commonly responsible for the Memorial Day picnic-type outbreaks of food poisoning. In the Northeastern United States alone, more than 2,000 cases of sickness and 11 deaths due to the ingestion of food contaminated with salmonella were reported in the 18-month period ending July 30, 1987.[36] Two-thirds of the cases were due to eating eggs that had been contaminated with salmonella bacteria.

Salmonella bacteria can cling to the outside of dirty egg shells or grow inside of eggs if hens that lay them are infected with the bacteria.[36] The best ways to prevent salmonella infection are to wash dirty eggs before using them and hands after touching them, to clean thoroughly all surfaces and equipment that came into contact with the eggs before they were cooked, and not to eat raw or undercooked eggs. Keeping potato, macaroni, and other salads that contain eggs cold will prevent the bacteria from growing.

Other Kinds of Food Poisoning

Food poisoning can be caused by substances in food other than bacteria. Other kinds of food poisoning can result from eating certain types of mushrooms, shellfish, and foods contaminated with mercury, lead, and various other toxic substances. Unlike bacterial infections, toxic substances in foods are not destroyed by high temperatures, and they cannot be removed by thoroughly cleaning the food.

The ingestion of foods containing unusually high amounts of herbicides or pesticides has also led to outbreaks of food poisoning. Rinsing fruits and vegetables with water (and washing them with soapy water if needed to remove dirt and other particles or coatings) removes most of the chemical residues on produce. The use of "organically" grown foods may reduce the risk of exposure to pesticides and herbicides, although the "organic" label does not guarantee that a product is pesticide- or herbicide-free. As states implement regulations on the use of the term *organically grown*, it will be more likely that foods labeled as such are indeed free of pesticides and herbicides.

The safety of food additives such as nitrates and preservatives and of other potentially toxic substances in foods was addressed in chapter 2, and Table 2-4 summarizes the discussion of potential toxicants.

■ ■ ■

EPILOGUE

This final chapter of the book has addressed a number of nutrition issues of importance to adults. Because it is likely that most readers of this book are adults, we end the discussion on a topic that is, or will become, important to every adult. That topic is how nutrition can help a person to achieve life-long weight control and vigorous health.

Excerpts from a Nutrition Lecture

Dr. Helmit Schmidt, Head of Obesity Research at the Max Plank Institute in Helsinki, delivered a lecture and shared the results of his research with an audience of more than 2,000 people at a convention in Rochester, Minnesota—the home of the prestigious Mayo Clinic. He reported research that identified a way of taking advantage of normal metabolic processes of the body in order to combat overweight and increase energy levels. As is the case for so many complex problems facing humankind, the solution that Dr. Schmidt identified is simple. It rests in a person's ability to increase the rate at which energy is produced from the carbohydrates, proteins, and fats contained in foods; that is, as more energy is produced, more calories are expended and less energy is stored. The net results are weight loss and increased energy levels. The metabolic key lies in the citric acid cycle, where **acetyl CoA**—broken-down bits of carbohydrates, proteins, and fats—enters this energy-formation pathway. Acetyl CoA is a derivative of acetic acid, a primary component of vinegar. Dr. Schmidt has found that when people consume vinegar, its acetic acid goes directly to the citric acid cycle and speeds up energy formation, and that the more vinegar a person consumes, the more rapidly the body produces energy.

acetyl CoA: (Latin *acetum*, "vinegar"; *CoA* abbreviates *coenzyme A*, a derivative of pantothenic acid) A molecule comprised of 2 atoms of carbon, 3 of hydrogen, 1 of oxygen, and coenzyme A. It is the first substance that enters the citric acid cycle. (See Appendix E.)

In Schmidt's studies, people consuming 4,000 calories a day have lost weight when they included two tablespoons or more of vinegar with each meal or snack. People who stuck with the vinegar regime—in spite of their dislike for the taste of the vinegar—lost weight, ate what they wanted, and had energy to spare.[37]

Dr. Schmidt's research has extended to include the effects on energy metabolism of consuming honey with the vinegar. The breakdown products of honey also enter the citric acid cycle rapidly and they further increase the rate at which energy is formed.[38]

Back to Reality

Does Dr. Schmidt's story sound too good to be true? It should, because it's *not* true! We offer this example to make a final point. Think critically about what you hear and read about nutrition. Investigate the information further. Peddlers of nutrition nonsense do not have to be right; they just attempt to be convincing. Who is Dr. Schmidt? Where were his results published? Has any other researcher found the same results? Is he proposing an easy solution to a tough problem for which there is no accepted, simple treatment? Vinegar and honey diets have been touted for centuries. The notion is still around because it can be *sold*.

So Where Do We Go from Here?

You now have a foundation of knowledge about human nutrition. Like any foundation, it is just the beginning. The finishing work will take continued study. As sure as the sun sets and rises, some of the diet and health relationships explained in this book will be modified, and new, important relationships will be identified. The science principles we have discussed will serve you as a base of knowledge because they will change very little with time. These principles will help you recognize the changing horizons of the human nutrition frontiers as they appear. To remain informed, stay tuned in and scrutinize your sources of nutrition information carefully. Most of all, keep up your healthy interest in nutrition.

REVIEW QUESTIONS

1. What is the fastest growing age segment of the U.S. population?
2. Life expectancy for males in the U.S. is ____ years, and for females it is ____ years.
3. Most of the gain in life expectancy for women and men in the U.S. has been due to improvements in ________.
4. Cite two major factors responsible for improvements in infant health and survival since the turn of the century.
5. What are the three major causes of death in adults?
6. List a key nutrition risk factor for each of the three major causes of death in adults.
7. Future gains in life expectancy in the U.S. will likely follow widespread improvements in ________, ________, ________, and other behaviors associated with the development of chronic disease.
8. Adults in which weight-status category tend to live the longest: very underweight, slightly underweight, normal weight, or overweight?
9. Based on studies of people who live long lives, three lifestyle factors appear to be significant. What are they?
10. True or false? The type of diet that tends to promote growth and development in laboratory animals is the same as the type of diet that promotes longevity.
11. Cite three problem areas in typical U.S. adult diets.
12. State two general rules about food safety.

Answers

1. 74 to 85 years.
2. 71, 78.
3. Infant survival.

4. Improved sanitation, control of infectious disease, and improved nutrition, housing, and hygiene.
5. Heart disease, cancer, stroke.
6. This question brings you back to content introduced in chapter 1. As summarized in Table 1-2, the major nutrition risk factors associated with disease development are
   Heart Disease: Diets that are high in saturated fat and cholesterol; obesity.
   Cancer: Diets that are high in fat and low in vitamin A, beta-carotene, dietary fiber, and certain types of vegetables (cabbage family).
   Stroke: Diets that are high in saturated fat, cholesterol, and sodium.
7. Diet, smoking, physical activity, weight control.
8. Slightly underweight.
9. Physical activity, low-fat diets, prevention of overweight.
10. False. Underfeeding appears to promote longevity but *not* growth and development.
11. Low-calorie diets (related to low levels of physical activity), lactose intolerance, low calcium and dietary fiber intakes, high fat and sodium intakes.
12. When in doubt, throw it (the food) out, and keep hot foods hot and cold foods cold.

■ ■ ■

PUTTING NUTRITION KNOWLEDGE TO WORK

1. Principle 4 discussed in chapter 2 stated: "Most health problems related to nutrition originate within cells." Many of the nutrition-related disease processes that occur as a person ages result from disruptions in nutrition that impair cell functions. Apply this principle to the development of hardening of the arteries, osteoporosis, and cancer. Note how high-fat diets can translate into high blood cholesterol levels and plaque formation, how habitually low calcium intakes may affect bone formation and maintenance, and how nutrients that act as antioxidants affect the body cells.
2. Fill in the minimum recommended number of servings for adults:

Food Group	Minimum Number of Servings per Day
Breads and cereals	
Vegetables and fruits	
Vitamin A-rich	
Vitamin C-rich	
Other	
Milk and milk products	
Meat or meat alternates	

(Refer to Table 16-3.)

3. You are in charge of the turkey and dressing for Thanksgiving dinner. You prepared the dressing from a recipe calling for dry bread cubes,

milk, eggs, and seasonings and stuffed the turkey with it. After 4 hours in the oven, the turkey is done, but the internal temperature of the stuffing has reached only 110°F. Is it sufficiently heated to assure that it's safe?

(*Refer to Figure 16-4.*)

■ ■ ■

NOTES

1. *The Surgeon General's Report on Nutrition and Health*, DHHS publication no. (PHS) 88-50210 (Washington, D.C.: U.S. Department of Health and Human Services, 1988).

2. *Women's Health*, volume II, DHHS publication no. (PHS) 85-50206 (Washington, D.C.: Public Health Service, 1985).

3. A. Leaf, Observations of a peripatetic gerontologist, *Nutrition Today*, September/October (1973): 4–12.

4. T. McKeown, *The Role of Medicine: Dream, Mirage, or Nemisus* (London: Nuffield Provential Hospital Trust, 1976). See also R. Cooper and C. Sempos, The price of progress, *Journal of the National Medical Association* 76 (1984): 163–166.

5. T. Cooper, *Report of the National Leadership Conference on American Health Policy*, Washington, D.C., 1976.

6. C. McCullough, *NIH Record*, 16 July 1985: 7.

7. T. Gordon, W. P. Castelli, et al., Diabetes, blood lipids, and the role of obesity in coronary heart disease risk for women, *Annals of Internal Medicine* 87 (1977): 393–397.

8. N. K. Wenger, Coronary disease in women, *Annual Review of Medicine* 36 (1985): 285–294.

9. Z. A. Menduedev, Caucasus and Altay longevity: A biological or social problem? *Gerontologist* 14 (1974): 381.

10. S. D. Morrison, Nutrition and longevity, *Nutrition Reviews* 41 (1983): 133–142.

11. M. H. Ross, Nutrition and longevity in experimental animals, in *Nutrition and Aging*, ed. M. Winick (New York: John Wiley and Sons, 1976), 43–57.

12. T. Harris, et al., Body mass index and mortality among nonsmoking older persons: The Framingham Heart Study, *Journal of the American Medical Association* 259 (1988): 1520–1524.

13. Severe malnutrition in a young man with AIDS, *Nutrition Reviews* 46 (1988): 126–132.

14. N. Fabris, AIDS, zinc deficiency, and thymic hormone failure (letter), *Journal of the American Medical Association* 259 (1988): 839–840.

15. S. S. Resler, Nutrition care of AIDS patients, *Journal of the American Dietetic Association* 88 (1988): 828.

16. A. E. Arntzenius, D. Kromhout, et al., Diet, lipoproteins, and the progression of coronary atherosclerosis: The Leiden Intervention Trial, *New England Journal of Medicine* 312 (1985): 805–811.

17. V. Matkovic, K. Kostial, et al., Bone status and fracture roles in two regions of Yugoslavia, *American Journal of Clinical Nutrition* 32 (1979): 540–549.

18. D. Rowe, Health care of the elderly, *New England Journal of Medicine* 312 (1985): 833–835.

19. *Healthy People: The Surgeon General's Report on Health Promotion and Disease Prevention*, DHEW publication no. (PHS) 79-55071 (Washington, D.C.: Public Health Service, 1979).

20. *Prevention '82*, Office of Disease Prevention and Health Promotion, DHHS publication no. (PHS) 82-50157 (Washington, D.C.: Public Health Service, 1982).

21. W. B. Kannel, Nutritional contributors to cardiovascular disease in the elderly, *Journal of the American Geriatric Society* 34 (1986): 27–36.

22. L. Hayflick, Theories of biological aging, *Experimental Gerontology* 20 (1985): 145–159.

23. L. H. Chen, S. Liu, et al., Survey of drug use by the elderly and possible impact of drugs on nutritional status, *Drug Nutrition Interactions* 3 (1985): 73–86.

24. S. C. Hartz, C. L. Otradovec, et al., Nutrient supplement use by healthy elderly, *Journal of the American College of Nutrition* 7 (1988): 119–128.

25. *Nationwide Food Consumption Survey*, Nutrition Monitoring Division, NFCS, CSFII (Washington, D.C.: U.S. Department of Agriculture, 1986).

26. *Nationwide Food Consumption Survey*, Nutrition Monitoring Division, NFCS, CSFII (Washington, D.C.: U.S. Department of Agriculture, 1987).

27. H. N. Munro, Nutrition and the elderly: A general overview, *Journal of the American College of Nutrition* 3 (1984): 341–350.

28. A. Kallner, D. Hartman, and D. Hornig, Steady-state turnover and body pool of ascorbic acid in man, *American Journal of Clinical Nutrition* 32 (1979): 530–539.

29. J. MacLaughlin and M. F. Hollic, Aging decreases the capacity of human skin to produce vitamin D_3, *Journal of Clinical Investigation* 76 (1985): 1536–1538.

30. R. P. Heaney, J. K. Gallagher, et al., Calcium nutrition and bone health in the elderly, *American Journal of Clinical Nutrition* 36 (1982): 986–1013.

31. M. F. Holick, Vitamin D requirements for the elderly, *Clinical Nutrition* 5 (1986): 121–129.

32. R. Marston and N. Raper, Nutrient content of the U.S. food supply, *National Food Review* 5 (1987): 27–33.

33. J. L. Omdahl, P. H. Garry, et al., Nutritional status in a healthy elderly population: Vitamin D, *American Journal of Clinical Nutrition* 36 (1982): 1225–1233.

34. N. Bilderbeck, M. D. Holdsworth, et al., Changing food habits among 100 elderly men and women in the United Kingdom, *Journal of Human Nutrition* 35 (1981): 448–455.

35. S. C. Hartz, C. L. Otradovec, et al., Nutrient supplement use by healthy elderly, *Journal of the American College of Nutrition* 7 (1988): 119–128.

36. M. E. St. Louis, D. L. Morse, et al., The emergence of Grade A eggs as a major source of *Salmonella enteritidis* infections, *Journal of the American Medical Association* 259 (1988): 2103–2107.

37. The reference to this documentation note was added purely for effect. Congratulations! You checked it! Read elsewhere, the research may have sounded credible enough, but sounding credible isn't enough, right? Right.

38. This reference was added in case you didn't check out documentation note 37.

APPENDIX A

DIETARY GUIDELINES FOR AMERICANS*

What should you eat to stay healthy?

The life expectancy, average body size, and general good health of the American population seem to indicate that most diets are adequate. Foods we have to choose from are varied, plentiful, and wholesome.

Even so, hardly a day goes by without someone trying to tell us what we should and should not eat. Newspapers, magazines, books, radio, and television give us lots of advice. Unfortunately, much of it is confusing.

Some of this confusion exists because we don't know enough about nutrition to identify an "ideal diet" for each individual. People differ—and their food needs differ depending on age, sex, body size, physical activity, and other conditions such as pregnancy and illness.

In those chronic conditions where diet may be important—heart disease, high blood pressure, strokes, tooth decay, diabetes, osteoporosis, and some forms of cancer—the roles of specific dietary substances have not deen defined fully.

Research seeks more information about the amounts of essential nutrients people need and diet's role in certain chronic disease. Much attention has been devoted recently, for example, to the possible effects of calcium intake on osteoporosis, and of dietary fat and fiber on certain forms of cancer and heart disease.

But what about advice for today? The following guidelines tell how to choose and prepare foods for you and your family. This advice is the best we can give based on the nutrition information we have now.

The first two guidelines form the framework for a good diet: "Eat a variety of foods" that provide enough of essential nutrients and energy

---

**Nutrition and Your Health: Dietary Guidelines for Americans*, 2nd edition, Home and Garden Bulletin No. 232 (U.S. Department of Agriculture and U.S. Department of Health and Human Services), August 1985.

These dietary guidelines are intended only for populations with food habits similar to those of people in the United States.

DIETARY GUIDELINES FOR AMERICANS

- Eat a variety of foods.
- Maintain desirable weight
- Avoid too much fat, saturated fat, and cholesterol.
- Eat foods with adequate starch and fiber.
- Avoid too much sugar.
- Avoid too much sodium.
- If you drink alcoholic beverages, do so in moderation.

(calories) to "maintain desirable weight." The next five guidelines describe special characteristics of good diets. They suggest that you get adequate starch and fiber and avoid too much fat, sugar, sodium, and alcohol.

The Recommended Dietary Allowances (RDA) are suggested amounts of energy, protein, and some minerals and vitamins for an adequate diet. For other dietary substances, specific goals must await further research. However, for the U.S. population as a whole, increasing starch and fiber in our diets and reducing calories (primarily from fats, sugars, and alcohol) is sensible. These suggestions are especially appropriate for people who have other risk factors for chronic diseases, such as family history of obesity, premature heart disease, diabetes, high blood pressure, high blood cholesterol levels, or for those who use tobacco, particularly cigarette smokers.

The guidelines are suggested for most Americans—those who are already healthy. They do not apply to people who need special diets because of diseases or conditions that interfere with normal nutritional requirements. These people may need special instruction from registered dietitians, in consultation with their own physicians.

No guidelines can guarantee health and well-being. Health depends on many things, including heredity, lifestyle, personality traits, mental health and attitudes, and environment, in addition to diet.

Food alone cannot make you healthy. But good eating habits based on moderation and variety can help keep you healthy and even improve your health.

EAT A VARIETY OF FOODS

You need more than 40 different nutrients for good health. These include vitamins and minerals, amino acids (from proteins), essential fatty acids (from fats and oils), and sources of energy (calories from carbohydrates, fats, and proteins). Adequate amounts of these nutrients are present in the foods in a well-balanced diet.

Most foods contain more than one nutrient. For example, milk provides protein, fats, sugar, riboflavin and other B vitamins, vitamin A, calcium, phosphorus, and other nutrients; meat provides protein, several B vitamins, iron, and zinc in important amounts.

Except for human milk during the first 4 to 6 months of life, no single food supplies all of the essential nutrients in the amounts that you need. Milk, for instance, contains very little iron and meat provides little calcium. Thus, you should eat a variety of foods to get an adequate diet. With a variety of foods, you are more likely to get all the nutrients you need.

One way to assure variety—and with it, a well-balanced diet—is to select foods each day from each of the major food groups. These groups include: fruits; vegetables; cereals and other foods made from grains, such as breads; milk and dairy products such as cheese and yogurt; and meats, fish, poultry, eggs, and dry beans and peas. Select different foods from within groups, too.

Fruits and vegetables are good sources of vitamin A, vitamin C, folic acid, fiber, and many minerals. Whole-grain and enriched breads, cereals, and other grain products provide B vitamins, iron, protein, calories, and fiber. Meats, poultry, fish, and eggs supply protein, fat, iron, and other minerals, as well as several B vitamins. Dairy products are major sources of calcium and many other nutrients. Recent research suggests that calcium may play a role in preventing osteoporosis.

The number and size of portions should be adjusted to reach and maintain your desirable body weight.

There are no known advantages and some potential harm in consuming excessive amounts of any nutrient. Large dose supplements of any nutrient should be avoided.

You will rarely need to take vitamin or mineral supplements if you eat a variety of foods. There are a few important exceptions to this general statement:

- **Women in their childbearing years** may need to take iron supplements to replace the iron they lose with menstrual bleeding. Women who are no longer menstruating should not take iron supplements routinely.
- **Women who are pregnant or who are breast-feeding** need more of many nutrients, especially iron, folic acid, vitamin A, calcium, and sources of energy. Detailed advice should come from their physicians and dietitians.
- **Infants** also have special nutritional needs. Infants should be breast-fed unless there are special problems. The nutrients in human breast milk tend to be absorbed by the body better than those in cow milk or infant formula. In addition, breast milk serves to transfer immunity to some diseases from the mother to the infant.

  Normally, most babies are not given solid foods until they are 4 to 6 months old. At that time, solid foods can be introduced gradually. Prolonged breast- or formula-feeding—without solid foods or supplemental iron—may result in iron deficiency.

  Salt or sugar should not be added to the baby's foods. Extra flavoring with salt and sugar is not necessary—infants do not need these inducements if they are really hungry.
- **Elderly people** may eat relatively little food. Thus, they need to eat less of foods that are high in calories and low in essential nutrients, such as fats and oils, sugars and sweets, and alcohol. (Alcohol often is not thought of as a food, but is high in calories.)

  Elderly people who eat a varied diet do not generally need vitamin and mineral supplements. However, some medications used for the treatment of diseases may interact with nutrients. In such instances, a physician may prescribe supplements.

MAINTAIN DESIRABLE WEIGHT

If you are too fat, your chances of developing some chronic disorders are increased. Obesity is associated with high blood pressure, increased levels of blood fats (triglycerides) and cholesterol, heart disease, strokes, the most common type of diabetes. certain cancers, and many other types of ill health. Thus, you should try to maintain a "desirable" weight.

But how do you determine what a desirable weight is for you?

There is no absolute answer. The table [Table A-1] shows desirable ranges for most adults. If you have been obese since childhood or adolescence, you may find it difficult to reach or maintain your weight within a desirable range. Generally, the weight of adults should not be much more than it was when they were younger—about 25 years old.

It is not well understood why some people can eat much more than others and still maintain desirable weight. However, one thing is definite—to lose weight, you must take in fewer calories than you burn. This means that you must either choose foods with fewer calories or you must increase your physical activity, preferably both.

For most people who decide to lose weight, a steady loss of 1 to 2 pounds a week—until you reach your goal—is safe.

TABLE A-1
Desirable body weight ranges

	Weight without Clothes	
Height without Shoes	Men (pounds)	Women (pounds)
4′10″		92–121
4′11″		95–124
5′0″		98–127
5′1″	105–134	101–130
5′2″	108–137	104–134
5′3″	111–141	107–138
5′4″	114–145	110–142
5′5″	117–149	114–146
5′6″	121–154	118–150
5′7″	125–159	122–154
5′8″	129–163	126–159
5′9″	133–167	130–164
5′10″	137–172	134–169
5′11″	141–177	
6′0″	145–182	
6′1″	149–187	
6′2″	153–192	
6′3″	157–197	

Note: For women 18–25 years, subtract one pound for each year under 25.
Source: Adapted from the 1959 Metropolitan Desirable Weight Table.

At the beginning of a weight-reduction diet, much of your weight loss comes from loss of water. Long-term success depends on new and better habits of eating and exercise. That is why so-called "crash" and "fad" diets usually fail in the long run.

Do not try to lose weight too rapidly. Avoid crash diets that are severely restricted in the variety of foods they allow. Diets containing fewer than 800 calories may be hazardous and should be followed only under medical supervision. Some people have developed kidney stones, disturbing psychological changes, and other complications while following such diets. A few people have died suddenly and without warning.

Also, do not attempt to lose weight by inducing vomiting or by using laxatives. Frequent vomiting and purging can cause chemical imbalance, which can lead to irregular heartbeats and even death. Frequent vomiting can also erode tooth enamel. Avoid these and other extreme means of losing weight.

A gradual increase of everyday physical activity like brisk walking can also be very helpful in losing weight and keeping it off. The chart [Table A-2] gives the approximate calories used per hour in different activities.

Do not attempt to reduce your weight below the desirable range. Severe weight loss may be associated with nutrient deficiencies, menstrual irregularities, infertility, hair loss, skin changes, cold intolerance, severe constipation, psychiatric disturbances, and other complications.

If you lose weight suddenly or for unknown reasons, see a physician. Unexplained weight loss may be an early clue to an unsuspected underlying disorder.

TABLE A-2

Approximate energy expenditure by a healthy adult weighing about 150 pounds

Activity	Calories per Hour
Lying quietly	80–100
Sitting quietly	85–105
Standing quietly	100–120
Walking slowly, 2½ mph	210–230
Walking quickly, 4 mph	315–345
Light work, such as ballroom dancing; cleaning house; office work; shopping	125–310
Moderate work, such as cycling, 9 mph; jogging, 6 mph, tennis; scrubbing floors; weeding garden	315–480
Hard work, such as aerobic dancing; basketball; chopping wood; cross-country skiing; running, 7 mph; shoveling snow; spading garden; swimming, "crawl"	480–625

Source: Based on material compiled by Robert E. Johnson, M.D., Ph.D., Professor Emeritus, University of Illinois.

AVOID TOO MUCH FAT, SATURATED FAT, AND CHOLESTEROL

If you have a high blood cholesterol level, you have a greater chance of having a heart attack. Other factors can also increase your risk of heart attack—high blood pressure and cigarette smoking, for example—but high blood cholesterol is clearly one of the major risk factors.

Populations like ours with diets relatively high in fat (especially saturated fat) and cholesterol tend to have high blood cholesterol levels. Individuals within these populations have a greater risk of having heart attacks than individuals within populations that have diets containing less fat.

Eating extra saturated fat, high levels of cholesterol, and excess calories will increase blood cholesterol in many people. Of these, saturated fat has the greatest influence. There are, however, wide variations among individuals—related to heredity and to the way each person's body uses cholesterol.

Some people can have diets high in saturated fats and cholesterol and still maintain desirable blood cholesterol levels. Other people, unfortunately, have high blood cholesterol levels even if they eat low-fat, low-cholesterol diets. However, as noted above, for many people, eating extra saturated fat, high levels of cholesterol, and excess calories will increase blood cholesterol.

There is controversy about what recommendations are appropriate for healthy Americans. But for the U.S. population as a whole, it is sensible to reduce daily consumption of fat. This suggestion is especially appropriate for individuals who have other cardiovascular risk factors, such as smokers or those with family histories of premature heart disease, high blood pressure, and diabetes.

The recommendations are not meant to prohibit you from using any specific food item or to prevent you from eating a variety of foods. Many foods that contain fat and cholesterol also provide high-quality protein and many essential vitamins and minerals. You can eat these foods in moderation as long as your overall fat and cholesterol intake is not excessive.

EAT FOODS WITH ADEQUATE STARCH AND FIBER

The major sources of energy (calories) in the American diet are carbohydrates and fats. (Protein and alcohol also supply calories.) Carbohydrates are especially helpful in weight-reduction diets because, ounce for ounce, they contain about half as many calories as fats do.

Simple carbohydrates, such as sugars, and complex carbohydrates, such as starches, have about the same caloric content. But most foods high in sugar, such as candies and other sweets, contain little or no vitamins and minerals. On the other hand, foods high in starch, such as breads and other grain products, dry beans and peas, and potatoes, contain many of these essential nutrients.

Eating more foods containing complex carbohydrates can also help to add dietary fiber to your diet. The American diet is relatively low in fiber.

TO AVOID TOO MUCH FAT, SATURATED FAT, AND CHOLESTEROL

- Choose lean meat, fish, poultry, and dry beans and peas as protein sources.
- Use skim or low-fat milk and milk products.
- Moderate your use of egg yolks and organ meats.
- Limit your intake of fats and oils, especially those high in saturated fat, such as butter, cream, lard, heavily hydrogenated fats (some margarines), shortenings, and foods containing palm and coconut oils.
- Trim fat off meats.
- Broil, bake, or boil rather than fry.
- Moderate your use of foods that contain fat, such as breaded and deep-fried foods.
- Read labels carefully to determine both amount and type of fat present in foods.

Dietary fiber is a term used to describe parts of plant foods which are generally not digestible by humans. There are several kinds of fiber with different chemical structures and biological effects. Because foods differ in the kinds of fiber they contain, it's best to include a variety of fiber-rich foods—whole-grain breads and cereals, fruits and vegetables, for example.

Eating foods high in fiber has been found to reduce symptoms of chronic constipation, diverticular disease, and some types of "irritable bowel." It has been suggested that diets low in fiber may increase the risk of developing colon cancer. Whether this is true is not yet known.

How dietary fiber relates to cancer is one of many fiber topics under study. Some others are the fiber content of foods and the amount of fiber we need in our diets. Also being studied are whether fiber extracted from food has the same effect as that from intact food and the extent to which high fiber intakes may lead to trace mineral deficiency.

Advice for today: A diet containing wholegrain breads and cereals, fruits, and vegetables should provide an adequate intake of dietary fiber. Increase your fiber intake by eating more of these foods that contain fiber naturally, not by adding fiber to foods that do not contain it.

■ ■ ■

AVOID TOO MUCH SUGAR

A significant health problem from eating too much sugar is tooth decay (dental caries). The risk of caries is not simply a matter of how much sugar and sugar-containing foods you eat but how often you eat them. The more frequently you eat sugar and sugar-containing foods, the greater the risk for tooth decay—especially if they are eaten between meals, and if they stick to your teeth.

Americans consume sugar in various forms in their diets. Common table sugar (sucrose) is only one form of sugar. Other sugars—such as glucose (dextrose), fructose, maltose, and lactose—occur naturally in foods and are added as ingredients in foods, e.g. corn sweeteners. Both starches and sugars appear to increase the risk of tooth decay when eaten between meals, but simple sugars appear to offer a higher risk. Thus, frequent in-between-meal snacks of foods such as cakes and pastries, candies, dried fruits, and soft drinks may be more harmful to your teeth than the sugars eaten in regular meals.

You cannot avoid all sugar because most of the foods we eat contain some sugar in one form or another. But keep the amount of sugars and sweet foods you eat moderate. And when you do eat them, brush your teeth afterwards, if possible.

Clearly, there is more to maintaining healthy teeth than avoiding sugars. Careful dental hygiene and exposure to adequate amounts of fluoride through fluoridated water are especially important. Fluoridated toothpastes or mouth rinses are helpful, particularly where there is no fluoridated water.

Contrary to widespread belief, too much sugar in your diet does not cause diabetes. The most common type of diabetes occurs in obese adults; avoiding sugar without correcting the overweight problem—which requires reduction in total caloric intake—will not solve the problem.

Sugars provide calories but few other nutrients. Thus, diets with large amounts of sugars should be avoided, especially by people with low calorie needs, such as those on weight-reducing diets and the elderly.

AVOID TOO MUCH SODIUM

Table salt contains sodium and choloride—both are essential in the diet. In addition, salt is often required for the preservation of certain foods.

Sodium is present in many beverages and foods that we eat, especially in certain processed foods, condiments, sauces, pickled foods, salty snacks, and sandwich meats. Baking soda, baking powder, monosodium glutamate (MSG), and even many medications (many antacids, for instance) contain sodium.

A major hazard of excess sodium is for persons who have high blood pressure. Not everyone is equally susceptible. In the United States, about one in four adults has elevated blood pressure. Sodium intake is but one of the factors known to affect high blood pressure. Several other nutrients may also be involved. Obesity plays a major role.

In populations with low sodium intakes, high blood pressure is rare. In contrast, in populations with high sodium intakes, high blood pressure is common. If people with high blood pressure severely restrict their sodium intakes, their blood pressure will usually fall, although not always to normal levels.

At present, there is no good way to predict who will develop high blood pressure, although certain groups such as blacks have a higher prevalence. Low-sodium diets may help some people avoid high blood pressure if they could be identified before they develop the condition.

Since most Americans eat more sodium than is needed, consider reducing your sodium intake. Use less table salt, read labels carefully, and eat sparingly those foods to which large amounts of sodium have been added.

Remember that a substantial amount of the sodium you eat may be "hidden"—either occurring naturally in foods or as part of a preservative or flavoring agent that has been added.

■ ■ ■

IF YOU DRINK ALCOHOLIC BEVERAGES, DO SO IN MODERATION

Alcoholic beverages are high in calories and low in nutrients. Thus, even moderate drinkers will need to drink less if they are overweight and wish to reduce.

Heavy drinkers frequently develop nutritional deficiencies as well as more serious diseases, such as cirrhosis of the liver and certain types of cancer, especially those who also smoke cigarettes. This is partly because of loss of appetite, poor food intake, and impaired absorption of nutrients.

Excessive consumption of alcoholic beverages by pregnant women may cause birth defects or other problems during pregnancy. The level of consumption at which risks to the unborn occur has not been established. Therefore, the National Institute on Alcohol Abuse and Alcoholism advises that pregnant women should refrain from the use of alcohol.

One or two standard-size drinks daily appear to cause no harm in normal, healthy, nonpregnant adults. Twelve ounces of regular beer, 5 ounces of wine, and 1½ ounces of distilled spirits contain about equal alcohol.

If you drink, be moderate in your intake and DO NOT DRIVE!

APPENDIX B

RELIABLE SOURCES OF NUTRITION INFORMATION

Many sources of nutrition information are available to consumers, but the quality of the information they provide varies widely. All of the sources listed here provide scientifically based information. Although this list is not all-encompassing, it can direct you to sources of nutrition information that you can trust.

■ ■ ■

HEALTH AND NUTRITION PROFESSIONALS

- Registered dietitians (hospitals)
- Public health nutritionists (public health departments)
- College nutrition instructors/professors (colleges and universities)
- Extension Service home economists (state and county U.S. Department of Agriculture Extension Service offices)
- Consumer affairs staff of the Food and Drug Administration (national, regional, and state FDA offices)

■ ■ ■

ORGANIZATIONS, ASSOCIATIONS, AND AGENCIES*

- American Dental Association
  211 East Chicago Avenue
  Chicago, IL 60611

*Many of these organizations and agencies have state offices that also can provide nutrition information.

- American Diabetes Association
18 East 48th Street
New York, NY 10017
- American Dietetics Association
216 West Jackson Boulevard, Suite 800
Chicago, IL 60606-6995
- American Heart Association
7320 Greenville Avenue
Dallas, TX 75231
- American Home Economics Association
2010 Massachusetts Avenue, N.W.
Washington, DC 20036
- American Institute of Nutrition
9650 Rockville Pike
Bethesda, MD 20014
- American Medical Association
Council on Food and Nutrition
535 North Dearborn Street
Chicago, IL 60610
- American National Red Cross
Nutrition Consultant
National Headquarters
Washington, DC 20005
- American Public Health Association
1015 Fifteenth Street, N.W.
Washington, DC 20005
- Food and Drug Administration *(for information on food safety)*
Consumer Inquiry Section
5600 Fishers Lane
Rockville, MD 20857
Phone: 800-426-3758
- Food and Nutrition Service *(for information on food stamps)*
U.S. Department of Agriculture
Washington, DC 20250
- Food and Nutrition Information Center
National Agriculture Library, Room 304
10301 Baltimore Boulevard
Beltsville, MD 20705
Phone: 301-344-3719
- La Leche League International *(for information on breast feeding)*
9616 Minneapolis Avenue
Franklin Park, IL 60131
Phone: 312-455-7730
- March of Dimes Birth Defects Foundation
1275 Mamaroneck Avenue
White Plains, NY 10605

- National Cancer Institute
  Office of Cancer Communication
  Building 31, Room 10A18
  Bethesda, MD 20205
  Phone: 800-422-6237
- National Cholesterol Education Program
  National Heart, Lung, and Blood Institute
  C-200
  Bethesda, MD 10892
- National High Blood Pressure Education Program
  120/80 National Institutes of Health
  Bethesda, MD 20892
- NHLBI Smoking Education Program
  Information Center
  4733 Bethesda Avenue, Suite 530
  Bethesda, MD 20814
- National Dairy Council
  6300 North River Road
  Rosemont, IL 60018-4233
- National Health Information Clearinghouse
  Post Office Box 1133
  Washington, DC 20013
  Phone: 800-336-4797
- National Maternal and Child Health Clearinghouse
  3520 Prospect Street, N.W., Suite 1
  Washington, DC 20057
  Phone: 202-625-8400
- Nutrition Foundation
  1122 Sixteenth Street, N.W.
  Washington, DC 20036
- Office of Disease Prevention and Health Promotion
  U.S. Department of Health and Human Services
  Mary E. Switze Building, Room 2132
  330 C Street, S.W.
  Washington, DC 20201
- School Lunch Program
  Food and Nutrition Service
  U.S. Department of Agriculture
  Washington, DC 20250
- Society for Nutrition Education
  1700 Broadway, Suite 300
  Oakland, CA 94612
  Phone: 415-444-7133
- Special Supplemental Food Program for Women, Infants, and Children (WIC)
  Supplemental Food Programs
  U.S. Department of Agriculture
  Washington, DC 20250

JOURNALS*

Nutrition Journals

- *American Journal of Clinical Nutrition*
- *British Journal of Nutrition*
- *Human Nutrition, Applied Nutrition*
- *Journal of the American College of Nutrition*
- *Journal of the American Dietetic Association*
- *Journal of Food Composition and Analysis*
- *Journal of Nutrition*
- *Journal of Nutrition Education*
- *Nutrition Abstracts and Reviews*
- *Nutrition and Metabolism*
- *Nutrition Reports International*
- *Nutrition Reviews*

Other Journals that Report on Nutrition Topics

- *American Journal of Epidemiology*
- *American Journal of Nursing*
- *American Journal of Public Health*
- *Annals of Internal Medicine*
- *Annals of Surgery*
- *Caries Research*
- *Food Technology*
- *Gastroenterology*
- *Journal of the American Dental Association*
- *Journal of the American Medical Association*
- *Journal of Clinical Investigation*
- *Journal of Home Economics*
- *Journal of Pediatrics*
- *Lancet*
- *New England Journal of Medicine*
- *Pediatrics*
- *Science*

---

*Many other scientific journals, such as those included in the documentation notes at the end of each chapter of this book, also are reliable sources of nutrition information.

APPENDIX C

DIGESTION: A CLOSER LOOK

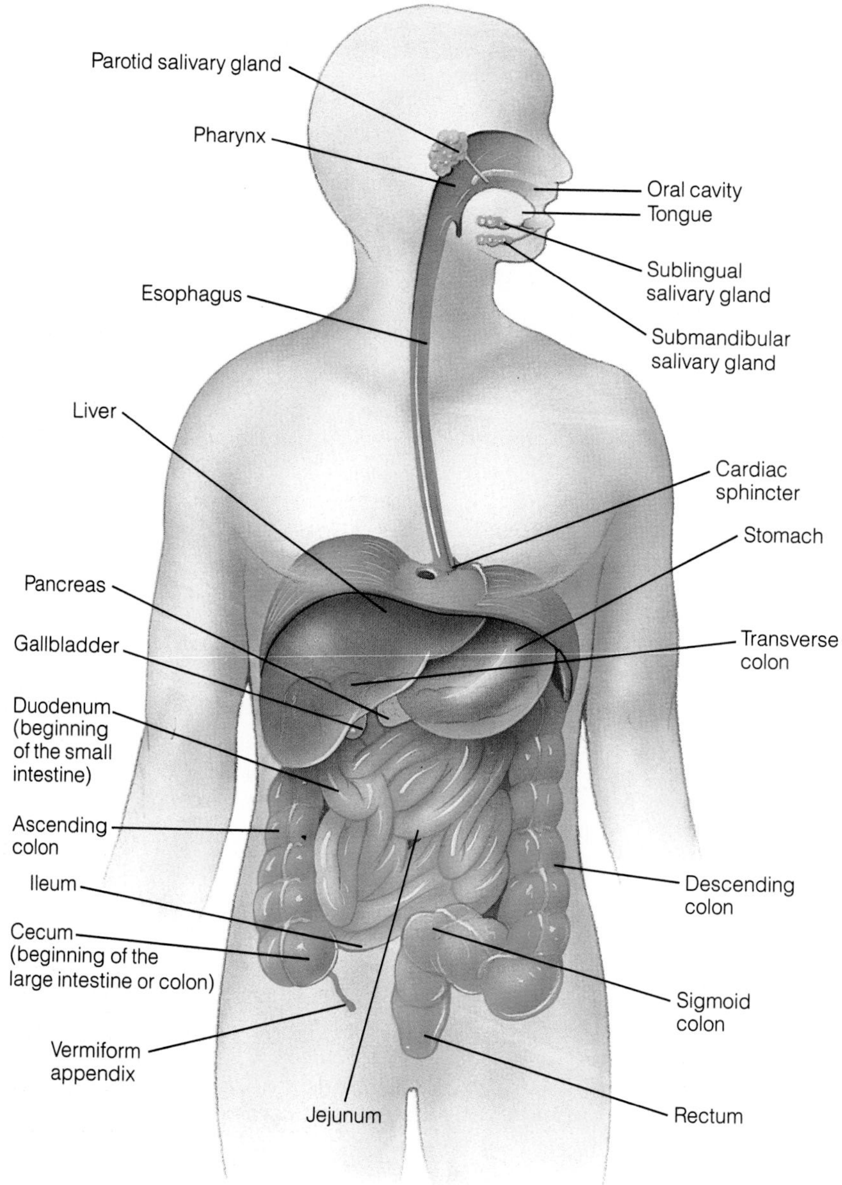

FIGURE C-1
The digestive system.

Foods are digested by a series of mechanical and chemical processes that break them down into particles that can be absorbed. In this appendix we will discuss the mechanical and chemical digestive processes according to where they occur in the digestive system. Figure C-1 presents a detailed view of the components of the digestive system. Key enzymes and other substances secreted in the digestive system that serve to break down carbohydrates, proteins, and fats are listed in Figure C-2.

MOUTH

Mechanical Processes

Food is physically separated into small pieces by chewing and the movement of the tongue, cheeks, lips, and lower jaw. Saliva is mixed with food during the chewing process, and the food becomes a moist, soft mass called the *bolus*. *Mucus*—a thick, slippery secretion of the mucous membranes that line the mouth—also helps moisten and soften food and to lubricate its passage from the mouth.

Chemical Processes

Only two enzymes participate in digestion in the mouth: salivary amylase and lingual lipase. Salivary amylase is secreted by the salivary glands and begins to break down starches. Lingual lipase, secreted by a gland located on the underside of the tongue, begins to break down short-chained fatty acids. Digestion of other carbohydrates and fats in the mouth is not extensive. Food does not remain in the mouth long enough for much digestion to occur.

FIGURE C-2
An overview of the participation of key enzymes, hydrochloric acid, and bile in the digestion of the energy nutrients.

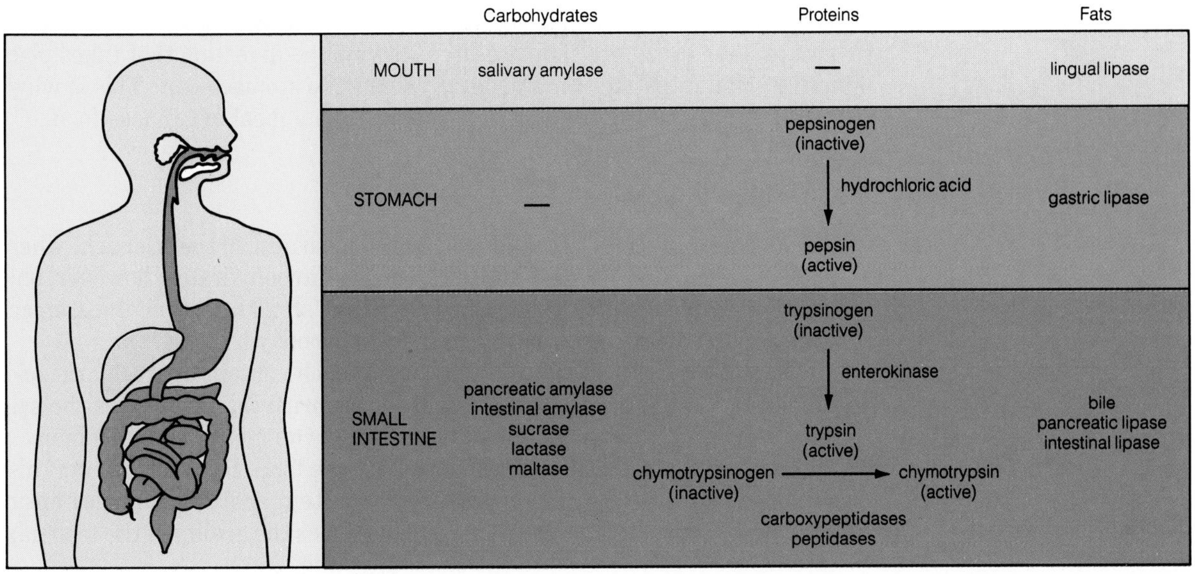

Carbohydrates
Proteins
Fats
MOUTH
salivary amylase
—
lingual lipase
STOMACH
—
pepsinogen (inactive)
hydrochloric acid
pepsin (active)
gastric lipase
SMALL INTESTINE
pancreatic amylase
intestinal amylase
sucrase
lactase
maltase
trypsinogen (inactive)
enterokinase
trypsin (active)
chymotrypsinogen (inactive)
chymotrypsin (active)
carboxypeptidases
peptidases
bile
pancreatic lipase
intestinal lipase

ESOPHAGUS

Mechanical Processes

Through coordinated contractions and relaxations, the 9- to 10-inch-long esophagus delivers the bolus of swallowed food to the stomach. At the end of the esophagus (or the beginning of the stomach) is the muscular valve called the *cardiac sphincter*, which relaxes to allow food to enter the stomach. The valve closes quickly after the bolus of food has been delivered, which prevents the highly acidic contents of the stomach from backing up into the esophagus. When the stomach contents spurt up into the esophagus due to vomiting or indigestion, the walls of the esophagus are irritated by stomach acid and the esophagus signals pain. Because the esophagus is close to the heart, this pain is commonly called "heartburn."

Chemical Processes

No chemical processes that aid digestion occur in the esophagus.

STOMACH

Mechanical Processes

chyme: (from Greek *chymos*, "juice") The semifluid mass of partly digested food that is expelled by the stomach into the duodenum.

Food is held and mixed in the stomach. Rhythmic contractions mix the food with stomach juices. After food is fully mixed and liquified the *pyloric sphincter* (pī lōr′ ik sfink′ tər) at the end of the stomach relaxes for an instant and allows about 1 to 2 teaspoons of the food, now called **chyme** (kīm), to enter the duodenum of the small intestine. This amount of chyme leaves the stomach about every 30 seconds when there is food in the stomach.

Whereas liquids are emptied from the stomach rapidly, solids and concentrated substances are released gradually. Because of the extent of mixing and liquifying required, carbohydrates tend to leave the stomach first. Proteins and fats remain in the stomach longer because they require extensive processing before they are prepared for the digestion that takes place in the small intestine. Fats generally leave the stomach last. This is why a high-fat meal "sticks to your ribs" longer than a meal of Chinese food.

Chemical Processes

The chemical processes of digestion begin in earnest in the stomach, where protein and fat digestion get fully underway. Carbohydrates, however, only pass through the stomach on their way to the small intestine; the stomach does not secrete enzymes that break down carbohydrates.

The digestive juices secreted in the stomach contain hydrochloric acid, bicarbonate (a base), and enzymes. Hydrochloric acid deactivates the salivary amylase that was combined with food in the mouth and kills many of the bacteria that were consumed along with the food. Hydrochloric acid also activates pepsinogen, the precursor of the protein-splitting enzyme pepsin. Bicarbonate secreted by the stomach neutralizes the acidity of the food mixture before it is delivered to the small intestine.

The fat-digestion enzyme secreted by the stomach is *gastric lipase.* Fats leave the stomach still requiring a good deal of digestion by enzymes and other substances in the small intestine.

Mucus secreted by the stomach protects its lining from its other secretions. Without this mucus, the stomach lining, too, would be digested.

A small amount of simple sugars, alcohol, and water are absorbed by the lining of the stomach and enter the blood stream.

SMALL INTESTINE

Mechanical Processes

The small intestine is 15 to 30 feet in length and consists of the *duodenum, jejunum,* and *ileum.* These components have different functions but are not separate, distinguishable compartments. Through rhythmic contractions of the muscles within the small intestine, chyme is mixed with digestive juices. The mixing and moving of chyme exposes food particles to the digestive processes that occur along the so-called *brush border*—consisting of microvilli—that lines the small intestine. Absorption also occurs at the brush border.

The digestive and absorptive capacity of the small intestine is dramatically increased by the microvilli in the brush border. The tiny, fingerlike projections act to increase the surface area of the lining of the small intestine, thus increasing the amount of contact between food substances and digestive enzymes. (See Figures 3-8a and 3-9 in chapter 3.)

Chemical Processes

Most digestion and nearly all absorption occur in the small intestine. The small intestine receives chyme from the stomach, enzymes from the pancreas, and bile from the gallbladder, and it produces enzymes as well. The presence of chyme in the small intestine stimulates the release of bile and of the enzymes produced by the pancreas and small intestine.

Bile is produced by the liver and stored in the gallbladder. It is released by the gallbladder when the small intestine signals that fat has arrived. Bile is not an enzyme, but an emulsifier; it makes fats partially soluble in water and thus more vulnerable to the action of enzymes.

Carbohydrates, proteins, and fat all are acted upon by enzymes in the small intestine. Some of the enzymes are manufactured in the pancreas and enter the duodenum by way of the *pancreatic duct.* The pancreas produces:

- *pancreatic amylase* for carbohydrate digestion,
- *trypsinogen, chymotrypsinogen,* and other substances for protein digestion, and
- *pancreatic lipase* for fat digestion.

Pancreatic amylase and lipase are used directly for digestion, but trypsinogen and chymotrypsinogen must first be activated by enzymes present in the small intestine. The ***-ogen*** suffix denotes "an agent that produces" an active substance; trypsinogen, for example, is activated by enterokinase

-ogen: "An agent that produces."

and forms trypsin, an active enzyme. Trypsin also converts chymotrypsinogen into the active enzyme chymotrypsin.

The small intestine produces enzymes that digest carbohydrates and fats. *Sucrase, lactase,* and *maltase* break down sugars, and *intestinal lipase* breaks down fats.

Components of foods that are incompletely digested or not digested in the small intestine are passed through the large intestine and excreted in feces. Little digestion occurs after food particles leave the small intestine.

LARGE INTESTINE

Mechanical Processes

The large intestine, or colon, is about five feet long. It serves to collect and transport waste products of digestion that will be excreted. As shown in Figure C-1, the large intestine begins with the cecum and ends with the sigmoid colon. In between the cecum and sigmoid colon are the ascending, transverse, and descending portions of the colon.

Chemical Processes

The lining of the large intestine absorbs water and a limited amount of vitamins and minerals. With the exception of water, nutrients that end up in the large intestine have almost totally missed their opportunity to be digested and absorbed. In people with normal digestive functions, 99% of carbohydrates, 92% of proteins, and 95% of fats consumed are absorbed. Normally, alcohol—which is absorbed directly into the blood stream—is completely (100%) absorbed. The body's efficient digestion mechanisms miss very little, regardless of how much of the energy nutrients are consumed.

The large intestine is home for many types of bacteria, which break down some types of dietary fiber and produce part of the body's supply of biotin and vitamin K. The end products of bacterial breakdown of dietary fiber are primarily fatty acids and gases. Although some of the fatty acids formed by bacteria from dietary fiber are absorbed, the amount appears to be too small to make a significant contribution to caloric intake.

APPENDIX D

ABSORPTION: A CLOSER LOOK

The main function of absorption is the transport of nutrients across cell membranes. Cell membranes act as sort of a "border patrol" in that they serve to maintain homeostasis within cells and in the fluids that surround cells. Some substances are able to pass through the cell membrane, whereas others are not; the membrane is selectively permeable. The physical and chemical properties of cell membranes control the processes of absorption.

Cell membranes are composed of lipids, proteins, and a small amount of carbohydrate (Figure D-1). The lipid portion comprises about half of the mass of the membrane and consists primarily of phospholipids. Cholesterol and other lipids are also present in the membrane, but in smaller amounts

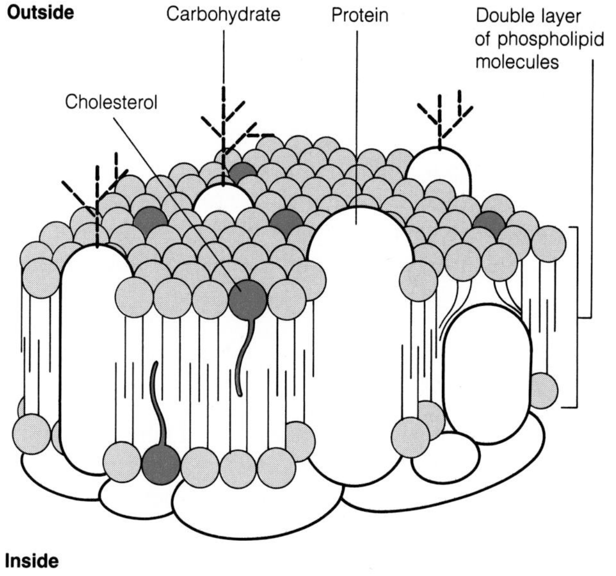

FIGURE D-1
Structure of a cell membrane. Proteins are embedded in a fluid lipid bilayer—some penetrating both surfaces, others embedded in one surface or the other. Most proteins and many lipids in the outer surface of the cell membrane are attached to chains of monosaccharides.

than the phospholipids. The phospholipids are arranged in a double layer, with their fatty acid chains directed toward the center of the membrane and their glycerol components oriented toward the surfaces of the membrane. The lipid portion of the cell membrane is in the form of oils, which gives cell membranes the property of being flexible. The flexibility of the membranes varies with the type of fatty acids present. Highly unsaturated fatty acids—such as the omega-3 fatty acids found in fish oils—tend to make cell membranes more flexible than saturated fatty acids do. Reduced flexibility of cell membranes can result in the inability of red blood cells to change shape and pass through narrow blood vessels. Such a situation can lead to the blockage of small vessels. Differences in the flexibility of cell membranes also affects the amount of time it takes blood to clot. The type of fatty acids found in cell membranes is influenced by diet. In recent years, identification of the types of fatty acids present in cell membranes has served as an indicator of dietary fat composition.

Proteins contained in cell membranes are usually embedded in the phospholipid layers, and some of them span the membrane from one side to the other. Because they are embedded and not bound to the phospholipids, the protein molecules essentially float in the oily phospholipid layers. The proteins in cell membranes provide structural support, transport molecules across the membrane, and serve as surface receptors for hormones and other regulatory substances. (This last function will be discussed later in this appendix.)

The carbohydrate portion of cell membranes accounts for 10% or less of the weight of the membrane. Composed of chains of monosaccharides attached to the outer surface of the membranes, these carbohydrates play an important role in the regulatory functions of cell membranes.

THE MECHANISMS OF ABSORPTION

Simple Diffusion

simple diffusion: The free movement of a substance across a cell membrane from an area of high concentration to an area of low concentration. The process equalizes the concentrations on either side of the membrane.

Nutrients are transported across cell membranes by four major mechanisms (Figure D-2). The most direct of these mechanisms is **simple diffusion**. Nutrients that are transported by simple diffusion pass freely into and out of cells. Water, oxygen, carbon dioxide, and some other substances are of the right size and chemical characteristics to cross membranes by simple diffusion. Because these chemicals pass freely into and out of cells, their concentrations in the fluid that surrounds cells and in the fluid within cells are equal.

Facilitated Diffusion

facilitated diffusion: Diffusion of a substance across a cell membrane with the help of carrier proteins.

Fructose ("fruit sugar") and certain vitamins and minerals require a carrier protein for passage and are thus transported by **facilitated diffusion**. Substances transported by facilitated diffusion may not be found in equal concentrations outside and inside of cells. Cells regulate the production of carrier proteins in proportion to their need for the substances transported.

| Fluid outside the cell | Cell membrane | Fluid inside the cell |

(a) **Simple Diffusion**

(b) **Facilitated Diffusion**

Carrier protein

(c) **Active Transport**

ATP
Carrier protein

(d) **Pinocytosis**

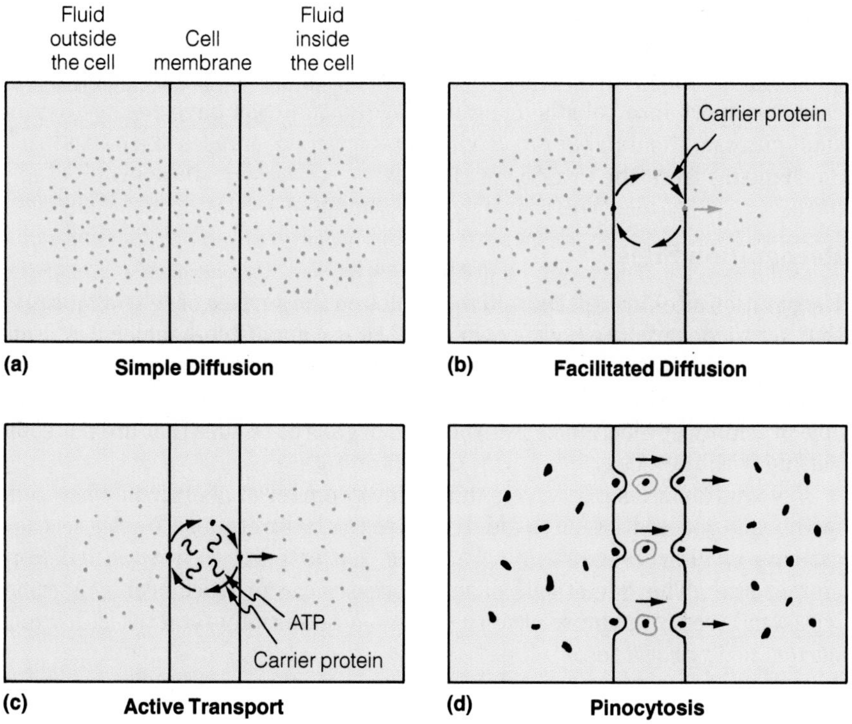

■
FIGURE D-2
The four major mechanisms of nutrient absorption across a cell membrane.

Active Transport

The third mechanism of absorption uses both a carrier protein and energy from ATP. This mechanism, referred to as **active transport**, is highly regulated. It is used to tightly control the concentration of particular nutrients within cells. Generally, glucose, amino acids, and certain vitamins and minerals are actively transported across cell membranes.

active transport: The transport of a substance across a cell membrane that involves a carrier protein and energy from ATP.

Pinocytosis

Pinocytosis, also called endocytosis, is the least common of the transport mechanisms. It is of special importance during early infancy, when large molecules of protein that confer immunity (immunoglobulins) are absorbed from the small intestine. Fluids and other substances that enter cells by pinocytosis do not simply pass through the cell membrane. They are surrounded and then enclosed by a portion of the cell membrane that moves into the interior of the cell with them. Once inside the cell, the engulfed substances are released, and the portion of the membrane that enclosed it disintegrates into the cell fluids. The lost part of the cell membrane is then replaced.

pinocytosis: (pī′ nō sī tō′ səs) The process by which a cell surrounds and then engulfs a substance.

■ ■ ■
CELL RECEPTORS AND RECOGNITION SITES

Cell Receptors

Cell membranes contain proteins that function as receptors for hormones and other chemical substances that trigger particular cell functions. The presence and activity of receptors on cell membranes is highly regulated. For example, insulin receptors are located in the membranes of fat, liver, and muscle cells. When receptors are present and occupied by insulin, glucose transport into cells is increased. When the cells have received sufficient glucose, the number or activity of receptors decreases due to feedback mechanisms from the interior of the cell.

Recognition Sites

Recognition sites are specialized molecules on the surface of cell membranes that act to identify the body's own—and thus compatible—molecules. Foreign molecules are detected by the recognition sites and rejected. Although the recognition sites protect cells from disruption in normal functions, they also precipitate rejection of transplanted organs or tissues that are not compatible with the body.

Recognition sites play a role in the development of allergies. When cell-membrane recognition sites identify a particular protein as "foreign," they activate an allergic reaction—processes that attempt to ward off the foreign protein. The side effects of the processes can produce problems ranging from hives or a runny nose to shock—a potentially fatal breakdown of normal body processes.

TRANSPORT OF ABSORBED NUTRIENTS

Specific nutrients are absorbed into either the lymph system or the blood system. Although all absorbed nutrients eventually make it into the general circulation, the routes they follow are different. Most fatty acids and fat-soluble vitamins are absorbed into the vessels of the lymph system. The network of small vessels that picks up fatty acids and vitamins from the small intestine combines and enlarges to form the *thoracic duct*. The thoracic duct empties into a large vein that leads to the heart. In the heart, lymph components are mixed with those of blood and pumped into the general circulation. After a person consumes a high-fat meal, his or her blood level of fat particles may be sufficiently high to give the blood a milky or cloudy appearance. High blood levels of fat normally decrease within a few hours, after the liver has had a chance to "clear" the excess fat. (Many people have been horrified by the results of blood tests taken after eating high-fat meals.)

Blood vessels in the intestinal walls transport water, glucose, glycerol, amino acids, and other substances to the liver via the *portal vein*. Fatty acids of a certain size also are absorbed into blood vessels, but this route of transportation is minor in comparison with the lymph system. While in the liver, nutrients are processed as described in chapter 3 and released into the general circulation. The transportation routes of carbohydrates, proteins, and fats are shown in Figure D-3.

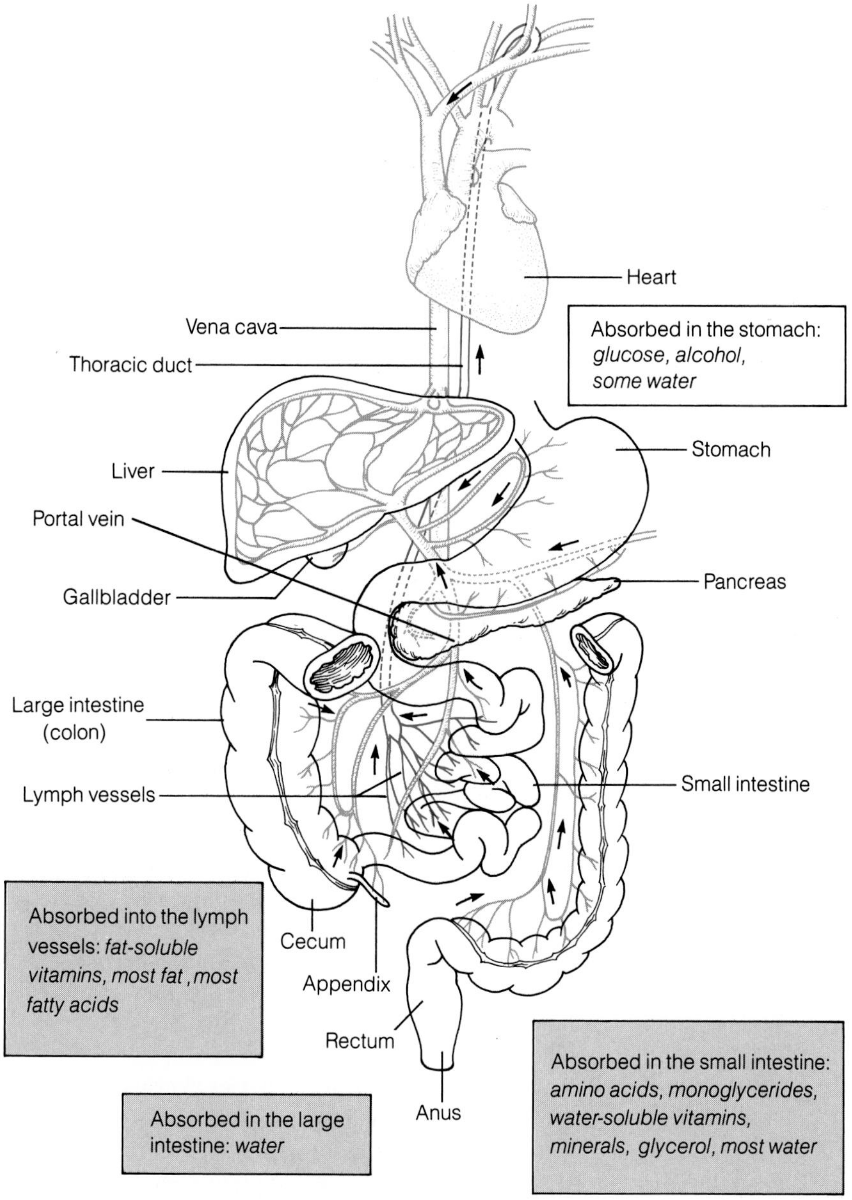

FIGURE D-3

Transportation systems for absorbed nutrients. Lymph vessels are shown in blue; blood vessels, in red.

APPENDIX

E

ENERGY METABOLISM: A CLOSER LOOK

Carbohydrates, proteins, and fats can have many different uses once they have been transported to the body's cells. One of the primary uses is in energy metabolism.

Glucose, glycogen, amino acids, fatty acids, and glycerol are the body's fuel sources. Of these, only glucose can enter directly into energy metabolism. The others must first be converted into substances that can enter either glycolysis or the citric acid cycle, the body's two major pathways of energy formation.

Glucose, glycogen, many amino acids, and glycerol are the raw ingredients that fuel glycolysis. Before glycogen, amino acids, and glycerol can be used for glycolysis, however, they must first be converted to glucose. (Remember that only glucose can be used to form energy by glycolysis.) The formation of glucose from glycogen, amino acids, and glycerol is called **gluconeogenesis**. The gluconeogenesis process is straightforward for glycogen and glycerol, but is a bit more complex for amino acids, because amino acids contain nitrogen. Their nitrogen component must be removed before they can be used to form glucose. **Deamination** is the process that separates the nitrogen group from the rest of the amino acid; see Figure E-1. The nitrogen released is either converted to urea and excreted in the urine or is used to create nonessential amino acids. With a few exceptions, deaminated amino acids can be converted to glucose and enter glycolysis. Amino acids that cannot be converted into glucose enter the citric acid cycle after they have been deaminated.

gluconeogenesis: (*gluco* = "glucose"; *neo* = "new"; *genesis* = "formation") The formation of "new" glucose by the body. Glucose can be formed from glycogen, glycerol, or a number of amino acids.

deamination: The removal of a nitrogen group from an amino acid. Amino acids must be deaminated before they can be used for glucose formation or converted to a nonessential amino acid.

Glucose—either obtained from glycogen, amino acids, or glycerol or supplied as is—forms energy when it is broken down into *pyruvic acid* (referred to as *glucose fragments* in chapter 3). The total amount of energy released by converting glucose into pyruvic acid is 2 ATP per glucose mole-

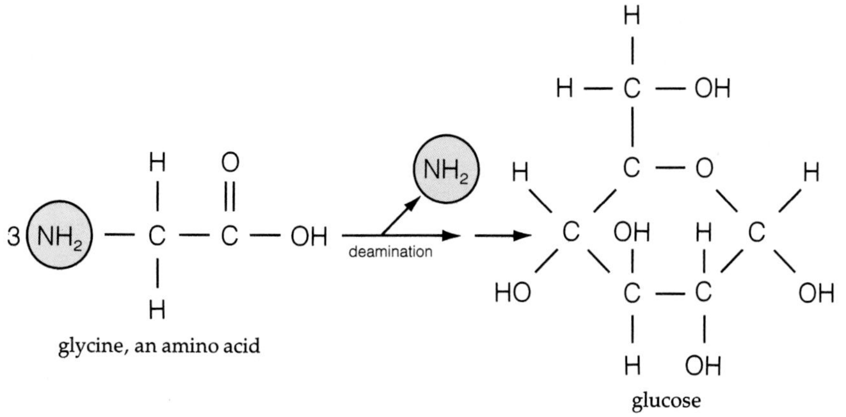

FIGURE E-1
An example of deamination.

cule. Although glycolysis does not yield a great deal of energy, it has the advantages of not requiring oxygen, of producing energy quickly, and of producing as its end product a substance that can be used to fuel the citric acid cycle.

The citric acid cycle forms energy from the glycolysis product pyruvic acid, from fatty acids, and from specific amino acids. Of these, fatty acids are the major raw material from which the citric acid cycle forms energy. The citric acid cycle is the primary pathway by which body fat stores are used and the supplier of the vast majority of energy formed by the body.

The singular of mitochondria *is* mitochondrion.

Pyruvic acid and fatty acids must be converted to *acetyl coenzyme A* (*acetyl CoA*) in order to be used for energy formation in the citric acid cycle. Before acetyl CoA can be used to form energy, however, it must enter the *mitochondria* of cells. (See Figure E-2.) Mitochondria are enzyme-packed

FIGURE E-2
Schematic representation of the formation of ATP from energy sources delivered in the blood.

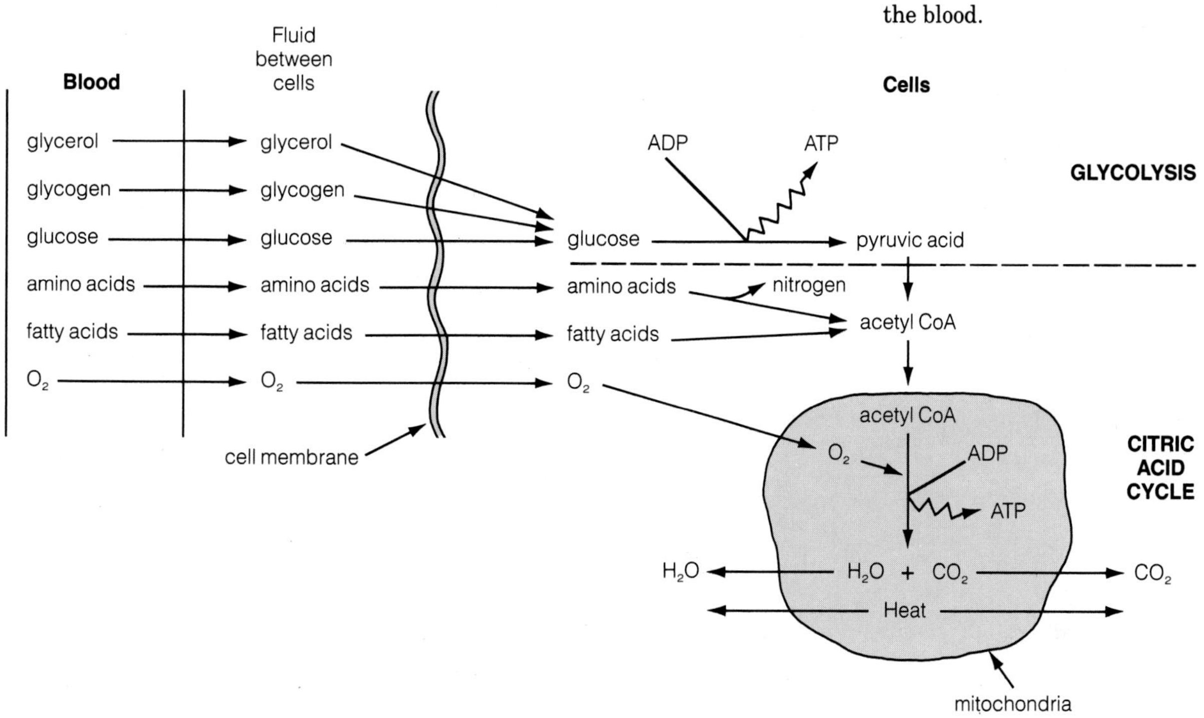

compartments of cells that specialize in energy metabolism, and they are especially numerous in muscle cells. Once inside the mitochondria, acetyl CoA begins its journey through the citric acid cycle. Oxygen entering the citric acid cycle combines with the hydrogen atoms that have been separated from acetyl CoA during its breakdown to form H_2O. Energy released when hydrogen atoms are separated from acetyl CoA and its breakdown products is used to convert ADP to ATP. Carbon dioxide (CO_2) is also formed from acetyl CoA during the citric acid cycle and it is another end product of this pathway of energy formation. Heat is the final end product of the citric acid cycle; it represents the energy that was released but not captured by ADP.

What if glycolysis or the citric acid cycle receives more fuel than is needed? Both pathways of energy metabolism form energy on an "as-needed" basis. Our bodies do not store ATP. Rather, they create the amount that is needed by our cells. Glucose—whether it comes straight from the blood or is formed from amino acids or glycerol—can be converted into fat or glycogen for storage (Figure E-3). When our glycogen stores are filled, excess glucose is converted to fat. Excess fuel in the form of fatty acids is generally converted to fat. Unlike glycogen, glycerol, and many amino acids, fatty acids cannot be converted to glucose. Only the glycerol component of fat molecules that makes up the 16% of their weight can be used to form glucose. Thus, the body quickly runs short of glucose for energy formation when body fat is the primary source of energy. The body needs a constant supply of glucose in order for energy metabolism to operate in peak condition. The consequences of overusing fatty acids as a source of fuel are discussed in chapter 7.

ROLES OF THE B-COMPLEX VITAMINS IN ENERGY FORMATION

Six of the eight B-complex vitamins act as *coenzymes* in reactions that lead to energy formation; that is, these six vitamins activate enzymes. (They are discussed in more detail in Chapter 8.) The enzymes that convert pyruvic acid to acetyl coenzyme A (acetyl CoA) are activated by coenzymes derived from thiamin, niacin, and biotin. The primary component of acetyl CoA is

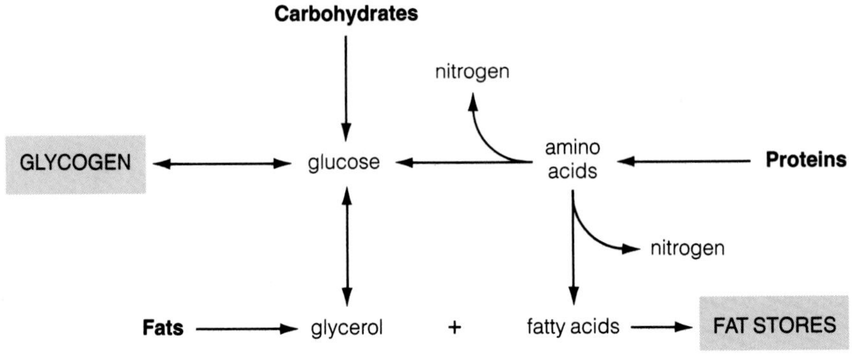

FIGURE E-3
Major routes to the formation of glycogen and fat stores.

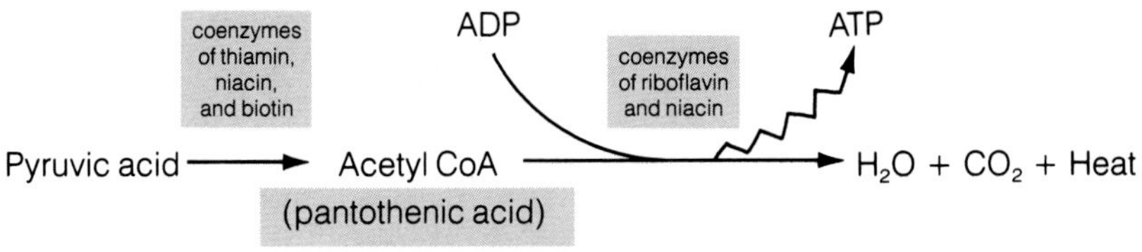

FIGURE E-4
Roles of the B-complex vitamins in energy formation.

pantothenic acid, another B-complex vitamin. Coenzymes derived from riboflavin and niacin play key roles in reactions that transfer energy released during the citric acid cycle to ATP. Figure E-4 summarizes these roles of the B-complex vitamins.

Many of the consequences of a deficiency of one or more of the B-complex vitamins involved in energy metabolism directly relate to inadequate energy formation. More information about the functions of these six B-complex vitamins is given in chapter 9.

APPENDIX

F

FOOD EXCHANGE LISTS

The two primary approaches to planning meals that meet nutrient needs are basic-food-group guides and food exchange lists. The food-group approach has been used throughout this book because it has broad applicability to normal nutrition. The exchange system is presented here, as an appendix, because it is commonly used in the dietary management of diabetes and for weight loss. Although food exchange lists are more complicated to use than the food-group guides, they come far closer to providing the desired levels of calories and percentages of total calories as carbohydrate, protein, and fat than does a food-group approach. With the food-exchange approach, the caloric, carbohydrate, protein, and fat contents of a diet are adjusted to the individual's needs by varying the number of exchanges. A dietician determines the servings and calorie intake for each individual. Both approaches can provide adequate levels of vitamins and minerals if caloric intake is not too restricted. The food exchange lists are generally most effectively translated into dietary practices when they are combined with advice and counseling from a registered dietitian.

HOW THE FOOD EXCHANGE SYSTEM WORKS

There are six food exchange lists (Table F-1). Each list contains foods that provide similar amounts of carbohydrate, protein, and fat in a standard serving. Because the content of each energy nutrient is similar, all foods within a particular list have a similar caloric content. As you read the exchange lists, you will notice that the serving sizes vary. This is necessary for standardizing the amounts of carbohydrate, protein, fat, and calories in the food items on a particular exchange list. Samples of each listed food have been weighed, measured, and analyzed to assure this standardization.

Foods within each list can be "exchanged" (traded) for each other, thus allowing for flexibility in food choices while meeting overall intake goals for calories, carbohydrates, protein, and fat. For example, oatmeal, crackers, noodles, and bread are included in the starch/bread exchange list. The standard serving size assigned to each of these foods provides a similar amount of calories (about 80), carbohydrates (15 grams), protein (3 grams), and fat (a trace to 1 gram). If a person's meal plan includes six starch/bread exchanges, he or she could select the six from the variety of foods included in the starch/bread list. The result is that the person's diet can provide a wide variety of foods.

Foods that contain more than 3 grams of dietary fiber and those that contain 400 mg or more of sodium are indicated by particular symbols in the exchange lists. This can help the user select foods to meet his or her particular needs. Alcohol-containing beverages and sugary foods such as jelly, candy, syrups, and soft drinks are not included in the exchange lists. The calories contributed by alcohol and sugary foods should be taken into account by reducing the number of fat exchanges included in the meal plan.

LIMITATIONS OF THE FOOD EXCHANGE LISTS

The food exchange lists are not a suitable guide for meal planning for all people or in all clinical situations. The system is relatively complex, and it does not provide exact levels of intake of calories, carbohydrate, protein, or fat. Furthermore, the lists fail to include the variety of ethnic foods consumed by people from various cultural backgrounds. Individualized approaches to meal planning may be required if the exchange system is not understood or if caloric and nutrient intakes need to be tightly controlled.

In addition to the six food exchange lists (Tables F-2 through F-7), we present a list of "free" foods (Table F-8), a list of exchanges for combination foods (Table F-9), and the exchange values for a selection of snack foods and desserts (Table F-10). All of the tables in this appendix are reprinted with permission from *Exchange Lists for Meal Planning* published by The American Diabetes Association and The American Dietetic Association (revised 1989 edition).

TABLE F-1

The amounts of carbohydrate, protein, fat, and calories in one serving from each exchange list

Exchange List	Carbohydrate, g	Protein, g	Fat, g	Calories
Starch/Bread	15	3	trace	80
Meat				
lean	—	7	3	55
medium-fat	—	7	5	75
high-fat	—	7	8	100
Vegetable	5	2	—	25
Fruit	15	—	—	60
Milk				
skim	12	8	trace	90
low-fat	12	8	5	120
whole	12	8	8	150
Fat	—	—	5	45

Source: Am. Diabetes Assoc., Amer. Dietetic Assoc., 1989.

■
TABLE F-2
Starch/bread exchange list

Each item in this list contains approximately 15 grams of carbohydrate, 3 grams of protein, a trace of fat, and 80 calories. Whole-grain products average about 2 grams of fiber per serving. Some foods are higher in fiber; those that contain 3 or more grams of fiber per serving are identified with the symbol ▨.

Select your starch exchanges from the items on this list. For starch foods not on this list, the general rule is that ½ cup of cereal, grain, or pasta or 1 ounce of a bread product is one serving. A dietitian can help you be more exact.

The starch foods prepared with fat count as 1 starch/bread exchange plus 1 fat exchange. All other items in this table count as 1 starch/bread exchange.

Cereals/Grains/Pasta	
▨ Bran cereals, concentrated (such as Bran Buds®, All Bran®)	⅓ c
▨ Bran cereals, flaked	½ c
Bulgur (cooked)	½ c
Cooked cereals	½ c
Cornmeal (dry)	2½ T
Grape-Nuts®	3 T
Grits (cooked)	½ c
Other ready-to-eat, unsweetened cereals	¾ c
Pasta (cooked)	½ c
Puffed cereal	1½ c
Rice, white or brown (cooked)	⅓ c
Shredded wheat	½ c
▨ Wheat germ	3 T

Dried Beans/Peas/Lentils	
▨ Beans and peas (cooked) (such as kidney, white, split, black-eyed)	⅓ c
▨ Lentils (cooked)	⅓ c
▨ Baked beans	¼ c

Starchy Vegetables	
▨ Corn	½ c
▨ Corn on cob, 6″	1
▨ Lima beans	½ c
▨ Peas, green (canned or frozen)	½ c
▨ Plantain	½ c
Potato, baked	1 sm. (3 oz)
Potato, mashed	½ c
▨ Squash, winter (acorn, butternut)	1 c
Yam/sweet potato, plain	⅓ c

TABLE F-2, *continued*

Bread	
Bagel	½ (1 oz)
Break sticks, crisp, 4″ × ½″	2 (⅔ oz)
Croutons, low-fat	1 c
English muffin	½
Frankfurter/hamburger bun	½ (1 oz)
Pita, 6″	½
Plain roll, sm.	1 (1 oz)
Raisin, unfrosted	1 slice (1 oz)
Rye, pumpernickel	1 slice (1 oz)
Tortilla, 6″	1
White (inc. French, Italian)	1 slice (1 oz)
Whole-wheat	1 slice (1 oz)
Crackers/Snacks	
Animal crackers	8
Graham crackers, 2½″ sq.	3
Matzoh	¾ oz
Melba toast	5 slices
Oyster crackers	24
Popcorn (popped, no fat added)	3 c
Pretzels	¾ oz
▨ RyKrisp®, 2″ × 3½″	4
Saltine-type crackers	6
▨ Whole-wheat crackers, no fat added (crisp breads, such as Finn®, Kavli®, Wasa®)	2–4 (¾ oz)
Starch Foods Prepared with Fat*	
Biscuit, 2½″	1
Chow mein noodles	½ c
Cornbread, 2″ cube	1 (2 oz)
Cracker, round butter-type	6
French fried potatoes, 2″–3½″ long	10 (1½ oz)
Muffin, plain	1 sm.
Pancake, 4″	2
Stuffing, bread (prepared)	¼ c
Taco shell, 6″	2
Waffle, 4½″ sq.	1
▨ Whole-wheat crackers, fat added (such as Triscuit®)	4–6 (1 oz)

Source: Am. Diabetes Assoc., Amer. Dietetic Assoc., 1989.

▨ 3 grams or more of fiber per exchange

*Starch foods prepared with fat count as 1 starch/bread exchange plus 1 fat exchange.

TABLE F-3
Meat Exchange List

Each service of meat or substitute on this list contains about 7 grams of protein. The amount of fat and number of calories vary, depending on the kind of meat or substitute.

Remember that the high-fat meats and substitutes are high in saturated fat, cholesterol, and calories; they should be used only 3 times per week.

With the exception of the beef/pork frankfurters on the high-fat list, all items in this table constitute one meat exchange.

Lean Meat and Substitutes

Beef	USDA Select or Choice grades of lean beef, such as round, sirloin, and flank steak; tenderloin; and chipped beef	1 oz
Pork	Lean pork, such as fresh ham; canned, cured, or boiled ham; Canadian bacon; tenderloin	1 oz
Veal	All cuts are lean except for veal cutlets (ground or cubed)	1 oz
Poultry	Chicken, turkey, cornish hen (without skin)	1 oz
Fish	All fresh and frozen fish	1 oz
	Crab, lobster, scallops, shrimp, clams (fresh or canned in water)	2 oz
	Oysters	6 med.
	Tuna (canned in water)	¼ c
	Herring (uncreamed or smoked)	1 oz
	Sardines (canned)	2 med.
Wild game	Venison, rabbit, squirrel	1 oz
	Pheasant, duck, goose (without skin)	1 oz
Cheese	Any cottage cheese	¼ c
	Parmesan, grated	2 T
	Diet cheeses (with less than 55 cal per oz)	1 oz
Other	95% fat-free luncheon meat	1½ oz
	Egg whites	3
	Egg substitutes with less than 55 cal per ½ c	½ c

Medium-Fat Meat and Substitutes

Beef	Most beef products; *examples:* all ground beef, roasts (rib, chuck, rump), steaks (cubed, Porterhouse, T-bone), meatloaf	1 oz
Pork	Most pork products; *examples:* chops, loin roast, Boston butt, cutlets	1 oz
Lamb	Most lamb products; *examples:* chops, leg, roast	1 oz

TABLE F-3, *continued*

Lean Meat and Substitutes, *continued*

Veal	Cutlet (ground or cubed, unbreaded)	1 oz
Poultry	Chicken (with skin), domestic duck or goose (well drained of fat), ground turkey	1 oz
Fish	Tuna ★ (canned in oil and drained)	¼ c
	Salmon ★ (canned)	¼ c
Cheese	Skim- or part-skim-milk cheeses, such as:	
	ricotta	¼ c
	mozzarella	1 oz
	diet cheeses ✎ (56–80 cal per oz)	1 oz
Other	86% fat-free luncheon meat ★	1 oz
	Egg (high in cholesterol; limit to 3 per week)	1
	Egg substitutes (56–80 cal per ¼ c)	¼ c
	Tofu (2½″ × 2¾″ × 1″)	4 oz
	Liver, heart, kidney, sweetbreads (high in cholesterol)	1 oz

High-Fat Meat and Substitutes*

Beef	Most USDA Prime cuts of beef, such as ribs, corned beef ★	1 oz
Pork	Spareribs, ground pork, pork sausage ✎ (patty or link)	1 oz
Lamb	Patties (ground lamb)	1 oz
Fish	Any fried fish product	1 oz
Cheese	All regular cheeses, such as American ✎, blue ✎, cheddar ★, Monterey Jack ★, Swiss	1 oz
Other	Luncheon meats ✎, such as bologna, salami, pimento loaf	1 oz
	Sausage ✎, such as Polish, Italian, smoked	1 oz
	Knockwurst ✎	1 oz
	Bratwurst ★	1 oz
	Frankfurter ✎ (turkey or chicken)	1 (10/lb)
	Peanut butter (contains unsaturated fat)	1 T
	Frankfurter ✎ (beef, pork, or combination)**	1 (10/lb)

Source: Am. Diabetes Assoc., Amer. Dietetic Assoc., 1989.

✎ 400 mg or more of sodium per exchange

★ 400 mg or more of sodium if two or more exchanges are eaten

*These items are high in saturated fat, cholesterol, and calories; they should be used only 3 times per week.

**count as 1 high-fat meat plus 1 fat exchange.

TABLE F-4
Vegetable exchange list

Each vegetable serving on this list contains about 5 grams of carbohydrate, 2 grams of protein, and 25 calories. Vegetables contain 2–3 grams of dietary fiber. Vegetables that contain 400 mg. of sodium per serving are identified with an asterisk.

Vegetables are a good source of vitamins and minerals. Fresh and frozen vegetables have more vitamins and less added salt. Rinsing canned vegetables will remove much of the salt.

Unless otherwise noted, the serving sizes for vegetables (one vegetable exchange) are ½ cup for cooked vegetables or vegetable juice and 1 cup for raw vegetables.

Starchy vegetables such as corn, peas, and potatoes are found on the starch/break list, Table F-2. For free vegetables, see the free food list, Table F-8.

Artichoke (½ med.)	Eggplant	Rutabaga
Asparagus	Greens (collard, mustard, turnip)	Sauerkraut ◼
Beans (green, wax, Italian)	Kohlrabi	Spinach, cooked
Bean sprouts	Leeks	Summer squash (crookneck)
Beets	Mushrooms, cooked	Tomato (1 lg.)
Broccoli	Okra	Tomato/vegetable juice ◼
Brussels sprouts	Onions	Turnips
Cabbage, cooked	Pea pods	Water chestnuts
Carrots	Peppers (green)	Zucchini, cooked
Cauliflower		

Source: Am. Diabetes Assoc., Amer. Dietetic Assoc., 1989.

◼ 400 mg or more of sodium per serving

TABLE F-5
Fruit exchange list

Each item on this list contains about 15 grams of carbohydrate and 60 calories. Fresh, frozen, and dried fruits have about 2 grams of fiber per serving. Fruits that have 3 or more grams of fiber per serving are indicated with a ◼ symbol. Fruit juices contain very little dietary fiber.

The carbohydrate and calorie content for a fruit serving are based on the usual serving of the most commonly eaten fruits. Use fresh fruits or fruits frozen or canned without sugar added. Whole fruit is more filling than fruit juice and may be a better choice for those who are trying to lose weight. Unless otherwise noted, the serving sizes for one fruit serving are ½ cup for fresh fruit or fruit juice and ¼ cup for dried fruit.

Fresh, Frozen, and Unsweetened Canned Fruit

	Apple (raw, 2″ diam.)	1
	Applesauce (unsweetened)	½ c
	Apricots (raw)	4 med.
	(canned)	½ c or 4 halves
	Banana (9″)	½
◼	Blackberries (raw)	¾ c

TABLE F-5, *continued*

▨ Blueberries (raw)	¾ c
Cantaloupe (5″ diam.)	⅓
(cubes)	1 c
Cherries (raw)	12 lg.
(canned)	½ c
Figs (raw, 2″ diam.)	2
Fruit cocktail (canned)	½ c
Grapefruit (med.)	½
(segments)	¾ c
Grapes (small)	15
Honeydew melon (med.)	⅛
(cubes)	1 c
Kiwi	1 lg.
Mandarin oranges	¾ c
Mango	½ sm.
▨ Nectarine (2½″ diam.)	1
Orange (2½″ diam.)	1
Papaya	1 c
Peaches (raw, 2¾ diam.)	1, or ¾ c
(canned)	½ c or 2 halves
Pears (raw)	½ lg. or 1 sm.
(canned)	½ c or 2 halves
Persimmon (native)	2 med.
Pineapple (raw)	¾ c
(canned)	⅓ c
Plums (raw, 2″ diam.)	2
▨ Pomegranate	½
▨ Raspberries (raw)	1 cu
▨ Strawberries (raw, whole)	1¼ c
▨ Tangerine (2½″ diam.)	2
Watermelon (cubes)	1¼
Dried Fruit	
▨ Apples	4 rings
▨ Apricots	7 halves
Dates	2½ med.
▨ Figs	1½
▨ Prunes	3 med.
Raisins	2 T
Fruit Juice	
Apple juice/cider	½ c
Cranberry juice cocktail	⅓ c
Grapefruit juice	½ c
Grape juice	⅓ c
Orange juice	½ c
Pineapple juice	½ c
Prune juice	⅓ c

Source: Am. Diabetes Assoc., Amer. Dietetic Assoc., 1989.

▨ 3 or more grams of fiber per exchange

TABLE F-6
Milk exchange list

Each serving of milk or milk products on this list contains about 12 grams of carbohydrate and 8 grams of protein. The amount of fat in milk is measured in percent of butterfat. Calories vary with the kind of milk. Skim and very low fat milk provide 90 calories; low-fat, 120 calories; whole milk, 150 calories.

Skim and Very Low Fat Milk	
Skim milk	1 c
½% milk	1 c
1% milk	1 c
Low-fat buttermilk	1 c
Evaporated skim milk	½ c
Dry nonfat milk	⅓ c
Plain nonfat yogurt	8 oz
Low-fat Milk	
2% milk	1 c fluid
Plain low-fat yogurt (with added nonfat milk solids)	8 oz
Whole Milk	
Whole milk	1 c
Evaporated whole milk	½ c
Plain whole-milk yogurt	8 oz

Source: Am. Diabetes Assoc., Amer. Dietetic Assoc., 1989.

TABLE F-7
Fat exchange list

Each serving on the fat exchange list contains about 5 grams of fat and 45 calories. The foods on the list contain mostly fat, although some items may also contain a small amount of protein. All fats are high in calories and should be measured carefully. Everyone should modify fat intake by eating unsaturated fats instead of saturated fats whenever possible. The sodium content of these foods varies widely; check the labels.

Unsaturated Fats

Avocado	⅛ med.
Margarine	1 t
★ Margarine, diet	1 T
Mayonnaise	1 t
★ Mayonnaise, reduced-calorie	1 T
Nuts and seeds	
Almonds, dry-roasted	6 whole
Cashews, dry-roasted	1 T
Pecans	2 whole
Peanuts	20 sm. or 10 lg.
Walnuts	2 whole
Other nuts	1 T
Seeds, pine nuts, sunflower (without shells)	1 T
Pumpkin seeds	2 t
Oil (corn, cottonseed, safflower, soybean, sunflower, olive, peanut)	1 t
★ Olives	10 sm. or 5 lg.
Salad dressing, mayonnaise-type	2 t
Salad dressing, reduced-calorie mayonnaise-type	1 T
★ Salad dressing (oil varieties)	1 T
✎ Salad dressing, reduced-calorie	2 T*

Saturated Fats

Butter	1 t
★ Bacon	1 slice
Chitterlings	½ oz
Coconut, shredded	2 T
Coffee whitener, liquid	2 T
Coffee whitener, powder	4 t
Cream (light, coffee, table)	2 T
Cream, sour	2 T
Cream (heavy, whipping)	1 T
Cream cheese	1 T
★ Salt pork	¼ oz

✎ 400 mg or more of sodium per exchange

★ 400 mg or more of sodium if two or more exchanges are eaten

*Two tablespoons of low-calorie salad dressing is a free food.

■

TABLE F-8

Free Foods

A "free" food is any food or beverage that contains less than 20 calories per serving. You may consume as much as you want of those items that have no serving size specified. You may eat 2 or 3 servings per day of those items for which a serving size is specified, but spread them out through the day.

Seasonings can be very helpful in making food taste better. Some of them, however, contain quite a bit of sodium. Read the labels and choose those that do not contain sodium or salt.

Drinks

Bouillon ◩ or broth without fat
Bouillon, low-sodium
Carbonated drinks, sugar-free
Carbonated water
Club soda
Cocoa powder, unsweetened, (1T)
Coffee/tea
Drink mixes, sugar-free
Tonic water, sugar-free

Fruits

Cranberries, unsweetened (½ c)
Rhubarb, unsweetened (½ c)

Vegetables (raw, 1 c)

Cabbage
Celery
Chinese cabbage ▧
Cucumber
Green onion
Hot peppers
Mushrooms
Radishes
Zucchini ▧

Salad greens

Endive
Escarole
Lettuce
Romaine
Spinach

Sweet Substitutes

Candy, hard, sugar-free
Gelatin, sugar-free
Gum, sugar-free
Jam/jelly, sugar-free (less than 20 cal/2 t.)
Pancake syrup, sugar-free (1–2 T)
Sugar substitutes (saccharin, aspartame)
Whipped topping (2 T)

Condiments

Catsup (1 T)
Horseradish
Mustard
Pickles ◩, dill, unsweetened
Salad dressing, low-calorie (2 T)
Taco sauce (3 T)
Vinegar

Other

Nonstick pan spray

Seasonings

Basil (fresh)
Celery seeds
Chili powder
Chives
Cinnamon
Curry
Dill
Flavoring extracts (vanilla, almond, walnut, peppermint, butter, lemon, etc.)
Garlic
Garlic powder
Herbs
Hot pepper sauce
Lemon
Lemon juice
Lemon pepper
Lime
Lime juice
Mint
Onion powder
Oregano
Paprika
Pepper
Pimento
Spices
Soy sauce ◩
Soy sauce ◩, low-sodium ("lite")
Wine, used in cooking (¼ c)
Worcestershire sauce

▧ 3 grams or more of fiber per exchange
◩ 400 mg or more of sodium per exchange

TABLE F-9

Exchanges for selected combination foods

Food	Amount	Exchange(s)
Casseroles, homemade	1 c (8 oz)	2 starch, 2 medium-fat meat, 1 fat
Cheese pizza ◪, thin crust	¼ of 15-oz or ¼ of 10″	2 starch, 1 medium-fat meat, 1 fat
Chili with beans (commercial) ▨, ◪	1 c (8 oz)	2 starch, 2 medium-fat meat, 2 fat
Chow mein ◪ (without noodles or rice)	2 c (16 oz)	1 starch, 2 vegetable, 2 lean meat
Macaroni and cheese ◪	1 c (8 oz)	2 starch, 1 medium-fat meat, 2 fat
Soups		
bean ▨, ◪	1 c (8 oz)	1 starch, 1 vegetable, 1 lean meat
chunky, all varieties ◪	10¾-oz can	1 starch, 1 vegetable, 1 medium-fat meat
cream ◪ (made with water)	1 c (8 oz)	1 starch, 1 fat
vegetable ◪ or broth-type ◪	1 c (8 oz)	1 starch
Spaghetti and meatballs (canned) ◪	1 c (8 oz)	2 starch, 1 medium-fat meat, 1 fat
Sugar-free pudding (made with skim milk)	½ c	1 starch
Dried beans ▨, peas ▨, lentils ▨ used as a meat substitute (cooked)	1 c	2 starch, 1 lean meat

▨ 3 grams or more of fiber per exchange

◪ 400 mg or more of sodium per exchange

TABLE F-10

Average exchange values for selected foods for occasional use

Food	Amount	Exchange(s)
Angel food cake	1/12 cake	2 starch
Cake, no icing	1/12 cake or a 3″ sq.	2 starch, 2 fat
Cookies	2 sm. (1¾″)	1 starch, 1 fat
Frozen fruit yogurt	⅓ c	1 starch
Gingersnaps	3	1 starch
Granola	¼ c	1 starch, 1 fat
Granola bars	1 sm.	1 starch, 1 fat
Ice cream, any flavor	½ c	1 starch, 2 fat
Ice milk, any flavor	½ c	1 starch, 1 fat
Sherbet, any flavor	¼ c	1 starch
Snack chips ✦, all varieties	1 oz	1 starch, 2 fat
Vanilla wafers	6 sm.	1 starch

✦ 400 mg or more of sodium if two or more exchanges are eaten

APPENDIX G

INSTRUCTIONS AND FORMAT FOR RECORDING DIETARY INTAKE

Please adhere to the following instructions when recording your dietary intake for analysis by the DAS™ software program. As is the case with all computer programs, the more accurate the input, the more reliable the output will be. Instructions for running the DAS program are contained in the manual that accompanies the program. The program is easy to run, but you will need to follow a few specific directions. Be sure to read the instructions before using the program.

After you have entered your dietary intake, you will receive a printout that lists your intake of 25 important food constituents and relates your intake to the recommended levels and to the food groups. The printout also identifies the percentages of calories in your diet contributed by carbohydrate, protein, and fat and compares those percentages with the recommended percentages.

Follow these instructions for recording your dietary intake:

1. For 3 days, record all of the foods, snacks, and beverages you consume. Include 2 weekdays and 1 weekend day.
2. Carry the Dietary Intake Recording Form with you. Write down each food, snack, and beverage you consume. Fully describe the foods and indicate the amounts or ingredients. (See the figure.) Since you will be entering food and beverage names into the computer, make certain you spell the names correctly.
3. Weigh, measure, or count food carefully. Use household measurement units. Refer to food labels if you are uncertain about amounts or ingredients.

Example of recording:

Day 1

What I ate and drank	How much I ate and drank
Egg McMuffin	1
coffee with	2 c
half & half	2 T
ham	3 oz
rye bread	2 slices
mustard	1 t
frozen yogurt	1 c
popcorn	3 c

DIETARY INTAKE RECORDING FORM

Day 1		Day 2		Day 3	
What I ate and drank	How much I ate and drank	What I ate and drank	How much I ate and drank	What I ate and drank	How much I ate and drank

APPENDIX H

COMPOSITION OF FOODS

TABLE H-1
Nutritive values of the edible part of foods

[Dashes in the columns for nutrients show that no suitable value could be found although there is reason to believe that a measurable amount of the nutrient may be present]

	Food, approximate measure, and weight (in grams)			Water	Food energy	Protein	Fat	Fatty acids: Saturated (total)	Fatty acids: Unsaturated: Oleic	Fatty acids: Unsaturated: Linoleic	Carbohydrate	Calcium	Iron	Vitamin A value	Thiamin	Riboflavin	Niacin	Ascorbic acid
	MILK, CHEESE, CREAM, IMITATION CREAM; RELATED PRODUCTS		*Grams*	*Per-cent*	*Calories*	*Grams*	*Grams*	*Grams*	*Grams*	*Grams*	*Grams*	*Milli-grams*	*Milli-grams*	*Inter-national units*	*Milli-grams*	*Milli-grams*	*Milli-grams*	*Milli-grams*
	Milk:																	
	Fluid:																	
1	Whole, 3.5% fat	1 cup	244	87	160	9	9	5	3	Trace	12	288	0.1	350	0.07	0.41	0.2	2
2	Nonfat (skim)	1 cup	245	90	90	9	Trace	------	------	------	12	296	.1	10	.09	.44	.2	2
3	Partly skimmed, 2% nonfat milk solids added.	1 cup	246	87	145	10	5	3	2	Trace	15	352	.1	200	.10	.52	.2	2
	Canned, concentrated, undiluted:																	
4	Evaporated, unsweetened.	1 cup	252	74	345	18	20	11	7	1	24	635	.3	810	.10	.86	.5	3
5	Condensed, sweetened.	1 cup	306	27	980	25	27	15	9	1	166	802	.3	1,100	.24	1.16	.6	3
	Dry, nonfat instant:																	
6	Low-density (1⅓ cups needed for reconstitution to 1 qt.).	1 cup	68	4	245	24	Trace	------	------	------	35	879	.4	[1]20	.24	1.21	.6	5
7	High-density (⅞ cup needed for reconstitution to 1 qt.).	1 cup	104	4	375	37	1	------	------	------	54	1,345	.6	[1]30	.36	1.85	.9	7
	Buttermilk:																	
8	Fluid, cultured, made from skim milk.	1 cup	245	90	90	9	Trace	------	------	------	12	296	.1	10	.10	.44	.2	2
9	Dried, packaged	1 cup	120	3	465	41	6	3	2	Trace	60	1,498	.7	260	.31	2.06	1.1	------
	Cheese:																	
	Natural:																	
	Blue or Roquefort type:																	
10	Ounce	1 oz.	28	40	105	6	9	5	3	Trace	1	89	.1	350	.01	.17	.3	0
11	Cubic inch	1 cu. in.	17	40	65	4	5	3	2	Trace	Trace	54	.1	210	.01	.11	.2	0

[1] Value applies to unfortified product; value for fortified low-density product would be 1500 I.U., and the fortified high-density product would be 2290 I.U.

TABLE H-1

Nutritive values of the edible part of foods, *continued*

[Dashes in the columns for nutrients show that no suitable value could be found although there is reason to believe that a measurable amount of the nutrient may be present]

No.	Food, approximate measure, and weight (in grams)			Water	Food energy	Protein	Fat	Fatty acids: Saturated (total)	Fatty acids: Unsaturated: Oleic	Fatty acids: Unsaturated: Linoleic	Carbohydrate	Calcium	Iron	Vitamin A value	Thiamin	Riboflavin	Niacin	Ascorbic acid
	MILK, CHEESE, CREAM, IMITATION CREAM; RELATED PRODUCTS—Con.																	
	Cheese—Continued																	
	Natural—Continued		*Grams*	*Per-cent*	*Calo-ries*	*Grams*	*Grams*	*Grams*	*Grams*	*Grams*	*Grams*	*Milli-grams*	*Milli-grams*	*Inter-national units*	*Milli-grams*	*Milli-grams*	*Milli-grams*	*Milli-grams*
12	Camembert, packaged in 4-oz. pkg. with 3 wedges per pkg.	1 wedge	38	52	115	7	9	5	3	Trace	1	40	0.2	380	0.02	0.29	0.3	0
	Cheddar:																	
13	Ounce	1 oz.	28	37	115	7	9	5	3	Trace	1	213	.3	370	.01	.13	Trace	0
14	Cubic inch	1 cu. in.	17	37	70	4	6	3	2	Trace	Trace	129	.2	230	.01	.08	Trace	0
	Cottage, large or small curd:																	
	Creamed:																	
15	Package of 12-oz., net wt.	1 pkg.	340	78	360	46	14	8	5	Trace	10	320	1.0	580	.10	.85	.3	0
16	Cup, curd pressed down.	1 cup	245	78	260	33	10	6	3	Trace	7	230	.7	420	.07	.61	.2	0
	Uncreamed:																	
17	Package of 12-oz., net wt.	1 pkg.	340	79	290	58	1	1	Trace	Trace	9	306	1.4	30	.10	.95	.3	0
18	Cup, curd pressed down.	1 cup	200	79	170	34	1	Trace	Trace	Trace	5	180	.8	20	.06	.56	.2	0
	Cream:																	
19	Package of 8-oz., net wt.	1 pkg.	227	51	850	18	86	48	28	3	5	141	.5	3,500	.05	.54	.2	0
20	Package of 3-oz., net wt.	1 pkg.	85	51	320	7	32	18	11	1	2	53	.2	1,310	.02	.20	.1	0
21	Cubic inch	1 cu. in.	16	51	60	1	6	3	2	Trace	Trace	10	Trace	250	Trace	.04	Trace	0
	Parmesan, grated:																	
22	Cup, pressed down	1 cup	140	17	655	60	43	24	14	1	5	1,893	.7	1,760	.03	1.22	.3	0
23	Tablespoon	1 tbsp.	5	17	25	2	2	1	Trace	Trace	Trace	68	Trace	60	Trace	.04	Trace	0
24	Ounce	1 oz.	28	17	130	12	9	5	3	Trace	1	383	.1	360	.01	.25	.1	0
	Swiss:																	
25	Ounce	1 oz.	28	39	105	8	8	4	3	Trace	1	262	.3	320	Trace	.11	Trace	0
26	Cubic inch	1 cu. in.	15	39	55	4	4	2	1	Trace	Trace	139	.1	170	Trace	.06	Trace	0
	Pasteurized processed cheese:																	
	American:																	
27	Ounce	1 oz.	28	40	105	7	9	5	3	Trace	1	198	.3	350	.01	.12	Trace	0
28	Cubic inch	1 cu. in.	18	40	65	4	5	3	2	Trace	Trace	122	.2	210	Trace	.07	Trace	0
	Swiss:																	
29	Ounce	1 oz.	28	40	100	8	8	4	3	Trace	1	251	.3	310	Trace	.11	Trace	0
30	Cubic inch	1 cu. in.	18	40	65	5	5	3	2	Trace	Trace	159	.2	200	Trace	.07	Trace	0
	Pasteurized process cheese food, American:																	
31	Tablespoon	1 tbsp.	14	43	45	3	3	2	1	Trace	1	80	.1	140	Trace	.08	Trace	0
32	Cubic inch	1 cu. in.	18	43	60	4	4	2	1	Trace	1	100	.1	170	Trace	.10	Trace	0
33	Pasteurized process cheese spread, American.	1 oz.	28	49	80	5	6	3	2	Trace	2	160	.2	250	Trace	.15	Trace	0
	Cream:																	
34	Half-and-half (cream and milk).	1 cup	242	80	325	8	28	15	9	1	11	261	.1	1,160	.07	.39	.1	2
35		1 tbsp.	15	80	20	1	2	1	1	Trace	1	16	Trace	70	Trace	.02	Trace	Trace
36	Light, coffee or table	1 cup	240	72	505	7	49	27	16	1	10	245	.1	2,020	.07	.36	.1	2
37		1 tbsp.	15	72	30	1	3	2	1	Trace	1	15	Trace	130	Trace	.02	Trace	Trace
38	Sour	1 cup	230	72	485	7	47	26	16	1	10	235	.1	1,930	.07	.35	.1	2
39		1 tbsp.	12	72	25	Trace	2	1	1	Trace	1	12	Trace	100	Trace	.02	Trace	Trace
40	Whipped topping (pressurized).	1 cup	60	62	155	2	14	8	5	Trace	6	67	------	570	------	.04	------	------
41		1 tbsp.	3	62	10	Trace	1	Trace	Trace	Trace	Trace	3	------	30	------	Trace	------	------
	Whipping, unwhipped (volume about double when whipped):																	
42	Light	1 cup	239	62	715	6	75	41	25	2	9	203	.1	3,060	.05	.29	.1	2
43		1 tbsp.	15	62	45	Trace	5	3	2	Trace	1	13	Trace	190	Trace	.02	Trace	Trace
44	Heavy	1 cup	238	57	840	5	90	50	30	3	7	179	.1	3,670	.05	.26	.1	2
45		1 tbsp.	15	57	55	Trace	6	3	2	Trace	1	11	Trace	230	Trace	.02	Trace	Trace

TABLE H-1

Nutritive values of the edible part of foods, *continued*

[Dashes in the columns for nutrients show that no suitable value could be found although there is reason to believe that a measurable amount of the nutrient may be present]

	Food, approximate measure, and weight (in grams)			Water	Food energy	Protein	Fat	Fatty acids: Saturated (total)	Fatty acids: Unsaturated: Oleic	Fatty acids: Unsaturated: Linoleic	Carbohydrate	Calcium	Iron	Vitamin A value	Thiamin	Riboflavin	Niacin	Ascorbic acid
	MILK, CHEESE, CREAM, IMITATION CREAM; RELATED PRODUCTS—Con.																	
	Cream—Continued		*Grams*	*Percent*	*Calories*	*Grams*	*Grams*	*Grams*	*Grams*	*Grams*	*Grams*	*Milligrams*	*Milligrams*	*International units*	*Milligrams*	*Milligrams*	*Milligrams*	*Milligrams*
	Imitation cream products (made with vegetable fat):																	
	Creamers:																	
46	Powdered	1 cup	94	2	505	4	33	31	1	0	52	21	.6	[2] 200	-----	-----	Trace	-----
47		1 tsp.	2	2	10	Trace	1	Trace	Trace	0	1	1	Trace	[2] Trace	-----	-----	-----	-----
48	Liquid (frozen)	1 cup	245	77	345	3	27	25	1	0	25	29	-----	[2] 100	0	0	-----	-----
49		1 tbsp.	15	77	20	Trace	2	1	Trace	0	2	2	-----	[2] 10	0	0	-----	-----
50	Sour dressing (imitation sour cream) made with nonfat dry milk.	1 cup	235	72	440	9	38	35	1	Trace	17	277	.1	10	.07	.38	.2	1
51		1 tbsp.	12	72	20	Trace	2	2	Trace	Trace	1	14	Trace	Trace	Trace	Trace	Trace	Trace
	Whipped topping:																	
52	Pressurized	1 cup	70	61	190	1	17	15	1	0	9	5	-----	[2] 340	-----	0	-----	-----
53		1 tbsp.	4	61	10	Trace	1	1	Trace	0	Trace	Trace	-----	[2] 20	-----	0	-----	-----
54	Frozen	1 cup	75	52	230	1	20	18	Trace	0	15	5	-----	[2] 560	-----	0	-----	-----
55		1 tbsp.	4	52	10	Trace	1	1	Trace	0	1	Trace	-----	[2] 30	-----	0	-----	-----
56	Powdered, made with whole milk.	1 cup	75	58	175	3	12	10	1	Trace	15	62	Trace	[2] 330	.02	.08	.1	Trace
57		1 tbsp.	4	58	10	Trace	1	1	Trace	Trace	1	3	Trace	[2] 20	Trace	Trace	Trace	Trace
	Milk beverages:																	
58	Cocoa, homemade	1 cup	250	79	245	10	12	7	4	Trace	27	295	1.0	400	.10	.45	.5	3
59	Chocolate-flavored drink made with skim milk and 2% added butterfat.	1 cup	250	83	190	8	6	3	2	Trace	27	270	.5	210	.10	.40	.3	3
	Malted milk:																	
60	Dry powder, approx. 3 heaping teaspoons per ounce.	1 oz.	28	3	115	4	2	-----	-----	-----	20	82	.6	290	.09	.15	.1	0
61	Beverage	1 cup	235	78	245	11	10	-----	-----	-----	28	317	.7	590	.14	.49	.2	2
	Milk desserts:																	
62	Custard, baked	1 cup	265	77	305	14	15	7	5	1	29	297	1.1	930	.11	.50	.3	1
	Ice cream:																	
63	Regular (approx. 10% fat).	½ gal.	1,064	63	2,055	48	113	62	37	3	221	1,553	.5	4,680	.43	2.23	1.1	11
64		1 cup	133	63	255	6	14	8	5	Trace	28	194	.1	590	.05	.28	.1	1
65		3 fl. oz. cup	50	63	95	2	5	3	2	Trace	10	73	Trace	220	.02	.11	.1	1
66	Rich (approx. 16% fat).	½ gal.	1,188	63	2,635	31	191	105	63	6	214	927	.2	7,840	.24	1.31	1.2	12
67		1 cup	148	63	330	4	24	13	8	1	27	115	Trace	980	.03	.16	.1	1
	Ice milk:																	
68	Hardened	½ gal.	1,048	67	1,595	50	53	29	17	2	235	1,635	1.0	2,200	.52	2.31	1.0	10
69		1 cup	131	67	200	6	7	4	2	Trace	29	204	.1	280	.07	.29	.1	1
70	Soft-serve	1 cup	175	67	265	8	9	5	3	Trace	39	273	.2	370	.09	.39	.2	2
	Yoghurt:																	
71	Made from partially skimmed milk.	1 cup	245	89	125	8	4	2	1	Trace	13	294	.1	170	.10	.44	.2	2
72	Made from whole milk	1 cup	245	88	150	7	8	5	3	Trace	12	272	.1	340	.07	.39	.2	2
	EGGS																	
	Eggs, large, 24 ounces per dozen:																	
	Raw or cooked in shell or with nothing added:																	
73	Whole, without shell	1 egg	50	74	80	6	6	2	3	Trace	Trace	27	1.1	590	.05	.15	Trace	0
74	White of egg	1 white	33	88	15	4	Trace	-----	-----	-----	Trace	3	Trace	0	Trace	.09	Trace	0
75	Yolk of egg	1 yolk	17	51	60	3	5	2	2	Trace	Trace	24	.9	580	.04	.07	Trace	0
76	Scrambled with milk and fat.	1 egg	64	72	110	7	8	3	3	Trace	1	51	1.1	690	.05	.18	Trace	0

[2] Contributed largely from beta-carotene used for coloring.

TABLE H-1

Nutritive values of the edible part of foods, *continued*

[Dashes in the columns for nutrients show that no suitable value could be found although there is reason to believe that a measurable amount of the nutrient may be present]

No.	Food, approximate measure, and weight (in grams)			Water	Food energy	Protein	Fat	Fatty acids: Saturated (total)	Fatty acids: Unsaturated: Oleic	Fatty acids: Unsaturated: Linoleic	Carbohydrate	Calcium	Iron	Vitamin A value	Thiamin	Riboflavin	Niacin	Ascorbic acid
	MEAT, POULTRY, FISH, SHELLFISH; RELATED PRODUCTS		Grams	Per-cent	Calo-ries	Grams	Grams	Grams	Grams	Grams	Grams	Milli-grams	Milli-grams	Inter-national units	Milli-grams	Milli-grams	Milli-grams	Milli-grams
77	Bacon, (20 slices per lb. raw), broiled or fried, crisp.	2 slices	15	8	90	5	8	3	4	1	1	2	.5	0	.08	.05	.8	------
	Beef,[3] cooked:																	
	Cuts braised, simmered, or pot-roasted:																	
78	Lean and fat	3 ounces	85	53	245	23	16	8	7	Trace	0	10	2.9	30	.04	.18	3.5	------
79	Lean only	2.5 ounces	72	62	140	22	5	2	2	Trace	0	10	2.7	10	.04	.16	3.3	------
	Hamburger (ground beef), broiled:																	
80	Lean	3 ounces	85	60	185	23	10	5	4	Trace	0	10	3.0	20	.08	.20	5.1	------
81	Regular	3 ounces	85	54	245	21	17	8	8	Trace	0	9	2.7	30	.07	.18	4.6	------
	Roast, oven-cooked, no liquid added:																	
	Relatively fat, such as rib:																	
82	Lean and fat	3 ounces	85	40	375	17	34	16	15	1	0	8	2.2	70	.05	.13	3.1	------
83	Lean only	1.8 ounces	51	57	125	14	7	3	3	Trace	0	6	1.8	10	.04	.11	2.6	------
	Relatively lean, such as heel of round:																	
84	Lean and fat	3 ounces	85	62	165	25	7	3	3	Trace	0	11	3.2	10	.06	.19	4.5	------
85	Lean only	2.7 ounces	78	65	125	24	3	1	1	Trace	0	10	3.0	Trace	.06	.18	4.3	------
	Steak, broiled:																	
	Relatively, fat, such as sirloin:																	
86	Lean and fat	3 ounces	85	44	330	20	27	13	12	1	0	9	2.5	50	.05	.16	4.0	------
87	Lean only	2.0 ounces	56	59	115	18	4	2	2	Trace	0	7	2.2	10	.05	.14	3.6	------
	Relatively, lean, such as round:																	
88	Lean and fat	3 ounces	85	55	220	24	13	6	6	Trace	0	10	3.0	20	.07	.19	4.8	------
89	Lean only	2.4 ounces	68	61	130	21	4	2	2	Trace	0	9	2.5	10	.06	.16	4.1	------
	Beef, canned:																	
90	Corned beef	3 ounces	85	59	185	22	10	5	4	Trace	0	17	3.7	20	.01	.20	2.9	------
91	Corned beef hash	3 ounces	85	67	155	7	10	5	4	Trace	9	11	1.7	-------	.01	.08	1.8	------
92	Beef, dried or chipped	2 ounces	57	48	115	19	4	2	2	Trace	0	11	2.9	-------	.04	.18	2.2	------
93	Beef and vegetable stew	1 cup	235	82	210	15	10	5	4	Trace	15	28	2.8	2,310	.13	.17	4.4	15
94	Beef potpie, baked, 4¼-inch diam., weight before baking about 8 ounces.	1 pie	227	55	560	23	33	9	20	2	43	32	4.1	1,860	0.25	0.27	4.5	7
	Chicken, cooked:																	
95	Flesh only, broiled	3 ounces	85	71	115	20	3	1	1	1	0	8	1.4	80	.05	.16	7.4	------
	Breast, fried, ½ breast:																	
96	With bone	3.3 ounces	94	58	155	25	5	1	2	1	1	9	1.3	70	.04	.17	11.2	------
97	Flesh and skin only	2.7 ounces	76	58	155	25	5	1	2	1	1	9	1.3	70	.04	.17	11.2	------
	Drumstick, fried:																	
98	With bone	2.1 ounces	59	55	90	12	4	1	2	1	Trace	6	.9	50	.03	.15	2.7	------
99	Flesh and skin only	1.3 ounces	38	55	90	12	4	1	2	1	Trace	6	.9	50	.03	.15	2.7	------
100	Chicken, canned, boneless	3 ounces	85	65	170	18	10	3	4	2	0	18	1.3	200	.03	.11	3.7	3
101	Chicken potpie, baked 4¼-inch diam., weight before baking about 8 ounces.	1 pie	227	57	535	23	31	10	15	3	42	68	3.0	3,020	.25	.26	4.1	5
	Chili con carne, canned:																	
102	With beans	1 cup	250	72	335	19	15	7	7	Trace	30	80	4.2	150	.08	.18	3.2	------
103	Without beans	1 cup	255	67	510	26	38	18	17	1	15	97	3.6	380	.05	.31	5.6	------
104	Heart, beef, lean, braised	3 ounces	85	61	160	27	5	------	------	------	1	5	5.0	20	.21	1.04	6.5	1
	Lamb,[3] cooked:																	
105	Chop, thick, with bone, broiled.	1 chop, 4.8 ounces.	137	47	400	25	33	18	12	1	0	10	1.5	-------	.14	.25	5.6	------
106	Lean and fat	4.0 ounces	112	47	400	25	33	18	12	1	0	10	1.5	-------	.14	.25	5.6	------
107	Lean only	2.6 ounces	74	62	140	21	6	3	2	Trace	0	9	1.5	-------	.11	.20	4.5	------
	Leg, roasted:																	
108	Lean and fat	3 ounces	85	54	235	22	16	9	6	Trace	0	9	1.4	-------	.13	.23	4.7	------
109	Lean only	2.5 ounces	71	62	130	20	5	3	2	Trace	0	9	1.4	-------	.12	.21	4.4	------

[3] Outer layer of fat on the cut was removed to within approximately ½-inch of the lean. Deposits of fat within the cut were not removed.

Nutritive values of the edible part of foods, *continued*

[Dashes in the columns for nutrients show that no suitable value could be found although there is reason to believe that a measurable amount of the nutrient may be present]

	Food, approximate measure, and weight (in grams)			Water	Food energy	Protein	Fat	Fatty acids: Saturated (total)	Fatty acids: Unsaturated: Oleic	Fatty acids: Unsaturated: Linoleic	Carbohydrate	Calcium	Iron	Vitamin A value	Thiamin	Riboflavin	Niacin	Ascorbic acid
	MEAT, POULTRY, FISH, SHELLFISH; RELATED PRODUCTS—Continued																	
	Lamb,[3] cooked—Continued		*Grams*	*Per-cent*	*Calo-ries*	*Grams*	*Grams*	*Grams*	*Grams*	*Grams*	*Grams*	*Milli-grams*	*Milli-grams*	*Inter-national units*	*Milli-grams*	*Milli-grams*	*Milli-grams*	*Milli-grams*
	Shoulder, roasted:																	
110	Lean and fat	3 ounces	85	50	285	18	23	13	8	1	0	9	1.0	------	.11	.20	4.0	------
111	Lean only	2.3 ounces	64	61	130	17	6	3	2	Trace	0	8	1.0	------	.10	.18	3.7	------
112	Liver, beef, fried	2 ounces	57	57	130	15	6	------	------	------	3	6	5.0	30,280	.15	2.37	9.4	15
	Pork, cured, cooked:																	
113	Ham, light cure, lean and fat, roasted.	3 ounces	85	54	245	18	19	7	8	2	0	8	2.2	0	.40	.16	3.1	------
	Luncheon meat:																	
114	Boiled ham, sliced	2 ounces	57	59	135	11	10	4	4	1	0	6	1.6	0	.25	.09	1.5	------
115	Canned, spiced or unspiced.	2 ounces	57	55	165	8	14	5	6	1	1	5	1.2	0	.18	.12	1.6	------
	Pork, fresh,[3] cooked:																	
116	Chop, thick, with bone	1 chop, 3.5 ounces.	98	42	260	16	21	8	9	2	0	8	2.2	0	.63	.18	3.8	------
117	Lean and fat	2.3 ounces	66	42	260	16	21	8	9	2	0	8	2.2	0	.63	.18	3.8	------
118	Lean only	1.7 ounces	48	53	130	15	7	2	3	1	0	7	1.9	0	.54	.16	3.3	------
	Roast, oven-cooked, no liquid added:																	
119	Lean and fat	3 ounces	85	46	310	21	24	9	10	2	0	9	2.7	0	.78	.22	4.7	------
120	Lean only	2.4 ounces	68	55	175	20	10	3	4	1	0	9	2.6	0	.73	.21	4.4	------
	Cuts, simmered:																	
121	Lean and fat	3 ounces	85	46	320	20	26	9	11	2	0	8	2.5	0	.46	.21	4.1	------
122	Lean only	2.2 ounces	63	60	135	18	6	2	3	1	0	8	2.3	0	.42	.19	3.7	------
	Sausage:																	
123	Bologna, slice, 3-in. diam. by 1/8 inch.	2 slices	26	56	80	3	7	------	------	------	Trace	2	.5	------	.04	.06	.7	------
124	Braunschweiger, slice 2-in. diam. by 1/4 inch.	2 slices	20	53	65	3	5	------	------	------	Trace	2	1.2	1,310	.03	.29	1.6	------
125	Deviled ham, canned	1 tbsp.	13	51	45	2	4	2	2	Trace	0	1	.3	------	.02	.01	.2	------
126	Frankfurter, heated (8 per lb. purchased pkg.).	1 frank	56	57	170	7	15	------	------	------	1	3	.8	------	.08	.11	1.4	------
127	Pork links, cooked (16 links per lb. raw).	2 links	26	35	125	5	11	4	5	1	Trace	2	.6	0	.21	.09	1.0	------
128	Salami, dry type	1 oz.	28	30	130	7	11	------	------	------	Trace	4	1.0	------	.10	.07	1.5	------
129	Salami, cooked	1 oz.	28	51	90	5	7	------	------	------	Trace	3	.7	------	.07	.07	1.2	------
130	Vienna, canned (7 sausages per 5-oz. can).	1 sausage	16	63	40	2	3	------	------	------	Trace	1	.3	------	.01	.02	.4	------
	Veal, medium fat, cooked, bone removed:																	
131	Cutlet	3 oz.	85	60	185	23	9	5	4	Trace	------	9	2.7	------	.06	.21	4.6	------
132	Roast	3 oz.	85	55	230	23	14	7	6	Trace	0	10	2.9	------	.11	.26	6.6	------
	Fish and shellfish:																	
133	Bluefish, baked with table fat.	3 oz.	85	68	135	22	4	------	------	------	0	25	.6	40	.09	.08	1.6	------
	Clams:																	
134	Raw, meat only	3 oz.	85	82	65	11	1	------	------	------	2	59	5.2	90	.08	.15	1.1	8
135	Canned, solids and liquid.	3 oz.	85	86	45	7	1	------	------	------	2	47	3.5	------	.01	.09	.9	------
136	Crabmeat, canned	3 oz.	85	77	85	15	2	------	------	------	1	38	.7	------	.07	.07	1.6	------
137	Fish sticks, breaded, cooked, frozen; stick 3 3/4 by 1 by 1/2 inch.	10 sticks or 8 oz. pkg.	227	66	400	38	20	5	4	10	15	25	0.9	------	0.09	0.16	3.6	------
138	Haddock, breaded, fried	3 oz.	85	66	140	17	5	1	3	Trace	5	34	1.0	------	.03	.06	2.7	2
139	Ocean perch, breaded, fried.	3 oz.	85	59	195	16	11	------	------	------	6	28	1.1	------	.08	.09	1.5	------
140	Oysters, raw, meat only (13–19 med. selects).	1 cup	240	85	160	20	4	------	------	------	8	226	13.2	740	.33	.43	6.0	------

[3] Outer layer of fat on the cut was removed to within approximately 1/2-inch of the lean. Deposits of fat within the cut were not removed.

TABLE H-1

Nutritive values of the edible part of foods, *continued*

[Dashes in the columns for nutrients show that no suitable value could be found although there is reason to believe that a measurable amount of the nutrient may be present]

No.	Food, approximate measure, and weight (in grams)			Water	Food energy	Protein	Fat	Fatty acids: Saturated (total)	Fatty acids: Unsaturated: Oleic	Fatty acids: Unsaturated: Linoleic	Carbohydrate	Calcium	Iron	Vitamin A value	Thiamin	Riboflavin	Niacin	Ascorbic acid
	MEAT, POULTRY, FISH, SHELLFISH; RELATED PRODUCTS—Continued		*Grams*	*Per cent*	*Calories*	*Grams*	*Grams*	*Grams*	*Grams*	*Grams*	*Grams*	*Milligrams*	*Milligrams*	*International units*	*Milligrams*	*Milligrams*	*Milligrams*	*Milligrams*
	Fish and shellfish—Continued																	
141	Salmon, pink, canned	3 oz.	85	71	120	17	5	1	1	Trace	0	[4]167	.7	60	.03	.16	6.8	------
142	Sardines, Atlantic, canned in oil, drained solids.	3 oz.	85	62	175	20	9	------	------	------	0	372	2.5	190	.02	.17	4.6	------
143	Shad, baked with table fat and bacon.	3 oz.	85	64	170	20	10	------	------	------	0	20	.5	20	.11	.22	7.3	------
144	Shrimp, canned, meat	3 oz.	85	70	100	21	1	------	------	------	1	98	2.6	50	.01	.03	1.5	------
145	Swordfish, broiled with butter or margarine.	3 oz.	85	65	150	24	5	------	------	------	0	23	1.1	1,750	.03	.04	9.3	------
146	Tuna, canned in oil, drained solids.	3 oz.	85	61	170	24	7	2	1	1	0	7	1.6	70	.04	.10	10.1	------
	MATURE DRY BEANS AND PEAS, NUTS, PEANUTS; RELATED PRODUCTS																	
147	Almonds, shelled, whole kernels.	1 cup	142	5	850	26	77	6	52	15	28	332	6.7	0	.34	1.31	5.0	Trace
	Beans, dry:																	
	Common varieties as Great Northern, navy, and others:																	
	Cooked, drained:																	
148	Great Northern	1 cup	180	69	210	14	1	------	------	------	38	90	4.9	0	.25	.13	1.3	0
149	Navy (pea)	1 cup	190	69	225	15	1	------	------	------	40	95	5.1	0	.27	.13	1.3	0
	Canned, solids and liquid:																	
	White with—																	
150	Frankfurters (sliced).	1 cup	255	71	365	19	18	------	------	------	32	94	4.8	330	.18	.15	3.3	Trace
151	Pork and tomato sauce.	1 cup	255	71	310	16	7	2	3	1	49	138	4.6	330	.20	.08	1.5	5
152	Pork and sweet sauce.	1 cup	255	66	385	16	12	4	5	1	54	161	5.9	------	.15	.10	1.3	------
153	Red kidney	1 cup	255	76	230	15	1	------	------	------	42	74	4.6	10	.13	.10	1.5	------
154	Lima, cooked, drained.	1 cup	190	64	260	16	1	------	------	------	49	55	5.9	------	.25	.11	1.3	------
155	Cashew nuts, roasted	1 cup	140	5	785	24	64	11	45	4	41	53	5.3	140	.60	.35	2.5	------
	Coconut, fresh, meat only:																	
156	Pieces, approx. 2 by 2 by ½ inch.	1 piece	45	51	155	2	16	14	1	Trace	4	6	.8	0	.02	.01	.2	1
157	Shredded or grated, firmly packed.	1 cup	130	51	450	5	46	39	3	Trace	12	17	2.2	0	.07	.03	.7	4
158	Cowpeas or blackeye peas, dry, cooked.	1 cup	248	80	190	13	1	------	------	------	34	42	3.2	20	.41	.11	1.1	Trace
159	Peanuts, roasted, salted, halves.	1 cup	144	2	840	37	72	16	31	21	27	107	3.0	------	.46	.19	24.7	0
160	Peanut butter	1 tbsp.	16	2	95	4	8	2	4	2	3	9	.3	------	.02	.02	2.4	0
161	Peas, split, dry, cooked	1 cup	250	70	290	20	1	------	------	------	52	28	4.2	100	.37	.22	2.2	------
162	Pecans, halves	1 cup	108	3	740	10	77	5	48	15	16	79	2.6	140	.93	.14	1.0	2
163	Walnuts, black or native, chopped.	1 cup	126	3	790	26	75	4	26	36	19	Trace	7.6	380	.28	.14	.9	------
	VEGETABLES AND VEGETABLE PRODUCTS																	
	Asparagus, green:																	
	Cooked, drained:																	
164	Spears, ½-in. diam. at base.	4 spears	60	94	10	1	Trace	------	------	------	2	13	.4	540	.10	.11	.8	16

[4] If bones are discarded, value will be greatly reduced.

TABLE H-1

Nutritive values of the edible part of foods, *continued*

[Dashes in the columns for nutrients show that no suitable value could be found although there is reason to believe that a measurable amount of the nutrient may be present]

	Food, approximate measure, and weight (in grams)			Water	Food energy	Protein	Fat	Fatty acids: Saturated (total)	Fatty acids: Unsaturated: Oleic	Fatty acids: Unsaturated: Linoleic	Carbohydrate	Calcium	Iron	Vitamin A value	Thiamin	Riboflavin	Niacin	Ascorbic acid
	VEGETABLES AND VEGETABLE PRODUCTS—Continued																	
	Asparagus, green—Continued																	
	Cooked, drained—Continued		*Grams*	*Percent*	*Calories*	*Grams*	*Grams*	*Grams*	*Grams*	*Grams*	*Grams*	*Milligrams*	*Milligrams*	*International units*	*Milligrams*	*Milligrams*	*Milligrams*	*Milligrams*
165	Pieces, 1½ to 2-in. lengths.	1 cup	145	94	30	3	Trace	------	------	------	5	30	.9	1,310	.23	.26	2.0	38
166	Canned, solids and liquid.	1 cup	244	94	45	5	1	------	------	------	7	44	4.1	1,240	.15	.22	2.0	37
	Beans:																	
167	Lima, immature seeds, cooked, drained.	1 cup	170	71	190	13	1	------	------	------	34	80	4.3	480	.31	.17	2.2	29
	Snap:																	
	Green:																	
168	Cooked, drained	1 cup	125	92	30	2	Trace	------	------	------	7	63	.8	680	.09	.11	.6	15
169	Canned, solids and liquid.	1 cup	239	94	45	2	Trace	------	------	------	10	81	2.9	690	.07	.10	.7	10
170	Cooked, drained	1 cup	125	93	30	2	Trace	------	------	------	6	63	0.8	290	0.09	0.11	0.6	16
171	Canned, solids and liquid.	1 cup	239	94	45	2	1	------	------	------	10	81	2.9	140	.07	.10	.7	12
172	Sprouted mung beans, cooked, drained.	1 cup	125	91	35	4	Trace	------	------	------	7	21	1.1	30	.11	.13	.9	8
	Beets:																	
	Cooked, drained, peeled:																	
173	Whole beets, 2-in. diam.	2 beets	100	91	30	1	Trace	------	------	------	7	14	.5	20	.03	.04	.3	6
174	Diced or sliced	1 cup	170	91	55	2	Trace	------	------	------	12	24	.9	30	.05	.07	.5	10
175	Canned, solids and liquid.	1 cup	246	90	85	2	Trace	------	------	------	19	34	1.5	20	.02	.05	.2	7
176	Beet greens, leaves and stems, cooked, drained.	1 cup	145	94	25	3	Trace	------	------	------	5	144	2.8	7,400	.10	.22	.4	22
	Blackeye peas. See Cowpeas.																	
	Broccoli, cooked, drained:																	
177	Whole stalks, medium size.	1 stalk	180	91	45	6	1	------	------	------	8	158	1.4	4,500	.16	.36	1.4	162
178	Stalks cut into ½-in. pieces.	1 cup	155	91	40	5	1	------	------	------	7	136	1.2	3,880	.14	.31	1.2	140
179	Chopped, yield from 10-oz. frozen pkg.	1⅜ cups	250	92	65	7	1	------	------	------	12	135	1.8	6,500	.15	.30	1.3	143
180	Brussels sprouts, 7–8 sprouts (1¼ to 1½ in. diam.) per cup, cooked.	1 cup	155	88	55	7	1	------	------	------	10	50	1.7	810	.12	.22	1.2	135
	Cabbage:																	
	Common varieties:																	
	Raw:																	
181	Coarsely shredded or sliced.	1 cup	70	92	15	1	Trace	------	------	------	4	34	.3	90	.04	.04	.2	33
182	Finely shredded or chopped.	1 cup	90	92	20	1	Trace	------	------	------	5	44	.4	120	.05	.05	.3	42
183	Cooked	1 cup	145	94	30	2	Trace	------	------	------	6	64	.4	190	.06	.06	.4	48
184	Red, raw, coarsely shredded.	1 cup	70	90	20	1	Trace	------	------	------	5	29	.6	30	.06	.04	.3	43
185	Savoy, raw, coarsely shredded.	1 cup	70	92	15	2	Trace	------	------	------	3	47	.6	140	.04	.06	.2	39
186	Cabbage, celery or Chinese, raw, cut in 1-in. pieces.	1 cup	75	95	10	1	Trace	------	------	------	2	32	.5	110	.04	.03	.5	19
187	Cabbage, spoon (or pakchoy), cooked.	1 cup	170	95	25	2	Trace	------	------	------	4	252	1.0	5,270	.07	.14	1.2	26
	Carrots:																	
	Raw:																	
188	Whole, 5½ by 1 inch, (25 thin strips).	1 carrot	50	88	20	1	Trace	------	------	------	5	18	.4	5,500	.03	.03	.3	4
189	Grated	1 cup	110	88	45	1	Trace	------	------	------	11	41	.8	12,100	.06	.06	.7	9

■

TABLE H-1

Nutritive values of the edible part of foods, *continued*

[Dashes in the columns for nutrients show that no suitable value could be found although there is reason to believe that a measurable amount of the nutrient may be present]

	Food, approximate measure, and weight (in grams)			Water	Food energy	Protein	Fat	Fatty acids: Saturated (total)	Fatty acids: Unsaturated: Oleic	Fatty acids: Unsaturated: Linoleic	Carbohydrate	Calcium	Iron	Vitamin A value	Thiamin	Riboflavin	Niacin	Ascorbic acid
	VEGETABLES AND VEGETABLE PRODUCTS—Continued																	
	Carrots—Continued		*Grams*	*Per-cent*	*Calories*	*Grams*	*Grams*	*Grams*	*Grams*	*Grams*	*Grams*	*Milligrams*	*Milligrams*	*International units*	*Milligrams*	*Milligrams*	*Milligrams*	*Milligrams*
190	Cooked, diced	1 cup	145	91	45	1	Trace	------	------	------	10	48	.9	15,220	.08	.07	.7	9
191	Canned, strained or chopped (baby food).	1 ounce	28	92	10	Trace	Trace	------	------	------	2	7	.1	3,690	.01	.01	.1	1
192	Cauliflower, cooked, flowerbuds.	1 cup	120	93	25	3	Trace	------	------	------	5	25	.8	70	.11	.10	.7	66
	Celery, raw:																	
193	Stalk, large outer, 8 by about 1½ inches, at root end.	1 stalk	40	94	5	Trace	Trace	------	------	------	2	16	.1	100	.01	.01	.1	4
194	Pieces, diced	1 cup	100	94	15	1	Trace	------	------	------	4	39	.3	240	.03	.03	.3	9
195	Collards, cooked	1 cup	190	91	55	5	1	------	------	------	9	289	1.1	10,260	.27	.37	2.4	87
	Corn, sweet:																	
196	Cooked, ear 5 by 1¾ inches.[5]	1 ear	140	74	70	3	1	------	------	------	16	2	.5	[6] 310	.09	.08	1.0	7
197	Canned, solids and liquid.	1 cup	256	81	170	5	2	------	------	------	40	10	1.0	[6] 690	.07	.12	2.3	13
198	Cowpeas, cooked, immature seeds.	1 cup	160	72	175	13	1	------	------	------	29	38	3.4	560	.49	.18	2.3	28
	Cucumbers, 10-ounce; 7½ by about 2 inches:																	
199	Raw, pared	1 cucumber	207	96	30	1	Trace	------	------	------	7	35	.6	Trace	.07	.09	.4	23
200	Raw, pared, center slice ⅛-inch thick.	6 slices	50	96	5	Trace	Trace	------	------	------	2	8	.2	Trace	.02	.02	.1	6
201	Dandelion greens, cooked	1 cup	180	90	60	4	1	------	------	------	12	252	3.2	21,060	.24	.29	------	32
202	Endive, curly (including escarole).	2 ounces	57	93	10	1	Trace	------	------	------	2	46	1.0	1,870	0.04	0.08	0.3	6
203	Kale, leaves including stems, cooked.	1 cup	110	91	30	4	1	------	------	------	4	147	1.3	8,140	------	------	------	68
	Lettuce, raw:																	
204	Butterhead, as Boston types; head, 4-inch diameter.	1 head	220	95	30	3	Trace	------	------	------	6	77	4.4	2,130	.14	.13	.6	18
205	Crisphead, as Iceberg; head, 4¾-inch diameter.	1 head	454	96	60	4	Trace	------	------	------	13	91	2.3	1,500	.29	.27	1.3	29
206	Looseleaf, or bunching varieties, leaves.	2 large	50	94	10	1	Trace	------	------	------	2	34	.7	950	.03	.04	.2	9
207	Mushrooms, canned, solids and liquid.	1 cup	244	93	40	5	Trace	------	------	------	6	15	1.2	Trace	.04	.60	4.8	4
208	Mustard greens, cooked	1 cup	140	93	35	3	1	------	------	------	6	193	2.5	8,120	.11	.19	.9	68
209	Okra, cooked, pod 3 by ⅝ inch.	8 pods	85	91	25	2	Trace	------	------	------	5	78	.4	420	.11	.15	.8	17
	Onions:																	
	Mature:																	
210	Raw, onion 2½-inch diameter.	1 onion	110	89	40	2	Trace	------	------	------	10	30	.6	40	.04	.04	.2	11
211	Cooked	1 cup	210	92	60	3	Trace	------	------	------	14	50	.8	80	.06	.06	.4	14
212	Young green, small, without tops.	6 onions	50	88	20	1	Trace	------	------	------	5	20	.3	Trace	.02	.02	.2	12
213	Parsley, raw, chopped	1 tablespoon	4	85	Trace	Trace	Trace	------	------	------	Trace	8	.2	340	Trace	.01	Trace	7
214	Parsnips, cooked	1 cup	155	82	100	2	1	------	------	------	23	70	.9	50	.11	.12	.2	16
	Peas, green:																	
215	Cooked	1 cup	160	82	115	9	1	------	------	------	19	37	2.9	860	.44	.17	3.7	33
216	Canned, solids and liquid.	1 cup	249	83	165	9	1	------	------	------	31	50	4.2	1,120	.23	.13	2.2	22

[5] Measure and weight apply to entire vegetable or fruit including parts not usually eaten.

[6] Based on yellow varieties; white varieties contain only a trace of cryptoxanthin and carotenes, the pigments in corn that have biological activity.

■

TABLE H-1

Nutritive values of the edible part of foods, *continued*

[Dashes in the columns for nutrients show that no suitable value could be found although there is reason to believe that a measurable amount of the nutrient may be present]

	Food, approximate measure, and weight (in grams)			Water	Food energy	Protein	Fat	Fatty acids: Saturated (total)	Fatty acids: Unsaturated: Oleic	Fatty acids: Unsaturated: Linoleic	Carbohydrate	Calcium	Iron	Vitamin A value	Thiamin	Riboflavin	Niacin	Ascorbic acid
	VEGETABLES AND VEGETABLE PRODUCTS—Continued																	
	Peas, green—Continued		Grams	Per-cent	Calo-ries	Grams	Grams	Grams	Grams	Grams	Grams	Milli-grams	Milli-grams	Inter-national units	Milli-grams	Milli-grams	Milli-grams	Milli-grams
217	Canned, strained (baby food).	1 ounce	28	86	15	1	Trace	-----	-----	-----	3	3	.4	140	.02	.02	.4	3
218	Peppers, hot, red, without seeds, dried (ground chili powder, added seasonings).	1 tablespoon	15	8	50	2	2	-----	-----	-----	8	40	2.3	9,750	.03	.17	1.3	2
	Peppers, sweet:																	
	Raw, about 5 per pound:																	
219	Green pod without stem and seeds.	1 pod	74	93	15	1	Trace	-----	-----	-----	4	7	.5	310	.06	.06	.4	94
220	Cooked, boiled, drained	1 pod	73	95	15	1	Trace	-----	-----	-----	3	7	.4	310	.05	.05	.4	70
	Potatoes, medium (about 3 per pound raw):																	
221	Baked, peeled after baking.	1 potato	99	75	90	3	Trace	-----	-----	-----	21	9	.7	Trace	.10	.04	1.7	20
	Boiled:																	
222	Peeled after boiling	1 potato	136	80	105	3	Trace	-----	-----	-----	23	10	.8	Trace	.13	.05	2.0	22
223	Peeled before boiling	1 potato	122	83	80	2	Trace	-----	-----	-----	18	7	.6	Trace	.11	.04	1.4	20
	French-fried, piece 2 by ½ by ½ inch:																	
224	Cooked in deep fat	10 pieces	57	45	155	2	7	2	2	4	20	9	.7	Trace	.07	.04	1.8	12
225	Frozen, heated	10 pieces	57	53	125	2	5	1	1	2	19	5	1.0	Trace	.08	.01	1.5	12
	Mashed:																	
226	Milk added	1 cup	195	83	125	4	1	-----	-----	-----	25	47	.8	50	.16	.10	2.0	19
227	Milk and butter added.	1 cup	195	80	185	4	8	4	3	Trace	24	47	.8	330	.16	.10	1.9	18
228	Potato chips, medium, 2-inch diameter.	10 chips	20	2	115	1	8	2	2	4	10	8	.4	Trace	.04	.01	1.0	3
229	Pumpkin, canned	1 cup	228	90	75	2	1	-----	-----	-----	18	57	.9	14,590	.07	.12	1.3	12
230	Radishes, raw, small, without tops.	4 radishes	40	94	5	Trace	Trace	-----	-----	-----	1	12	.4	Trace	.01	.01	.1	10
231	Sauerkraut, canned, solids and liquid.	1 cup	235	93	45	2	Trace	-----	-----	-----	9	85	1.2	120	.07	.09	.4	33
	Spinach:																	
232	Cooked	1 cup	180	92	40	5	1	-----	-----	-----	6	167	4.0	14,580	.13	.25	1.0	50
233	Canned, drained solids	1 cup	180	91	45	5	1	-----	-----	-----	6	212	4.7	14,400	.03	.21	.6	24
	Squash:																	
	Cooked:																	
234	Summer, diced	1 cup	210	96	30	2	Trace	-----	-----	-----	7	52	.8	820	.10	.16	1.6	21
235	Winter, baked, mashed.	1 cup	205	81	130	4	1	-----	-----	-----	32	57	1.6	8,610	.10	.27	1.4	27
	Sweetpotatoes:																	
	Cooked, medium, 5 by 2 inches, weight raw about 6 ounces:																	
236	Baked, peeled after baking.	1 sweet-potato.	110	64	155	2	1	-----	-----	-----	36	44	1.0	8,910	.10	.07	.7	24
237	Boiled, peeled after boiling.	1 sweet-potato.	147	71	170	2	1	-----	-----	-----	39	47	1.0	11,610	.13	.09	.9	25
238	Candied, 3½ by 2¼ inches.	1 sweet-potato.	175	60	295	2	6	2	3	1	60	65	1.6	11,030	0.10	0.08	0.8	17
239	Canned, vacuum or solid pack.	1 cup	218	72	235	4	Trace	-----	-----	-----	54	54	1.7	17,000	.10	.10	1.4	30
	Tomatoes:																	
240	Raw, approx. 3-in. diam. 2⅛ in. high; wt., 7 oz.	1 tomato	200	94	40	2	Trace	-----	-----	-----	9	24	.9	1,640	.11	.07	1.3	[7] 42
241	Canned, solids and liquid.	1 cup	241	94	50	2	1	-----	-----	-----	10	14	1.2	2,170	.12	.07	1.7	41

[7] Year-round average. Samples marketed from November through May, average 20 milligrams per 200-gram tomato; from June through October, around 52 milligrams.

Nutritive values of the edible part of foods, *continued*

[Dashes in the columns for nutrients show that no suitable value could be found although there is reason to believe that a measurable amount of the nutrient may be present]

No.	Food, approximate measure, and weight (in grams)			Water	Food energy	Protein	Fat	Fatty acids: Saturated (total)	Fatty acids: Unsaturated: Oleic	Fatty acids: Unsaturated: Linoleic	Carbohydrate	Calcium	Iron	Vitamin A value	Thiamin	Riboflavin	Niacin	Ascorbic acid
	VEGETABLES AND VEGETABLE PRODUCTS—Continued		*Grams*	*Percent*	*Calories*	*Grams*	*Grams*	*Grams*	*Grams*	*Grams*	*Grams*	*Milligrams*	*Milligrams*	*International units*	*Milligrams*	*Milligrams*	*Milligrams*	*Milligrams*
	Tomato catsup:																	
242	Cup	1 cup	273	69	290	6	1	------	------	------	69	60	2.2	3,820	.25	.19	4.4	41
243	Tablespoon	1 tbsp.	15	69	15	Trace	Trace	------	------	------	4	3	.1	210	.01	.01	.2	2
	Tomato juice, canned:																	
244	Cup	1 cup	243	94	45	2	Trace	------	------	------	10	17	2.2	1,940	.12	.07	1.9	39
245	Glass (6 fl. oz.)	1 glass	182	94	35	2	Trace	------	------	------	8	13	1.6	1,460	.09	.05	1.5	29
246	Turnips, cooked, diced	1 cup	155	94	35	1	Trace	------	------	------	8	54	.6	Trace	.06	.08	.5	34
247	Turnip greens, cooked	1 cup	145	94	30	3	Trace	------	------	------	5	252	1.5	8,270	.15	.33	.7	68
	FRUITS AND FRUIT PRODUCTS																	
248	Apples, raw (about 3 per lb.).[5]	1 apple	150	85	70	Trace	Trace	------	------	------	18	8	.4	50	.04	.02	.1	3
249	Apple juice, bottled or canned.	1 cup	248	88	120	Trace	Trace	------	------	------	30	15	1.5	------	.02	.05	.2	2
	Applesauce, canned:																	
250	Sweetened	1 cup	255	76	230	1	Trace	------	------	------	61	10	1.3	100	.05	.03	.1	[8] 3
251	Unsweetened or artificially sweetened.	1 cup	244	88	100	1	Trace	------	------	------	26	10	1.2	100	.05	.02	.1	[8] 2
	Apricots:																	
252	Raw (about 12 per lb.)[5]	3 apricots	114	85	55	1	Trace	------	------	------	14	18	.5	2,890	.03	.04	.7	10
253	Canned in heavy sirup	1 cup	259	77	220	2	Trace	------	------	------	57	28	.8	4,510	.05	.06	.9	10
254	Dried, uncooked (40 halves per cup).	1 cup	150	25	390	8	1	------	------	------	100	100	8.2	16,350	.02	.23	4.9	19
255	Cooked, unsweetened, fruit and liquid.	1 cup	285	76	240	5	1	------	------	------	62	63	5.1	8,550	.01	.13	2.8	8
256	Apricot nectar, canned	1 cup	251	85	140	1	Trace	------	------	------	37	23	.5	2,380	.03	.03	.5	[8] 8
	Avocados, whole fruit, raw:[5]																	
257	California (mid- and late-winter; diam. 3⅛ in.).	1 avocado	284	74	370	5	37	7	17	5	13	22	1.3	630	.24	.43	3.5	30
258	Florida (late summer, fall; diam. 3⅝ in.).	1 avocado	454	78	390	4	33	7	15	4	27	30	1.8	880	.33	.61	4.9	43
259	Bananas, raw, medium size.[5]	1 banana	175	76	100	1	Trace	------	------	------	26	10	.8	230	.06	.07	.8	12
260	Banana flakes	1 cup	100	3	340	4	1	------	------	------	89	32	2.8	760	.18	.24	2.8	7
261	Blackberries, raw	1 cup	144	84	85	2	1	------	------	------	19	46	1.3	290	.05	.06	.5	30
262	Blueberries, raw	1 cup	140	83	85	1	1	------	------	------	21	21	1.4	140	.04	.08	.6	20
263	Cantaloups, raw; medium, 5-inch diameter about 1⅔ pounds.[5]	½ melon	385	91	60	1	Trace	------	------	------	14	27	.8	[9] 6,540	.08	.06	1.2	63
264	Cherries, canned, red, sour, pitted, water pack.	1 cup	244	88	105	2	Trace	------	------	------	26	37	.7	1,660	.07	.05	.5	12
265	Cranberry juice cocktail, canned.	1 cup	250	83	165	Trace	Trace	------	------	------	42	13	.8	Trace	.03	.03	.1	[10] 40
266	Cranberry sauce, sweetened, canned, strained.	1 cup	277	62	405	Trace	1	------	------	------	104	17	.6	60	.03	.03	.1	6
267	Dates, pitted, cut	1 cup	178	22	490	4	1	------	------	------	130	105	5.3	90	.16	.17	3.9	0
268	Figs, dried, large, 2 by 1 in.	1 fig	21	23	60	1	Trace	------	------	------	15	26	.6	20	.02	.02	.1	0
269	Fruit cocktail, canned, in heavy sirup.	1 cup	256	80	195	1	Trace	------	------	------	50	23	1.0	360	.05	.03	1.3	5

[5] Measure and weight apply to entire vegetable or fruit including parts not usually eaten.

[8] This is the amount from the fruit. Additional ascorbic acid may be added by the manufacturer. Refer to the label for this information.

[9] Value for varieties with orange-colored flesh; value for varieties with green flesh would be about 540 I.U.

[10] Value listed is based on products with label stating 30 milligrams per 6 fl. oz. serving.

TABLE H-1

Nutritive values of the edible part of foods, *continued*

[Dashes in the columns for nutrients show that no suitable value could be found although there is reason to believe that a measurable amount of the nutrient may be present]

	Food, approximate measure, and weight (in grams)			Water	Food energy	Protein	Fat	Fatty acids: Saturated (total)	Fatty acids: Unsaturated: Oleic	Fatty acids: Unsaturated: Linoleic	Carbohydrate	Calcium	Iron	Vitamin A value	Thiamin	Riboflavin	Niacin	Ascorbic acid
	FRUITS AND FRUIT PRODUCTS—Con.		*Grams*	*Per-cent*	*Calo-ries*	*Grams*	*Grams*	*Grams*	*Grams*	*Grams*	*Grams*	*Milli-grams*	*Milli-grams*	*Inter-national units*	*Milli-grams*	*Milli-grams*	*Milli-grams*	*Milli-grams*
	Grapefruit:																	
	Raw, medium, 3¾-in. diam.[5]																	
270	White	½ grapefruit.	241	89	45	1	Trace	------	------	------	12	19	0.5	10	0.05	0.02	0.2	44
271	Pink or red	½ grapefruit.	241	89	50	1	Trace	------	------	------	13	20	0.5	540	0.05	0.02	0.2	44
272	Canned, sirup pack	1 cup	254	81	180	2	Trace	------	------	------	45	33	.8	30	.08	.05	.5	76
	Grapefruit juice:																	
273	Fresh	1 cup	246	90	95	1	Trace	------	------	------	23	22	.5	([11])	.09	.04	.4	92
	Canned, white:																	
274	Unsweetened	1 cup	247	89	100	1	Trace	------	------	------	24	20	1.0	20	.07	.04	.4	84
275	Sweetened	1 cup	250	86	130	1	Trace	------	------	------	32	20	1.0	20	.07	.04	.4	78
	Frozen, concentrate, unsweetened:																	
276	Undiluted, can, 6 fluid ounces.	1 can	207	62	300	4	1	------	------	------	72	70	.8	60	.29	.12	1.4	286
277	Diluted with 3 parts water, by volume.	1 cup	247	89	100	1	Trace	------	------	------	24	25	.2	20	.10	.04	.5	96
278	Dehydrated crystals	4 oz.	113	1	410	6	1	------	------	------	102	100	1.2	80	.40	.20	2.0	396
279	Prepared with water (1 pound yields about 1 gallon).	1 cup	247	90	100	1	Trace	------	------	------	24	22	.2	20	.10	.05	.5	91
	Grapes, raw:[5]																	
280	American type (slip skin).	1 cup	153	82	65	1	1	------	------	------	15	15	.4	100	.05	.03	.2	3
281	European type (adherent skin).	1 cup	160	81	95	1	Trace	------	------	------	25	17	.6	140	.07	.04	.4	6
	Grapejuice:																	
282	Canned or bottled	1 cup	253	83	165	1	Trace	------	------	------	42	28	.8	------	.10	.05	.5	Trace
	Frozen concentrate, sweetened:																	
283	Undiluted, can, 6 fluid ounces.	1 can	216	53	395	1	Trace	------	------	------	100	22	.9	40	.13	.22	1.5	([12])
284	Diluted with 3 parts water, by volume.	1 cup	250	86	135	1	Trace	------	------	------	33	8	.3	10	.05	.08	.5	([12])
285	Grapejuice drink, canned.	1 cup	250	86	135	Trace	Trace	------	------	------	35	8	.3	------	.03	.03	.3	([12])
286	Lemons, raw, 2⅛-in. diam., size 165.[5] Used for juice.	1 lemon	110	90	20	1	Trace	------	------	------	6	19	.4	10	.03	.01	.1	39
287	Lemon juice, raw	1 cup	244	91	60	1	Trace	------	------	------	20	17	.5	50	.07	.02	.2	112
	Lemonade concentrate:																	
288	Frozen, 6 fl. oz. per can.	1 can	219	48	430	Trace	Trace	------	------	------	112	9	.4	40	.04	.07	.7	66
289	Diluted with 4⅓ parts water, by volume.	1 cup	248	88	110	Trace	Trace	------	------	------	28	2	Trace	Trace	Trace	.02	.2	17
	Lime juice:																	
290	Fresh	1 cup	246	90	65	1	Trace	------	------	------	22	22	.5	20	.05	.02	.2	79
291	Canned, unsweetened	1 cup	246	90	65	1	Trace	------	------	------	22	22	.5	20	.05	.02	.2	52
	Limeade concentrate, frozen:																	
292	Undiluted, can, 6 fluid ounces.	1 can	218	50	410	Trace	Trace	------	------	------	108	11	.2	Trace	.02	.02	.2	26
293	Diluted with 4⅓ parts water, by volume.	1 cup	247	90	100	Trace	Trace	------	------	------	27	2	Trace	Trace	Trace	Trace	Trace	5
294	Oranges, raw, 2⅝-in. diam., all commercial, varieties.[5]	1 orange	180	86	65	1	Trace	------	------	------	16	54	.5	260	.13	.05	.5	66

[5] Measure and weight apply to entire vegetable or fruit including parts not usually eaten.

[11] For white-fleshed varieties value is about 20 I.U. per cup; for red-fleshed varieties, 1,080 I.U. per cup.

[12] Present only if added by the manufacturer. Refer to the label for this information.

TABLE H-1

Nutritive values of the edible part of foods, *continued*

[Dashes in the columns for nutrients show that no suitable value could be found although there is reason to believe that a measurable amount of the nutrient may be present]

	Food, approximate measure, and weight (in grams)			Water	Food energy	Protein	Fat	Fatty acids: Saturated (total)	Fatty acids: Unsaturated: Oleic	Fatty acids: Unsaturated: Linoleic	Carbohydrate	Calcium	Iron	Vitamin A value	Thiamin	Riboflavin	Niacin	Ascorbic acid
	FRUITS AND FRUIT PRODUCTS—Con.		*Grams*	*Percent*	*Calories*	*Grams*	*Grams*	*Grams*	*Grams*	*Grams*	*Grams*	*Milligrams*	*Milligrams*	*International units*	*Milligrams*	*Milligrams*	*Milligrams*	*Milligrams*
295	Orange juice, fresh, all varieties.	1 cup	248	88	110	2	1	------	------	------	26	27	.5	500	.22	.07	1.0	124
296	Canned, unsweetened	1 cup	249	87	120	2	Trace	------	------	------	28	25	1.0	500	.17	.05	.7	100
	Frozen concentrate:																	
297	Undiluted, can, 6 fluid ounces.	1 can	213	55	360	5	Trace	------	------	------	87	75	.9	1,620	.68	.11	2.8	360
298	Diluted with 3 parts water, by volume.	1 cup	249	87	120	2	Trace	------	------	------	29	25	.2	550	.22	.02	1.0	120
299	Dehydrated crystals	4 oz.	113	1	430	6	2	------	------	------	100	95	1.9	1,900	.76	.24	3.3	408
300	Prepared with water (1 pound yields about 1 gallon).	1 cup	248	88	115	2	1	------	------	------	27	25	.5	500	.20	.07	1.0	109
301	Orange-apricot juice drink	1 cup	249	87	125	1	Trace	------	------	------	32	12	.2	1,440	.05	.02	.5	[10] 40
	Orange and grapefruit juice:																	
	Frozen concentrate:																	
302	Undiluted, can, 6 fluid ounces.	1 can	210	59	330	4	1	------	------	------	78	61	0.8	800	0.48	0.06	2.3	302
303	Diluted with 3 parts water, by volume.	1 cup	248	88	110	1	Trace	------	------	------	26	20	.2	270	.16	.02	.8	102
304	Papayas, raw, ½-inch cubes.	1 cup	182	89	70	1	Trace	------	------	------	18	36	.5	3,190	.07	.08	.5	102
	Peaches:																	
	Raw:																	
305	Whole, medium, 2-inch diameter, about 4 per pound.[5]	1 peach	114	89	35	1	Trace	------	------	------	10	9	.5	[13]1,320	.02	.05	1.0	7
306	Sliced	1 cup	168	89	65	1	Trace	------	------	------	16	15	.8	[13]2,230	.03	.08	1.6	12
	Canned, yellow-fleshed, solids and liquid:																	
	Sirup pack, heavy:																	
307	Halves or slices	1 cup	257	79	200	1	Trace	------	------	------	52	10	.8	1,100	.02	.06	1.4	7
308	Water pack	1 cup	245	91	75	1	Trace	------	------	------	20	10	.7	1,100	.02	.06	1.4	7
309	Dried, uncooked	1 cup	160	25	420	5	1	------	------	------	109	77	9.6	6,240	.02	.31	8.5	28
310	Cooked, unsweetened, 10–12 halves and juice.	1 cup	270	77	220	3	1	------	------	------	58	41	5.1	3,290	.01	.15	4.2	6
	Frozen:																	
311	Carton, 12 ounces, not thawed.	1 carton	340	76	300	1	Trace	------	------	------	77	14	1.7	2,210	.03	.14	2.4	[14] 135
	Pears:																	
312	Raw, 3 by 2½-inch diameter.[5]	1 pear	182	83	100	1	1	------	------	------	25	13	.5	30	.04	.07	.2	7
	Canned, solids and liquid:																	
	Sirup pack, heavy:																	
313	Halves or slices	1 cup	255	80	195	1	1	------	------	------	50	13	.5	Trace	.03	.05	.3	4
	Pineapple:																	
314	Raw, diced	1 cup	140	85	75	1	Trace	------	------	------	19	24	.7	100	.12	.04	.3	24
	Canned, heavy sirup pack, solids and liquid:																	
315	Crushed	1 cup	260	80	195	1	Trace	------	------	------	50	29	.8	120	.20	.06	.5	17
316	Sliced, slices and juice.	2 small or 1 large.	122	80	90	Trace	Trace	------	------	------	24	13	.4	50	.09	.03	.2	8
317	Pineapple juice, canned	1 cup	249	86	135	1	Trace	------	------	------	34	37	.7	120	.12	.04	.5	[9] 22

[5] Measure and weight apply to entire vegetable or fruit including parts not usually eaten.

[9] This is the amount from the fruit. Additional ascorbic acid may be added by the manufacturer. Refer to the label for this information.

[10] Value listed is based on product with label stating 30 milligrams per 6 fl. oz. serving.

[13] Based on yellow-fleshed varieties; for white-fleshed varieties value is about 50 I.U. per 114-gram peach and 80 I.U. per cup of sliced peaches.

[14] This value includes ascorbic acid added by manufacturer.

TABLE H-1

Nutritive values of the edible part of foods, *continued*

[Dashes in the columns for nutrients show that no suitable value could be found although there is reason to believe that a measurable amount of the nutrient may be present]

	Food, approximate measure, and weight (in grams)			Water	Food energy	Protein	Fat	Fatty acids: Saturated (total)	Fatty acids: Unsaturated: Oleic	Fatty acids: Unsaturated: Linoleic	Carbohydrate	Calcium	Iron	Vitamin A value	Thiamin	Riboflavin	Niacin	Ascorbic acid
	FRUITS AND FRUIT PRODUCTS—Con.		*Grams*	*Percent*	*Calories*	*Grams*	*Grams*	*Grams*	*Grams*	*Grams*	*Grams*	*Milligrams*	*Milligrams*	*International units*	*Milligrams*	*Milligrams*	*Milligrams*	*Milligrams*
	Plums, all except prunes:																	
318	Raw, 2-inch diameter, about 2 ounces.[5]	1 plum	60	87	25	Trace	Trace	----	----	----	7	7	.3	140	.02	.02	.3	3
	Canned, sirup pack (Italian prunes):																	
319	Plums (with pits) and juice.[5]	1 cup	256	77	205	1	Trace	----	----	----	53	22	2.2	2,970	.05	.05	.9	4
	Prunes, dried, "softenized", medium:																	
320	Uncooked[5]	4 prunes	32	28	70	1	Trace	----	----	----	18	14	1.1	440	.02	.04	.4	1
321	Cooked, unsweetened, 17–18 prunes and ⅓ cup liquid.[5]	1 cup	270	66	295	2	1	----	----	----	78	60	4.5	1,860	.08	.18	1.7	2
322	Prune juice, canned or bottled.	1 cup	256	80	200	1	Trace	----	----	----	49	36	10.5	----	.03	.03	1.0	[8]5
	Raisins, seedless:																	
323	Packaged, ½ oz. or 1½ tbsp. per pkg.	1 pkg.	14	18	40	Trace	Trace	----	----	----	11	9	.5	Trace	.02	.01	.1	Trace
324	Cup, pressed down	1 cup	165	18	480	4	Trace	----	----	----	128	102	5.8	30	.18	.13	.8	2
	Raspberries, red:																	
325	Raw	1 cup	123	84	70	1	1	----	----	----	17	27	1.1	160	.04	.11	1.1	31
326	Frozen, 10-ounce carton, not thawed.	1 carton	284	74	275	2	1	----	----	----	70	37	1.7	200	.06	.17	1.7	59
327	Rhubarb, cooked, sugar added.	1 cup	272	63	385	1	Trace	----	----	----	98	212	1.6	220	.06	.15	.7	17
	Strawberries:																	
328	Raw, capped	1 cup	149	90	55	1	1	----	----	----	13	31	1.5	90	.04	.10	1.0	88
329	Frozen, 10-ounce carton, not thawed.	1 carton	284	71	310	1	1	----	----	----	79	40	2.0	90	.06	.17	1.5	150
330	Tangerines, raw, medium, 2⅜-in. diam., size 176.[5]	1 tangerine	116	87	40	1	Trace	----	----	----	10	34	.3	360	.05	.02	.1	27
331	Tangerine juice, canned, sweetened.	1 cup	249	87	125	1	1	----	----	----	30	45	.5	1,050	.15	.05	.2	55
332	Watermelon, raw, wedge, 4 by 8 inches (1/16 of 10 by 16-inch melon, about 2 pounds with rind).[5]	1 wedge	925	93	115	2	1	----	----	----	27	30	2.1	2,510	.13	.13	.7	30
	GRAIN PRODUCTS																	
	Bagel, 3-in. diam.:																	
333	Egg	1 bagel	55	32	165	6	2	----	----	----	28	9	1.2	30	0.14	0.10	1.2	0
334	Water	1 bagel	55	29	165	6	2	----	----	----	30	8	1.2	0	.15	.11	1.4	0
335	Barley, pearled, light, uncooked.	1 cup	200	11	700	16	2	Trace	1	1	158	32	4.0	0	.24	.10	6.2	0
336	Biscuits, baking powder from home recipe with enriched flour, 2-in. diam.	1 biscuit	28	27	105	2	5	1	2	1	13	34	.4	Trace	.06	.06	.1	Trace
337	Biscuits, baking powder from mix, 2-in. diam.	1 biscuit	28	28	90	2	3	1	1	1	15	19	.6	Trace	.08	.07	.6	Trace
338	Bran flakes (40% bran), added thiamin and iron.	1 cup	35	3	105	4	1	----	----	----	28	25	12.3	0	.14	.06	2.2	0
339	Bran flakes with raisins, added thiamin and iron.	1 cup	50	7	145	4	1	----	----	----	40	28	13.5	Trace	.16	.07	2.7	0
	Breads:																	
340	Boston brown bread, slice 3 by ¾ in.	1 slice	48	45	100	3	1	----	----	----	22	43	.9	0	.05	.03	.6	0
	Cracked-wheat bread:																	
341	Loaf, 1 lb.	1 loaf	454	35	1,190	40	10	2	5	2	236	399	5.0	Trace	.53	.41	5.9	Trace

[5] Measure and weight apply to entire vegetable or fruit including parts not usually eaten.

[8] This is the amount from the fruit. Additional ascorbic acid may be added by the manufacturer. Refer to the label for this information.

Nutritive values of the edible part of foods, *continued*

[Dashes in the columns for nutrients show that no suitable value could be found although there is reason to believe that a measurable amount of the nutrient may be present]

	Food, approximate measure, and weight (in grams)			Water	Food energy	Protein	Fat	Fatty acids: Saturated (total)	Fatty acids: Unsaturated: Oleic	Fatty acids: Unsaturated: Linoleic	Carbohydrate	Calcium	Iron	Vitamin A value	Thiamin	Riboflavin	Niacin	Ascorbic acid
	GRAIN PRODUCTS—Continued																	
	Bread—Continued		*Grams*	*Per-cent*	*Calo-ries*	*Grams*	*Grams*	*Grams*	*Grams*	*Grams*	*Grams*	*Milli-grams*	*Milli-grams*	*Inter-national units*	*Milli-grams*	*Milli-grams*	*Milli-grams*	*Milli-grams*
342	Slice, 18 slices per loaf.	1 slice	25	35	65	2	1	-----	-----	-----	13	22	.3	Trace	.03	.02	.3	Trace
	French or vienna bread:																	
343	Enriched, 1 lb. loaf	1 loaf	454	31	1,315	41	14	3	8	2	251	195	10.0	Trace	1.27	1.00	11.3	Trace
344	Unenriched, 1 lb. loaf.	1 loaf	454	31	1,315	41	14	3	8	2	251	195	3.2	Trace	.36	.36	3.6	Trace
	Italian bread:																	
345	Enriched, 1 lb. loaf	1 loaf	454	32	1,250	41	4	Trace	1	2	256	77	10.0	0	1.32	.91	11.8	0
346	Unenriched, 1 lb. loaf.	1 loaf	454	32	1,250	41	4	Trace	1	2	256	77	3.2	0	.41	.27	3.6	0
	Raisin bread:																	
347	Loaf, 1 lb.	1 loaf	454	35	1,190	30	13	3	8	2	243	322	5.9	Trace	.23	.41	3.2	Trace
348	Slice, 18 slices per loaf.	1 slice	25	35	65	2	1	-----	-----	-----	13	18	.3	Trace	.01	.02	.2	Trace
	Rye bread:																	
	American, light (⅓ rye, ⅔ wheat):																	
349	Loaf, 1 lb.	1 loaf	454	36	1,100	41	5	-----	-----	-----	236	340	7.3	0	.82	.32	6.4	0
350	Slice, 18 slices per loaf.	1 slice	25	36	60	2	Trace	-----	-----	-----	13	19	.4	0	.05	.02	.4	0
351	Pumpernickel, loaf, 1 lb.	1 loaf	454	34	1,115	41	5	-----	-----	-----	241	381	10.9	0	1.04	.64	5.4	0
	White bread, enriched: [15]																	
	Soft-crumb type:																	
352	Loaf, 1 lb.	1 loaf	454	36	1,225	39	15	3	8	2	229	381	11.3	Trace	1.13	.95	10.9	Trace
353	Slice, 18 slices per loaf.	1 slice	25	36	70	2	1	-----	-----	-----	13	21	.6	Trace	.06	.05	.6	Trace
354	Slice, toasted	1 slice	22	25	70	2	1	-----	-----	-----	13	21	.6	Trace	.06	.05	.6	Trace
355	Slice, 22 slices per loaf.	1 slice	20	36	55	2	1	-----	-----	-----	10	17	.5	Trace	.05	.04	.5	Trace
356	Slice, toasted	1 slice	17	25	55	2	1	-----	-----	-----	10	17	.5	Trace	.05	.04	.5	Trace
357	Loaf, 1½ lbs.	1 loaf	680	36	1,835	59	22	5	12	3	343	571	17.0	Trace	1.70	1.43	16.3	Trace
358	Slice, 24 slices per loaf.	1 slice	28	36	75	2	1	-----	-----	-----	14	24	.7	Trace	.07	.06	.7	Trace
359	Slice, toasted	1 slice	24	25	75	2	1	-----	-----	-----	14	24	.7	Trace	.07	.06	.7	Trace
360	Slice, 28 slices per loaf.	1 slice	24	36	65	2	1	-----	-----	-----	12	20	.6	Trace	.06	.05	.6	Trace
361	Slice, toasted	1 slice	21	25	65	2	1	-----	-----	-----	12	20	.6	Trace	.06	.05	.6	Trace
	Firm-crumb type:																	
362	Loaf, 1 lb.	1 loaf	454	35	1,245	41	17	4	10	2	228	435	11.3	Trace	1.22	.91	10.9	Trace
363	Slice, 20 slices per loaf.	1 slice	23	35	65	2	1	-----	-----	-----	12	22	.6	Trace	.06	.05	.6	Trace
364	Slice, toasted	1 slice	20	24	65	2	1	-----	-----	-----	12	22	.6	Trace	.06	.05	.6	Trace
365	Loaf, 2 lbs.	1 loaf	907	35	2,495	82	34	8	20	4	455	871	22.7	Trace	2.45	1.81	21.8	Trace
366	Slice, 34 slices per loaf.	1 slice	27	35	75	2	1	-----	-----	-----	14	26	.7	Trace	.07	.05	.6	Trace
367	Slice, toasted	1 slice	23	35	75	2	1	-----	-----	-----	14	26	.7	Trace	.07	.05	.6	Trace
	Whole-wheat bread, soft-crumb type:																	
368	Loaf, 1 lb.	1 loaf	454	36	1,095	41	12	2	6	2	224	381	13.6	Trace	1.36	.45	12.7	Trace
369	Slice, 16 slices per loaf.	1 slice	28	36	65	3	1	-----	-----	-----	14	24	.8	Trace	.09	.03	.8	Trace
370	Slice, toasted	1 slice	24	24	65	3	1	-----	-----	-----	14	24	.8	Trace	.09	.03	.8	Trace
371	Loaf, 1 lb.	1 loaf	454	36	1,100	48	14	3	6	3	216	449	13.6	Trace	1.18	0.54	12.7	Trace

[15] Values for iron, thiamin, riboflavin, and niacin per pound of unenriched white bread would be as follows:

	Iron	Thiamin	Riboflavin	Niacin
	Milligrams	*Milligrams*	*Milligrams*	*Milligrams*
Soft crumb	3.2	.31	.39	5.0
Firm crumb	3.2	.32	.59	4.1

TABLE H-1

Nutritive values of the edible part of foods, *continued*

[Dashes in the columns for nutrients show that no suitable value could be found although there is reason to believe that a measurable amount of the nutrient may be present]

	Food, approximate measure, and weight (in grams)			Water	Food energy	Protein	Fat	Fatty acids: Saturated (total)	Fatty acids: Unsaturated: Oleic	Fatty acids: Unsaturated: Linoleic	Carbohydrate	Calcium	Iron	Vitamin A value	Thiamin	Riboflavin	Niacin	Ascorbic acid
	GRAIN PRODUCTS—Continued																	
	Bread—Continued		*Grams*	*Percent*	*Calories*	*Grams*	*Grams*	*Grams*	*Grams*	*Grams*	*Grams*	*Milligrams*	*Milligrams*	*International units*	*Milligrams*	*Milligrams*	*Milligrams*	*Milligrams*
	Whole-wheat bread, firm-crumb type:																	
372	Slice, 18 slices per loaf.	1 slice	25	36	60	3	1	-----	-----	-----	12	25	.8	Trace	.06	.03	.7	Trace
373	Slice, toasted	1 slice	21	24	60	3	1	-----	-----	-----	12	25	.8	Trace	.06	.03	.7	Trace
374	Breadcrumbs, dry, grated	1 cup	100	6	390	13	5	1	2	1	73	122	3.6	Trace	.22	.30	3.5	Trace
375	Buckwheat flour, light, sifted.	1 cup	98	12	340	6	1	-----	-----	-----	78	11	1.0	0	.08	.04	.4	0
376	Bulgur, canned, seasoned	1 cup	135	56	245	8	4	-----	-----	-----	44	27	1.9	0	.08	.05	4.1	0
	Cakes made from cake mixes:																	
	Angelfood:																	
377	Whole cake	1 cake	635	34	1,645	36	1	-----	-----	-----	377	603	1.9	0	.03	.70	.6	0
378	Piece, 1/12 of 10-in. diam. cake.	1 piece	53	34	135	3	Trace	-----	-----	-----	32	50	.2	0	Trace	.06	.1	0
	Cupcakes, small, 2½ in. diam.:																	
379	Without icing	1 cupcake	25	26	90	1	3	1	1	1	14	40	.1	40	.01	.03	.1	Trace
380	With chocolate icing	1 cupcake	36	22	130	2	5	2	2	1	21	47	.3	60	.01	.04	.1	Trace
	Devil's food, 2-layer, with chocolate icing:																	
381	Whole cake	1 cake	1,107	24	3,755	49	136	54	58	16	645	653	8.9	1,660	.33	.89	3.3	1
382	Piece, 1/16 of 9-in. diam. cake.	1 piece	69	24	235	3	9	3	4	1	40	41	.6	100	.02	.06	.2	Trace
383	Cupcake, small, 2½ in. diam.	1 cupcake	35	24	120	2	4	1	2	Trace	20	21	.3	50	.01	.03	.1	Trace
	Gingerbread:																	
384	Whole cake	1 cake	570	37	1,575	18	39	10	19	9	291	513	9.1	Trace	.17	.51	4.6	2
385	Piece, 1/9 of 8-in. square cake.	1 piece	63	37	175	2	4	1	2	1	32	57	1.0	Trace	.02	.06	.5	Trace
	White, 2-layer, with chocolate icing:																	
386	Whole cake	1 cake	1,140	21	4,000	45	122	45	54	17	716	1,129	5.7	680	.23	.91	2.3	2
387	Piece, 1/16 of 9-in. diam. cake.	1 piece	71	21	250	3	8	3	3	1	45	70	.4	40	.01	.06	.1	Trace
	Cakes made from home recipes: [16]																	
388	Boston cream pie; piece 1/12 of 8-in. diam.	1 piece	69	35	210	4	6	2	3	1	34	46	.3	140	.02	.08	.1	Trace
	Fruitcake, dark, made with enriched flour:																	
389	Loaf, 1-lb.	1 loaf	454	18	1,720	22	69	15	37	13	271	327	11.8	540	.59	.64	3.6	2
390	Slice, 1/30 of 8-in. loaf.	1 slice	15	18	55	1	2	Trace	1	Trace	9	11	.4	20	.02	.02	.1	Trace
	Plain sheet cake:																	
	Without icing:																	
391	Whole cake	1 cake	777	25	2,830	35	108	30	52	21	434	497	3.1	1,320	.16	.70	1.6	2
392	Piece, 1/9 of 9-in. square cake.	1 piece	86	25	315	4	12	3	6	2	48	55	.3	150	.02	.08	.2	Trace
393	With boiled white icing, piece, 1/9 of 9-in. square cake.	1 piece	114	23	400	4	12	3	6	2	71	56	.3	150	.02	.08	.2	Trace
	Pound:																	
394	Loaf, 8½ by 3½ by 3in.	1 loaf	514	17	2,430	29	152	34	68	17	242	108	4.1	1,440	.15	.46	1.0	0
395	Slice, ½-in. thick	1 slice	30	17	140	2	9	2	4	1	14	6	.2	80	.01	.03	.1	0
	Sponge:																	
396	Whole cake	1 cake	790	32	2,345	60	45	14	20	4	427	237	9.5	3,560	.40	1.11	1.6	Trace
397	Piece, 1/12 of 10-in. diam. cake.	1 piece	66	32	195	5	4	1	2	Trace	36	20	.8	300	.03	.09	.1	Trace
	Yellow, 2-layer, without icing:																	
398	Whole cake	1 cake	870	24	3,160	39	111	31	53	22	506	618	3.5	1,310	.17	.70	1.7	2

[16] Unenriched cake flour used unless otherwise specified.

■
TABLE H-1
Nutritive values of the edible part of foods, *continued*

[Dashes in the columns for nutrients show that no suitable value could be found although there is reason to believe that a measurable amount of the nutrient may be present]

No.	Food, approximate measure, and weight (in grams)			Water	Food energy	Protein	Fat	Fatty acids: Saturated (total)	Fatty acids: Unsaturated: Oleic	Fatty acids: Unsaturated: Linoleic	Carbohydrate	Calcium	Iron	Vitamin A value	Thiamin	Riboflavin	Niacin	Ascorbic acid
			Grams	*Per-cent*	*Calories*	*Grams*	*Grams*	*Grams*	*Grams*	*Grams*	*Grams*	*Milli-grams*	*Milli-grams*	*Inter-national units*	*Milli-grams*	*Milli-grams*	*Milli-grams*	*Milli-grams*
	Cakes made from home recipes—Continued																	
	Yellow, 2-layer, without icing—Continued																	
399	Piece, 1/16 of 9-in. diam. cake.	1 piece	54	24	200	2	7	2	3	1	32	39	.2	80	.01	.04	.1	Trace
	Yellow, 2-layer, with chocolate icing:																	
400	Whole cake	1 cake	1,203	21	4,390	51	156	55	69	23	727	818	7.2	1,920	.24	.96	2.4	Trace
401	Piece, 1/16 of 9-in. diam. cake.	1 piece	75	21	275	3	10	3	4	1	45	51	.5	120	.02	.06	.2	Trace
	Cake icings. See Sugars, Sweets.																	
	Cookies:																	
	Brownies with nuts:																	
402	Made from home recipe with enriched flour.	1 brownie	20	10	95	1	6	1	3	1	10	8	.4	40	.04	.02	.1	Trace
403	Made from mix	1 brownie	20	11	85	1	4	1	2	1	13	9	.4	20	.03	.02	.1	Trace
	Chocolate chip:																	
404	Made from home recipe with enriched flour.	1 cookie	10	3	50	1	3	1	1	1	6	4	0.2	10	0.01	0.01	0.1	Trace
405	Commercial	1 cookie	10	3	50	1	2	1	1	Trace	7	4	.2	10	Trace	Trace	Trace	Trace
406	Fig bars, commercial	1 cookie	14	14	50	1	1	----	----	----	11	11	.2	20	Trace	.01	.1	Trace
407	Sandwich, chocolate or vanilla, commercial.	1 cookie	10	2	50	1	2	1	1	Trace	7	2	.1	0	Trace	Trace	.1	0
	Corn flakes, added nutrients:																	
408	Plain	1 cup	25	4	100	2	Trace	----	----	----	21	4	.4	0	.11	.02	.5	0
409	Sugar-covered	1 cup	40	2	155	2	Trace	----	----	----	36	5	.4	0	.16	.02	.8	0
	Corn (hominy) grits, degermed, cooked:																	
410	Enriched	1 cup	245	87	125	3	Trace	----	----	----	27	2	.7	[17] 150	.10	.07	1.0	0
411	Unenriched	1 cup	245	87	125	3	Trace	----	----	----	27	2	.2	[17] 150	.05	.02	.5	0
	Cornmeal:																	
412	Whole-ground, unbolted, dry.	1 cup	122	12	435	11	5	1	2	2	90	24	2.9	[17] 620	.46	.13	2.4	0
413	Bolted (nearly whole-grain) dry.	1 cup	122	12	440	11	4	Trace	1	2	91	21	2.2	[17] 590	.37	.10	2.3	0
	Degermed, enriched:																	
414	Dry form	1 cup	138	12	500	11	2	----	----	----	108	8	4.0	[17] 610	.61	.36	4.8	0
415	Cooked	1 cup	240	88	120	3	1	----	----	----	26	2	1.0	[17] 140	.14	.10	1.2	0
	Degermed, unenriched:																	
416	Dry form	1 cup	138	12	500	11	2	----	----	----	108	8	1.5	[17] 610	.19	.07	1.4	0
417	Cooked	1 cup	240	88	120	3	1	----	----	----	26	2	.5	[17] 140	.05	.02	.2	0
418	Corn muffins, made with enriched degermed cornmeal and enriched flour; muffin 2⅜-in. diam.	1 muffin	40	33	125	3	4	2	2	Trace	19	42	.7	[17] 120	.08	.09	.6	Trace
419	Corn muffins, made with mix, egg, and milk; muffin 2⅜-in. diam.	1 muffin	40	30	130	3	4	1	2	1	20	96	.6	100	.07	.08	.6	Trace
420	Corn, puffed, presweetened, added nutrients.	1 cup	30	2	115	1	Trace	----	----	----	27	3	.5	0	.13	.05	.6	0
421	Corn, shredded, added nutrients.	1 cup	25	3	100	2	Trace	----	----	----	22	1	.6	0	.11	.05	.5	0
	Crackers:																	
422	Graham, 2½-in. square	4 crackers	28	6	110	2	3	----	----	----	21	11	.4	0	.01	.06	.4	0
423	Saltines	4 crackers	11	4	50	1	1	----	1	----	8	2	.1	0	Trace	Trace	.1	0
	Danish pastry, plain (without fruit or nuts):																	
424	Packaged ring, 12 ounces.	1 ring	340	22	1,435	25	80	24	37	15	155	170	3.1	1,050	.24	.51	2.7	Trace

[17] This value is based on product made from yellow varieties of corn; white varieties contain only a trace.

TABLE H-1
Nutritive values of the edible part of foods, *continued*

[Dashes in the columns for nutrients show that no suitable value could be found although there is reason to believe that a measurable amount of the nutrient may be present]

No.	Food, approximate measure, and weight (in grams)			Water	Food energy	Protein	Fat	Fatty acids: Saturated (total)	Fatty acids: Unsaturated: Oleic	Fatty acids: Unsaturated: Linoleic	Carbohydrate	Calcium	Iron	Vitamin A value	Thiamin	Riboflavin	Niacin	Ascorbic acid
	GRAIN PRODUCTS—Continued																	
	Danish pastry—Continued		*Grams*	*Per-cent*	*Calo-ries*	*Grams*	*Grams*	*Grams*	*Grams*	*Grams*	*Grams*	*Milli-grams*	*Milli-grams*	*Inter-national units*	*Milli-grams*	*Milli-grams*	*Milli-grams*	*Milli-grams*
425	Round piece, approx. 4¼-in. diam. by 1 in.	1 pastry	65	22	275	5	15	5	7	3	30	33	.6	200	.05	.10	.5	Trace
426	Ounce	1 oz.	28	22	120	2	7	2	3	1	13	14	.3	90	.02	.04	.2	Trace
427	Doughnuts, cake type	1 doughnut	32	24	125	1	6	1	4	Trace	16	13	[18].4	30	[18].05	[18].05	[18].4	Trace
428	Farina, quick-cooking, enriched, cooked.	1 cup	245	89	105	3	Trace	------	------	------	22	147	[19].7	0	[19].12	[19].07	[19]1.0	0
	Macaroni, cooked:																	
	Enriched:																	
429	Cooked, firm stage (undergoes additional cooking in a food mixture).	1 cup	130	64	190	6	1	------	------	------	39	14	[19]1.4	0	[19].23	[19].14	[19]1.8	0
430	Cooked until tender	1 cup	140	72	155	5	1	------	------	------	32	8	[19]1.3	0	[19].20	[19].11	[19]1.5	0
	Unenriched:																	
431	Cooked, firm stage (undergoes additional cooking in a food mixture).	1 cup	130	64	190	6	1	------	------	------	39	14	.7	0	.03	.03	.5	0
432	Cooked until tender	1 cup	140	72	155	5	1	------	------	------	32	11	.6	0	.01	.01	.4	0
433	Macaroni (enriched) and cheese, baked.	1 cup	200	58	430	17	22	10	9	2	40	362	1.8	860	.20	.40	1.8	Trace
434	Canned	1 cup	240	80	230	9	10	4	3	1	26	199	1.0	260	.12	.24	1.0	Trace
435	Muffins, with enriched white flour; muffin, 3-inch diam.	1 muffin	40	38	120	3	4	1	2	1	17	42	.6	40	.07	.09	.6	Trace
	Noodles (egg noodles), cooked:																	
436	Enriched	1 cup	160	70	200	7	2	1	1	Trace	37	16	[19]1.4	110	[19].22	[19].13	[19]1.9	0
437	Unenriched	1 cup	160	70	200	7	2	1	1	Trace	37	16	1.0	110	.05	.03	.6	0
438	Oats (with or without corn) puffed, added nutrients.	1 cup	25	3	100	3	1	------	------	------	19	44	1.2	0	0.24	0.04	0.5	0
439	Oatmeal or rolled oats, cooked.	1 cup	240	87	130	5	2	------	------	1	23	22	1.4	0	.19	.05	.2	0
	Pancakes, 4-inch diam.:																	
440	Wheat, enriched flour (home recipe).	1 cake	27	50	60	2	2	Trace	1	Trace	9	27	.4	30	.05	.06	.4	Trace
441	Buckwheat (made from mix with egg and milk).	1 cake	27	58	55	2	2	1	1	Trace	6	59	.4	60	.03	.04	.2	Trace
442	Plain or buttermilk (made from mix with egg and milk).	1 cake	27	51	60	2	2	1	1	Trace	9	58	.3	70	.04	.06	.2	Trace
	Pie (piecrust made with unenriched flour):																	
	Sector, 4-in., ⅐ of 9-in. diam. pie:																	
443	Apple (2-crust)	1 sector	135	48	350	3	15	4	7	3	51	11	.4	40	.03	.03	.5	1
444	Butterscotch (1-crust)	1 sector	130	45	350	6	14	5	6	2	50	98	1.2	340	.04	.13	.3	Trace
445	Cherry (2-crust)	1 sector	135	47	350	4	15	4	7	3	52	19	.4	590	.03	.03	.7	Trace
446	Custard (1-crust)	1 sector	130	58	285	8	14	5	6	2	30	125	.8	300	.07	.21	.4	0
447	Lemon meringue (1-crust).	1 sector	120	47	305	4	12	4	6	2	45	17	.6	200	.04	.10	.2	4
448	Mince (2-crust)	1 sector	135	43	365	3	16	4	8	3	56	38	1.4	Trace	.09	.05	.5	1
449	Pecan (1-crust)	1 sector	118	20	490	6	27	4	16	5	60	55	3.3	190	.19	.08	.4	Trace
450	Pineapple chiffon (1-crust).	1 sector	93	41	265	6	11	3	5	2	36	22	.8	320	.04	.08	.4	1
451	Pumpkin (1-crust)	1 sector	130	59	275	5	15	5	6	2	32	66	.7	3,210	.04	.13	.7	Trace

[18] Based on product made with enriched flour. With unenriched flour, approximate values per doughnut are: Iron, 0.2 milligram; thiamin, 0.01 milligram; riboflavin, 0.03 milligram; niacin, 0.2 milligram.

[19] Iron, thiamin, riboflavin, and niacin are based on the minimum levels of enrichment specified in standards of identity promulgated under the Federal Food, Drug, and Cosmetic Act.

TABLE H-1

Nutritive values of the edible part of foods, *continued*

[Dashes in the columns for nutrients show that no suitable value could be found although there is reason to believe that a measurable amount of the nutrient may be present]

No.	Food, approximate measure, and weight (in grams)			Water	Food energy	Protein	Fat	Fatty acids: Saturated (total)	Fatty acids: Unsaturated: Oleic	Fatty acids: Unsaturated: Linoleic	Carbohydrate	Calcium	Iron	Vitamin A value	Thiamin	Riboflavin	Niacin	Ascorbic acid
	GRAIN PRODUCTS—Continued																	
	Pie—Continued		*Grams*	*Percent*	*Calories*	*Grams*	*Grams*	*Grams*	*Grams*	*Grams*	*Grams*	*Milligrams*	*Milligrams*	*International units*	*Milligrams*	*Milligrams*	*Milligrams*	*Milligrams*
	Piecrust, baked shell for pie made with:																	
452	Enriched flour	1 shell	180	15	900	11	60	16	28	12	79	25	3.1	0	.36	.25	3.2	0
453	Unenriched flour	1 shell	180	15	900	11	60	16	28	12	79	25	.9	0	.05	.05	.9	0
	Piecrust mix including stick form:																	
454	Package, 10-oz., for double crust.	1 pkg.	284	9	1,480	20	93	23	46	21	141	131	1.4	0	.11	.11	2.0	0
455	Pizza (cheese) 5½-in. sector; ⅛ of 14-in. diam. pie.	1 sector	75	45	185	7	6	2	3	Trace	27	107	.7	290	.04	.12	.7	4
	Popcorn, popped:																	
456	Plain, large kernel	1 cup	6	4	25	1	Trace	----	----	----	5	1	.2	----	----	.01	.1	0
457	With oil and salt	1 cup	9	3	40	1	2	1	Trace	Trace	5	1	.2	----	----	.01	.2	0
458	Sugar coated	1 cup	35	4	135	2	1	----	----	----	30	2	.5	----	----	.02	.4	0
	Pretzels:																	
459	Dutch, twisted	1 pretzel	16	5	60	2	1	----	----	----	12	4	.2	0	Trace	Trace	.1	0
460	Thin, twisted	1 pretzel	6	5	25	1	Trace	----	----	----	5	1	.1	0	Trace	Trace	Trace	0
461	Stick, small, 2¼ inches	10 sticks	3	5	10	Trace	Trace	----	----	----	2	1	Trace	0	Trace	Trace	Trace	0
462	Stick, regular, 3⅛ inches.	5 sticks	3	5	10	Trace	Trace	----	----	----	2	1	Trace	0	Trace	Trace	Trace	0
	Rice, white:																	
	Enriched:																	
463	Raw	1 cup	185	12	670	12	1	----	----	----	149	44	[20]5.4	0	[20].81	[20].06	[20]6.5	0
464	Cooked	1 cup	205	73	225	4	Trace	----	----	----	50	21	[20]1.8	0	[20].23	[20].02	[20]2.1	0
465	Instant, ready-to-serve.	1 cup	165	73	180	4	Trace	----	----	----	40	5	[20]1.3	0	[20].21	[20]---	[20]1.7	0
466	Unenriched, cooked	1 cup	205	73	225	4	Trace	----	----	----	50	21	.4	0	.04	.02	.8	0
467	Parboiled, cooked	1 cup	175	73	185	4	Trace	----	----	----	41	33	[20]1.4	0	[20].19	[20]---	[20]2.1	0
468	Rice, puffed, added nutrients.	1 cup	15	4	60	1	Trace	----	----	----	13	3	.3	0	.07	.01	.7	0
	Rolls, enriched:																	
	Cloverleaf or pan:																	
469	Home recipe	1 roll	35	26	120	3	3	1	1	1	20	16	.7	30	.09	.09	.8	Trace
470	Commercial	1 roll	28	31	85	2	2	Trace	1	Trace	15	21	.5	Trace	.08	.05	.6	Trace
471	Frankfurter or hamburger.	1 roll	40	31	120	3	2	1	1	1	21	30	.8	Trace	.11	.07	.9	Trace
472	Hard, round or rectangular.	1 roll	50	25	155	5	2	Trace	1	Trace	30	24	1.2	Trace	.13	.12	1.4	Trace
473	Rye wafers, whole-grain, 1⅞ by 3½ inches.	2 wafers	13	6	45	2	Trace	----	----	----	10	7	.5	0	.04	.03	.2	0
474	Spaghetti, cooked, tender stage, enriched.	1 cup	140	72	155	5	1	----	----	----	32	11	[19]1.3	0	[19].20	[19].11	[19]1.5	0
	Spaghetti with meat balls, and tomato sauce:																	
475	Home recipe	1 cup	248	70	330	19	12	4	6	1	39	124	3.7	1,590	0.25	0.30	4.0	22
476	Canned	1 cup	250	78	260	12	10	2	3	4	28	53	3.3	1,000	.15	.18	2.3	5
	Spaghetti in tomato sauce with cheese:																	
477	Home recipe	1 cup	250	77	260	9	9	2	5	1	37	80	2.3	1,080	.25	.18	2.3	13
478	Canned	1 cup	250	80	190	6	2	1	1	1	38	40	2.8	930	.35	.28	4.5	10
479	Waffles, with enriched flour, 7-in. diam.	1 waffle	75	41	210	7	7	2	4	1	28	85	1.3	250	.13	.19	1.0	Trace
480	Waffles, made from mix, enriched, egg and milk added, 7-in. diam.	1 waffle	75	42	205	7	8	3	3	1	27	179	1.0	170	.11	.17	.7	Trace

[19] Iron, thiamin, riboflavin, and niacin are based on the minimum levels of enrichment specified in standards of identity promulgated under the Federal Food, Drug, and Cosmetic Act.

[20] Iron, thiamin, and niacin are based on the minimum levels of enrichment specified in standards of identity promulgated under the Federal Food, Drug, and Cosmetic Act. Riboflavin is based on unenriched rice. When the minimum level of enrichment for riboflavin specified in the standards of identity becomes effective the value will be 0.12 milligram per cup of parboiled rice and of white rice.

TABLE H-1

Nutritive values of the edible part of foods, *continued*

[Dashes show that no basis could be found for imputing a value although there was some reason to believe that a measurable amount of the constituent might be present]

	Food, approximate measure, and weight (in grams)			Water	Food energy	Protein	Fat	Fatty acids: Saturated (total)	Fatty acids: Unsaturated: Oleic	Fatty acids: Unsaturated: Linoleic	Carbohydrate	Calcium	Iron	Vitamin A value	Thiamin	Riboflavin	Niacin	Ascorbic acid
	GRAIN PRODUCTS—Continued		*Grams*	*Per-cent*	*Calories*	*Grams*	*Grams*	*Grams*	*Grams*	*Grams*	*Grams*	*Milligrams*	*Milligrams*	*International units*	*Milligrams*	*Milligrams*	*Milligrams*	*Milligrams*
481	Wheat, puffed, added nutrients.	1 cup	15	3	55	2	Trace	-----	-----	-----	12	4	.6	0	.08	.03	1.2	0
482	Wheat, shredded, plain	1 biscuit	25	7	90	2	1	-----	-----	-----	20	11	.9	0	.06	.03	1.1	0
483	Wheat flakes, added nutrients.	1 cup	30	4	105	3	Trace	-----	-----	-----	24	12	1.3	0	.19	.04	1.5	0
	Wheat flours:																	
484	Whole-wheat, from hard wheats, stirred.	1 cup	120	12	400	16	2	Trace	1	1	85	49	4.0	0	.66	.14	5.2	0
	All-purpose or family flour, enriched:																	
485	Sifted	1 cup	115	12	420	12	1	-----	-----	-----	88	18	[19]3.3	0	[19].51	[19].30	[19]4.0	0
486	Unsifted	1 cup	125	12	455	13	1	-----	-----	-----	95	20	[19]3.6	0	[19].55	[19].33	[19]4.4	0
487	Self-rising, enriched	1 cup	125	12	440	12	1	-----	-----	-----	93	331	[19]3.6	0	[19].55	[19].33	[19]4.4	0
488	Cake or pastry flour, sifted.	1 cup	96	12	350	7	1	-----	-----	-----	76	16	.5	0	.03	.03	.7	0
	FATS, OILS																	
	Butter:																	
	Regular, 4 sticks per pound:																	
489	Stick	½ cup	113	16	810	1	92	51	30	3	1	23	0	[21]3,750	-----	-----	-----	0
490	Tablespoon (approx. ⅛ stick).	1 tbsp.	14	16	100	Trace	12	6	4	Trace	Trace	3	0	[21]470	-----	-----	-----	0
491	Pat (1-in. sq. ⅓-in. high; 90 per lb.).	1 pat	5	16	35	Trace	4	2	1	Trace	Trace	1	0	[21]170	-----	-----	-----	0
	Whipped, 6 sticks or 2, 8-oz. containers per pound:																	
492	Stick	½ cup	76	16	540	1	61	34	20	2	Trace	15	0	[21]2,500	-----	-----	-----	0
493	Tablespoon (approx. ⅛ stick).	1 tbsp.	9	16	65	Trace	8	4	3	Trace	Trace	2	0	[21]310	-----	-----	-----	0
494	Pat (1¼-in. sq. ⅓-in. high; 120 per lb.).	1 pat	4	16	25	Trace	3	2	1	Trace	Trace	1	0	[21]130	-----	-----	-----	0
	Fats, cooking:																	
495	Lard	1 cup	205	0	1,850	0	205	78	94	20	0	0	0	0	0	0	0	0
496		1 tbsp.	13	0	115	0	13	5	6	1	0	0	0	0	0	0	0	0
497	Vegetable fats	1 cup	200	0	1,770	0	200	50	100	44	0	0	0	-----	0	0	0	0
498		1 tbsp.	13	0	110	0	13	3	6	3	0	0	0	-----	0	0	0	0
	Margarine:																	
	Regular, 4 sticks per pound:																	
499	Stick	½ cup	113	16	815	1	92	17	46	25	1	23	0	[22]3,750	-----	-----	-----	0
500	Tablespoon (approx. ⅛ stick).	1 tbsp.	14	16	100	Trace	12	2	6	3	Trace	3	0	[22]470	-----	-----	-----	0
501	Pat (1-in. sq. ⅓-in. high; 90 per lb.).	1 pat	5	16	35	Trace	4	1	2	1	Trace	1	0	[22]170	-----	-----	-----	0
	Whipped, 6 sticks per pound:																	
502	Stick	½ cup	76	16	545	1	61	11	31	17	Trace	15	0	[22]2,500	-----	-----	-----	0
	Soft, 2 8-oz. tubs per pound:																	
503	Tub	1 tub	227	16	1,635	1	184	34	68	68	1	45	0	[22]7,500	-----	-----	-----	0
504	Tablespoon	1 tbsp.	14	16	100	Trace	11	2	4	4	Trace	3	0	[22]470	-----	-----	-----	0
	Oils, salad or cooking:																	
505	Corn	1 cup	220	0	1,945	0	220	22	62	117	0	0	0	-----	0	0	0	0
506		1 tbsp.	14	0	125	0	14	1	4	7	0	0	0	-----	0	0	0	0
507	Cottonseed	1 cup	220	0	1,945	0	220	55	46	110	0	0	0	-----	0	0	0	0
508		1 tbsp.	14	0	125	0	14	4	3	7	0	0	0	-----	0	0	0	0
509	Olive	1 cup	220	0	1,945	0	220	24	167	15	0	0	0	-----	0	0	0	0
510		1 tbsp.	14	0	125	0	14	2	11	1	0	0	0	-----	0	0	0	0

[19] Iron, thiamin, riboflavin, and niacin are based on the minimum levels of enrichment specified in standards of identity promulgated under the Federal Food, Drug, and Cosmetic Act.

[21] Year-round average.

[22] Based on the average vitamin A content of fortified margarine. Federal specifications for fortified margarine require a minimum of 15,000 I.U. of vitamin A per pound.

TABLE H-1

Nutritive values of the edible part of foods, *continued*

[Dashes in the columns for nutrients show that no suitable value could be found although there is reason to believe that a measurable amount of the nutrient may be present]

	Food, approximate measure, and weight (in grams)			Water	Food energy	Protein	Fat	Fatty acids: Saturated (total)	Fatty acids: Unsaturated: Oleic	Fatty acids: Unsaturated: Linoleic	Carbohydrate	Calcium	Iron	Vitamin A value	Thiamin	Riboflavin	Niacin	Ascorbic acid
	FATS, OILS—Continued																	
	Oils, salad or cooking—Continued		*Grams*	*Per-cent*	*Calories*	*Grams*	*Grams*	*Grams*	*Grams*	*Grams*	*Grams*	*Milli-grams*	*Milli-grams*	*Inter-national units*	*Milli-grams*	*Milli-grams*	*Milli-grams*	*Milli-grams*
511	Peanut	1 cup	220	0	1,945	0	220	40	103	64	0	0	0	-----	0	0	0	0
512		1 tbsp.	14	0	125	0	14	3	7	4	0	0	0	-----	0	0	0	0
513	Safflower	1 cup	220	0	1,945	0	220	18	37	165	0	0	0	-----	0	0	0	0
514		1 tbsp.	14	0	125	0	14	1	2	10	0	0	0	-----	0	0	0	0
515	Soybean	1 cup	220	0	1,945	0	220	33	44	114	0	0	0	-----	0	0	0	0
516		1 tbsp.	14	0	125	0	14	2	3	7	0	0	0	-----	0	0	0	0
	Salad dressings:																	
517	Blue cheese	1 tbsp.	15	32	75	1	8	2	2	4	1	12	Trace	30	Trace	0.02	Trace	Trace
	Commercial, mayonnaise type:																	
518	Regular	1 tbsp.	15	41	65	Trace	6	1	1	3	2	2	Trace	30	Trace	Trace	Trace	-----
519	Special dietary, low-calorie.	1 tbsp.	16	81	20	Trace	2	Trace	Trace	1	1	3	Trace	40	Trace	Trace	Trace	-----
	French:																	
520	Regular	1 tbsp.	16	39	65	Trace	6	1	1	3	3	2	.1	-----	-----	-----	-----	-----
521	Special dietary, low-fat with artificial sweeteners.	1 tbsp.	15	95	Trace	Trace	Trace	-----	-----	-----	Trace	2	.1	-----	-----	-----	-----	-----
522	Home cooked, boiled	1 tbsp.	16	68	25	1	2	1	1	Trace	2	14	.1	80	.01	.03	Trace	Trace
523	Mayonnaise	1 tbsp.	14	15	100	Trace	11	2	2	6	Trace	3	.1	40	Trace	.01	Trace	-----
524	Thousand island	1 tbsp.	16	32	80	Trace	8	1	2	4	3	2	.1	50	Trace	Trace	Trace	Trace
	SUGARS, SWEETS																	
	Cake icings:																	
525	Chocolate made with milk and table fat.	1 cup	275	14	1,035	9	38	21	14	1	185	165	3.3	580	.06	.28	.6	1
526	Coconut (with boiled icing).	1 cup	166	15	605	3	13	11	1	Trace	124	10	.8	0	.02	.07	.3	0
527	Creamy fudge from mix with water only.	1 cup	245	15	830	7	16	5	8	3	183	96	2.7	Trace	.05	.20	.7	Trace
528	White, boiled	1 cup	94	18	300	1	0	-----	-----	-----	76	2	Trace	0	Trace	.03	Trace	0
	Candy:																	
529	Caramels, plain or chocolate.	1 oz.	28	8	115	1	3	2	1	Trace	22	42	.4	Trace	.01	.05	.1	Trace
530	Chocolate, milk, plain	1 oz.	28	1	145	2	9	5	3	Trace	16	65	.3	80	.02	.10	.1	Trace
531	Chocolate-coated peanuts.	1 oz.	28	1	160	5	12	3	6	2	11	33	.4	Trace	.10	.05	2.1	Trace
532	Fondant; mints, uncoated; candy corn.	1 oz.	28	8	105	Trace	1	-----	-----	-----	25	4	.3	0	Trace	Trace	Trace	0
533	Fudge, plain	1 oz.	28	8	115	1	4	2	1	Trace	21	22	.3	Trace	.01	.03	.1	Trace
534	Gum drops	1 oz.	28	12	100	Trace	Trace	-----	-----	-----	25	2	.1	0	0	Trace	Trace	0
535	Hard	1 oz.	28	1	110	0	Trace	-----	-----	-----	28	6	.5	0	0	0	0	0
536	Marshmallows	1 oz.	28	17	90	1	Trace	-----	-----	-----	23	5	.5	0	0	Trace	Trace	0
	Chocolate-flavored sirup or topping:																	
537	Thin type	1 fl. oz.	38	32	90	1	1	Trace	Trace	Trace	24	6	.6	Trace	.01	.03	.2	0
538	Fudge type	1 fl. oz.	38	25	125	2	5	3	2	Trace	20	48	.5	60	.02	.08	.2	Trace
	Chocolate-flavored beverage powder (approx. 4 heaping teaspoons per oz.):																	
539	With nonfat dry milk	1 oz.	28	2	100	5	1	Trace	Trace	Trace	20	167	.5	10	.04	.21	.2	1
540	Without nonfat dry milk.	1 oz.	28	1	100	1	1	Trace	Trace	Trace	25	9	.6	-----	.01	.03	.1	0
541	Honey, strained or extracted.	1 tbsp.	21	17	65	Trace	0	-----	-----	-----	17	1	.1	0	Trace	.01	.1	Trace
542	Jams and preserves	1 tbsp.	20	29	55	Trace	Trace	-----	-----	-----	14	4	.2	Trace	Trace	.01	Trace	Trace
543	Jellies	1 tbsp.	18	29	50	Trace	Trace	-----	-----	-----	13	4	.3	Trace	Trace	.01	Trace	1
	Molasses, cane:																	
544	Light (first extraction)	1 tbsp.	20	24	50	-----	-----	-----	-----	-----	13	33	.9	-----	.01	.01	Trace	-----
545	Blackstrap (third extraction).	1 tbsp.	20	24	45	-----	-----	-----	-----	-----	11	137	3.2	-----	.02	.04	.4	-----
	Sirups:																	
546	Sorghum	1 tbsp.	21	23	55	-----	-----	-----	-----	-----	14	35	2.6	-----	-----	.02	Trace	-----

TABLE H-1

Nutritive values of the edible part of foods, *continued*

[Dashes in the columns for nutrients show that no suitable value could be found although there is reason to believe that a measurable amount of the nutrient may be present]

	Food, approximate measure, and weight (in grams)			Water	Food energy	Protein	Fat	Fatty acids: Saturated (total)	Fatty acids: Unsaturated: Oleic	Fatty acids: Unsaturated: Linoleic	Carbohydrate	Calcium	Iron	Vitamin A value	Thiamin	Riboflavin	Niacin	Ascorbic acid
	FRUITS AND FRUIT PRODUCTS—Con.																	
	Sirups—Continued		*Grams*	*Percent*	*kCalories*	*Grams*	*Grams*	*Grams*	*Grams*	*Grams*	*Grams*	*Milligrams*	*Milligrams*	*International units*	*Milligrams*	*Milligrams*	*Milligrams*	*Milligrams*
547	Table blends, chiefly corn, light and dark.	1 tbsp.	21	24	60	0	0	----	----	----	15	9	.8	0	0	0	0	0
	Sugars:																	
548	Brown, firm packed	1 cup	220	2	820	0	0	----	----	----	212	187	7.5	0	.02	.07	.4	0
	White:																	
549	Granulated	1 cup	200	Trace	770	0	0	----	----	----	199	0	.2	0	0	0	0	0
550		1 tbsp.	11	Trace	40	0	0	----	----	----	11	0	Trace	0	0	0	0	0
551	Powdered, stirred before measuring.	1 cup	120	Trace	460	0	0	----	----	----	119	0	.1	0	0	0	0	0
	MISCELLANEOUS ITEMS																	
552	Barbecue sauce	1 cup	250	81	230	4	17	2	5	9	20	53	2.0	900	.03	.03	.8	13
	Beverages, alcoholic:																	
553	Beer	12 fl. oz.	360	92	150	1	0	----	----	----	14	18	Trace	----	.01	.11	2.2	----
	Gin, rum, vodka, whiskey:																	
554	80-proof	1½ fl. oz. jigger.	42	67	100	----	----	----	----	----	Trace	----	----	----	----	----	----	----
555	86-proof	1½ fl. oz. jigger.	42	64	105	----	----	----	----	----	Trace	----	----	----	----	----	----	----
556	90-proof	1½ fl. oz. jigger.	42	62	110	----	----	----	----	----	Trace	----	----	----	----	----	----	----
557	94-proof	1½ fl. oz. jigger.	42	60	115	----	----	----	----	----	Trace	----	----	----	----	----	----	----
558	100-proof	1½ fl. oz. jigger.	42	58	125	----	----	----	----	----	Trace	----	----	----	----	----	----	----
	Wines:																	
559	Dessert	3½ fl. oz. glass.	103	77	140	Trace	0	----	----	----	8	8	----	----	.01	.02	.2	----
560	Table	3½ fl. oz. glass.	102	86	85	Trace	0	----	----	----	4	9	.4	----	Trace	.01	.1	----
	Beverages, carbonated, sweetened, nonalcoholic:																	
561	Carbonated water	12 fl. oz.	366	92	115	0	0	----	----	----	29	----	----	0	0	0	0	0
562	Cola type	12 fl. oz.	369	90	145	0	0	----	----	----	37	----	----	0	0	0	0	0
563	Fruit-flavored sodas and Tom Collins mixes.	12 fl. oz.	372	88	170	0	0	----	----	----	45	----	----	0	0	0	0	0
564	Ginger ale	12 fl. oz.	366	92	115	0	0	----	----	----	29	----	----	0	0	0	0	0
565	Root beer	12 fl. oz.	370	90	150	0	0	----	----	----	39	----	----	0	0	0	0	0
566	Bouillon cubes, approx. ½ in.	1 cube	4	4	5	1	Trace	----	----	----	Trace	----	----	----	----	----	----	----
	Chocolate:																	
567	Bitter or baking	1 oz.	28	2	145	3	15	8	6	Trace	8	22	1.9	20	.01	.07	.4	0
568	Semi-sweet, small pieces.	1 cup	170	1	860	7	61	34	22	1	97	51	4.4	30	.02	.14	.9	0
	Gelatin:																	
569	Plain, dry powder in envelope.	1 envelope	7	13	25	6	Trace	----	----	----	0	----	----	----	----	----	----	----
570	Dessert powder, 3-oz. package.	1 pkg.	85	2	315	8	0	----	----	----	75	----	----	----	----	----	----	----
571	Gelatin dessert, prepared with water.	1 cup	240	84	140	4	0	----	----	----	34	----	----	----	----	----	----	----
	Olives, pickled:																	
572	Green	4 medium or 3 extra large or 2 giant.	16	78	15	Trace	2	Trace	2	Trace	Trace	8	.2	40	----	----	----	----
573	Ripe: Mission	3 small or 2 large.	10	73	15	Trace	2	Trace	2	Trace	Trace	9	.1	10	Trace	Trace	----	----
	Pickles, cucumber:																	
574	Dill, medium, whole, 3¾ in. long, 1¼ in. diam.	1 pickle	65	93	10	1	Trace	----	----	----	1	17	.7	70	Trace	.01	Trace	4

TABLE H-1

Nutritive values of the edible part of foods, *continued*

[Dashes in the columns for nutrients show that no suitable value could be found although there is reason to believe that a measurable amount of the nutrient may be present]

No.	Food, approximate measure, and weight (in grams)	Measure	Weight	Water	Food energy	Protein	Fat	Fatty acids: Saturated (total)	Fatty acids: Unsaturated: Oleic	Fatty acids: Unsaturated: Linoleic	Carbohydrate	Calcium	Iron	Vitamin A value	Thiamin	Riboflavin	Niacin	Ascorbic acid
	MISCELLANEOUS ITEMS—Continued																	
	Pickles, cucumber–Continued		*Grams*	*Per-cent*	*kCalories*	*Grams*	*Grams*	*Grams*	*Grams*	*Grams*	*Grams*	*Milli-grams*	*Milli-grams*	*Inter-national units*	*Milli-grams*	*Milli-grams*	*Milli-grams*	*Milli-grams*
575	Fresh, sliced, 1½ in. diam., ¼ in. thick.	2 slices	15	79	10	Trace	Trace	------	------	------	3	5	.3	20	Trace	Trace	Trace	1
576	Sweet, gherkin, small, whole, approx. 2½ in. long, ¾ in. diam.	1 pickle	15	61	20	Trace	Trace			------	6	2	.2	10	Trace	Trace	Trace	1
577	Relish, finely chopped, sweet.	1 tbsp.	15	63	20	Trace	Trace	------	------	------	5	3	.1	------	------	------	------	------
	Popcorn. See Grain Products.																	
578	Popsicle, 3 fl. oz. size	1 popsicle	95	80	70	0	0	0	0	0	18	0	Trace	0	0	0	0	0
	Pudding, home recipe with starch base:																	
579	Chocolate	1 cup	260	66	385	8	12	7	4	Trace	67	250	1.3	390	.05	.36	.3	1
580	Vanilla (blanc mange)	1 cup	255	76	285	9	10	5	3	Trace	41	298	Trace	410	.08	.41	.3	2
581	Pudding mix, dry form, 4-oz. package.	1 pkg.	113	2	410	3	2	1	1	Trace	103	23	1.8	Trace	.02	.08	.5	0
582	Sherbet	1 cup	193	67	260	2	2	------	------	------	59	31	Trace	120	.02	.06	Trace	4
	Soups:																	
	Canned, condensed, ready-to-serve:																	
	Prepared with an equal volume of milk:																	
583	Cream of chicken	1 cup	245	85	180	7	10	3	3	3	15	172	.5	610	.05	.27	.7	2
584	Cream of mushroom.	1 cup	245	83	215	7	14	4	4	5	16	191	.5	250	.05	.34	.7	1
585	Tomato	1 cup	250	84	175	7	7	3	2	1	23	168	.8	1,200	.10	.25	1.3	15
	Prepared with an equal volume of water:																	
586	Bean with pork	1 cup	250	84	170	8	6	1	2	2	22	63	2.3	650	.13	.08	1.0	3
587	Beef broth, bouillon consomme.	1 cup	240	96	30	5	0	------	------	------	3	Trace	.5	Trace	Trace	.02	1.2	------
588	Beef noodle	1 cup	240	93	70	4	3	1	1	1	7	7	1.0	50	.05	.07	1.0	Trace
589	Clam chowder, Manhattan type (with tomatoes, without milk).	1 cup	245	92	80	2	3	------	------	------	12	34	1.0	880	.02	.02	1.0	------
590	Cream of chicken	1 cup	240	92	95	3	6	1	2	3	8	24	.5	410	.02	.05	.5	Trace
591	Cream of mushroom.	1 cup	240	90	135	2	10	1	3	5	10	41	.5	70	.02	.12	.7	Trace
592	Minestrone	1 cup	245	90	105	5	3	------	------	------	14	37	1.0	2,350	.07	.05	1.0	------
593	Split pea	1 cup	245	85	145	9	3	1	2	Trace	21	29	1.5	440	0.25	0.15	1.5	1
594	Tomato	1 cup	245	90	90	2	3	Trace	1	1	16	15	.7	1,000	.05	.05	1.2	12
595	Vegetable beef	1 cup	245	92	80	5	2	------	------	------	10	12	.7	2,700	.05	.05	1.0	------
596	Vegetarian	1 cup	245	92	80	2	2	------	------	------	13	20	1.0	2,940	.05	.05	1.0	------
	Dehydrated, dry form:																	
597	Chicken noodle (2-oz. package).	1 pkg.	57	6	220	8	6	2	3	1	33	34	1.4	190	.30	.15	2.4	3
598	Onion mix (1½-oz. package).	1 pkg.	43	3	150	6	5	1	2	1	23	42	.6	30	.05	.03	.3	6
599	Tomato vegetable with noodles (2½-oz. pkg.).	1 pkg.	71	4	245	6	6	2	3	1	45	33	1.4	1,700	.21	.13	1.8	18
	Frozen, condensed:																	
	Clam chowder, New England type (with milk, without tomatoes):																	
600	Prepared with equal volume of milk.	1 cup	245	83	210	9	12	------	------	------	16	240	1.0	250	.07	.29	.5	Trace
601	Prepared with equal volume of water.	1 cup	240	89	130	4	8	------	------	------	11	91	1.0	50	.05	.10	.5	------
	Cream of potato:																	
602	Prepared with equal volume of milk.	1 cup	245	83	185	8	10	5	3	Trace	18	208	1.0	590	.10	.27	.5	Trace

TABLE H-1

Nutritive values of the edible part of foods, *continued*

[Dashes in the columns for nutrients show that no suitable value could be found although there is reason to believe that a measurable amount of the nutrient may be present]

	Food, approximate measure, and weight (in grams)			Water	Food energy	Protein	Fat	Fatty acids: Saturated (total)	Fatty acids: Unsaturated: Oleic	Fatty acids: Unsaturated: Linoleic	Carbohydrate	Calcium	Iron	Vitamin A value	Thiamin	Riboflavin	Niacin	Ascorbic acid
	MISCELLANEOUS ITEMS—Continued																	
	Soups—Continued																	
	Frozen, condensed—Continued																	
	Cream of Potato—Continued		*Grams*	*Per-cent*	*Calories*	*Grams*	*Grams*	*Grams*	*Grams*	*Grams*	*Grams*	*Milli-grams*	*Milli-grams*	*Inter-national units*	*Milli-grams*	*Milli-grams*	*Milli-grams*	*Milli-grams*
603	Prepared with equal volume of water.	1 cup	240	90	105	3	5	3	2	Trace	12	58	1.0	410	.05	.05	.5	------
	Cream of shrimp:																	
604	Prepared with equal volume of milk.	1 cup	245	82	245	9	16	------	------	------	15	189	.5	290	.07	.27	.5	Trace
605	Prepared with equal volume of water.	1 cup	240	88	160	5	12	------	------	------	8	38	.5	120	.05	.05	.5	------
	Oyster stew:																	
606	Prepared with equal volume of milk.	1 cup	240	83	200	10	12	------	------	------	14	305	1.4	410	.12	.41	.5	Trace
607	Prepared with equal volume of water.	1 cup	240	90	120	6	8	------	------	------	8	158	1.4	240	.07	.19	.5	------
608	Tapioca, dry, quick-cooking.	1 cup	152	13	535	1	Trace	------	------	------	131	15	.6	0	0	0	0	0
	Tapioca desserts:																	
609	Apple	1 cup	250	70	295	1	Trace	------	------	------	74	8	.5	30	Trace	Trace	Trace	Trace
610	Cream pudding	1 cup	165	72	220	8	8	4	3	Trace	28	173	.7	480	.07	.30	.2	2
611	Tartar sauce	1 tbsp.	14	34	75	Trace	8	1	1	4	1	3	.1	30	Trace	Trace	Trace	Trace
612	Vinegar	1 tbsp.	15	94	Trace	Trace	0	------	------	------	1	1	.1	------	------	------	------	------
613	White sauce, medium	1 cup	250	73	405	10	31	16	10	1	22	288	.5	1,150	.10	.43	.5	2
	Yeast:																	
614	Baker's, dry, active	1 pkg.	7	5	20	3	Trace	------	------	------	3	3	1.1	Trace	.16	.38	2.6	Trace
615	Brewer's, dry	1 tbsp.	8	5	25	3	Trace	------	------	------	3	17	1.4	Trace	1.25	.34	3.0	Trace
	Yoghurt. See Milk, Cheese, Cream, Imitation Cream.																	

TABLE H-2

Nutritional analyses of fast foods

(Dashes indicate no data available. X = Less than 2% US RDA; tr=trace.)

	Wt (g)	Energy (kcal)	PRO (g)	CHO (g)	Fat (g)	Chol (mg)	Vitamins: A (IU)	B_1 (mg)	B_2 (mg)	Nia. (mg)	B_6 (mg)	B_{12} (μg)	C (mg)	D (IU)	Minerals: Ca (mg)	Cu (mg)	Fe (mg)	K (mg)	Mg (mg)	P (mg)	Na (mg)	Zn (mg)	Moisture (g)	Crude Fiber (g)
ARBY'S®																								
Roast Beef	140	350	22	32	15	45	X	0.30	0.34	5	-	-	X	-	80	-	3.6	-	-	-	880	-	-	-
Beef and Cheese	168	450	27	36	22	55	X	0.38	0.43	6	-	-	X	-	200	-	4.5	-	-	-	1220	-	-	-
Super Roast Beef	263	620	30	61	28	85	X	0.53	0.43	7	-	-	X	-	100	-	5.4	-	-	-	1420	-	-	-
Junior Roast Beef	74	220	12	21	9	35	X	0.15	0.17	3	-	-	X	-	40	-	1.8	-	-	-	530	-	-	-
Ham & Cheese	154	380	23	33	17	60	X	0.75	0.34	5	-	-	X	-	200	-	2.7	-	-	-	1350	-	-	-
Turkey Deluxe	236	510	28	46	24	70	X	0.45	0.34	8	-	-	X	-	80	-	2.7	-	-	-	1220	-	-	-
Club Sandwich	252	560	30	43	30	100	X	0.68	0.43	7	-	-	X	-	200	-	3.6	-	-	-	1610	-	-	-
Source: Consumer Affairs, Arby's, Inc. Atlanta, Georgia. Nutritional analysis by Technological Resources, Camden, New Jersey																								
BURGER CHEF®																								
Hamburger	91	244	11	29	9	27	114	0.17	0.16	2.7	0.16	0.26	1.2	-	45	0.08	2.0	208	9	106	-	1.6	41	0.2
Cheeseburger	104	290	14	29	13	39	267	0.18	0.21	2.8	0.17	0.36	1.2	-	132	0.08	2.2	218	9	202	-	1.9	46	0.2
Double Cheeseburger	145	420	24	30	22	77	431	0.20	0.32	4.4	0.31	0.73	1.2	-	223	0.10	3.2	360	15	355	-	3.6	67	0.2
Fish Filet	179	547	21	46	31	43	400	0.23	0.22	2.7	0.04	0.10	1.0	-	145	0.04	2.2	271	19	302	-	1.2	72	0.4
Super Shef® Sandwich	252	563	29	44	30	105	754	0.31	0.40	6.0	0.45	0.87	9.3	-	205	0.21	4.5	578	25	377	-	4.5	143	0.5
Big Shef® Sandwich	186	569	23	38	36	81	279	0.26	0.31	4.7	0.31	0.63	1.0	-	152	0.05	3.6	382	14	280	-	3.4	80	0.3
TOP Shef® Sandwich	138	661	41	36	38	134	273	0.35	0.47	8.1	0.56	1.16	0	-	194	0.13	5.4	612	26	445	-	5.9	91	0.1

TABLE H-2

Nutritional analyses of fast foods, *continued*

(Dashes indicate no data available. X = Less than 2% US RDA; tr = trace.)

							Vitamins								Minerals									
	Wt (g)	Energy (kcal)	PRO (g)	CHO (g)	Fat (g)	Chol (mg)	A (IU)	B_1 (mg)	B_2 (mg)	Nia. (mg)	B_6 (mg)	B_{12} (μg)	C (mg)	D (IU)	Ca (mg)	Cu (mg)	Fe (mg)	K (mg)	Mg (mg)	P (mg)	Na (mg)	Zn (mg)	Moisture (g)	Crude Fiber (g)
Funmeal* Feast	-	545	15	55	30	27	123	0.25	0.21	4.6	0.16	0.26	12.8	-	61	0.24	2.8	688	26	183	-	1.6	70	0.8
Rancher® Platter*	316	640	32	33	42	106	1750*	0.29	0.38	8.6	0.61	1.01	23.5	-	66	0.38	5.3	1237	53	326	-	5.6	209	1.3
Mariner® Platter*	373	734	29	78	34	35	2069*	0.34	0.23	5.2	0.09	0.56	23.5	-	63	0.32	3.3	996	49	397	-	1.2	195	1.8
French Fries, small	68	250	2	20	19	0	0	0.07	0.04	1.7	-	0	11.5	-	9	0.16	0.7	473	16	62	-	<0.1	29	0.6
French Fries, large	85	351	3	28	26	0	0	0.10	0.06	2.4	-	0	16.2	-	13	0.23	0.9	661	22	86	-	<0.1	40	0.9
Vanilla Shake (12 oz)	336	380	13	60	10	40	387	0.10	0.66	0.5	0.1	1.77	0	-	497	-	0.3	622	40	392	-	1.3	-	-
Chocolate Shake (12 oz)	336	403	10	72	9	36	292	0.16	0.76	0.4	0.1	1.07	0	-	449	-	1.1	762	54	429	-	1.6	-	-
Hot Chocolate	-	198	8	23	8	30	288	0.93	0.39	0.3	0.1	0.79	2.1	-	271	0.09	0.7	436	50	245	-	1.1	-	-

*Includes salad. Source: Burger Chef Systems, Inc, Indianapolis, Indiana. Nutritional analysis from *Handbook No. 8*, Washington, US Dept of Agriculture

CHURCH'S FRIED CHICKEN®	Wt (g)	Energy (kcal)	PRO (g)	CHO (g)	Fat (g)	Chol (mg)	A (IU)	B_1 (mg)	B_2 (mg)	Nia. (mg)	B_6 (mg)	B_{12} (μg)	C (mg)	D (IU)	Ca (mg)	Cu (mg)	Fe (mg)	K (mg)	Mg (mg)	P (mg)	Na (mg)	Zn (mg)	Moisture (g)	Crude Fiber (g)
White Chicken Portion	100	327	21	10	23	-	160	0.10	0.18	7.2	-	-	0.7	-	94	-	1.00	186	-	-	498	-	45	0.10
Dark Chicken Portion	100	305	22	7	21	-	140	0.10	0.27	5.3	-	-	1.0	-	15	-	1.3	206	-	-	475	-	48	0.20

Source: Church's Fried Chicken, San Antonio, Texas. Nutritional analysis by Medallion Laboratories, Minneapolis, Minnesota

DAIRY QUEEN®	Wt (g)	Energy (kcal)	PRO (g)	CHO (g)	Fat (g)	Chol (mg)	A (IU)	B_1 (mg)	B_2 (mg)	Nia. (mg)	B_6 (mg)	B_{12} (μg)	C (mg)	D (IU)	Ca (mg)	Cu (mg)	Fe (mg)	K (mg)	Mg (mg)	P (mg)	Na (mg)	Zn (mg)	Moisture (g)	Crude Fiber (g)
Frozen Dessert	113	180	5	27	6	20	100	0.09	0.17	X	-	0.6	X	-	150	-	X	-	-	100	-	-	-	-
DQ Cone, small	71	110	3	18	3	10	100	0.03	0.14	X	-	0.4	X	X	100	-	X	-	-	60	-	-	-	-
DQ Cone, regular	142	230	6	35	7	20	300	0.09	0.26	X	-	0.6	X	X	200	-	X	-	-	150	-	-	-	-
DQ Cone, large	213	340	10	52	10	30	400	0.15	0.43	X	-	1.2	X	8	300	-	X	-	-	200	-	-	-	-
DQ Dip Cone, small	78	150	3	20	7	10	100	0.03	0.17	X	-	0.4	X	X	100	-	X	-	-	80	-	-	-	-
DQ Dip Cone, regular	156	300	7	40	13	20	300	0.09	0.34	X	-	0.6	X	X	200	-	0.4	-	-	150	-	-	-	-
DQ Dip Cone, large	234	450	10	58	20	30	400	0.12	0.51	X	-	0.9	X	8	300	-	0.4	-	-	200	-	-	-	-
DQ Sundae, small	106	170	4	30	4	15	100	0.03	0.17	X	-	0.5	X	X	100	-	0.7	-	-	100	-	-	-	-
DQ Sundae, regular	177	290	6	51	7	20	300	0.06	0.26	X	-	0.6	X	X	200	-	1.1	-	-	150	-	-	-	-
DQ Sundae, large	248	400	9	71	9	30	400	0.09	0.43	0.4	-	1.2	X	8	300	-	1.8	-	-	250	-	-	-	-
DQ Malt, small	241	340	10	51	11	30	400	0.06	0.34	0.4	-	1.2	2.4	60	300	-	1.8	-	-	200	-	-	-	-
DQ Malt, regular	418	600	15	89	20	50	750	0.12	0.60	0.8	-	1.8	3.6	100	500	-	3.6	-	-	400	-	-	-	-
DQ Malt, large	588	840	22	125	28	70	750	0.15	0.85	1.2	-	2.4	6	140	600	-	5.4	-	-	600	-	-	-	-
DQ Float	397	330	6	59	8	20	100	0.12	0.17	X	-	0.6	X	X	200	-	X	-	-	200	-	-	-	-
DQ Banana Split	383	540	10	91	15	30	750	0.60	0.60	0.8	-	0.9	18	X	350	-	1.8	-	-	250	-	-	-	-
DQ Parfait	284	460	10	81	11	30	400	0.12	0.43	0.4	-	1.2	X	8	300	-	1.8	-	-	250	-	-	-	-
DQ Freeze	397	520	11	89	13	35	200	0.15	0.34	X	-	1.2	X	X	300	-	X	-	-	250	-	-	-	-
Mr. Misty* Freeze	411	500	10	87	12	35	200	0.15	0.34	X	-	0.12	X	X	300	-	X	-	-	200	-	-	-	-
Mr. Misty* Float	404	440	6	85	8	20	100	0.12	0.17	X	-	0.6	X	X	200	-	X	-	-	200	-	-	-	-
"Dilly"* Bar	85	240	4	22	15	10	100	0.06	0.17	X	-	0.5	X	X	100	-	0.4	-	-	100	-	-	-	-
DQ Sandwich	60	140	3	24	4	10	100	0.03	0.14	0.4	-	0.2	X	X	60	-	0.4	-	-	60	-	-	-	-
Mr. Misty Kiss*	89	70	0	17	0	0	X	X	X	X	-	X	X	X	X	-	X	-	-	X	-	-	-	-
Brazier* Cheese Dog	113	330	15	24	19	-	-	-	0.18	3.3	0.07	1.22	-	23	168	0.08	1.6	-	24	182	-	1.9	-	-
Brazier* Chili Dog	128	330	13	25	20	-	-	0.15	0.23	3.9	0.17	1.29	11.0	20	86	0.13	2.0	-	38	139	939	1.8	-	-
Brazier* Dog	99	273	11	23	15	-	-	0.12	0.15	2.6	0.08	1.05	11.0	23	75	0.79	1.5	-	21	104	868	1.4	-	-
Fish Sandwich	170	400	20	41	17	-	tr	0.15	0.26	3.0	0.16	1.20	tr	40	60	0.08	1.1	-	24	200	-	0.3	-	-
Fish Sandwich w/Ch	177	440	24	39	21	-	100	0.15	0.26	3.0	0.16	1.50	tr	40	150	0.08	0.4	-	24	250	-	0.3	-	-
Super Brazier* Dog	182	518	20	41	30	-	tr	0.42	0.44	7.0	0.17	2.09	14.0	44	158	0.18	4.3	-	37	195	1552	2.8	-	-
Super Brazier* Dog w/Ch	203	593	26	43	36	-	-	0.43	0.48	8.1	0.18	2.34	14.0	44	297	0.18	4.4	-	42	312	1986	3.5	-	-
Super Brazier* Chili Dog	210	555	23	42	33	-	-	0.42	0.48	8.8	0.27	2.67	18.0	32	158	0.21	4.0	-	48	231	1640	2.8	-	-
Brazier* Fries, small	71	200	2	25	10	-	tr	0.06	tr	0.8	0.16	-	3.6	16	tr	0.04	0.4	-	16	100	-	tr	-	-
Brazier* Fries, large	113	320	3	40	16	-	tr	0.09	0.03	1.2	0.30	-	4.8	24	tr	0.08	0.4	-	24	150	-	0.3	-	-
Brazier* Onion Rings	85	300	6	33	17	-	tr	0.09	tr	0.4	0.08	-	2.4	8	20	0.08	0.4	-	16	60	-	0.3	-	-

Source: International Dairy Queen, Inc, Minneapolis, Minnesota. Nutritional analysis by Raltech Scientific Services, Inc (formerly WARF), Madison, Wisconsin. (Nutritional analysis not applicable in the state of Texas.)

JACK IN THE BOX®	Wt (g)	Energy (kcal)	PRO (g)	CHO (g)	Fat (g)	Chol (mg)	A (IU)	B_1 (mg)	B_2 (mg)	Nia. (mg)	B_6 (mg)	B_{12} (μg)	C (mg)	D (IU)	Ca (mg)	Cu (mg)	Fe (mg)	K (mg)	Mg (mg)	P (mg)	Na (mg)	Zn (mg)	Moisture (g)	Crude Fiber (g)
Hamburger	97	263	13	29	11	26	49	0.27	0.18	5.6	0.11	0.73	1.1	20	82	0.10	2.3	165	20	115	566	1.8	43	0.2
Cheeseburger	109	310	16	28	15	32	338	0.27	0.21	5.4	0.12	0.87	<1.1	20	172	0.10	2.6	177	22	194	877	2.3	47	0.2
Jumbo Jack* Hamburger	246	551	28	45	29	80	246	0.47	0.34	11.6	0.30	2.68	3.7	42	134	0.22	4.5	492	44	261	1134	4.2	139	0.7
Jumbo Jack* Hamburger w/Ch	272	628	32	45	35	110	734	0.52	0.38	11.3	0.31	3.05	4.9	41	273	0.24	4.6	499	49	411	1666	4.8	153	0.8
Regular Taco	83	189	8	15	11	22	356	0.07	0.08	1.8	0.14	0.5	<0.9	6	116	0.11	1.2	264	36	150	460	1.3	47	0.6
Super Taco	146	285	12	20	17	37	599	0.10	0.12	2.8	0.22	0.77	1.6	9	196	0.18	1.9	415	53	235	968	2.1	92	1.0
Moby Jack* Sandwich	141	455	17	38	26	56	240	0.30	0.21	4.5	0.12	1.1	1.4	24	167	0.08	1.7	246	30	263	837	1.1	57	0.1
Breakfast Jack* Sandwich	121	301	18	28	13	182	442	0.41	0.47	5.1	0.14	1.1	3.4	51	177	0.11	2.5	190	24	310	1037	1.8	59	0.1
French Fries	80	270	3	31	15	13	-	0.12	0.02	1.9	0.22	0.17	3.7	<1	19	0.10	0.7	423	27	88	128	0.3	29	0.6
Onion Rings	85	351	5	32	23	24	-	0.24	0.12	3.1	0.07	0.26	<1.2	<1	26	0.07	1.4	109	16	69	318	0.4	24	0.3
Apple Turnover	119	411	4	45	24	17	-	0.23	0.12	2.5	0.03	0.17	<1.2	1	11	0.06	1.4	69	10	33	352	0.2	45	0.2
Vanilla Shake*	317	317	10	57	6	26	-	0.16	0.38	0.5	0.20	1.36	<3.2	41	349	0.06	0.2	599	38	312	229	1.0	243	0.3
Strawberry Shake*	328	323	11	55	7	26	-	0.16	0.46	0.6	0.15	1.25	<3.3	43	371	0.10	0.6	613	40	328	241	1.1	253	0.3
Chocolate Shake*	322	325	11	55	7	26	-	0.16	0.64	0.6	0.19	1.55	<3.2	45	348	0.13	0.7	676	53	328	270	1.1	247	0.3
Vanilla Shake	314	342	10	54	9	36	440	0.16	0.47	0.5	0.18	1.1	3.5	44	349	0.06	0.4	536	48	318	263	1.0	238	0.3
Strawberry Shake	328	380	11	63	10	33	426	0.16	0.62	0.5	0.18	0.92	<3.3	30	351	0.07	0.3	556	47	316	268	1.0	242	0.3
Chocolate Shake	317	365	11	59	10	35	380	0.16	0.60	0.6	0.18	0.98	<3.2	38	350	0.16	1.2	633	57	332	294	1.2	235	0.3
Ham & Cheese Omelette	174	425	21	32	23	355	766	0.45	0.70	3.0	0.18	1.44	<1.7	64	260	0.14	4.0	237	29	397	975	2.3	94	0.2
Double Cheese Omelette	166	423	19	30	25	370	797	0.33	0.68	2.5	0.14	1.33	1.7	61	276	0.13	3.6	208	26	370	899	2.1	88	0.2
Ranchero Style Omelette	196	414	20	33	23	343	853	0.33	0.74	2.6	0.18	1.51	<2.0	78	278	0.14	3.8	260	29	372	1098	2.0	117	0.4
French Toast	180	537	15	54	29	115	522	0.56	0.30	4.4	0.47	1.62	9.2	22	119	0.11	3.0	194	27	256	1130	1.8	78	0.9
Pancakes	232	626	16	79	27	87	488	0.63	0.44	4.6	0.19	0.56	<26.2	23	105	0.12	2.8	237	36	633	1670	1.9	104	0.7
Scrambled Eggs	267	719	26	55	44	259	694	0.69	0.56	5.2	0.34	1.31	<12.8	80	257	0.24	5.0	635	55	483	1110	3.0	137	1.3

*Special formula for shakes sold in California, Arizona, Texas and Washington. Source: Jack-in-the-Box, Foodmaker, Inc, San Diego, California. Nutritional analysis by Raltech Scientific Services, Inc (formerly WARF), Madison, Wisconsin

KENTUCKY FRIED CHICKEN®	Wt (g)	Energy (kcal)	PRO (g)	CHO (g)	Fat (g)	Chol (mg)	A (IU)	B_1 (mg)	B_2 (mg)	Nia. (mg)	B_6 (mg)	B_{12} (μg)	C (mg)	D (IU)	Ca (mg)	Cu (mg)	Fe (mg)	K (mg)	Mg (mg)	P (mg)	Na (mg)	Zn (mg)	Moisture (g)	Crude Fiber (g)
Original Recipe* Dinner*																								
Wing & Rib	322	603	30	48	32	133	25.5	0.22	0.19	10.0	-	-	36.6	-	-	-	-	-	-	-	-	-	-	-
Wing & Thigh	341	661	33	48	38	172	25.5	0.24	0.27	8.4	-	-	36.6	-	-	-	-	-	-	-	-	-	-	-
Drum & Thigh	346	643	35	46	35	180	25.5	0.25	0.32	8.5	-	-	36.6	-	-	-	-	-	-	-	-	-	-	-
Extra Crispy Dinner*																								
Wing & Rib	349	755	33	60	43	132	25.5	0.31	0.29	10.4	-	-	36.6	-	-	-	-	-	-	-	-	-	-	-
Wing & Thigh	371	812	36	58	48	176	25.5	0.31	0.35	10.3	-	-	36.6	-	-	-	-	-	-	-	-	-	-	-
Drum & Thigh	376	765	38	55	44	183	25.5	0.32	0.38	10.4	-	-	36.6	-	-	-	-	-	-	-	-	-	-	-
Mashed Potatoes	85	64	2	12	1	0	<18	<0.01	0.02	0.8	-	-	4.9	-	-	-	-	-	-	-	-	-	-	-
Gravy	14	23	0	1	2	0	<3	0.00	0.01	0.1	-	-	<0.2	-	-	-	-	-	-	-	-	-	-	-
Cole Slaw	91	122	1	13	8	7	-	-	-	-	-	-	-	-	-	-	-	-	-	-	-	-	-	-
Rolls	21	61	2	11	1	1	<5	0.10	0.04	1.0	-	-	0.3	-	-	-	-	-	-	-	-	-	-	-
Corn (5.5-inch ear)	135	169	5	31	3	X	162	0.12	0.07	1.2	-	-	2.6	-	-	-	-	-	-	-	-	-	-	-

* Includes two pieces of chicken, mashed potato and gravy, cole slaw, and roll. Source: Kentucky Fried Chicken, Inc, Louisville, Kentucky. Nutritional analysis by Raltech Scientific Services, Inc (formerly WARF), Madison, Wisconsin

APPENDIX I

GLOSSARY

Definitions given in this book were obtained from three sources: *Taber's Cyclopedic Medical Dictionary*, 12th edition (Philadelphia: F. A. Davis Company, 1973); R. T. Lagua, V. S. Claudio, and V. F. Thiele, *Nutrition and Diet Therapy Reference Dictionary* (St. Louis: C. V. Mosby Company, 1974); and *The Random House Dictionary of the English Language*, unabridged edition (New York: Random House, 1979).

absorption: The process by which nutrients and other substances are transported from the gastrointestinal tract into the body proper.

acetyl CoA: (Latin *acetum*, "vinegar"; *CoA* abbreviates *coenzyme A*, a derivative of pantothenic acid) A molecule comprised of 2 atoms of carbon, 3 of hydrogen, 1 of oxygen, and coenzyme A. It is the first substance that enters the citric acid cycle. (See Appendix E.)

actin: One of the two major proteins found in muscle. It combines with myosin, the other major protein, when muscles contract.

adaptive mechanisms: In the context of nutrition, body processes that act to maintain a constant supply of nutrients for cells.

adequate diet: A diet that supplies approximately the RDAs for essential nutrients and enough calories to meet the person's need for energy.

active transport: The transport of a substance across a cell membrane that involves a carrier protein and energy from ATP.

adolescence: 12 to 18 years of age.

aerobic: "With oxygen"; the pathway of energy formation that requires oxygen is the citric acid cycle.

albumin: One of the most common proteins in blood. It is a relatively small polypeptide that carries certain nutrients in blood and serves as a source of amino acids for cells.

alcohol: A chemical substance primarily derived from carbohydrates.

alcohol sugars: Monosaccharides whose chemical structures contain an alcohol group.

amino acid score: An estimate of protein quality derived by comparing the amino acid composition of a food with that of a high-quality protein such as egg white or milk or with an established amino acid reference pattern.

amniotic fluid: Fluid that surrounds the fetus in the uterus. It and the fetus are contained in a thick membrane called the *amniotic sac*.

anabolism: The constructive, or build-up, phase of metabolism; also called *synthesis*. The formation of muscle tissue is an example of an anabolic process. Anabolic processes generally require energy in addition to "building" materials.

anaerobic: "Without oxygen"; the pathway of energy formation that does not require oxygen is glycolysis.

anemia: A condition in which the body's content of red blood cells, or the amount of hemoglobin within the cells, is lower than normal. There are many types of anemia, including the genetic sickle-cell anemia and those caused by deficiencies in vitamin B_{12} and folic acid. Iron-deficiency anemia, however, is the most common.

anorexia nervosa: (*an*, "not"; *orexis*, "appetite"; *nervosa*, "assumed to have psychological origins") A condition in which a person *appears* to have no appetite. People with anorexia nervosa do have appetite, but they don't eat in response to it because they have a pathological fear of gaining weight.

antibodies: Substances secreted in response to the presence of a foreign protein (antigen). They counteract the harmful effects of bacteria, viruses, and other sources of foreign protein that enter the body. Immunizations protect against specific infectious diseases by supplying the body with antibodies that ward off invading germs.

antigens: Bacteria, viruses, and other "foreign" proteins that enter the body and interfere with normal body processes. The presence of antigens prompts the body to produce antibodies, which attempt to destroy the antigens. The body's ability to produce antibodies varies with the type and amount of the antigen, the person's nutritional status, and other factors.

antioxidant: A substance that delays or prevents oxidation.

appetite: The desire to eat; a pleasant sensation that is aroused by thoughts of the taste and enjoyment of food.

ariboflavinosis: (*a-*, "without"; *-osis*, "abnormal condition") The riboflavin-deficiency disease.

association: Relationship that exists when one condition accompanies another condition. An association does not show a cause-and-effect relationship. High-fat diets, high blood pressure, and smoking are all *associated with* the development of heart disease, for example, but it is not clear at this time that any of them *causes* heart disease.

atherosclerosis: A type of "hardening of the arteries" in which plaque (cholesterol and other blood components) builds up in the walls of arteries. As the condition progresses, the arteries narrow, and the supply of blood to the heart, brain, muscles, and other organs and tissues is reduced.

balanced diet: A diet that consists of a variety of foods that together provide calories and nutrients in amounts that promote health; it contains neither too little nor too much energy (calories), fat, protein, vitamins, minerals, water, and fiber.

basal metabolic rate (BMR): The amount of energy used for basal metabolic processes over a 24-hour period.

basal metabolism: Energy used to support the body's ongoing metabolic processes while the body is in a state of complete physical, digestive, and emotional rest. Basal metabolism represents the energy the body expends to keep the heart beating, the lungs working, the body temperature normal, and a variety of other processes operating.

beriberi: The thiamin-deficiency disease.

bioavailability: The percentage of the total amount of a mineral consumed that is absorbed.

biological value: The percentage of absorbed protein that is retained by the body for use in growth and tissue maintenance.

binge: With regard to nutrition, consumption of excessive quantities of food in a short period of time.

bulimia: (literally, "ox hunger"; also referred to as *bulimia nervosa*) Condition characterized by alternating episodes of dieting and binging on food.

bran: The outermost covering of a whole grain. It is removed during refining.

calorie: A unit of measure for energy. The nutrition "calorie" refers to the kilo-

calorie *(continued)*
calorie (kcal), the amount of energy needed to raise the temperature of a kilogram of water from 15°C to 16°C.

carotenemia: Yellowish discoloration of the skin caused by excessive intake of carotene; also called *hypercarotenemia.*

catabolism: The breakdown phase of metabolism. The release of energy from the energy nutrients is an example of a catabolic process. (Memory aid: Just as a *Cat*erpillar tractor can break down buildings, a *cat*abolic reaction breaks down molecules.)

cause-and-effect relationship: Relationship that exists when one condition produces another. For example, bacteria *causes* wounds to become infected, and vitamin C deficiency *causes* scurvy.

chemical bonds: Energy in the form of electrons that hold atoms within a molecule together (see Figure 3-10).

childhood: 1 to 11 years of age.

cholesterol: A fat-soluble, colorless liquid found in animals but not in plants. Cholesterol is used by the body to form steroid hormones such as testosterone and estrogen and is a component of animal cell membranes.

chylomicrons: (kī lō mī'krän) Tiny droplets containing triglycerides, phospholipids, cholesterol, and protein that are manufactured in the cells that line the small intestine. They serve to transport some of the end products of fat digestion to the heart and general circulation by way of the lymph system. They are just barely soluble in water.

chyme: (from Greek *chymos*, "juice") The semifluid mass of partly digested food that is expelled by the stomach into the duodenum.

citric acid cycle: A complex series of chemical reactions that leads to the formation of energy from fatty acids, certain amino acids, and glucose fragments. The citric acid cycle requires oxygen; it is aerobic. Also called the *Kreb's cycle* and the *tricarboxylic acid cycle.*

coenzyme: A form of a B-complex vitamin that activates an enzyme. Each B-complex vitamin has one or more coenzyme forms that activate specific enzymes.

cofactor: A chemical substance that activates a particular enzyme. Many minerals act as cofactors.

collagen: Protein found in connective tissue in bones, skin, ligaments, and cartilage. Collagen accounts for about 30% of the total body protein.

colostrum: The milk produced during the first few days after delivery. It contains more antibodies, protein, and certain minerals than *mature milk*, milk that is produced later. It is thicker than mature milk and has a yellowish color.

complementary proteins: Two or more incomplete proteins that produce a complete protein when combined. The limiting amino acid in one food is complemented by the presence of that amino acid in the other food(s).

complete proteins: Proteins that contain all of the essential amino acids in amounts sufficient to support growth and tissue maintenance.

cretinism: A condition in which the thyroid fails to function normally in a fetus and infant. Cretinism is characterized by small stature and mental retardation. When related to iodine deficiency, it is called *endemic cretinism.*

critical period: Pertaining to growth, a specific interval of time during which the cells of a tissue or organ are programmed to multiply. If the supply of nutrients to cells is not adequate during a critical period of growth, cell division does not occur and the affected tissues or organs remain smaller than they would otherwise.

deamination: The removal of a nitrogen group from an amino acid. Amino acids must be deaminated before they can be used for glucose formation or converted to a nonessential amino acid.

dehydration: A condition that occurs when water excretion exceeds water intake.

dementia: (from Latin *dementare*, "to make insane") A deteriorative mental state.

dermatitis: (*dermis*, "skin"; *-itis*, "inflammation") Inflammation of the skin.

development: The processes involved in enhancing the capabilities of a human; the maturation of humans to more advanced and complex stages of functioning. (The brain *grows* in size, whereas the ability to reason *develops*.)

diabetes: A disorder of carbohydrate metabolism characterized by high blood-glucose levels. It results from the inadequate production of insulin by the body, or more commonly, from abnormal utilization of insulin. Two major types of diabetes are recognized: insulin-dependent and non-insulin-dependent diabetes.

diet: Foods and fluids regularly consumed in the course of living.

dietary fiber: Polysaccharides and carbohydratelike substances that, because of their chemical structure, cannot be digested by enzymes in the human digestive tract.

differentiation: The development of cells that function differently than the parent cells.

diffusion, facilitated: Diffusion of a substance across a cell membrane with the help of carrier proteins.

diffusion, simple: The free movement of a substance across a cell membrane from an area of high concentration to an area of low concentration. The process equalizes the concentrations on either side of the membrane.

digestion: The process by which ingested food is prepared for use by the body. It occurs in the digestive system and involves several mechanical processes and thousands of chemical reactions.

diglyceride: A fat in which the glycerol molecule has two fatty acids attached to it; also called *diacylglycerol*.

dipeptides: Proteins consisting of two amino acids.

disaccharide: (*di-*, "two"; *saccharide*, "sugar") A sugar consisting of two monosaccharide molecules.

dopamine: (dō′pə mēn′) A neurotransmitter formed from the amino acid tyrosine. It is thought to be involved with emotions, motor functions, and hormone release.

double bond: Bond formed by the sharing of four electrons between two adjacent atoms.

edema: Condition in which fluid accumulates in the spaces between cells; swelling.

elastin: Protein found in elastic connective tissue such as blood vessels and ligaments.

electrolytes: Chemical substances that form charged particles and conduct an electrical current when in solution. The chief electrolytes in body fluids are sodium, potassium, and chloride.

empty-calorie foods: Foods that provide an excess of calories in relation to nutrients. Commercial soft drinks, candy, sugar, alcohol, and fats such as butter, margarine, and oil are considered empty-calorie foods.

emulsifying agent: A substance that will cause two liquids that are not soluble in each other to mix. An emulsifying agent allows a fat to mix with water, such as happens when bile causes the mixing of fat with digestive juices.

endemic: Descriptive of a disease or condition that recurs continuously among a significant number of people within a population. Protein–calorie malnutrition and goiter are examples of endemic problems in some countries. Iron deficiency and obesity are endemic problems in the U.S.

energy balance: Condition that exists when the amount of energy consumed in foods equals the amount used by the body.

enrichment: The replacement of thiamin, riboflavin, niacin, and iron lost during the refining of grains. The term applies only to grain products, and the levels of enrichment are regulated.

environmental conditions: Physical, economic, psychosocial, and dietary factors that determine the circumstances under which people live.

enzymes: Complex protein substances that increase the rate of chemical reactions without being permanently changed themselves in the process; sometimes referred to as *catalysts*. The body contains hundreds of enzymes. They are found in particularly high amounts in the gastrointestinal tract. They are specific in their action, each acting only upon a particular chemical substance. The suffix *-ase* is common for enzyme names; amyl*ase* and sucr*ase* are examples. The suffix *-in* also is common—as in tryps*in* and peps*in*.

epidemic: The appearance of a disease or condition that attacks many people within a population at the same time. Outbreaks of polio earlier in this century and the recent spread of acquired immune deficiency syndrome (AIDS) are examples of epidemics in the U.S.

epinephrine: (also called *adrenalin*) A chemical messenger derived from an amino acid, it increases blood pressure, the force of the contractions of the heart, and the pulse rate. It is the "fight or flight" chemical that surges into the blood stream in times of stress.

epithelial tissue: The outermost layer of cells that form the surface of the skin and eyes and the lining of the respiratory, reproductive, and gastrointestinal tracts.

essential amino acids: Amino acids that cannot be synthesized in adequate amounts by humans and therefore must be obtained from the diet.

essential fatty acid: A fatty acid that is required but cannot be produced by the body; it must be provided in the diet. (See *linoleic acid.*)

essential hypertension: Hypertension of no known cause; also called *primary* or *idiopathic hypertension*, it accounts for over 95% of all cases of hypertension.

essential nutrients: Substances required by the body for normal growth and health that cannot be manufactured in sufficient amounts by the body; they must be obtained in the diet.

facilitated diffusion: Diffusion of a substance across a cell membrane with the help of carrier proteins.

fatty acids: fat-soluble molecules containing carbon, hydrogen, and an acid group (COOH). When combined with glycerol, they form a fat. Fatty acids come in many forms. They may be short-, medium-, or long-chained, and saturated, monounsaturated, or polyunsaturated.

ferritin: The storage form of iron. Most of the body's iron is stored in the liver and bone marrow.

fertility: The biological ability to conceive and maintain a pregnancy.

fetus: A baby in the womb from the eighth week of pregnancy until birth. Before then, it is referred to as an *embryo*.

fibrous proteins: Long, thin strands of polypeptides.

fluorosis: Fluoride overdose characterized by discolored ("mottled") teeth in children. Fluorosis generally results from water supplies that contain over 1 part per million of fluoride.

food additive: Any substance put into a food that becomes part of the food and/or affects the characteristics of the food. The term applies both to substances intentionally added to foods and to substances added inadvertently, such as packaging materials.

food allergy: The development of immune-system reactions in response to the presence of an offending food substance in the body. True allergies can be diagnosed by the abnormally high presence of antibodies in the blood following ingestion and absorption of an antigen—the offending component of food. Common food antigens include wheat gluten, egg-white protein, and cow's-milk protein.

food intolerance: Any adverse reaction caused by the consumption of a food or a particular component of food that does not involve the body's immune system. Lactose intolerance, adverse reactions to monosodium glutamate (MSG), and the gas and intestinal cramps related to the consumption of dried beans, cabbage, cauliflower, and certain other vegetables are examples of food intolerances.

food poisoning: An imprecise term for an illness resulting from ingestion of foods containing a harmful substance such as bacteria, a bacterial toxin, a poisonous insecticide, or a toxic material such as mercury or lead.

fore milk: Milk that accumulates in the milk-collection ducts of the breast. It makes up about one-third of the total amount of milk available to an infant during a normal feeding.

fortification: The addition of nutrients to foods. Nutrients used in fortification may or may not have been present in the food originally. There are no regulations governing the types of foods that may be fortified or the fortifying nutrients.

free radicals: Atoms within molecules that have become highly reactive because they have lost electrons due to oxidation by singlet oxygen or another oxidizing agent. The double bonds in unsaturated fatty acids are particularly susceptible to oxidation and, therefore, to free radical formation.

fruitarian: Person whose dietary staples are fruits.

gastrointestinal tract: The portion of the digestive system that consists of the stomach and intestines. Although the mouth and esophagus are parts of the digestive system and are involved in digestion, the vast majority of digestive processes occur in the stomach and intestines. (The gastrointestinal tract is sometimes referred to as the *gut.*)

germ: The nutrient- and fat-dense component of a whole grain. Because the unsaturated fats in the germ may break down during storage and cause the grain to become rancid, the germ is removed during refining.

globular proteins: Tightly folded strands of polypeptides.

globulins: Polypeptides that constitute a component of blood (e.g., gamma globulin). They help protect the body from infectious diseases.

glucagon: A hormone secreted by the pancreas that acts to raise blood glucose levels. Glucagon stimulates the breakdown of glycogen and the release of glucose by the liver, thereby increasing blood glucose levels. It helps to maintain normal blood glucose levels between meals and during periods of fasting.

gluconeogenesis: (*gluco*, "glucose"; *neo*, "new"; *genesis*, "formation") The formation of "new" glucose by the body. Glucose can be formed from glycogen, glycerol, or a number of amino acids.

glycerol: Water-soluble, glucoselike component of fats; accounts for about 16% of the weight of a fat molecule.

glycolysis: The lysis (splitting) of glucose to yield energy. Glucose, which has 6 carbon atoms, is split by a series of enzymes into two smaller molecules having 3 carbons each. The process releases energy that is then trapped by ADP. Unlike energy formation from fatty acids and certain types of amino acids, glycolysis does not require oxygen; it is anaerobic.

goiter: Enlargement of the thyroid gland. When it is caused by a dietary lack of iodine, the disease is called *iodine-deficiency goiter.*

GRAS: "***G***enerally ***r***ecognized ***a***s ***s***afe," a category of food additives that have not been specifically tested for safety but are assumed to be safe because of their long-term use without apparent connections to health problems. The vast majority of food additives used today are on the GRAS list.

growth: An increase in size due to increases in the number of cells and the sizes of cells.

heat cramps: Muscle spasms caused by a deficiency of water and sodium in the body resulting from prolonged physical exertion in a hot environment.

heat exhaustion: A condition marked by weakness, dizziness, nausea, and profuse sweating resulting from excessive exposure to heat; also called *heat prostration* and *heat collapse.*

heatstroke: A condition characterized by cessation of sweating, extremely high body temperature, and collapse resulting from prolonged exposure to high temperature; called *sunstroke* if caused by direct exposure to the sun.

heme iron: Iron attached to the hemoglobin and myoglobin in animal tissues. About 40% of the total amount of iron in meats is in this form.

hemoglobin: The iron-containing protein of red blood cells.

hind milk: Milk that is stored in the milk-producing cells of the breast. It is released by hormonal stimulation about a minute after sucking begins and makes up about two-thirds of the total amount of milk available to an infant during a normal feeding.

homeostasis: (hō′ mē ō stā′ sis) The state of equilibrium of the body's internal environment. Homeostatic mechanisms act to maintain a constant balance among fluid, nutrients, and other substances in the body.

hormones: Chemical substances produced by specific glands in the body that affect the functions of particular cells.

hunger: Unpleasant physical sensation resulting from the lack of food; may be accompanied by weakness, an overwhelming desire to eat, and "hunger pangs" in the lower part of the chest that coincide with powerful contractions of the stomach.

hydrogenation: The addition of hydrogen to unsaturated fatty acids; the process converts double bonds to single bonds.

hypercalcemia: Above-normal levels of calcium in the blood.

hypertension: A condition in which blood pressure is higher than normal; also referred to as *high blood pressure.*

hypervitaminosis A: The vitamin-A toxicity disease.

hypoglycemia: (*hypo*, "low"; *glyc*, "glucose"; *emia*, "in the blood") A condition in which blood glucose levels are abnormally low. It can be caused by certain tumors, an excessive level of insulin secretion, or other processes that interfere with the body's utilization of glucose or insulin.

hypothesis: (hī päth′ ə sis) An educated guess about the anticipated result of an experiment. A hypothesis is formulated during the planning stage of a research study in order to focus the research on a specific issue. The research then proves or disproves the hypothesis.

immunity: Resistance to a disease generally conferred by the presence of specific antibodies that destroy disease-generating bacteria and viruses.

incomplete proteins: Proteins that are deficient in one or more essential amino acids.

infancy: Birth to 1 year of age.

infertility: Biological inability to conceive or to maintain a pregnancy.

inorganic substances: Chemical substances that may occur in nature but that cannot be produced by living matter.

insoluble fiber: Dietary fiber that is not soluble in water. This type of fiber "holds" water and is found in the fibrous components of plant cell walls. Most whole grains and seeds are good dietary sources of insoluble fiber.

insulin: A hormone secreted by the pancreas that acts to lower blood glucose levels. Insulin helps to transport glucose into cells and to return blood glucose levels to normal after a meal. Inadequate secretion, or a lack of cell sensitivity to the presence of insulin, results in inadequate cell supply of glucose and overutilization of fatty acids for energy. Inadequate "clearing" of blood glucose due to depressed insulin activity leads to an elevation in blood glucose level and diabetes.

intrinsic factor: A protein produced by the stomach that facilitates the absorption of vitamin B_{12} in the small intestine.

ion: An atom that carries an electric charge (positive or negative).

keratins: Proteins in skin, hair, and nails that provide external protection.

ketone bodies: A group of chemical by-products formed by incomplete utilization of fat for energy.

ketosis: A condition in which *ketone bodies*—breakdown products from fats used in energy formation—accumulate in the blood and urine; it results when people depend primarily on dietary fat or body fat stores for energy.

kwashiorkor: (kwä′ shē ôr′ kôr) A deficiency disease primarily caused by a lack of complete protein in the diet. It usually occurs after children are taken off breast milk and given solid foods that have protein of low biologic value.

lacto-ovovegetarian diet: Diet that includes plants, milk products, and eggs.

lactovegetarian diet: Diet that includes plants and milk products.

legumes: Seeds such as peas, various beans, and peanuts that split into two parts.

let-down reflex: The release of the hind milk. It is stimulated by the hormone oxytocin, which causes the milk-producing cells to contract.

limiting amino acid: The essential amino acid whose concentration is lowest in a given food.

linoleic acid: The only known essential fatty acid for adults.

lipids: Compounds that are insoluble in water and soluble in fat; commonly referred to as *fats*.

lipoprotein: (*lipo* = "lipid" = fat) Water-soluble substance containing fat and protein molecules. The vast majority of lipids found in blood are lipoproteins.

low birth weight: Birth weight below 5½ pounds.

lymphatic system: A network of vessels that absorb some of the products of digestion and transport them to the heart, where they are mixed with the substances contained in blood.

macrobiotic diet: A vegan diet that is restricted to unprocessed, unrefined foods and foods believed to be endowed with special health properties.

malnutrition: "Poor" nutrition caused by an inadequate or excessive intake of calories or one or more nutrients. Protein–calorie malnutrition is caused by a lack of protein and calories. Obesity is a form of malnutrition related to excessive intake of calories.

maximal oxygen consumption: The largest potential amount of oxygen available to cells for use in the citric acid cycle of energy formation; also referred to as *VO_2 max*.

megadose: Dosage level of a vitamin or mineral that exceeds 10 times the U.S. RDA.

megaloblasts: Large, irregularly shaped red blood cells. They are found in cases of folacin deficiency and vitamin-B_{12} deficiency.

menopause: The period of a woman's life when her physiological ability to reproduce ends; generally occurs between the ages of 45 and 52 and is accompanied by decreased levels of estrogen.

menses: (Latin, "monthly") Periodic uterine bleeding accompanied by a shedding of the endometrium (the lining of the uterus). On average, it occurs every 27 to 28 days and lasts 4 to 5 days. Also called *menstruation*.

menstrual cycle: The interval between the start of one menses and the start of the next.

metabolism: The chemical changes that take place within the body.

micelles: (mī sel′) Loosely bound molecules containing long-chain fatty acids, monoglycerides, phospholipids, and cholesterol. They are soluble in water.

Minimum Daily Requirements (MDRs): Standards of nutrient intake levels based on amounts of nutrients needed to prevent deficiency diseases. *These standards are no longer recognized as appropriate for labeling purposes.*

molecules: Chemical substances formed from the union of two or more atoms. For example, oxygen and hydrogen atoms bond together to form H_2O molecules (water).

monoglyceride: A fat in which the glycerol molecule has one fatty acid attached to it; also called *monoacylglycerol*.

monosaccharide: (*mono-*, "one"; *saccharide*, "sugar") A carbohydrate whose chemical structure contains one sugar molecule. Monosaccharides are the basic chemical units from which all sugars are built.

monounsaturated fatty acid: Fatty acid that contains one double bond between carbons.

muscular dystrophy: A condition characterized by a wasting away and weakening of muscles.

myoglobin: The iron-containing protein in muscle cells.

myosin: A protein present in muscle. Myosin accounts for about 65% of total muscle protein and is responsible for the elastic property of muscles. (See *actin.*)

naturally occurring toxicant: Substance that is a natural part of foods that can have a harmful effect on health if it is consumed in excessive quantities.

negative energy balance: Condition that exists when energy intake is less than energy output; results in use of the body's energy stores.

neurotransmitters: Small molecules most often formed from amino acids that direct cells to perform specific chemical reactions. Epinephrine (adrenalin) and serotonin are two examples.

nitrogen balance: Nitrogen intake minus nitrogen excretion.

nonessential amino acids: Amino acids that can be readily produced by humans from components of the diet. Because the body can produce them, there are no dietary requirements for them and no deficiency diseases associated with inadequate intakes of them.

nonessential nutrients: Nutrients the body can manufacture in sufficient quantities from components of the diet.

nonheme iron: Iron that is not bound to hemoglobin or myoglobin. In plants, iron is usually bound to phytates.

norepinephrine: (nôr′ ep′ ə nef′ rin) A neurotransmitter formed from tyrosine that is involved in motor function and hormone release.

nutrient-dense foods: Foods that contain relatively high amounts of nutrients relative to their content of calories. Broccoli, collards, bread, and cantaloupe are examples of nutrient-dense foods.

nutrients: Chemical substances found in food that are used by the body to maintain health. The six categories of nutrients are carbohydrates, proteins, fats, vitamins, minerals, and water.

nutrition: Simply stated, the study of the effects of substances in food on the body and health.

***-ogen*:** "An agent that produces."

organic substances: Chemical substances that arise from living matter. Almost all organic substances contain carbon.

osteoblasts: (*osteo*, "bone"; *blast*, "germinating, growing") Bone cells that cause bone to form.

osteoclasts: (*clast*, "breaking, destroying") Bone cells that cause the breakdown of bone.

osteomalacia: The vitamin-D deficiency disease in adults.

osteoporosis: (*osteo*, "bone"; *poro*, "porous"; *osis*, "abnormal condition") A condition characterized by porous bones; it is due to the loss of minerals from the bones.

oxidation: The addition of oxygen to (or the removal of electrons from) a molecule.

oxytocin: The hormone that causes the release of hind milk from the milk-producing cells in the breast. Oxytocin release is stimulated by the infant's sucking and in some cases by the mother's psychological response to her baby's cry or thoughts about breast feeding.

pellagra (*pelle*, "skin"; *agra*, "rash") The niacin-deficiency disease, which is accompanied by characteristic changes in the skin.

percentile: Point on a scale of 100 that represents the percentage of measurements equal to or below a particular measurement. For example, 15% of children have growth measurements that place them between the 75th and 90th percentiles on growth curves. If a child is at the 50th percentile, 50% of children are smaller than the child and 50% are bigger.

pernicious anemia: (pernicious means destructive, fatal) A severe form of anemia characterized by an increase in the size, and a decrease in the number of red blood cells. Symptoms include degenerative changes in nerve cells and impaired functioning of the nervous system.

pH: A measure of how acidic or basic (alkaline) a solution is. The neutral point—where a solution is neither acidic nor basic—is pH 7. Acidity increases as pH drops from 7 to 0, and basicity increases as pH rises from 7 to 14. Reference points:
lemon juice 2.2
tomato juice 4.2
milk 6.6
water 7.0 (neutral)
seawater 8.0
ammonia 11.1

phospholipids: (*phospho-*, "phosphorus") Fatlike substances that contain fatty acids and phosphorus, and sometimes nitrogen. They are soluble in both water and fat. Lecithin is the most common phospholipid in the body.

pica: The regular ingestion of a nonfood substance, such as laundry starch, clay, or dirt; most commonly occurs during pregnancy and childhood.

pinocytosis: (pī′ nō si tō′ səs) The process by which a cell surrounds and then engulfs a substance.

placebo: (plə sē′ bō) A substance having no medical properties that is used as a control in an experiment to test the effects of a biologically active substance. Also, a "sugar pill" or other substance with no medicinal effect that is given to a patient as though it were a medication.

placebo effect: An improvement in physical health or sense of well being in response to the use of a placebo. It is often observed among control subjects in experiments that employ placebos.

placenta: The organ that connects the fetus with the mother's uterus and through which nutrients pass from the mother to the fetus.

plaque: A soft, white, sticky material that forms on the surface of teeth and contains a dense collection of bacteria.

polypeptides: Proteins consisting of four or more amino acids. (Most proteins contain at least 50 amino acids.)

polysaccharides: (*poly-*, "many") Complex carbohydrates (starches, dietary fibers, and glycogen) consisting of three or more monosaccharides or monosaccharidelike substances.

polyunsaturated fatty acid: Fatty acid that contains two or more double bonds between carbons.

positive energy balance: Energy intake exceeds energy output; the excess energy is stored in the body as fat.

preterm infant: Infant born at or before 37 weeks of pregnancy. Infants born between 38 and 42 weeks of pregnancy are considered to be "term."

primary malnutrition: Malnutrition directly resulting from inadequate or excessive dietary intakes; vitamin-A deficiency and toxicity are examples.

prolactin: The hormone that initiates milk production. Its release is stimulated by an infant's sucking and the emptying of milk from the breasts.

prostaglandins: (präs′ tə glan′ din) Hormonelike substances derived from specific types of fatty acids. More than 90 types of prostaglandins are found in the human body.

protein efficiency ratio: A measure of the growth-promoting effect of dietary protein sources.

provitamin: A vitaminlike substance that is converted to a vitamin by metabolic reactions in the body.

puberty: The stage in life during which humans become biologically capable of reproduction.

purge: Self-induced vomiting or laxative use intended to prevent weight gain.

radioactive particles: Atoms whose nuclei emit rays of energy. Atoms of iodine-131 (^{131}I), strontium-90 (^{90}Sr), and uranium are examples of radioactive particles; the energy emitted by the nuclei of these atoms can damage human cells.

remodeling: The breakdown and build up of bone tissue.

rhodopsin: The light-sensitive component of the rods in the retina. It is produced when retinal, a form of vitamin A, combines with the protein opsin. It is also called *visual purple.*

rickets: The vitamin-D deficiency disease in children.

risk factors: Conditions that increase the likelihood that a particular disease or condition will develop. For example, since diets that are high in animal fat have been found to increase the likelihood of developing heart disease, they are said to be a risk factor for heart disease.

rooting reflex: Instinctive movement of an infant's mouth to the nipple when his or her face touches a breast.

satiety: (sə tī′ ə tē) Being full to the point of satisfaction; occurs when a person no longer feels a need for food and loses interest in eating.

saturated fat: A fat that contains glycerol and saturated fatty acids.

saturated fatty acid: Fatty acid that contains only single bonds between adjacent carbons. The carbons are "saturated" with hydrogens; they contain the maximum possible number of hydrogens.

secondary malnutrition: Malnutrition resulting from a condition not directly related to dietary intake; weight loss due to a gastrointestinal-tract infection is an example.

selenosis: The selenium-toxicity disease.

semivegetarian diet: Diet that includes some meats in addition to plants, generally excluding "red" meats.

serotonin: (sir′ ə tō′ nin) A neurotransmitter formed from the amino acid tryptophan. It is involved in the processes of sleep, pain, appetite, and perception of well-being.

simple diffusion: The free movement of a substance across a cell membrane from an area of high concentration to an area of low concentration. The process equalizes the concentrations on either side of the membrane.

single bond: Bond formed by the sharing of an electron by two adjacent atoms within a molecule.

singlet oxygen: A high-energy, highly reactive form of oxygen. Singlet oxygen participates in reactions that yield free radicals.

soluble fiber: Dietary fiber that dissolves in water and results in the production of a gel. Soluble fibers are mainly found in the pulp part of fruits and vegetables. Oat bran and pectin, a substance found in fruits and used to make jelly "gel," are examples of soluble fibers.

starch: A polysaccharide produced by plants from glucose; the plant storage form of glucose.

steroid hormones: (stir′ oid) Hormones such as estrogen and testosterone that are synthesized from cholesterol.

stillborn: Infant that is not alive when delivered.

substrate: The substance acted upon by enzymes. Food particles are the *substrate* of digestive enzymes.

tetany: A condition in which muscles contract but fail to relax.

thermogenesis: (*thermo*, "heat"; *genesis*, "production") The rise in metabolic rate that occurs as a result of eating. It represents the energy the body expends in digesting foods and absorbing and processing nutrients. The elevation in metabolism due to thermogenesis is greatest two hours after a meal and lasts for three to four hours. Also referred to as *dietary thermogenesis* and *specific dynamic action.*

thyroxine: A hormone secreted by the thyroid gland that increases the rate at which energy is formed in the body. Thyroxine plays a major role in stimulating energy formation during times of growth. Adults who produce too little or too much thyroxine have trouble maintaining a constant body weight because of disruptions in energy metabolism.

toxemia: Condition characterized by abnormally high blood pressure and extensive swelling throughout the body. Women who develop toxemia during pregnancy are at high risk of delivering a small infant early. The condition is now referred to as *pregnancy-induced hypertension (PIH).*

toxic: Poisonous; harmful to the body.

triglyceride: A fat in which the glycerol molecule has three fatty acids attached to it; also called *triacylglycerol.*

tripeptides: Proteins consisting of three amino acids.

unsaturated fat: A fat that contains glycerol and one to three unsaturated fatty acids.

unsaturated fatty acid: Fatty acid that contains one or more double bonds between adjacent carbons. The carbons are not saturated with hydrogens; they contain fewer than the maximum possible number of hydrogens.

U.S. RDAs: Standards by which the nutrient composition of food products are assessed and reported on food labels. They are based on the 1968 RDA table.

uterus: The womb; a pear-shaped, muscular organ for containing the fetus during pregnancy.

vegan diet: Diet that excludes all animal products.

water balance: The ratio of the amount of water outside of cells to the amount inside of cells; this balance is needed for normal cell functioning.

water intoxication: A condition that occurs when water intake exceeds water losses. Water intoxication can result from consuming too much water or from drugs and diseases that decrease the concentration of minerals in body fluids.

waxes: Fat-soluble substances composed of long-chain fatty acids and alcohol.

xerophthalmia: (zir′ äf thal′ mē ə) "Dry eyes"; a condition caused by vitamin-A deficiency. If not corrected in its early stages, it can lead to permanent blindness; generally accompanied by chronic infections of the eyes.

APPENDIX J

MAJOR RECENT GOVERNMENT REPORTS ON NUTRITION AND HEALTH

The late 1980s was a busy time for professionals working in nutrition. Between 1988–1989, three major reports were published:

1. The Surgeon General's Report on Nutrition and Health
2. Promoting Health/Preventing Disease: Year 2000 Objectives for the Nation
3. The 1989 RDAs

The first two are summarized here. The 1989 RDAs were not available to us at press time. The 1989 RDAs should be released in December, 1989. Please review them with your students and let them know how they differ from the 1980 RDAs. You should be able to obtain a copy of the 1989 RDAs by writing:

- Food and Nutrition Board
  National Academy of Sciences
  National Research Council
  2101 Constitution Avenue
  Washington, D.C. 20418

THE SURGEON GENERAL'S REPORT ON NUTRITION AND HEALTH

This is the first Surgeon General's Report devoted to the subject of nutrition. It is intended for professionals in the field of nutrition, and documents the rationale for the Dietary Guidelines for Americans. Although a wealth of literature is reviewed, very little new information is presented and very few new recommendations are made in this book. However, if you would like to have access to a general reference book on nutrition and heart disease, hypertension, cancer, diabetes, obesity, skeletal diseases, dental diseases, kidney diseases, gastrointestinal diseases, infections and immunity, anemia, neurologic disorders, behavior, maternal and child nutrition, aging, alcohol, drug-nutrient interactions, and dietary fads and frauds, this book will be helpful.

Students should be made aware of this resource and may want to use it for reference. It is available from the U.S. Government Printing Office:

- Superintendent of Documents
  U.S. Government Printing Office
  Washington, D.C. 20402

Ask for stock number 017-001-00465-1, (PHS) Publication No. 88-50210. You may be able to get a free copy by a request for information from your representative in congress or a senator from your state. Ask for information from the Surgeon General about nutrition and health.

■ ■ ■

PROMOTING HEALTH/PREVENTING DISEASE: YEAR 2000 OBJECTIVES FOR THE NATION

Year 2000 Objectives for the Nation, published by the Department of Health and Human Services, represents a follow-up to the *1990 Objectives for the Nation*. It is a much more detailed and thought-out publication than the first version released in 1980. Included are summaries of graphs, tables, and research material that support the stated objectives. An enumerated summary of the report's findings follows.

Health Status

1. Reduce growth retardation to less than 10 percent in children five years old and younger. (Baseline: 4.5 to 19.4 percent in 1987)

Risk Reduction

2. Reduce iron deficiency among children ages 1 through 2 years old to less than 5 percent and among children ages 3 through 4 years old to less than 2 percent. (Baseline: 9.4 percent for children ages 1 through 2 years and 3.9 percent for children ages 3 through 4 years in 1976–1980)
3. Reduce iron deficiency among women ages 20 through 44 years to less than 3 percent. (Baseline: 5.4 percent in 1976–1980)
   —*Special Population Targets:*
   a. Reduce iron deficiency among low-income women to less than 4 percent. (Baseline: 7.8 percent in 1976–1980)
4. Reduce iron deficiency anemia, as measured by hemoglobin or hematocrit in the third trimester of pregnancy, among low-income pregnant women age 20 years and older to less than 15 percent. (Baselines 24.2 percent as measured by hemoglobin and 22.4 percent as measured by hematocrit in 1987

—*Special Population Targets:*

a. Reduce iron deficiency anemia among black low-income pregnant women to 20 percent. (Baseline: 41.5 percent by hemoglobin and 35.6 percent by hematocrit in 1987)

b. Reduce iron deficiency anemia among teenage, low-income, pregnant women ages 15 through 19 years to 15 percent. (33.9 percent by hemoglobin and 31.0 percent by hematocrit in 1987)

5. Reduce the percentage of overweight individuals among people ages 20 through 74 years to a prevalence of no more than 20 percent. (Baseline: 25.7 percent in 1976–1980; 24.2 percent for men and 27.1 percent for women)

   —*Special Population Targets:*

   a. Reduce the precentage of overweight low-income women to 25 percent. (Baseline: 37 percent in 1976–1980)

   b. Reduce the percentage of overweight black women to 30 percent. (Baseline: 43.5 percent in 1976–1980)

   c. Reduce the percentage of overweight Hispanic women to 25 percent. (Baseline: 39.1 percent for Mexican-American women; 34.1 percent for Cuban women; 37.3 percent for Puerto Rican women in 1982–1984)

6. Reduce the percentage of overweight adolescents ages 12 through 17 years to a prevalence of less than 15 percent. (Baseline: 15 percent in 1976–1980)

7. Increase to at least 75 percent the proportion of overweight people age 12 years and older who have adopted sound dietary practices combined with physical activity to achieve weight reduction. (Baseline: 30 percent of overweight women and 25 percent of overweight men for people age 18 and older in 1985)

8. Among people ages 2 years and older, reduce average dietary fat intake to no more than 30 percent of a day's total calories and average saturated fat intake to no more than 10 percent. (Baseline: 36.4 percent of calories from total fat and 13.2 percent from saturated fat in 1985)

9. Increase to at least 50 percent the proportion of people age 12 years and older who consume at least three servings daily of foods rich in calcium. (Baseline: 20 percent in 1985–1986)

10. Increase average intake of dietary fiber and complex carbohydrates in the diets of adults to five or more daily servings for vegetables and fruits and to six or more daily servings for grain products and legumes to provide between 20 and 30 grams daily of dietary fiber. (Baseline: 2½ servings of vegetables and fruits and 3 servings of grain products and legumes for women ages 19 through 50 years in 1985; an average of 10 grams of dietary fiber in 1987, 11.5 grams for men and 8.8 grams for women)

11. Reduce to less than 5 percent the proportion of people age 21 years and older who consume more than two drinks of beverage alcohol per day. (Baseline: 9 percent in 1985)

12. Increase to at least 50 percent the proportion of households purchasing foods low in sodium, preparing foods without adding salt, and avoiding salt at the table. (Baseline: 20 percent of women ages 19 through 50

years regularly purchased foods with reduced salt and sodium content, 46 percent who served as the main food planner or preparer used salt in food preparation, and 32 percent used salt at the table in 1985)

13. Increase to at least 75 percent the proportion of mothers who exclusively or partially breast feed their babies in the early postpartum period and to at least 50 percent the proportion who continue breast feeding until their babies are 5 to 6 months old. (Baseline: 54.3 percent at discharge from birth site and 21.1 percent at 5 to 6 months in 1988)
    —*Special Population Targets:*
    a. Increase to at least 75 percent the proportion of low-income mothers who exclusively or partially breast feed their babies until 5 to 6 months old. (Baseline: 31.6 percent in 1988)
    b. Increase to at least 75 percent the proportion of black mothers who exclusively or partially breast feed their babies until 5 to 6 months old. (Baseline: 24.9 and 7.7 percent in 1988)

Public Awareness

14. Increase to at least 90 percent the proportion of people ages 12 years and older who can identify the principal dietary factors that are associated with heart disease, hypertension, cancer, and osteoporosis. (Baseline: 74 percent for fat and heart disease; 70 percent for cholesterol and heart disease; 64 percent for sodium and hypertension; 43 percent for calcium and osteoporosis; 25 percent for fiber and cancer among adults in 1988)
15. Increase to at least 75 percent the proportion of people age 12 years and older who can identify the major food sources of fat, saturated fat, cholesterol, calories, sodium, calcium, and fiber. (Baseline: 62 percent for saturated fats; 55 percent for polyunsaturated fats; and 3 to 46 percent for fiber, in 1988)
16. Increase to at least 80 percent the proportion of people ages 21 years and older who use food labels to make food selections. (Baseline: 74 percent used labels to make nutritious food selections among people age 18 years and older in 1988)

Professional Education and Awareness

17. Extend the requirement of courses in human nutrition to all medical and dental schools. (Baseline: Approximately 33 percent of medical schools in 1985 and 55 to 57 percent of dental schools in 1987–88)
18. Increase to at least 50 percent the proportion of primary care providers who provide nutrition counseling and/or referral to qualified nutritionists and dietitians. (Baseline data unavailable)

Services and Protection

19. Increase to at least 95 percent the proportion of school lunch and breakfast services with menus that are consistent with the *Dietary Guidelines for Americans*. (Baseline data unavailable)

20. Increase to at least 75 percent the proportion of institutional food service operations with menus that are consistent with the *Dietary Guidelines for Americans*. (Baseline data unavailable)
21. Increase to at least 5,000 brand items the availability of processed food products that are reuced in fat, saturated fat, and cholesterol. (Baseline: 2,500 items in 1986)
22. Increase to at least 5,000 brand items the availability of processed foods with lowered sodium. (Baseline: 2,150 items in 1986)
23. Increase nutrition labeling that provides information to facilitate choosing foods consistent with the *Dietary Guidelines for Americans* to at least 80 percent of processed foods and 40 percent of fresh meats, poultry, fruits, vegetables, baked goods, and ready-to-eat foods. (Baseline: 55 percent of processed foods in 1988; baseline data on fresh and ready-to-eat foods unavailable)
24. Extend to all states required nutrition education from preschool through grade 12, preferably as part of comprehensive school health education. (Baseline: 12 states in 1985)

APPENDIX K

THE 1989 RDAs

Along with the new 1989 RDA Tables, 1980 Tables are included to allow you to compare the "old" values with the "new."

Vitamin K and Selenium were moved from Table 2 of the 1980 RDAs (Estimated Safe and Adequate Daily Dietary Intakes) to Table 1 (Recommended Dietary Allowances), and sodium was deleted from Table 2. RDAs for protein, vitamin B_{12}, iron, biotin, copper, and molybdenum are generally lower in the 1989 than in the 1980 Tables. RDA levels for calcium have been increased for young adults.

Please refer to the 1989 Tables when it is important to know the latest values. RDA values will continue to change as more is learned about nutrients and health.

1980 TABLE 1

Food and Nutrition Board, National Academy of Sciences–National Research Council Recommended Daily Dietary Allowances,[a] Revised 1980

	Age, years	Weight		Height		Protein, g	Fat-Soluble Vitamins		
		kg	lb	cm	in		Vitamin A, μg RE[b]	Vitamin D, μg[c]	Vitamin E, mg α-TE[d]
Infants	0.0–0.5	6	13	60	24	kg ×	420	10	3
	0.5–1.0	9	20	71	28	2.2	400	10	4
Children	1–3	13	29	90	35	kg ×	400	10	5
	4–6	20	44	112	44	2.0	500	10	6
	7–10	28	62	132	52	23	700	10	7
Males	11–14	45	99	157	62	30	1000	10	8
	15–18	66	145	176	69	34	1000	10	10
	19–22	70	154	177	70	45	1000	7.5	10
	23–50	70	154	178	70	56	1000	5	10
	51+	70	154	178	70	56	1000	5	10
Females	11–14	46	101	157	62	56	800	10	8
	15–18	55	120	163	64	56	800	10	8
	19–22	55	120	163	64	46	800	7.5	8
	23–50	55	120	163	64	46	800	5	8
	51+	55	120	163	64	44	800	5	8
Pregnant						+30	+200	+5	+2
Lactating						+20	+400	+5	+3

[a]The allowances are intended to provide for individual variations among most normal persons as they live in the United States under usual environmental stresses. Diets should be based on a variety of common foods in order to provide other nutrients for which human requirements have been less well defined.
[b]Retinol equivalents. 1 retinol equivalent = 1 μg retinol or 6 μg β carotene.
[c]As cholecalciferol. 10 μg cholecalciferol = 400 IU of vitamin D.
[d]α-tocopherol equivalents. 1 mg *d*-α tocopherol = 1 α-TE.

Water-Soluble Vitamins							Minerals						
Vitamin C, mg	Thiamin, mg	Riboflavin, mg	Niacin, mg NE[e]	Vitamin B-6, mg	Folacin[f], μg	Vitamin B-12, μg	Calcium, mg	Phosphorus, mg	Magnesium, mg	Iron, mg	Zinc, mg	Iodine, μg
35	0.3	0.4	6	0.3	30	0.5[g]	360	240	50	10	3	40
35	0.5	0.6	8	0.6	45	1.5	540	360	70	15	5	50
45	0.7	0.8	9	0.9	100	2.0	800	800	150	15	10	70
45	0.9	1.0	11	1.3	200	2.5	800	800	200	10	10	90
45	1.2	1.4	16	1.6	300	3.0	800	800	250	10	10	120
50	1.4	1.6	18	1.8	400	3.0	1200	1200	350	18	15	150
60	1.4	1.7	18	2.0	400	3.0	1200	1200	400	18	15	150
60	1.5	1.7	19	2.2	400	3.0	800	800	350	10	15	150
60	1.4	1.6	18	2.2	400	3.0	800	800	350	10	15	150
60	1.2	1.4	16	2.2	400	3.0	800	800	350	10	15	150
50	1.1	1.3	15	1.8	400	3.0	1200	1200	300	18	15	150
60	1.1	1.3	14	2.0	400	3.0	1200	1200	300	18	15	150
60	1.1	1.3	14	2.0	400	3.0	800	800	300	18	15	150
60	1.0	1.2	13	2.0	400	3.0	800	800	300	18	15	150
60	1.0	1.2	13	2.0	400	3.0	800	800	300	10	15	150
+20	+0.4	+0.3	+2	+0.6	+400	+1.0	+400	+400	+150	*h*	+5	+25
+40	+0.5	+0.5	+5	+0.5	+100	+1.0	+400	+400	+150	*h*	+10	+50

[a]The allowances are intended to provide for individual variations among most normal persons as they live in the United States under usual environmental stresses. Diets should be based on a variety of common foods in order to provide other nutrients for which human requirements have been less well defined.
[b]Retinol equivalents. 1 retinol equivalent = 1 μg retinol or 6 μg β carotene.
[c]As cholecalciferol. 10 μg cholecalciferol = 400 IU of vitamin D.
[d]α-tocopherol equivalents. 1 mg *d*-α tocopherol = 1 α-TE.
[e]1 NE (niacin equivalent) is equal to 1 mg of niacin or 60 mg of dietary tryptophan.
[f]The folacin allowances refer to dietary sources as determined by *Lactobacillus casei* assay after treatment with enzymes (conjugases) to make polyglutamyl forms of the vitamin available to the test organism.
[g]The recommended dietary allowance for vitamin B-12 in infants is based on average concentration of the vitamin in human milk. The allowances after weaning are based on energy intake (as recommended by the American Academy of Pediatrics) and consideration of other factors, such as intestinal absorption.
[h]The increased requirement during pregnancy cannot be met by the iron content of habitual American diets nor by the existing iron stores of many women; therefore the use of 30–60 mg of supplemental iron is recommended. Iron needs during lactation are not substantially different from those of nonpregnant women, but continued supplementation of the mother for 2–3 months after parturition is advisable in order to replenish stores depleted by pregnancy.

1989 TABLE 1

Food and Nutrition Board, National Academy of Sciences–National Research Council Recommended Dietary Allowances,[a] Revised 1989

		Weight[b]		Height[b]			Fat-Soluble Vitamins			
Category	Age (years) or Condition	kg	lb	cm	in	Protein, g	Vitamin A, μg RE[c]	Vitamin D, μg[d]	Vitamin E, mg α-TE[e]	Vitamin K, μg
Infants	0.0–0.5	6	13	60	24	13	375	7.5	3	5
	0.5–1.0	9	20	71	28	14	375	10	4	10
Children	1–3	13	29	90	35	16	400	10	6	15
	4–6	20	44	112	44	24	500	10	7	20
	7–10	28	62	132	52	28	700	10	7	30
Males	11–14	45	99	157	62	45	1,000	10	10	45
	15–18	66	145	176	69	59	1,000	10	10	65
	19–24	72	160	177	70	58	1,000	10	10	70
	25–50	79	174	176	70	63	1,000	5	10	80
	51+	77	170	173	68	63	1,000	5	10	80
Females	11–14	46	101	157	62	46	800	10	8	45
	15–18	55	120	163	64	44	800	10	8	55
	19–24	58	128	164	65	46	800	10	8	60
	25–50	63	138	163	64	50	800	5	8	65
	51+	65	143	160	63	50	800	5	8	65
Pregnant						60	800	10	10	65
Lactating	1st 6 months					65	1,300	10	12	65
	2nd 6 months					62	1,200	10	11	65

[a]The allowances, expressed as average daily intakes over time, are intended to provide for individual variations among most normal persons as they live in the United States under usual environmental stresses. Diets should be based on a variety of common foods in order to provide other nutrients for which human requirements have been less well defined.

[b]Weights and heights of Reference Adults are actual medians for the U.S. population of the designated age, as reported by NHANES II. The median weights and heights of those under 19 years of age were taken from Hamill et al. (1979) (see pages 16–17). The use of these figures does not imply that the height-to-weight ratios are ideal.

[c]Retinol equivalents. 1 retinol equivalent = 1 μg retinol or 6 μg β-carotene. See text for calculation of vitamin A activity of diets as retinol equivalents.

[d]As cholecalciferol. 10 μg cholecalciferol = 400 IU of vitamin D.

[e]α-Tocopherol equivalents. 1 mg d-α tocopherol = 1 α-TE. See text for variation in allowances and calculation of vitamin E activity of the diet as α-tocopherol equivalents.

Water-Soluble Vitamins							Minerals						
Vitamin C, mg	Thiamin, mg	Riboflavin, mg	Niacin, mg NE[f]	Vitamin B_6, mg	Folate, μg	Vitamin B_{12}, μg	Calcium, mg	Phosphorus, mg	Magnesium, mg	Iron, mg	Zinc, mg	Iodine, μg	Selenium μg
30	0.3	0.4	5	0.3	25	0.3	400	300	40	6	5	40	10
35	0.4	0.5	6	0.6	35	0.5	600	500	60	10	5	50	15
40	0.7	0.8	9	1.0	50	0.7	800	800	80	10	10	70	20
45	0.9	1.1	12	1.1	75	1.0	800	800	120	10	10	90	20
45	1.0	1.2	13	1.4	100	1.4	800	800	170	10	10	120	30
50	1.3	1.5	17	1.7	150	2.0	1,200	1,200	270	12	15	150	40
60	1.5	1.8	20	2.0	200	2.0	1,200	1,200	400	12	15	150	50
60	1.5	1.7	19	2.0	200	2.0	1,200	1,200	350	10	15	150	70
60	1.5	1.7	19	2.0	200	2.0	800	800	350	10	15	150	70
60	1.2	1.4	15	2.0	200	2.0	800	800	350	10	15	150	70
50	1.1	1.3	15	1.4	150	2.0	1,200	1,200	280	15	12	150	45
60	1.1	1.3	15	1.5	180	2.0	1,200	1,200	300	15	12	150	50
60	1.1	1.3	15	1.6	180	2.0	1,200	1,200	280	15	12	150	55
60	1.1	1.3	15	1.6	180	2.0	800	800	280	15	12	150	55
60	1.0	1.2	13	1.6	180	2.0	800	800	280	10	12	150	55
70	1.5	1.6	17	2.2	400	2.2	1,200	1,200	320	30	15	175	65
95	1.6	1.8	20	2.1	280	2.6	1,200	1,200	355	15	19	200	75
90	1.6	1.7	20	2.1	260	2.6	1,200	1,200	340	15	16	200	75

[f] 1 NE (niacin equivalent) is equal to 1 mg of niacin or 60 mg of dietary tryptophan.

1980 TABLE 2

Estimated Safe and Adequate Daily Dietary Intakes of Selected Vitamins and Minerals[a]

	Age, years	Vitamins: Vitamin K, μg	Biotin, μg	Pantothenic Acid, mg
Infants	0–0.5	12	35	2
	0.5–1	10–20	50	3
Children and Adolescents	1–3	15–30	65	3
	4–6	20–40	85	3–4
	7–10	30–60	120	4–5
	11+	50–100	100–200	4–7
Adults		70–140	100–200	4–7

	Age, years	Trace Elements[b]: Copper, mg	Manganese, mg	Fluoride, mg	Chromium, mg	Selenium, mg	Molybdenum, mg
Infants	0–0.5	0.5–0.7	0.5–0.7	0.1–0.5	0.01–0.04	0.01–0.04	0.03–0.06
	0.5–1	0.7–1.0	0.7–1.0	0.2–1.0	0.02–0.06	0.02–0.06	0.04–0.08
Children and Adolescents	1–3	1.0–1.5	1.0–1.5	0.5–1.5	0.02–0.08	0.02–0.08	0.05–0.1
	4–6	1.5–2.0	1.5–2.0	1.0–2.5	0.03–0.12	0.03–0.12	0.06–0.15
	7–10	2.0–2.5	2.0–3.0	1.5–2.5	0.05–0.2	0.05–0.2	0.10–0.3
	11+	2.0–3.0	2.5–5.0	1.5–2.5	0.05–0.2	0.05–0.2	0.15–0.5
Adults		2.0–3.0	2.5–5.0	1.5–4.0	0.05–0.2	0.05–0.2	0.15–0.5

	Age, years	Electrolytes: Sodium, mg	Potassium, mg	Chloride, mg
Infants	0–0.5	115–350	350–925	275–700
	0.5–1	250–750	425–1275	400–1200
Children and Adolescents	1–3	325–975	550–1650	500–1500
	4–6	450–1350	775–2325	700–2100
	7–10	600–1800	1000–3000	925–2775
	11+	900–2700	1525–4575	1400–4200
Adults		1100–3300	1875–5625	1700–5100

[a]Because there is less information on which to base allowances, these figures are not given in the main table of RDA and are provided here in the form of ranges of recommended intakes.

[b]Since the toxic levels for many trace elements may be only several times usual intakes, the upper levels for the trace elements given in this table should not be habitually exceeded.

1989 TABLE 2

Estimated Safe and Adequate Daily Dietary Intakes of Selected Vitamins and Minerals[a]

		Vitamins	
Category	**Age, years**	Biotin, μg	Pantothenic Acid, mg
Infants	0–0.5	10	2
	0.5–1	15	3
Children and Adolescents	1–3	20	3
	4–6	25	3–4
	7–10	30	4–5
	11+	30–100	4–7
Adults		30–100	4–7

		Trace Elements[b]				
Category	**Age, years**	Copper, mg	Manganese, mg	Fluoride, mg	Chromium, μg	Molybdenum, μg
Infants	0–0.5	0.4–0.6	0.3–0.6	0.1–0.5	10–40	15–30
	0.5–1	0.6–0.7	0.6–1.0	0.2–1.0	20–60	20–40
Children and Adolescents	1–3	0.7–1.0	1.0–1.5	0.5–1.5	20–80	25–50
	4–6	1.0–1.5	1.5–2.0	1.0–2.5	30–120	30–75
	7–10	1.0–2.0	2.0–3.0	1.5–2.5	50–200	50–150
	11+	1.5–2.5	2.0–5.0	1.5–2.5	50–200	75–250
Adults		1.5–3.0	2.0–5.0	1.5–4.0	50–200	75–250

[a]Because there is less information on which to base allowances, these figures are not given in the main table of RDA and are provided here in the form of ranges of recommended intakes.
[b]Since the toxic levels for many trace elements may be only several times usual intakes, the upper levels for the trace elements given in this table should not be habitually exceeded.

1980 TABLE 3

Mean Heights and Weights and Recommended Energy Intake[a]

Category	Age, years	Weight kg	Weight lb	Height cm	Height in.	Energy Needs (with range) kcal		MJ
Infants	0.0–0.5	6	13	60	24	kg × 115	(95–145)	kg × 0.48
	0.5–1.0	9	20	71	28	kg × 105	(80–135)	kg × 0.44
Children	1–3	13	29	90	35	1300	(900–1800)	5.5
	4–6	20	44	112	44	1700	(1300–2300)	7.1
	7–10	28	62	132	52	2400	(1650–3300)	10.1
Males	11–14	45	99	157	62	2700	(2000–3700)	11.3
	15–18	66	145	176	69	2800	(2100–3900)	11.8
	16–22	70	154	177	70	2900	(2500–3300)	12.2
	23–50	70	154	178	70	2700	(2300–3100)	11.3
	51–75	70	154	178	70	2400	(2000–2800)	10.1
	76+	70	154	178	70	2050	(1650–2450)	8.6
Females	11–14	46	101	157	62	2200	(1500–3000)	9.2
	15–18	55	120	163	64	2100	(1200–3000)	8.8
	19–22	55	120	163	64	2100	(1700–2500)	8.8
	23–50	55	120	163	64	2000	(1600–2400)	8.4
	51–75	55	120	163	64	1800	(1400–2200)	7.6
	76+	55	120	163	64	1600	(1200–2000)	6.7
Pregnancy						+300		
Lactation						+500		

[a]The data in this table have been assembled from the observed median heights and weights of children together with desirable weights for adults for the mean heights of men (70 in.) and women (64 in.) between the ages of 18 and 34 years as surveyed in the U.S. population (HEW/NCHS data).

The energy allowances for the young adults are for men and women doing light work. The allowances for the two older age groups represent mean energy needs over these age spans, allowing for a 2-percent decrease in basal (resting) metabolic rate per decade and a reduction in activity of 200 kcal/day for men and women between 51 and 75 years, 500 kcal for men over 75 years, and 400 kcal for women over 75 years.

The customary range of daily energy output is shown in parentheses for adults and is based on a variation in energy needs of ±400 kcal at any one age, emphasizing the wide range of energy intakes appropriate for any group of people.

Energy allowances for children through age 18 are based on median energy intakes of children of these ages followed in longitudinal growth studies. The values in parentheses are 10th and 90th percentiles of energy intake, to indicate the range of energy consumption among children of these ages.

1989 TABLE 3

Median Heights and Weights and Recommended Energy Intake

		Weight		Height			Average Energy Allowance, kcal[b]		
Category	Age (years) or Condition	kg	lb	cm	in	REE[a] kcal/day	Multiples of REE	Per kg	Per day[c]
Infants	0.0–0.5	6	13	60	24	320		108	650
	0.5–1.0	9	20	71	28	500		98	850
Children	1–3	13	29	90	35	740		102	1,300
	4–6	20	44	112	44	950		90	1,800
	7–10	28	62	132	52	1,130		70	2,000
Males	11–14	45	99	157	62	1,440	1.70	55	2,500
	15–18	66	145	176	69	1,760	1.67	45	3,000
	19–24	72	160	177	70	1,780	1.67	40	2,900
	25–50	79	174	176	70	1,800	1.60	37	2,900
	51+	77	170	173	68	1,530	1.50	30	2,300
Females	11–14	46	101	157	62	1,310	1.67	47	2,200
	15–18	55	120	163	64	1,370	1.60	40	2,200
	19–24	58	128	164	65	1,350	1.60	38	2,200
	25–50	63	138	163	64	1,380	1.55	36	2,200
	51+	65	143	160	63	1,280	1.50	30	1,900
Pregnant	1st trimester								+0
	2nd trimester								+300
	3rd trimester								+300
Lactating	1st 6 months								+500
	2nd 6 months								+500

[a]Calculation based on FAO equations (Table 3-1), then rounded.
[b]In the range of light to moderate activity, the coefficient of variation is ±20%.
[c]Figure is rounded.

COPYRIGHTS AND ACKNOWLEDGMENTS

Text

Table 5-9: Reproduced by permission of the American Diabetes Association, Inc.

Appendix F: The exchange lists are the basis of a meal planning system designed by a committee of the American Diabetes Association and The American Dietetic Association. While designed primarily for people with diabetes and others who must follow special diets, the exchange lists are based on principles of good nutrition that apply to everyone. © 1986 American Diabetes Association, The American Dietetic Association.

Appendix G: Reprinted with permission of Ross Laboratories, Columbus OH 43216, from *Dietetic Currents*, Vol. 13, #6, © 1986 Ross Laboratories.

Illustrations

CHAPTER 1

Page 6: Division of Vital Statistics, National Center for Health Statistics, 1988. **9:** Division of Vital Statistics, National Vital Statistics System. Projections computed by Division of Epidemiology from data compiled by Division of Vital Statistics, 1986. **11:** American Chemical Society.

CHAPTER 2

Page 35: From Mertz, Walter, The essential trace elements, *Science* 213 (Sept. 18, 1981): 1332–38, fig. 2; copyright 1981 by the AAAS.

CHAPTER 3

Page 66 (top): Katch, F. I., and McArdle, W. D.; *Nutrition, Weight Control, and Exercise*; Lea & Febiger, Philadelphia, 1988. **69:** Figure adapted from *Human Anatomy and Physiology* by Gaudin and Jones; copyright © 1989 by Harcourt Brace Jovanovich, Inc., reprinted by permission of the publisher. **70:** From Horowitz, M., et al. in *British Journal of Surgery* 71 (1984): 435 by permission of the publishers, Butterworth & Co. **71:** Figure from *Living Chemistry*, second edition, by David A. Ucko; copyright © 1986 by Harcourt Brace Jovanovich, Inc., reprinted by permission of the publisher. **72 (top):** Figure adapted from *Human Anatomy and Physiology* by Gaudin and Jones, copyright © 1989 by Harcourt Brace Jovanovich, Inc., reprinted by permission of the publisher. **73:** Figure adapted from *Human Anatomy and Physiology* by Gaudin and Jones; copyright © by Harcourt Brace Jovanovich, Inc., reprinted by permission of the publisher. **77:** Reproduced from the *Journal of Clinical Investigation* 68 (1981): 388–404 by copyright permission of the American Society for Clinical Investigation.

CHAPTER 4

Page 103: From Van Itallie, T. B., *Food Technology*, December 1979, pp. 43–47, and from Van Itallie, T. B., paper presented at the Fourth International Congress on Obesity, New York, October 3–5, 1983. **104:** Data from the Ten-State Nutrition Survey. **114 (top):** Johnson, D., et al. in *Archives of Internal Medicine* 137 (1977): 1381; copyright 1977, American Medical Association.

CHAPTER 5

Page 144: Adapted from Sreebny, L. M., in *Community Dentistry and Oral Epidemiology* 10 (1982): 1–7. **151 (bottom):** From *Alcohol and Health*, DHHS pub. no. (ADM) 84-1291. National Institute on Alcohol Abuse and Alcoholism; Alcohol, Drug Abuse, and Mental Health Administration, Washington, D.C., U.S. Government Printing Office, 1983. **163:** Data obtained from Jenkins, D. J. A., in *Diabetes Care* 5 (1982): 634–41; reproduced with permission of the American Diabetes Association, Inc.

CHAPTER 7

Page 210: From Grundy, Cholesterol and heart disease, *Journal of the American Medical Association* 256 (1986): 2851; copyright 1986, American Medical Association. **211:** From Blackburn, H., et al., Heart disease, in J. Last, ed., *Public Health and Preventive Medicine*, Appleton-Century-Crofts, 1985, p. 1184. **222:** USDA, 1986. **223:** From Wynder, E. L., et al., Dietary fat and fiber and colon cancer, *Seminars in Oncology* 10, (1983): 264–72; W. B. Saunders Co.

CHAPTER 10

Page 284 (bottom): Figure from *Human Anatomy and Physiology* by Gaudin and Jones; copyright © 1989 by Harcourt Brace Jovanovich, Inc., reprinted by permission of the publisher. **289 (bottom):** Adapted from information appearing in Goodman, D. S., Vitamin A and retinoids in health and disease, *The New England Journal of Medicine* 310 (1984): 1023–31, 1984.

CHAPTER 11

Page 309: Figure adapted from *Human Anatomy and Physiology* by Gaudin and Jones; copyright © 1989 by Harcourt Brace Jovanovich, Inc., reprinted by permission of the publisher. **312:** Data from Spencer, H., and Kramer, L., NIH Consensus Conference: Osteoporosis, *Journal of Nutrition* 116 (1986): 316–19. **326 (top):** Adapted from data of Graham, Caesar, and Burger, *Metabolism: Clinical and Experimental* 9 (1960): 646; W. B. Saunders Co. **330:** From Monsen, E. R., Hallberg, M., et al. Estimation of available dietary iron, *American Journal of Clinical Nutrition* 31 (1978): 134–41; © *Am. J. Clin. Nutr.* American Society for Clinical Nutrition. **332:** U.S. Interdepartmental Committee for National Defense, *Nutrition Survey of the Armed Forces* (Washington, D.C.: Department of Defense, 1956–1961).

CHAPTER 12

Page 351 (bottom): Reprinted with permission from De Pola, P. F., et al., A dental survey of Massachusetts school children, *Journal of Dental Research* 61 (1982): 356–60. **352:** From *Nutrition Today*, May/June 1977; © Williams & Wilkins. **362:** From Dahl, L. K., Salt and hypertension, *American Journal of Clinical Nutrition* 25 (1972): 231; © *Am. J. Clin. Nutr.* American Society for Clinical Nutrition. **363:** Adapted from MacGregor, G. A., Dietary sodium and potassium intake and blood pressure, *Lancet*, i (1983): 750–52.

CHAPTER 14

Page 392: Adapted from Van der Spuy, Z. M., in *Clinical Obstetrics and Gynecology* 12 (1985): 579–604. **411:** Reproduced by permission from *Pediatrics* 76 (1985): 1004–1008, copyright 1985. **418:** Figure from *Human Anatomy and Physiology* by Gaudin and Jones; copyright © 1989 by Harcourt Brace Jovanovich, Inc., reprinted by permission of the publisher.

CHAPTER 15

Page 439: Tanner, J. M., and Davies, P. S. W., courtesy of Serono Laboratories, Inc., Norwell, Mass. **441:** Adapted from Smith, D. W., *Growth and Its Disorders*, p. 69; W. B. Saunders Co., 1974. **442:** From Lifshitz, in *Clinical Nutrition* 44 (1985): 44, fig. 4; C. V. Mosby Co. **444 (top):** Adapted from Fomon, S. J., *Infant Nutrition*, second edition, p. 69; W. B. Saunders Co., 1974. **445:** National Center for Health Statistics, Rockville, Md., 1976. **446:** Used with permission of Ross Laboratories, © 1982. **447:** Used with permission of Ross Laboratories, © 1982. **448:** Reproduced by permission from *Pediatrics* 75 (1985): 807–12, copyright 1985.

CHAPTER 16

Page 485: *Statistical Abstracts of the United States*, Bureau of the Census, 1986. **488:** U.S. Department of Commerce, Bureau of the Census, *United Nations Demographic Year Book*. **497:** Adapted from publication of Agricultural Extension Service, University of Minnesota.

APPENDIX

Page XXX: Figure adapted from *Human Anatomy and Physiology* by Gaudin and Jones; copyright © 1989 by Harcourt Brace Jovanovich, Inc., reprinted by permission of the publisher. **XXX** Figure from *Human Anatomy and Physiology* by Gaudin and Jones; copyright © 1989 by Harcourt Brace Jovanovich, Inc., reprinted by permission of the publisher.

Photographs

CHAPTER 1

Page 3 (left and right): © Irven DeVore/Anthro-Photo. **4 (left):** Brown Brothers. **4 (right):** © J. L. Barkan/The Picture Cube. **5:** © Judith E. Brown. **7:** © L. L. T. Rhodes/Taurus Photos. **16 (left):** Photo by Nathan Holtz. **17:** Linda L. Creighton, *U.S. News & World Report.*

CHAPTER 2

Page 26: © Mark Antman/The Image Works. **34:** Photo by Lennart Nilsson, *The Body Victorious*, Dell Publishing Company, Inc., © Boehringer Ingelheim International GmbH. **39:** © Katsutoshi Ito/Nature Production, Tokyo. **42 (top):** © W. B. Finch/Stock, Boston. **42 (bottom):** © D. Gutekunst/Gamma-Liason. **44:** Mark Antman/The Image Works. **46:** © Dave Black/AllSport. **60:** United States Department of Agriculture, Human Nutrition Information Service.

CHAPTER 3

Page 72 (bottom left and right): From *Tissues and Organs: A Text-Atlas of Scanning Electron Microscopy* by Richard G. Kessel and Randy H. Kardon. Copyright © 1979 W. H. Freeman and Co. Reprinted with permission. **79:** © Dean Abramson/Stock, Boston. **81:** © Therese Frare/The Picture Cube. **82:** © Frank Siteman/The Picture Cube. **89:** © Charles Gupton/Stock, Boston. **91 (left and right):** NASA. **92:** Courtesy of Exercise Physiology Lab, San Diego State University.

CHAPTER 4

Page 100: © Martin Rotker/Taurus Photos. **101 (top):** Photo courtesy of Neal E. Miller. **101 (bottom):** © Sally Weigand/The Picture Cube. **105:** © Linda L. Legaspi/Photo Researchers. **106 (top):** © Steve Takatsumo/The Picture Cube. **106 (middle):** Courtesy of Exercise Physiology Lab, San Diego State University. **106 (bottom):** © Bart Bartholomew/Black Star. **110 (left and right):** Van Itallie, T. B., *Food Technology* (December 1979): 46. Photographs by S. K. Gale. Courtesy T. B. Van Itallie, M.D., St. Luke's/Roosevelt Hospital Center, New York. **113:** © The Photo Works/Photo Researchers. **114 (bottom):** © Ray Ellis/Photo Researchers. **119:** © Edward Lettau/Science Source/Photo Researchers. **121 (right):** © Sarah Putnam/The Picture Cube. **122:** Wallace Kirkland, *Life* Magazine © Time Inc. **125:** © Susan Rosenberg/Photo Researchers.

CHAPTER 5

Page 42: Photo by Nathan Holtz. **145 (bottom):** © David Scharf/Peter Arnold, Inc. **147 (top):** Courtesy Dr. Arthur J. Nowak, University of Iowa, Iowa City, Iowa. **151 (top):** © Richard Wood/Taurus Photos. **157:** Courtesy Lactaid, Inc. **160:** © John Griffin/The Image Works. **165 (bottom):** © Marty Heitner/The Picture Cube.

CHAPTER 6

Page 173: © Dan Bernstein/Photo Researchers. **176 (top):** Emil Bernstein and Eila Kairinen, Gillette Co. Research Institute, Rockville, Md. **179:** Van Steenbergen, William, et al., *Tropical and Geographical Medicine* 30 (1978): 407. **182:** © Dion Ogust/The Image Works. **189:** © Tom Hollyman/Photo Researchers. **190:** F.A.O.

CHAPTER 7

Page 195: From *Tissues and Organs: A Text-Atlas of Scanning Electron Microscopy* by Richard G. Kessel and Randy H. Kardon. Copyright © 1979 W. H. Freeman and Co. Reprinted with permission. **197:** © Topham/The Image Works. **204 (bottom):** Photo by Mark Ristau. **205:** © Tom Wolfe. **206:** © Charles Gatewood/The Image Works. **209 (all):** Photos by Lennart Nilsson, *The Body Victorious*, Dell Publishing Company, Inc., © Boehringer Ingelheim International GmbH. **217 (top):** Courtesy Daniel J. Kieffer, Biomedical Graphics, University of Minnesota. **218:** © Steve McCutcheon.

CHAPTER 8

Page 240: © Charles Gatewood/The Image Works.

CHAPTER 9

Page 255 (top): With permission of editor *Nutrition Today.* **258:** © Carroll H. Weiss/Camera M. D. Studios. **264 (top left):** © Martin Rotker/Phototake. **264 (top right):** © Carroll H. Weiss/Camera M.D. Studios. **276:** © N.M.S./Custom Medical Stock Photos.

CHAPTER 10

Page 284 (bottom right): From *Tissues and Organs: A Text-Atlas of Scanning Electron Microscopy* by Richard G. Kessel and Randy H. Kardon. Copyright © 1979 W. H. Freeman and Co. Reprinted with permission. **286:** © John Kaprielian/Photo Researchers. **289 (top):** From Alfred Sommer, *Nutritional Blindness*. Oxford University Press, 1982. **292:** © Wally McNamee/Woodfin Camp and Associates. **293 (bottom):** © Jerry Wachter/Photo Researchers. **294:** © Biophoto Associates /Science Source /Photo Researchers. **295:** The Bettmann Archive. **300:** © Therese Frare/The Picture Cube. **301:** Photo by Lennart Nilsson, *The Body Victorious*, Dell Publishing Company, Inc., © Boehringer Ingelheim International GmbH. **302:** From *Tissues and Organs: A Text-Atlas of Scanning Electron Microscopy* by Richard G. Kessel and Randy H. Kardon. Copyright © 1979 by W. H. Freeman and Co. Reprinted with permission.

CHAPTER 11

Page 308: Photo by Susan Holtz. **310:** © Phototake. **313 (bottom):** © Jacques Chenet/Woodfin Camp and Associates. **317:** Karl Eric Steinbrenner/TIME Magazine. **334 (left):** © Martin Rotker/Phototake. **334 (right):** © Josquin Carrillo/Photo Researchers. **342 (bottom):** © John Paul Kay/Peter Arnold, Inc.

CHAPTER 12

Page 353: Courtesy Dr. Arthur J. Nowak, University of Iowa, Iowa City, Iowa.

CHAPTER 13

Page 377: © Lawrence Migdale/Stock, Boston. **382:** © IPA/The Image Works. **384:** Van Steenbergen, William, et al., *Tropical and Geographical Medicine* 30 (1978): 397. **385:** © Richard Pasley/Stock, Boston.

CHAPTER 14

Page 391: Photo by Lennart Nilsson, *A Child is Born*, Dell Publishing Company, Inc. **393:** © Marjorie Shostak/Anthro-Photo. **396:** Courtesy Diane Pella. **397:** © Elizabeth Crews/The Image Works. **400:** Courtesy Maggie and Kate Porter. **402:** © Dion Ogust/The Image Works. **405:** © David Brownell. **407 (top):** Kenneth L. Jones, University of California Medical Center. **407 (bottom):** Courtesy Beth Pugh. **420 (left):** © Francine Manning/The Picture Cube. **420 (right):** © Bruce McAllister/The Image Works. **421 (bottom):** © Bernard Pierre Wolff/Photo Researchers.

CHAPTER 15

Page 438 (top): National Archives Neg. #90-G-5-20. **438 (bottom):** © Lawrence Migdale. **440 (both):** © V. Williams, M. D./Custom Medical Stock Photo. **449 (bottom):** © Bob Daemmrich/The Image Works. **452:** © Robert Eckert/Stock, Boston. **453:** *American Journal of Diseases of Children* 36 (1928): 660, fig. 6; copyright 1928, American Medical Association. **465:** © Suzanne Szasz/Photo Researchers. **471:** Courtesy Colin Young and Lindsay Snead. **474:** © Bob Daemmrich/The Image Works. **476:** © Ellis Herwig/Stock, Boston.

CHAPTER 16

Page 484: Photo by Nathan Holtz. **487:** © Smithsonian Institution Neg. #79-10265. **489 (bottom left and right):** © John Launois/Black Star. **491:** © Peter Menzel/Stock, Boston. **496:** © B. B. Norton/The Picture Cube.

Photos on pp. 87, 146, 154, 165 (top), 214, 238, 252, 274, 290 (both), 293, 322, 342 (top), 395, 400, 407 (bottom), 454, and 471 by McClain/Pennett Photography.

▪ INDEX ▪

A

B

C

E

G

H

I

R

S

T

W

X

Y

Z

A 9
B 0
C 1
D 2
E 3
F 4
G 5
H 6
I 7
J 8